HANDBOOK OF CRITICAL CARE PAIN MANAGEMENT

NOTICE

Medicine is an ever-changing science. As new research and clinical experience broaden our knowledge, changes in treatment and drug therapy are required. The editors and the publisher of this work have checked with sources believed to be reliable in their efforts to provide information that is complete and generally in accord with the standards accepted at the time of publication. However, in view of the possibility of human error or changes in medical sciences, neither the editors nor the publisher nor any other party who has been involved in the preparation or publication of this work warrants that the information contained herein is in every respect accurate or complete, and they are not responsible for any errors or omissions or for the results obtained from use of such information. Readers are encouraged to confirm the information contained herein with other sources. For example and in particular, readers are advised to check the product information sheet included in the package of each drug they plan to administer to be certain that the information contained in this book is accurate and that changes have not been made in the recommended dose or in the contraindications for administration. This recommendation is of particular importance in connection with new or infrequently used drugs.

HANDBOOK OF CRITICAL CARE PAIN MANAGEMENT

EDITORS

Robin J. Hamill, M.D.

*Assistant Professor of Anesthesiology and Critical Care Medicine
Associate Director, Surgical Intensive Care Unit
Staff Physician, Pain Management Center
University of Virginia Health Sciences Center
Charlottesville, Virginia*

John C. Rowlingson, M.D.

*Professor of Anesthesiology
Director, Pain Management Center
University of Virginia Health Sciences Center
Charlottesville, Virginia*

McGraw-Hill, Inc.
Health Professions Division
New York St. Louis San Francisco Auckland Bogotá Caracas
Lisbon London Madrid Mexico City Milan Montreal New Delhi
Paris San Juan Singapore Sydney Tokyo Toronto

*Dedicated to those we care for and about
—patients, friends, and family—
who suffer as we struggle to truly understand pain.*

*And to the lights of my life,
John, Laura, and Jamie,
for their humor, courage, patience, and love.
rjh*

This book is printed on acid-free paper.

HANDBOOK OF CRITICAL CARE PAIN MANAGEMENT

Copyright © 1994 by McGraw-Hill, Inc. All rights reserved. Printed in the United States of America. Except as permitted under the United States Copyright Act of 1976, no part of this publication may be reproduced or distributed in any form or by any means, or stored in a data base or retrieval system, without the prior written permission of the publisher.

1 2 3 4 5 6 7 8 9 0 DOC DOC 9 8 7 6 5 4 3

ISBN 0-07-025814-7

This book was set in Times Roman by University Graphics, Inc.
The editors were Mariapaz Englis and Michael J. Houston
the production supervisor was Richard Ruzycka;
the project was managed by Hockett Editorial Service;
the cover was designed by Michele Simari;
the index was prepared by Patricia Couser
R. R. Donnelley and Sons Company was printer and binder.

Library of Congress Cataloging-in-Publication Data

Handbook of critical care pain management / edited by Robin J. Hamill,
  John C. Rowlingson.
     p. cm.
  Includes bibliographical references and index.
  ISBN 0-07-025814-7
  1. Pain—Handbooks, manuals, etc. 2. Critical care medicine-
Handbooks, manuals, etc. 3. Analgesia—Handbooks, manuals, etc.
4. Anesthesia—Handbooks, manuals, etc. 5. Intractable pain-
-Handbooks, manuals, etc. I. Hamill, Robin J. II. Rowlingson,
John C.
   [DNLM: 1. Pain—therapy—handbooks. 2.Critical Illness-
handbooks. 3. Critical care—methods—handbooks. 4. Anesthesia-
-handbooks. 5. Analgesia—handbooks. WL 39 H2365 1994]
RB127.H3534 1994
618'.0472—dc20
DNLM/DLC
for Library of Congress   93-26996
                                                                 CIP

Contents

Contributors   ix
Preface   xiii

PART ONE   INTRODUCTION   1

1   The Philosophy and Economics of Pain Management   3
William Sibbald / Ravi Gill

PART TWO   THE ANATOMY, PHYSIOLOGY, AND ASSESSMENT OF PAIN   11

2   The Assessment of Pain   13
John C. Rowlingson

3   Pain Mechanisms and Pathways   27
John C. Rowlingson

4   The Physiologic and Metabolic Response to Pain and Stress   39
Robin J. Hamill

5   A Matrix Model for the Psychological Assessment and Treatment of Acute Pain   53
Joseph R. Dane / Rodger S. Kessler

PART THREE   PHARMACOLOGIC AGENTS   83

6   Phamacokinetic and Pharmacodynamic Concerns in the Critically Ill   85
Robb McGory

7   Nonsteroidal Analgesic and Anti-inflammatory Agents   103
Victor C. Lee / John C. Rowlingson / Robin J. Hamill

8	Opiate Pharmacology Richard L. Noren	117
9	General Anesthetics in the Intensive Care Unit Charles G. Durbin, Jr.	143
10	Pharmacology of Local Anesthetics Cosmo DiFazio / Andrew M. Woods	157
11	Sedatives, Anxiolytics, and Other Adjunct Medications Marcia L. Buck	169
12	Neuromuscular Blocking Agents John Campbell	191

PART FOUR APPLICATIONS OF MODALITIES AND TREATMENT OPTIONS 205

13	Techniques of Narcotic and Local Anesthetic Administration John C. Rowlingson / Robin J. Hamill	207
14	Adjunctive Therapy for Pain John C. Rowlingson / Rodger S. Kessler / Joseph R. Dane / Robin J. Hamill	229
15	Physical and Occupational Therapy in the Prevention and Management of Pain in the Intensive Care Unit Kathleen Henahan / Leslie D. Baruch	251

PART FIVE CLINICAL PROBLEMS 269

16	Neurologic Injury and Disease Karen J. Schwenzer / Robin J. Hamill	271
17	Pain and Cardiovascular Disease Kenneth R. Greer / John W. Hoyt	301

18	Respiratory Disease Richard B. Becker	319
19	Renal Diseases Timothy B. Gilbert / John F. Williams	339
20	Hepatobiliary Disease Catherine K. Lineberger	361
21	Pain Management in Patients with Hemostatic Failure Susan Anderson	373
22	Sepsis and Multiple System Organ Failure Mark O. Daugherty	389
23	Pain Management for the Patient with Burns or Integument Failure Sherry T. Sutton / Harvey N. Himel	405
24	Pain Management After Trauma Roger Cicala / Douglas B. Coursin	425
25	Issues in Postoperative Pain Control John C. Rowlingson / Robin J. Hamill	443
26	Transplantation Glenn Murray / Kyle Tipton	455
27	Pain Management in the Patient with HIV Terrance Calder / Michael Frank	469

PART SIX SPECIAL CONCERNS 479

28	Pain Management in the Terminally Ill Sherry T. Sutton / Margot L. White / Richard F. Edlich	481
29	Tolerance, Dependence, and Addiction in the ICU Patient Charles G. Durbin, Jr.	495

30	**Pain Management in the Critically Ill Child** *Madelyn Kahana*	**507**
31	**The Critically Ill Obstetric Patient** *Robert B. Lechner*	**523**
32	**Concomitant Chronic Pain Syndromes** *John C. Rowlingson / Robin J. Hamill*	**543**
33	**Nursing Issues** *Ann Gill Taylor*	**555**

PART SEVEN   APPENDIXES — **569**
  Appendix A   Pain Terminology — 571
  Appendix B   Common Drugs, Doses, and Metabolism — 573

INDEX — **587**

Contributors

Susan Anderson, B.M., F.R.C.A. [21]
Assistant Professor of Anesthesiology
University of Virginia Health Sciences Center
Charlottesville, Virginia

Leslie D. Baruch, R.O.T. [15]
Department of Occupational Therapy
University of Virginia Health Sciences Center
Charlottesville, Virginia

Richard B. Becker, M.D. [18]
Assistant Professor of Anesthesiology
Director of Obstetric Anesthesia
Co-Director of the Intensive Care Unit
George Washington University Hospital
Washington, D.C.

Marcia L. Buck. Pharm.D. [11]
Pediatric Clinical Pharmacy Specialist
Department of Pharmacy
Clinical Assistant Professor
Department of Pediatrics
University of Virginia Health Sciences Center
Charlottesville, Virginia

Terrance Calder, M.D. [27]
Head Pain Management Division
Department of Anesthesiology
National Naval Medical Center
Bethesda, Maryland

John C. Campbell, M.B., B.S., F.R.C.A. [12]
Specialist Anesthetist
Private Practice
Frankston, Victoria, Australia

Roger Cicala, M.D. [24]
Associate Professor
Department of Anesthesiology
Director of University of Tennessee Pain Center
Memphis, Tennessee

Douglas B. Coursin, M.D. [24]
Professor of Anethesiology and Internal Medicine
Associate Director of the Trauma and Life Support Center
University of Wisconsin Clinical Science Center
Madison, Wisconsin

Joseph R. Dane, Ph.D. [5, 14]
Assistant Professor of Anesthesiology
Staff Psychologist, Pain Management Center
University of Virginia Health Sciences Center
Charlottesville, Virginia

Cosmo DiFazio, M.D., Ph.D. [10]
Professor of Anesthesiology
University of Virginia Health Sciences Center
Charlottesville, Virginia

Mark O. Daugherty, M.B.B.Ch., F.R.C.A.
Assistant Professor of Anesthesiology
University of Virginia Health Sciences Center
Charlottesville, Virginia

Charles G. Durbin, Jr., M.D., F.C.C.M. [9, 29]
Professor of Anesthesiology and Critical Care Medicine
Medical Director, Surgical Intensive Care Unit
University of Virginia Health Sciences Center
Charlottesville, Virginia

Richard F. Edlich, M.D., Ph.D. [28]
Distinguished Professor of Plastic Surgery and Biomedical Engineering
Department of Plastic Surgery
University of Virginia Health Sciences Center
Charlottesville, Virginia

*The numbers in brackets following the contributor name refer to chapter(s) authored or co-authored by the contributor.

CONTRIBUTORS

Michael Frank, M.D. [27]
Department of Medicine
Fellow, Division of Infectious Disease
University of Virginia Health Sciences Center
Charlottesville, Virginia

Timothy B. Gilbert, M.D. [19]
Assistant Professor of Anesthesiology
Director of Cardiothoracic Anesthesiology
Division of Cardiothoracic Anesthesia and Critical Care Medicine
University of Maryland at Baltimore
Baltimore, Maryland

Ravi Gill, B.M., F.R.C.A. [1]
Senior Fellow in Critical Care
Division of Critical Care Medicine
University of Western Ontario
London, Ontario

Kenneth R. Greer, M.D. [17]
Assistant Clinical Professor of Anesthesiology and Critical Care Medicine
University of Pittsburgh
Director Critical Care Transport Team
St. Francis Medical Center
Pittsburgh, Pennsylvania

Robin J. Hamill, M.D. [4, 7, 13, 14, 16, 25, 32]
Assistant Professor of Anesthesiology
Associate Director, Surgical Intensive Care Unit
Staff Physician, Pain Management Center
University of Virginia Health Sciences Center
Charlottesville, Virginia

Kathleen Henahan, R.P.T. [15]
Department of Physical Therapy
University of Virginia Health Sciences Center
Charlottesville, Virginia

Harvey N. Himel, M.D. [23]
Assistant Professor of Surgery
Department of Plastic Surgery
Director, DeCamp Burn Center
University of Virginia Health Sciences Center
Charlottesville, Virginia

John W. Hoyt, M.D. [17]
Clinical Professor of Anesthesiology and Critical Care Medicine
University of Pittsburgh School of Medicine
Chairman, Department of Critical Care Medicine
St. Francis Medical Center
Pittsburgh, Pennsylvania

Madelyn Kahana, M.D. [30]
Associate Professor of Anesthesiology
Attending Physician, Pediatric Intensive Care Unit
Children's Hospital Medical Center
Cincinnati, Ohio

Rodger S. Kessler, Ph.D. [5, 14]
Director of Behavioral Medicine
Copley Hospital
Morrisville, VT
Department of Anesthesiology & Surgery
Central VT Medical Center
Montpelier, VT

Robert B. Lechner, M.D., Ph.D. [31]
Assistant Professor of Anesthesiology
University of Virginia Health Sciences Center
Charlottesville, Virginia

Victor C. Lee, M.D. [7]
Assistant Professor of Anesthesiology
Pain Management Center
University of Virginia Health Sciences Center
Charlottesville, Virginia

Catherine K. Lineberger, M.D. [20]
Assistant Professor
Department of Anesthesiology
Duke Medical Center
Durham, North Carolina

Robb McGory, Pharm.D. [6]
Pharmacy Clinical Specialist, Surgical Intensive Care Unit
Department of Pharmacy
University of Virginia Health Sciences Center
Charlottesville, Virginia

Glen Murray, M.D. [26]
Assistant Professor of Anesthesiology and Critical Care Medicine
Department of Anesthesiology
University of Pittsburgh Medical Center
Pittsburgh, PA 15213-2582

Richard L. Noren, M.D. [8]
Assistant Professor of Anesthesiology
Emory University Hospital
Atlanta, Georgia

John C. Rowlingson, M.D. [2, 3, 7, 13, 14, 25, 32]
Professor of Anesthesiology
Director, Pain Management Center
University of Virginia Health Sciences Center
Charlottesville, Virginia

Karen J. Schwenzer, M.D. [16]
Assistant Professor of Anesthesiology and Critical Care Medicine
Associate Director, Surgical Intensive Care Unit
Staff Physician, Nerancy Neuroscience Intensive Care Unit
University of Virginia Health Sciences Center
Charlottesville, Virginia

William Sibbald, M.D., F.R.C.P.(C.), F.C.C.P., F.A.C.P. [1]
Professor of Medicine
Director, Critical Care Trauma Center
University of Western Ontario
Victoria Hospital
London, Ontario

Sherry T. Sutton, Pharm.D. [23, 28]
Pharmacy Clinical Specialist, Burn and Neurosciences
Department of Pharmacy
University of Virginia Health Sciences Center
Charlottesville, Virginia

Ann Gill Taylor, R.N., Ed.N., F.A.A.N. [33]
Professor of Nursing
Director, Child/Adult Health Division
School of Nursing
University of Virginia Health Sciences Center
Charlottesville, Virginia

Kyle Tipton, M.D. [26]
Assistant Professor of Anesthesiology and Critical Care Medicine
Department of Anesthesiology
University of Pittsburgh Medical Center
Pittsburgh, Pennsylvania

Margot L. White, J.D. [28]
Assistant Professor of Biomedical Ethics and Health Law
Director, Program on Law in Medicine
University of Virginia School of Medicine
University of Virginia Health Sciences Center
Charlottesville, Virginia

John F. Williams, M.D. M.P.H., F.C.C.M. [19]
Associate Professor of Anesthesiology
Division of Critical Care Medicine
Assistant Dean of Admissions
Co-Director, Intensive Care Unit
The George Washington University Medical Center
Washington, D.C.

Andrew M. Woods, M.D. [10]
Associate Professor of Anesthesiology
Director, Surgical Admission Suite
Medical Director, Post Anesthesia Care Unit
University of Virginia Health Sciences Center
Charlottesville, Virginia

PREFACE

Pain is a universal experience of the human condition and is the complaint that most frequently prompts patients to see physicians. The diagnostic process that leads to a therapeutic plan depends upon more than data gleaned from this history and physical examination. The behavioral interaction between the patient and the health-care professional reveals significant information regarding the patient's level of distress *and* the unique meaning that the pain experience has for that particular person.

A vital source of discriminatory information regarding the pain is lost when the health-care professional's interaction with the patient is compromised, whether because of acute injury, critical illness, cognitive deficits, or the extremes of age. The caretaker must then rely more on the clinical findings, diagnostic tests, and his or her experience in assessing the pain. The "incomplete" data base that this affords is often frustrating and disquieting to the practitioner. In addition, the critically ill patient often has a long problem list, headed by life-threatening conditions. In this situation, the significance of pain pales when compared with hypoxia or hemorrhage. Review of most of the major critical care texts supports this philosophy, as there is little attention given to pain management in this patient population while life-maintaining therapy is provided.

Our contemporary understanding of pain has been generated by intriguing anatomic, neuropharmacologic, and physiologic discoveries, an appreciation of the impact of the neuroendocrine response to stress, as well as an awareness of the detrimental effect that pain and stress have on coagulation and immunocompetence. This broadened knowledge elevates pain from its designation as an unfortunate inconvenience to the realistic status of a significant factor with the potential to affect the morbidity and mortality of patients in the particularly tenuous circumstances of critical illness. The *Handbook of Critical Care Pain Management* was conceived in an attempt to raise our collective level of consciousness with regard to the importance of pain *and* the benefits of effective pain management in these high-risk patients. The primary pain texts are aimed at practitioners who have received some formal training in pain management. This handbook, on the other hand, is intended as a ready source of information for practitioners in many health-care disciplines who may well lack extensive experience with pain medicine. By providing basic information about pain management in a simple, easily accessible format, it is our hope that the *Handbook* will help health-care professionals (with little or no formal training in the specialty) to develop a respect for the potential adverse effects of inadequately treated pain and, at the same time, that it will proffer additional tools and strategies with which to assess and manage pain.

Acute pain in the face of critical illness or injury requires decisive action. With this in mind, we chose a succinct outline format with key ideas highlighted for quick reference. Multiple tables and the appendix of common drugs further enhance the ready access to information. The book addresses the essentials of assessment of patients with acute pain and critical illness and reviews sedative and analgesic pharmacology. An overview of analgesic techniques and modalities is provided in order to facilitate an understanding of the indications, contraindications, and complications associated with the various treatment options. In the system-by-system clinical problems section, we discuss pain syndromes specific to each organ system as well as how dysfunction of that system influences pain management choices. This section also includes case presentations and pertinent discussions, to enhance the clinical relevance of the commentary. Finally, several special concerns, including terminal care, tolerance and addiction, and analgesia in pediatric and obstetrical ICU patients, are addressed in order to provide information across the spectrum of critically ill patients. The vital issues specific to nursing care are also presented. A chapter that briefly reviews common chronic pain syndromes is provided to expand the practitioner's understanding of preexisting painful conditions that may still be of concern *to the patient* despite the presence of a critical illness.

Pain is often underrecognized. Even when appreciated, pain is frequently undertreated because of our fears, prejudices, and the perception that we have a limited armamentarium. It is our hope that the *Handbook of Critical Care Pain Management* will be practical and useful for many practitioners, including intensivists, surgeons, emergency physicians, internists, physicians in training, and nursing personnel. By providing core information about assessment and treatment, the *Handbook* will allow health-care providers to feel better equipped to provide *complete care* to their patients, gain greater satisfaction in dealing with these patients, and reduce morbidity and mortality.

ACKNOWLEDGEMENTS

An undertaking such as this is always a larger task than one anticipates and the creative process depends on the efforts and talents of many people. There is the role of our esteemed mentors, including Bill Sibbald and the late Harold Carron, who have taught us to think, to question, and to seek medically sound but also humane ways to care for patients. We would be remiss if we didn't express our gratitude to Michael Houston and Mariapaz Ramos-Englis of McGraw-Hill for their direction and encouragement as we forged our way through unfamiliar territory. Thanks to Rachel Youngman of Hockett Editorial Service for sharing her editorial expertise and calmly accepting the scarred proofs and last-minute phone calls. We also appreciate the contributions from our authors, many of whom were friends until they realized how little information was available in the literature about pain management in the critically ill to facilitate their writing efforts, making the research for their chapters a bit like a scavenger hunt. Invaluable technical assistance was provided by a number of people including Pat Meté, Kim Jenner, Sue Herndon, Rhonda Taylor, Robert Bland, Patty Jenkins, and Jackie Roe, all of whom deserve our heartfelt thanks for their contributions.

Robin J. Hamill
John C. Rowlingson

PART ONE

INTRODUCTION

CHAPTER 1

THE PHILOSOPHY AND ECONOMICS OF PAIN MANAGEMENT

William J. Sibbald
Ravi Gill

I. Implications of Pain in the Critically Ill Patient
II. Benefits of Effective Pain Management
III. Economic Implications of Pain Management
IV. Technology Evaluation
V. Conclusions
References

> Pain is perfect misery,
> The worse of all evils; and
> excessive, overturns all patients.
>
> John Milton, *Paradise Lost*

Pain is as old as humankind. In the book of Genesis, it is written that pain came to man through the Fall from Grace. Early myths speak of pain suffered even by the gods. The Sun God, Apollo, was afflicted by the painful infirmities of old age; Isis (the Goddess of the Underworld) had an inflammation of the heart; Dionysus and Aesculapius could not be born by natural means, but only by a primitive cesarean section on their *conscious* mother.

I. IMPLICATIONS OF PAIN IN THE CRITICALLY ILL PATIENT

Pain has been defined as an unpleasant sensory and emotional experience associated with actual or potential tissue damage or described in terms of such damage.[1] Critical illness presents as a complicated physiologic and psychosocial predicament which is frequently associated with pain. Discomfort and distress may be due to the primary insult, care-related interventions, or simply prolonged bed rest. In addition, chronic pain syndromes may coexist with acute pain and further confound assessment and treatment.

Often, the acuity of illness causes pain to be underappreciated by the health-care team and, subsequently, to be inadequately treated. Organ system dysfunction, commonly seen in critically ill patients, can carry significant implications with regard to pain management. Inappropriate analgesic dosing is common in the very ill patient due to the caretaker's inability to assess pain severity accurately coupled with concerns about hemodynamic instability, excessive drug accumulation, and iatrogenic addiction. Chronic pain problems are relegated to an even lower priority status than are acute pain generators.

Acute pain is associated with a distinct disease or injury, and is the most commonly treated type of pain in the setting of the intensive care unit (ICU). Caretakers often think in terms of the sensory experience of pain, yet acute pain is a complex experience that extends well beyond simple nociceptor stimulation. Pain alone can initiate a cascade of hormonal changes termed the suprasegmental response. As the contemporary definition of pain implies, neuronal input is altered by emotive elements such as fear, anxiety, and depression. These modifiers of pain are common in critically ill patients who are exposed to the unfamiliar, confusing, noisy, and threatening environs of the ICU, where they are also frequently unable to express the extent of their distress.

While pain and fear can activate the metabolic stress response, the critically ill patient also experiences substantial stress from the primary disease or injury. Disrupted sleep patterns and repeated invasive and/or painful procedures augment the patient's distress and precipitate disorientation and confusion. These patients are also intensely dependent upon their caregivers for the most basic of needs. All of these factors impel the critically ill patient toward an emotionally regressed state, magnifying the distress that sometimes exceeds the limits of his or her ability to cope effectively.

Concern for appropriate treatment of pain in the ICU environment has generally lagged behind the practitioner's concern about managing the altered physiology which is threatening the patient's life. Such inattention to pain management is deep seated. Colin MacInnes wrote of "the nonchalant attitude of the medical profession toward quite unnecessary suffering—so much so that one place in the country where you can get least relief is a hospital itself."[2] He considered the management of postoperative pain to be "a cruel and callous disgrace." The critically ill patient, often having an impaired ability to communicate, is at particular risk of suffering from inadequately treated pain.

Difficulties with pain management in the critically ill cannot be explained by a lack of appropriate analgesics. We need to increase our appreciation of when to treat pain and of how much of what to give. Analgesic medications, traditionally prescribed in fixed doses and administered on an "as needed" basis, are usually given at the discretion of a nurse and/or upon the request of the patient *(in whom the pain threshold has been exceeded)*. We now appreciate that this type of regimen is frequently ineffective. Caregivers vary widely in their degree of rapport with the patient, their interpretation of nonverbal cues that indicate "pain," their level of concern about narcotic dependence or addiction, and their ability or desire to attend to a request in a timely fashion. In the absence of a personal experience with severe pain or in situations where painful therapy is necessary for the patient's well-being, as with burn debridements, it is often difficult *(threatening)* for a caregiver to acknowledge the extent of a patient's suffering. Inter- and intrapatient pain thresholds cover a wide spectrum and depend upon such factors as the pain's history and significance (e.g., malignant versus benign), the patient's cultural background and level of education, and the presence of fatigue or anxiety.

For these reasons, it is not surprising that many patients complain about pain management in the ICU. Bion[3] interviewed 60 patients after their discharge from a general ICU, and found that 40 percent could recall painful experiences despite the well-known fact that ICU patients have poor recall of events occurring during their critical illness. A growing appreciation of the positive impact of effective analgesia on outcome and cost has led the Agency for Health Care Policy and Research (U.S.A.) and the Royal College of Surgeons (England) to issue guidelines for the management of acute pain.[4,5]

II. BENEFITS OF EFFECTIVE PAIN MANAGEMENT

Whereas patients on general wards can usually discuss their pain and cooperate in its assessment, one of the main problems faced in the ICU setting is the glaring lack of a satisfactory, objective, readily applied measure of analgesia. Changes in heart rate and blood pressure may be misleading indices of the response to pain due to the effects of the patient's illness on these parameters. Both sympathetically and vagally mediated cardiovascular changes may suggest a reflex response to intermittent painful stimuli. Hypovolemia, sepsis, or cardiac failure confuses the interpretation of hemodynamic changes, and pain all too often is used as an endogenous inotrope.

Despite our limited ability to measure pain, an increasing awareness of the problem should lead eventually to an improvement in pain assessment, and this in turn to more effective pain control. Notwithstanding the ethics and humanism of providing good analgesia, other benefits that accrue from adequate pain control include:

- Improvement in postoperative pulmonary function.[6,15]
- Decreased length of postoperative ventilation and ICU stay.[7]
- Decreased mortality in patients with traumatic thoracic injuries.[8]
- Attenuation of the stress response to surgery.[9]
- Associated improvement in the metabolic response to injury.[10]
- Maintenance of immunocompetence.[11]
- Earlier mobilization, which may lead to a decreased incidence of thrombotic sequelae.[12]

III. ECONOMIC IMPLICATIONS OF PAIN MANAGEMENT

The disadvantages of conventional methods of analgesic administration are daunting. An awareness of the inadequacies of earlier practices has led to the development of new technologies to combat the formidable problem of pain control in patients with critical illness and acute pain. However, the economic stresses posed by soaring health-care costs require that new technologies be utilized widely only after there has been a *clear* demonstration of effectiveness. Increasingly, an economic analysis is required while evaluating new technologies. Therefore, future reports should not only discuss the application of analgesic techniques, but also examine their effect on morbidity, mortality, and the costs of hospitalization.

Patient-controlled analgesia (PCA) is a technique that allows the patient to manipulate his or her own plasma concentrations of analgesic medications through self-administration. In acute pain management, evaluations of PCA have documented its safety and effectiveness.[13] Hecker and Albert[14] have shown that PCA offers greater efficacy and patient satisfaction at a lower total narcotic dose than does conventional therapy. While the PCA technique was found to be 23 percent to 33 percent more expensive (depending on the type of pump) than conventional therapy, Hecker and Albert also noted that if the pumps were purchased by the hospital, the cost over time would decrease.

Central neural blockade using epidural analgesia is becoming increasingly popular for acute and postoperative pain management. In high-risk surgical patients admitted to the ICU, postoperative pulmonary function is improved and leads to earlier extubation. The economic benefit of this technique has been elegantly summarized by Yeager, Glass, Neff, and Brinck-Johnsen.[15] Thoracic epidural techniques reduce mortality in patients with traumatic chest injury and associated pulmonary insufficiency because the need for assisted ventilation may be avoided.[8] Some studies also suggest that stress depresses immune competence. Can we then infer that good pain management will minimize the adverse impact of pain on the stress response, and thereby decrease ICU complications such as nosocomial infection? Rem, Brant, and Kehlet[11] have demonstrated that epidural analgesia prevents postoperative lymphopenia. Brant, Fernandes, Mordhorst, and Kehlet[10] have shown improvement in postoperative nitrogen balance when epidural anesthesia is employed. Thus there are data suggesting that we can affect the extent and ramifications of the stress response in a positive manner. Intuitively, this should improve outcome. Pain is a trigger of the metabolic stress response that *can* be treated and managed effectively, even in homeostatically tenuous patients. Just as antibiotics are used to treat infection, sedatives and analgesics should be used to manage anxiety, discomfort, and the resultant hypermetabolic state.

IV. TECHNOLOGY EVALUATION

Traditional discussions about technology evaluation in critical care emphasize such components of the program as drugs and medical devices. In the past two decades, regulations surrounding the introduction of new drugs have become more stringent. At the same time, however, there has been an abject lack of similar processes to guide the evaluation of new medical devices. *Technology assessment* is the process of designing and conducting investigations which enable reasoned judgment regarding effective and efficient patient care.[16,17] Evaluation of the efficacy of new therapeutic technologies is a process which requires demonstration that the patient benefits from the use of the technology. Methods for determining this vary in both credibility and cost. Randomized controlled trials, while expensive, are still the gold standard. Unfortunately, many investigations stop with a demonstration of clinical benefit. After determining that a therapeutic modality improves health-care outcome, an economic evaluation should be required to establish its efficiency or cost-per-patient benefit in comparison with other health-care services. Although there is a growing body of literature on the clinical assessment of critical care technologies, only recently have economic analyses been considered important in the overall study design of this work.

A significant question for the future will be, "Are the tools for economic assessment appropriate to analyze the benefits of adequate pain control?" *(The balance of evidence would refute this premise.)* It is likely that a well-constructed study using new analgesic technologies in appropriate patients would show benefit in terms of improved patient outcome and/or cost containment, and preferably both.

V. CONCLUSIONS

Acute pain management has assumed an increasingly important role in the ICU. We now understand that patients' needs for pain relief can be better met than they have been in the past. Simultaneously, morbidity and its attendant emotional and financial cost may be avoided. Much remains to be done, both in the realm of research ("How can we do better?") and in educating caregivers about the importance of adequate pain control in the critically ill patient ("*Why* should we do better?"). This text contributes significantly to this latter process—educating the caregiver. Improved understanding of the importance of effective pain management in the critically ill patient, it is hoped, will give birth to a strong commitment to research and the development of technologies for the assessment and treatment of pain.

REFERENCES

1. IASP Subcommittee on Taxonomy: Pain terms: a list with definitions and notes on usage. *Pain* 8:249, 1980.
2. MacInnes C: Cancer ward. *New Society* April 29:232, 1976.
3. Bion JF: Sedation and analgesia in the intensive care unit. *Hosp Update* 14:1272, 1988.
4. Jarrett J: From the Agency for Health Care Policy and Research. *JAMA* 267(editorial)19:2850, 1992.
5. Royal College of Surgeons of England and College of Anaesthetists' Commission on the Provision of Surgical Services: Report of the working party on pain after surgery. London, RCS, 1990.
6. Coleman DL: Control of postoperative pain: nonnarcotic and narcotic alternatives and their effect on pulmonary fuction. *Chest* 92:520, 1987.
7. Rawal N, Sjostrand U, Dahlstrom B, et al: Epidural morphine for postoperative pain relief: a comparative study with intramuscular narcotic and intercostal nerve block. *Anes Analg* 61(1):93, 1982.
8. Tinkle JK, Richardson JD, Franz JL, et al: Management of flail chest without mechanical ventilation. *Ann Thoracic Surg* 19:355, 1975.
9. Pflug AE, Halter JB: Effect of spinal anaesthesia on adrenergic tone and the neuroendocrine response to surgical stress in humans. *Anesthesiology* 55:120, 1981.
10. Brant MR, Fernandes A, Mordhorst R, Kehlet H: Epidural anaesthesia improves postoperative nitrogen balance. *Br Med J* 1:1106, 1981.
11. Rem J, Brant MR, Kehlet H: Prevention of postoperative lymphopenia and granulocytosis by epidural analgesia. *Lancet* 1:283, 1980.
12. Tuman KJ, McCarthy RJ, March RJ, et al: Effects of epidural anesthesia and analgesia on coagulation and outcome after major vascular surgery. *Anesth Analg* 73:696, 1991.
13. Bedder MD, Soifer BE, Mulhall JJV: A comparison of patient controlled analgesia and bolus prn intravenous morphine in the intensive care environment. *Clin J Pain* 7:205, 1991.
14. Hecker B, Albert L: Patient-controlled analgesia: a randomized, prospective comparison between two commercially available PCA pumps and conventional analgesic therapy for postoperative pain. *Pain* 35:115, 1988.

15. Yeager MP, Glass DD, Neff RK, Brinck-Johnsen T: Epidural anesthesia and analgesia in high-risk patients. *Anesthesiology* 66:729, 1987.
16. Guyatt GH, Tugwell PX, Feeny DH, et al: A framework for clinical evaluation of diagnostic technologies. *Can Med Assoc J* 134:587, 1986.
17. Laupacis A, Fenny D, Detsky AS, Tugwell PX: How attractive does a new technology have to be to warrant adoption and utilization? Tentative guidelines for using clinical economic evaluations. *Can Med Assoc J* 146(4):473, 1992.

PART TWO

THE ANATOMY, PHYSIOLOGY, AND ASSESSMENT OF PAIN

CHAPTER 2

THE ASSESSMENT OF PAIN

John C. Rowlingson

I. Introduction
    A. Definition of Assessment
    B. Definition of Pain
II. Why Is Assessment Important?
    A. Goals of Assessment
    B. Barriers to Assessment
III. What to Assess
    A. Requirements of Assessment Tools
    B. Components of the Pain Experience
    C. Physiologic Data
    D. Psychological Data
IV. How to Assess the Patient
    A. Introductory Comments
    B. History
    C. Physical Examination
    D. Behavioral Assessment
    E. Laboratory Studies
V. Assessment Instruments
    A. Desirable Characteristics
    B. Common Assessment Techniques
    C. Less Common Techniques
VI. Issues Specific to Pediatric Patients
    A. Introductory Comments
    B. History
    C. Physical Examination
    D. Laboratory Study
    E. Psychosocial Issues
    F. Assessment Tools
VII. Conclusions
Suggested Readings

I. INTRODUCTION

A. Definition of Assessment

Assessment is a process of evaluation with the purpose of making a decision or developing an opinion. In medicine, the usual goal of patient assessment is **to establish a diagnosis.** In patients who have been acutely injured or who are critically ill, this process is essential because a patient's status can change quickly and decisive action may be required to regain physiologic stability or provide lifesaving care.

B. Definition of Pain

In specific reference to pain, the **etiology and consequences of the painful injury or illness must be evaluated.** This is *not* the same as simply measuring the amount of pain, even though this is a literal definition of assessment. Assessment implies a more extensive investigation into such associated issues as the patient's concurrent medical history, the circumstances of the injury or illness, his or her background and usual environment, and the reaction to the acute situation.

Pain is defined as "an unpleasant sensory and emotional experience associated with actual or potential tissue damage or described in terms of such damage." This description embraces the crucial concept that *both* the physical *and* the nonphysical aspects of pain must be assessed. **Pain is a dynamic, multidimensional experience** that must be examined entirely so that no possible etiology for the pain, or a factor that is influencing its expression or perception, is missed.

II. WHY IS ASSESSMENT IMPORTANT?

A. Goals of Assessment

The **goals of assessment** include the following.

1. What the current pain complaints mean to the patient must be accurately identified.

2. Information collected from many sources will lead to the **diagnosis of the cause(s) of the "pain."** What is wrong is *not* always obvious by simply observing the patient. The caretaker must address the patient's interpretation of the pain, as well as other psychological factors that may be altering the patient's perception of the pain. These issues are particularly important for patients who appear to be responding to their pain "inappropriately."

3. **Procuring the diagnosis** is paramount to providing appropriate therapy, and doing so in a timely fashion. This will also enhance the quality of patient care and improve the outcome.

4. Once **treatment** is being provided, its **effect must be assessed repeatedly,** as this information is the basis upon which decisions are made to continue or alter therapy.

B. Barriers to Assessment

In critically ill and acutely injured patients, the barriers to assessment include:

1. Adherence to an outdated definition of pain and a lack of appreciation that assessment must include both physical and nonphysical factors,
2. The absence of ways to quantitate scientifically or mathematically the subjective experience of pain. This factor is further complicated in critically ill patients who may not be able to articulate their complaints or cooperate with assessment or treatment,
3. The fact that observational skills for pain behaviors require clinical experience, and yet can be biased by the observer's attitudes, prejudices, and beliefs,
4. A vast variation in patients' presentations of their pain (e.g., the stoic versus the histrionic patient) and the staff's reaction to the presentation.
5. The absolute need for communication among doctors, nurses, ancillary staff, patients, and family members, particularly in the critical care setting,
6. The impact of circadian rhythms and chronobiologic patterns (e.g., the menstrual cycle, diurnal variation in cortisol level, wake–sleep cycles) on the results of assessment. Stress and critical illness can alter even some of these very basic cycles, making the patient's response to pain assessment vary over an even wider range.

III. WHAT TO ASSESS

A. Requirements of Assessment Tools

Methods, techniques, and/or systems are needed that are patient friendly, can efficiently combine data in different formats and from multiple sources, are sensitive to changes in pain intensity, and show reliability in a variety of clinical settings. The tools for assessment must be free of bias and capable of accentuating the dual nature of the pain experience. This is problematic because pain is a dynamic psychophysiologic event that is affected by many extraneous factors. The data so generated must be readily available for clinical use, so that momentous therapeutic and ethical decisions, let alone the day-to-day management choices, can be made based upon it.

B. Components of the Pain Experience

Given the contemporary definition of pain, attention must be paid to the pain's sensory aspect, its unpleasantness, the patient's illness or injury and the associated tissue damage (whether real or only perceived by the patient), the premorbid emotional status and coping style, and the patient's reaction to current affairs. Information about preexisting pain syndromes should be sought from the patient and/or family, as this may raise pertinent issues such as past pain experiences, coping strategies used in the past, and drug history, among others.

C. Physiologic Data

1. That pain has a sensory component is a well-accepted premise. Patients with acute injuries and/or critical illness will have obvious physical sources for their pain. There is a hazard in attributing the severity of pain to the amount or degree of tissue injury. Some idea of the **distress** a patient is suffering may be gained by reviewing the **vital signs,** including blood pressure, heart rate, and respiratory rate. This is reasonable, though the anxiety and sympathetic nervous system stimulation associated with acute illness or injury confound a literal translation.

2. Other variables that can be assessed include the patient's general appearance, his or her posture, the reaction to touch and examination, the presence of sweating, and the movement in response to stimulation.

3. Communication barriers are prominent in the intensive care unit (ICU) due to the presence of endotracheal or tracheostomy tubes, sedative drugs or muscle relaxants, and encephalopathy or other pathology of the central nervous system (CNS). Patients may well be nonverbal and/or immobile due to their primary injuries or the coincident effects of necessary treatment. These conditions will make assessment a greater challenge.

D. Psychological Data

1. Behavior is a form of communication, and a patient's behavior is likely to reflect the presence of pain.

2. Pain has an inherent unpleasant quality. Its **perceived intensity and severity** will be influenced by a medley of physical *and* emotional factors. The significant factors that lower pain threshold, listed in Table 3-1 in Chapter 3, to which an ICU patient could be subject include discomfort, insomnia, fatigue, fear, isolation, loss of control, and anxiety (due to the threat to health and/or life, the projected implications of the illness/injury for the future, and the interruption of daily routine).

   3. **Observation** is one form of psychological assessment. Numerous studies have documented a discrepancy between a patient's stated level of pain and that projected onto the patient, even by trained observers. There is a consensus that **pain behaviors** such as grimacing, crying, and immobility connote distress within the patient, but no quantitation of the complaints is possible from these general data.

   4. **Interviewing** the patient to establish his or her self-assessment is the best method for evaluating the pain, but this modality may not be feasible for some patients in the ICU. The arousal of negative emotions can increase the awareness of pain, whereas positive emotions can decrease pain.

IV. HOW TO ASSESS THE PATIENT

A. Introductory Comments

It is obvious that a **systematic yet individualized approach** to assessment is absolutely necessary so that the goal of deciphering the diagnosis based on an appreciation of the unique circumstances of the patient can be achieved. Any technique or instrument used must be reliable (this reflects the repeatability and trustworthiness) and valid (this is a measure of the ability of a test to identify patients with the characteristic being screened for; its sensitivity and specificity affect its validity).

B. History

The history of the acute injury or the evolution of the critical illness is vital to understanding the chronologic events surrounding the patient's current problem(s). **Review of the pertinent records,** whether of past admissions for a similar illness or of past medical history, will afford some insight. This may provide an outline of the patient's story such that the actual interview time can be kept short and focused. The history and mechanism of the injury must be elicited, as well as the presence of chronic medical problems, including chronic pain syndromes, preexisting conditions that will affect the physical consequences or physiologic reserve of the patient, psychosocial features, and current medications.

C. Physical Examination

   1. The **area of injury** and the **associated physiologic systems** must be evaluated. Body systems not directly related to the trauma or critical illness may be obscurely involved, so it is optimal to perform a complete physical examination when circumstances allow.

2. **Vital signs** do not necessarily correlate with the intensity or the seriousness of the pain. It may be useful to discriminate between complaints of pain and the anxiety related to the acute situation. Causes of sympathetic stimulation, such as hypoxia, hypercarbia, and a full bladder, must be ruled out.

3. Use of the **Glasgow coma scale** is routine in assessing patients suspected of intracranial pathology of many types, though its original application was for assessing coma.

4. **Observation** for signs of distress, body posturing, and the cooperation with verbal responses is important.

5. It is critical that all health-care professionals acknowledge that **infants and children** feel pain. Definite reactions are noted in physiologic and behavioral parameters, and though these are indirect measures, they are the primary sources of information about pain in all nonverbal patients.

D. Behavioral Assessment

1. Because pain is both a sensory *and* an emotional experience, attention must be directed to the **psychosocial ramifications** of the acute injury or disease. We must know how the injury has changed the patient's attitudes, behavior, and lifestyle. The impact of the injury on subsequent **functional abilities,** be they physical or psychological, is also becoming a contemporary issue.

2. The **perceived consequences of the pain** will influence the related behavior.

3. Features that are important to evaluate early in the illness include the **patient's understanding** and **degree of acceptance** of his or her situation, his or her **attitudes,** and the **premorbid emotional status** of the patient.

4. After a period of hospitalization, signs of **depression,** such as irritability, decreased energy, poor concentration, and decreased appetite, should be sought.

5. The issue of **loss of control** due to hospitalization for acute injury or critical illness is a particular area for investigation, as it may markedly affect the patient's cooperation with and participation in therapy.

6. The assessment may identify patients for whom **psychological therapies** may be an option (see Chapters 5 and 14).

E. Laboratory Studies

1. Positive laboratory results may aid in the attainment of a diagnosis, but they are but one piece of the diagnosis equation (a history and a physical examination are the others).

2. Negative laboratory results do *not* mean that there is no "real" pain or that psychopathology is dominant.

3. Many of the studies requested in the presence of acute injury or critical illness are done for the specific purpose of confirming a presumptive diagnosis or to rule out items of the differential diagnosis.

4. Indices that track the stress response (e.g., catecholamine release, protein wasting, negative nitrogen balance, corticosteroid levels, renin–angiotensin–aldosterone release, and sodium/water retention) may be of benefit.

5. Measures of specific organ system function (e.g., vital capacity, functional residual capacity, and liver function tests) can be done on a serial basis to guide therapy and the response to it.

6. Somatosensory evoked potential (SSEP) studies are being used to assess the degree of CNS reactivity in patients with diminished levels of consciousness.

V. ASSESSMENT INSTRUMENTS

A. Desirable Characteristics

Given the variety of presentations of pain and the innumerable combinations of physical and psychosocial circumstances, it is not surprising that many tests have been recommended for assessing pain. They range from simple linear scales to complex machines. Patients in an ICU may be difficult to assess using these techniques, because most require a verbal patient whose cognitive function is intact. These patients may have neither the attentional ability nor the stamina to complete even the simple tests. Some require hand–eye coordination, and that can be an additional issue for the ICU patient.

The characteristics of an ideal assessment test would include:

1. Relative freedom from bias.
2. Provision of immediate feedback.
3. Applicability in both clinical and research conditions and with a variety of patients.
4. Reliability.
5. Sensitivity to changes in pain intensity.
6. Inclusion of the physical *and* nonphysical aspects of pain.

B. Common Assessment Techniques

1. The Visual Analogue Scale (VAS)   This scale (Fig. 2-1*A*) is the most common pain assessment tool used in pain medicine today. There is a large body of literature that supports its validity. The scale is usually a 10-cm line with the anchors of "no pain" and "the worst pain imaginable" at either end.

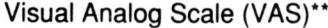

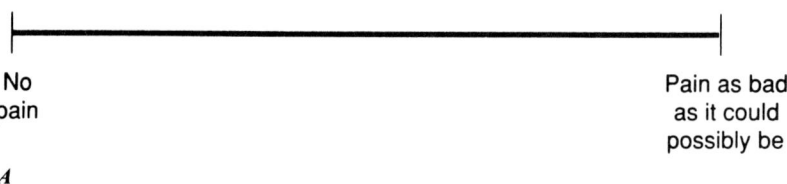

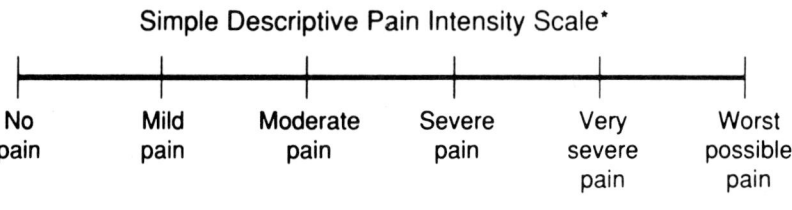

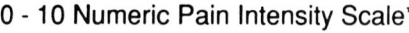

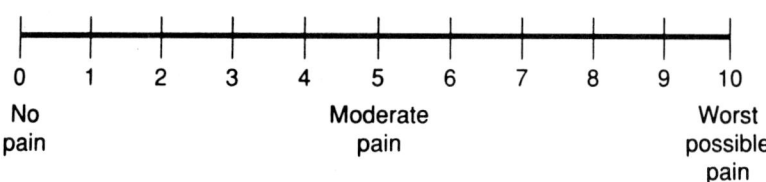

*If used as a graphic rating scale, a 10-cm baseline is recommended.
**A 10-cm baseline is recommended for VAS scales.

Figure 2-1 Simple assessment instruments that provide information about pain quickly. *(From Acute Pain Management Panel:* Acute Pain Management: Operative or Medical Procedures and Trauma. Clinical Practice Guideline. *AHCPR Pub No. 92-0032. Rockville, Maryland: Agency for Health Care Policy and Research, Public Health Service, U.S. Department of Health and Human Services, February 1992.)

     a. The advantages of the VAS include a positive association with other self-report measures, good sensitivity to treatment effects, scores that can be statistically analyzed, and a high number of response options, so that it is sensitive to changes in pain intensity, its use is simple, information is quickly obtained, the results are reproducible, and it is useful in a wide range of clinical and research conditions.
     b. The disadvantages of the VAS include a lack of quantitation of

pain between the end points, the necessity that the patient have a certain level of cognitive functioning to cooperate with it, its use being limited to patients older than approximately 8 years of age, and the linear measurement of the patient's response, which adds time and a potential source of error.

2. Verbal scales The patient's self-report is the best verbal test, but this option may be severely limited in the ICU patient. **Verbal scales** ask the patient to pick a word that reflects the intensity of the pain from a list of words (Fig. 2-2) or from words spaced along a horizontal or vertical line (Fig. 2-1*B*). This concept can be used to assess not only the intensity of pain, but also its relief after treatment, or symptom intensity and/or relief, depending on the grouping of words chosen.

   a. The advantages of verbal scales are that they are easy to administer and score and that there is good evidence of their validity.

   b. The disadvantages include the demand on the patient to choose a word that may not be exactly descriptive of the pain, the need for education to understand the words and the concept, there being only as many response categories as there are words, and the fact that the data are only somewhat amenable to statistical review.

3. Numerical scales These scales require the patient to pick a number from 0 to 10 or 0 to 100 that represents his or her pain (Fig. 2-1*C*). Some patients find it easier to assign a monetary value to their pain, perhaps because it offers a slightly more concrete image of the 0 to 100 scale. The

CIRCLE THE NUMBER IN EACH COLUMN THAT BEST DESCRIBES YOUR PAIN THE PAST MONTH

INTENSITY	REACTION	SENSATION
1. EXCRUCIATING	1. AGONIZING	1. PIERCING
2. INTOLERABLE	2. INTOLERABLE	2. STABBING
3. VERY INTENSE	3. UNBEARABLE	3. SHOOTING
4. EXTREMELY STRONG	4. AWFUL	4. BURNING
5. SEVERE	5. MISERABLE	5. GRINDING
6. VERY STRONG	6. DISTRESSING	6. THROBBING
7. INTENSE	7. UNPLEASANT	7. CRAMPING
8. STRONG	8. DISTRACTING	8. ACHING
9. UNCOMFORTABLE	9. UNCOMFORTABLE	9. STINGING
10. MODERATE	10. TOLERABLE	10. SQUEEZING
11. MILD	11. BEARABLE	11. NUMBING
12. WEAK	12. NONE	12. ITCHING
13. VERY WEAK		13. TINGLING
14. JUST NOTICEABLE		14. NONE
15. EXTREMELY WEAK		
16. NONE		

Figure 2-2 Verbal scale word lists—lists of descriptive terms from which the patient can choose to characterize his/her pain. This is similar to the concept of the McGill Pain Questionaire. *(From University of Virginia Health Sciences Center, Department of Anesthesiology, Pain Management Center:* Patient Assessment Inventory and Narrative.*)*

patient is asked, "If 0 = no pain and $1.00 = the worst pain imaginable, how much is your pain worth?"

    a. The **advantages** of numerical scales include their being easy to score and administer, the high number of response categories possible, good patient cooperation, and support of their validity.

    b. The **disadvantages** relate to the weak statistical basis of the data and the low treatment sensitivity. Additionally, like the VAS, numerical scales demand a requisite level of mental functioning and abstract thinking to be usable.

    4. Drawings Drawing on body figures is a technique that provides more data about the location of pain than anything else. In general, the more widespread the drawing of the pain, the more intense, frequent, and disruptive the pain is (see Fig. 2-3). While a picture can be worth a thousand words, this modality requires coordination, visual integrity, and, depending on the task given, a variable level of cognitive functioning.

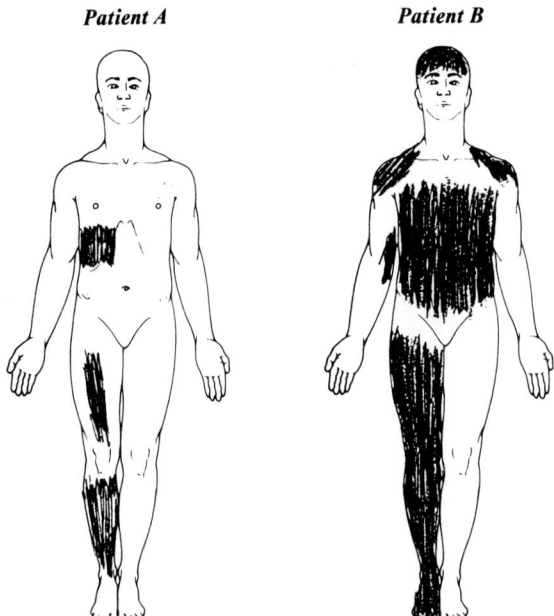

Figure 2-3 Draw-your-pain tests: Both patients (A and B) have suffered broken ribs, a femur fracture, and tibial-fibular fracture in a motor vehicle accident. *A* is the depiction of a 44-year-old male whose car skidded on the ice and hit a utility pole. *B* represents the same injuries in a 35-year-old male whose car was hit by a drunken driver and whose wife and children were killed in the accident. There is a great deal more "pain" reflected in drawing *B*, reflecting the associated emotional distress this patient feels over the loss of his family.

5. **Affective measures** Tests that assess the affective component of pain are numerous, but are not as well studied as those mentioned above. The **McGill Pain Questionnaire** is a traditional test that demands that the patient choose descriptive words from long lists. It takes both time and education, and can be influenced by repeat testing, past experience, and unrelated events. The **Minnesota Multiphasic Personality Inventory** (MMPI) is an even longer test and requires the patient to be fully alert. Neither of these is practical for most acutely injured or critically ill patients.

C. Less Common Techniques

Less common tests include choosing pictures, facial expressions (see Chapter 30), or colors; grouping poker chips (proportional to the amount of pain—a concrete VAS); and completing diaries and questionnaires.

VI. ISSUES SPECIFIC TO PEDIATRIC PATIENTS

A. Introductory Comments

Children require patience and understanding during the assessment process. Their cooperation will depend on their age, stage of cognitive development, and communication skills. Even their age is only a relative indicator of the likely success of interactive assessment given the propensity for children to regress behaviorally in response to stress. We can make inferences about pain in nonverbal infants and children only on the basis of their behavioral and physiologic responses (see Chapter 30).

B. History

The **history-taking** process may be complicated by the child's ability to understand the questions or to express his or her feelings. He or she may be inhibited by fear of the accident, the hospital, and/or the interviewer. There may be a reluctance to discuss psychosocial issues. The quality of information obtained may be enhanced or impaired by the presence of family members, depending on the age of the patient; the patient's rapport with the family member present; the nature of the injury or illness; and the type of information being sought. The history taker needs to use sensitivity in determining the impact of family members on the effectiveness of the interview.

C. Physical Examination

The physical examination may be confounded by the child's reluctance to cooperate. Observational data relative to facial expression, crying, verbalization, movement, and withdrawal may be useful.

D. Laboratory Tests

There may be a reticence to order **laboratory tests,** so information from this source may not be available during the assessment process.

E. Psychosocial Issues

The **psychosocial assessment** process may be difficult due to the child's emotional immaturity and the presence or absence of the parents. The family's values and belief systems can have a strong influence on the child's responses.

F. Assessment Tools

Assessment tests are useful in children who are old enough to understand their purpose and cooperate in their completion. **Drawing** is a form of play for children, and can be used alone or in combination with colors to evaluate the presence and severity of pain. The child must choose the color for pain before the testing, so this may not be applicable in the unexpectedly hospitalized child. This technique, although labor intensive, does let the child set his or her own individual scale, and it enhances the communication between the staff and the patient.

VII. CONCLUSIONS

   A. The assessment of the patient with pain requires an appreciation for the reality that "pain" is a diverse psychophysiologic experience which is felt by the patient. His or her presentation thereof must be blended with data from physical examinations and laboratory studies to create a diagnosis.
   B. Assessment is partly a clinical art, but it is also partly intuitive. There has to be a place in medicine where the experience of day-to-day practice gives one the ability to accurately project where the trend of findings is going and to act preemptively.
   C. The most valuable information about the pain is the patient's self-report. Addressing the needs of the patient is always important, but may have to be relegated temporarily to a lower priority, while attention is paid to critical, life-threatening problems.
   D. There are many supplemental assessment techniques that have utility, but none of them is perfect. Assessment must be performed in a serial manner to gauge the patient's response to injury and/or treatment.
   E. Whenever possible, the patient should participate in management decisions. The patient who perceives himself or herself as a partner on the

pain management team is likely to experience less distress over pain and to be more cooperative with treatment and care than the patient who feels victimized by his or her discomfort.

SUGGESTED READINGS

Craig KD, Whitfield MF, Grunau RVE, et al.: Pain in the preterm neonate: behavioral and physiological indices. *Pain* 52:287–299, 1993.
Ferrell BR, McCaffery M, Grant M: Clinical decision making and pain. *Cancer Nursing* 14(6):289–297, 1991.
Holroyd KA, Holm JE, Keefe FJ, et al.: A multi-center evaluation of the McGill Pain Questionnaire: results from more than 1700 chronic pain patients. *Pain* 48:301–311, 1992.
Manne SL, Jacobsen PB, Redd WH: Assessment of acute pediatric pain: do child self reports, parent ratings and nurse ratings measure the same phenomenon? *Pain* 48:45–52, 1992.
Merskey H: Classification of chronic pain. Descriptions of chronic pain syndromes and definitions of pain terms. *Pain* suppl 3, 1986.
Ness TJ, Gebhart GF: Visceral pain: A review of experimental studies. *Pain* 41:167–234, 1990.
Paige D, Cioffi AM: Pain assessment and measurement, in Sinatra RS, Hord AH, Ginsberg B, Preble LM (eds): *Acute Pain Mechanisms and Management.* St. Loius, Mosby, 1992, pp 70–77.
Price DD, Harkins SW, Baker C: Sensory-affective relationships among different types of clinical and experimental pain. *Pain* 28:297–307, 1987.
Toomey TC, Mann JD, Abashian S, et al: Relationship of pain drawing scores to rating of pain description and function. *Clin J Pain* 7:269–274, 1991.
Turk DC, Melzack R (eds.): *Handbook of Pain Assessment.* New York, Guilford Press, 1992.
Zelter LK, Barr RG, McGrath PA, et al: Pediatric pain: interacting behavioral and physical factors. *Pediatrics* 90:816–821, 1992.

CHAPTER
3

PAIN MECHANISMS AND PATHWAYS

John C. Rowlingson

I. Introduction
II. Understanding Pain
III. Types of Pain
   A. Definition
   B. Acute pain
   C. Chronic pain
   D. Cancer pain
   E. Comparison of Acute and Chronic Pain
   F. Pain in Pediatric Patients
IV. The Circuitry of Pain
   A. Peripheral Receptors
   B. Chemicals
   C. Nerve Fibers
   D. Dorsal Horn of the Spinal Cord
   E. Ascending Tracts
   F. Descending Circuits
V. Postoperative and Traumatic Pain
VI. Sympathetically Maintained Pain
VII. Myofascial Pain
VIII. Neuralgic Pain
IX. Cancer Pain
X. Conclusions
Suggested Readings

I. INTRODUCTION

A. Why is this subject important?
   1. One answer is that when we understand the possible mechanisms of pain, we will be more exacting in our diagnosis of its cause.
   2. By knowing the mechanism, we can provide specific therapy that treats the pain by managing its cause rather than just the symptoms.

II. UNDERSTANDING PAIN

A. Pain is defined as **"a sensory and emotional experience associated with actual or potential tissue damage or described in terms of such damage."**

B. All pain is a **combination of physical and nonphysical factors.** Each patient has his or her own personal and "environmental" factors that powerfully influence the "pain."

C. One's concept of pain is influenced by specialty training and clinical experience such that health care professionals bring a bias to their assessment and treatment of patients.

D. Pain has different meanings and significance to different patients, depending on their understanding of it, the circumstances under which it occurs, and its cause.

    1. For example, a patient with an acute and painful injury is likely to experience anxiety as well as the pain.

    2. The patient in the intensive care unit (ICU) must deal with that environment, as well as the consequences and the discomfort of an injury or operation.

    3. Pain known to be due to malignancy after an operation will be perceived as more intense than that due to benign disease.

    4. Pain after an amputation carried out to abolish cancer will be perceived differently than when the amputation is performed for peripheral arterial insufficiency, after which the loss of function may be the patient's major focus.

E. Patients of **all ages** experience pain.

F. Factors that influence the **threshold for pain** are listed in Table 3-1.

    1. These factors increase or decrease the intensity and perception of the pain.

    2. The workup of the patient must identify whether they are present or not, as they must be considered in therapeutic decisions.

III. TYPES OF PAIN

A. All pain is *not* the same.

B. Acute pain is a biologically necessary, physiologic response that provokes an escape/protection reaction.

C. Chronic pain has less physiologic correlation with tissue damage. It can have a devastating effect on a patient and his or her family. The original injury may resolve, but the consequences of the pain linger.

    1. Physical deconditioning is due to inactivity.
    2. Morphologic changes in the nervous system persist.

Table 3-1 Factors that influence pain threshold*

Lower	Raise
Discomfort	Relief of symptoms/analgesics
Insomnia	Sleep
Fatigue	Rest
Anxiety	Sympathy/anxiolytics
Fear	Understanding
Anger	Diversion
Sadness/depression	Elevation of mood/antidepressants
Mental isolation	
Introversion	
Past experience	

*With permission from Twycross R: The relief of pain in far-advanced cancer. *Reg Anesth* 5(3):2–11, 1980 (July–September).

    3. Changes in behavior, productivity, lifestyle, and attitudes toward becoming healthy again become entrenched.

  D. Cancer pain is often a combination of the features of both acute and chronic pain (see Chapters 28 and 32).

  E. The comparison of Acute and Chronic Pain is highlighted in Table 3-2.

    1. Each type of pain has a different warning/signal function.

    2. Different evaluation protocols are called for.

      a. use history taking, a physical examination, and laboratory testing as a database.

      b. the evaluation must acknowledge the potential for the emotional component of the pain to interplay with its clinical presentation and response to therapy, as well as for "pain" to become a lifestyle for the patient with chronic pain.

    3. Different therapeutic modalities are used because most treatments that effectively curtail acute pain are not appropriate for the long duration of treatment that is usually necessary for patients with chronic pain.

    4. Different expectations of therapy are realistic:

      a. acute pain should be eliminated;

      b. chronic pain should be maximally controlled, and the patient given help in coping with the residual pain.

    5. In the setting of chronic pain, superimposed acute pain should be aggressively treated.

Table 3-2 Differences between acute and chronic pain

Acute	Chronic
Ample training and experience gained	Less so
Evaluation and treatment take less time	Time-consuming process
Pain is a useful physiologic signal	Pain is a disease that affects attitudes, lifestyles, and behavior
Pain plus anxiety	Pain plus frustration
Short, self-limiting treatment course	Prolonged therapy needed
Expect to cure the pain	Hope to control the pain
Success rate of therapy is high	Success rate is moderate

   6. Frequently the pain is more manageable when the patient understands its etiology and significance. Thus repeated explanations to the patient are critical.

F. Pain in Pediatric Patients

   1. There is a false impression that children feel less pain and necessarily "heal quicker" than do adults.
   2. Children understand and describe pain according to their age, cognitive and developmental level, sex, and previous experience with pain. Stress-related emotional regression may demand communication at a very basic and concrete level.
   3. The pain is difficult to evaluate because the ability to communicate and obtain the history varies, children lack the vocabulary to describe the pain, doing a physical examination can be problematic, there may be a reticence to do laboratory testing and/or invasive procedures, and 'psychological' issues may be ignored.
   4. See Chapter 30 for a more detailed discussion of pain management in the critically ill child.

IV. THE CIRCUITRY OF PAIN

A. Peripheral Receptors

   1. Free nerve endings are stimulated and code pain to the central nervous system (CNS). The pain receptors in the periphery are called **nociceptors.** These are different from the receptors that are activated by temperature and pressure (Fig. 3-1).
   2. There are specific receptors for sensing damaging temperature and pressure throughout the body.

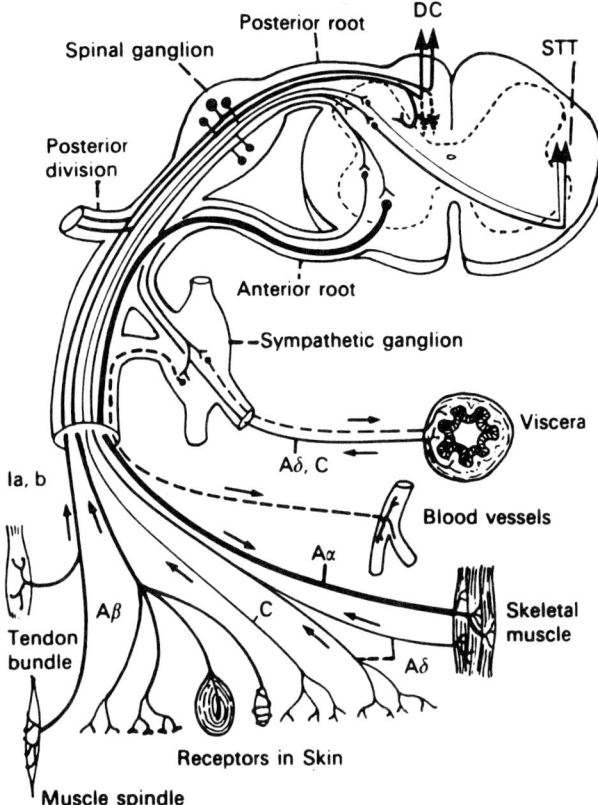

Figure 3-1 The connections from the peripheral receptors to the dorsal horn of the spinal cord. *(From Bonica J:* The Management of Pain, *2nd ed. Philadelphia, Lea & Febiger, 1990.)*

3. The peripheral receptors may be sensitized by the sympathetic nervous system.

B. Chemicals

1. Chemicals act on the receptors to change their thresholds. **Histamine, serotonin, and bradykinin** that are released when tissues are injured sensitize the receptors, as well as stimulate them.

2. **Arachidonic acid derivatives,** such as prostaglandins, leukotrienes, and thromboxanes, sensitize without stimulating the receptors.

C. Nerve Fibers

Nerve fibers connect the receptors to the dorsal horn (Fig. 3-1).

1. **A-delta fibers** transmit impulses quickly because they are myelinated. They carry so-called "first pain," which is sharp and localized.

2. C fibers are not myelinated. They conduct impulses slowly. They carry so-called "second pain," which is diffuse, burning, throbbing, and aching in character.

3. A-alpha and A-beta fibers can become involved through recruitment and plasticity in the injured nervous system. Their input does not undergo the same checks and balances as does that of the A-delta and C fibers in the CNS, so their pain may be episodic, sharp, stabbing, and difficult to control.

D. Dorsal Horn of the Spinal Cord

The dorsal horn of the spinal cord is the site of first entry for pain impulses.

1. The substantia gelatinosa is the crucial relay station where there is a layering of function-specific cells.

2. It makes a difference as to which level of the substantia gelatinosa the A-delta, C, A-alpha, or A-beta fiber steps in.

3. This is where opioids work primarily; there is a high concentration of opiate receptors in the second and third layers. Opioids exert both a pre- and postsynaptic effect in causing inhibition/modification of nociceptive input.

  a. **Mu$_1$ receptors** mediate somatic and visceral analgesia.

  b. **Mu$_2$ receptors** mediate respiratory depression.

  c. **Delta receptors** mediate somatic but not visceral analgesia and some respiratory depression.

  d. **Kappa receptors** mediate visceral analgesia.

  e. **Sigma receptors** are involved with the psychotomimetic effects of opioids.

4. Many other substances contribute to excitation or inhibition of neural input at this level, such as clonidine, epinephrine, serotonin, and substance P.

E. Ascending Tracts

Ascending tracts (Fig. 3-2) carry pain information to the thalamus and cortex. The **paleospinothalamic system** transmits pain that is dull in character and poorly localized. It feeds the limbic system, the reticular formation, and the brain stem, with the combined input causing vasomotor, autonomic, motivational, adversive, and suffering reactions in the organism.

The **neospinothalamic system** carries discrete, sharp, localized pain messages. It is not the primary nociceptive pathway, but rather an alternate for discriminating somatosensory information.

1. The dorsolateral funiculus ascends ipsilaterally.

2. The lateral spinothalamic tract carries information that has crossed the midline.

3. The sympathetic nervous system can contribute to abnormalities in

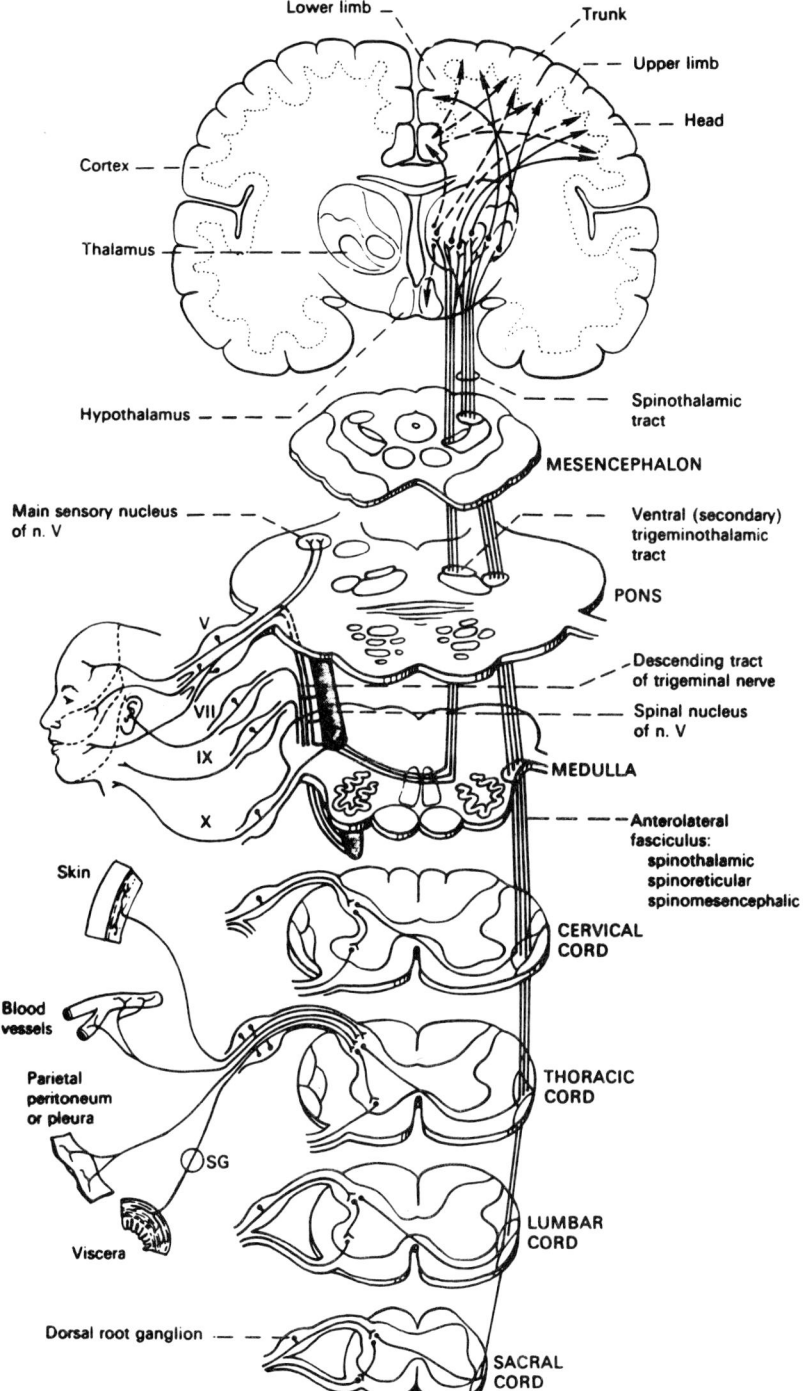

Figure 3-2 The ascending pain pathways. *(From Bonica J:* The Management of Pain, *2nd ed. Philadelphia, Lea & Febiger, 1990.)*

the central processing of noxious afferent input by mechanisms that are as yet unclear.

F. Descending Circuits

Descending circuits from many levels of the CNS play a vital role in modifying the transmission and processing of pain input through chemical messengers. The descending modulation system can be triggered by drugs or by hypnosis.

V. POSTOPERATIVE AND TRAUMATIC PAIN

    A. Tissue incision and manipulation cause the release of **algesic mediators** that stimulate and/or sensitize the nociceptors.
    B. This input bombards the CNS and triggers reflex responses (see Chapter 4).
        1. **Segmental spinal reflexes** result in muscle spasm and vasoconstriction.
        2. **Suprasegmental reflex responses** are the result of noxious input from a number of spinal segments accumulating to cause the release of catecholamines, steroids, and renin-angiotensin, all of which result in metabolic and physiologic effects.
        3. The patient will have a **cortical reaction** to the seemingly inescapable pain. What the patient thinks and believes about the pain will strongly influence the effectiveness of the other therapy provided.
    C. The **summation of** the spinal, suprasegmental, and cortical **responses puts a patient at risk** for developing the pathophysiologic consequences of acute pain, as listed in Table 3-3, and also discussed in Chapter 4.
        1. Note that *all* body systems can be *adversely* affected.
        2. Overstressing one physiologic system can create excessive demands on and compensatory changes in another, and put the already compromised, critically ill patient at risk for multisystem organ failure.
        3. These factors directly influence the patient's morbidity and mortality; thus the pain *must be* effectively treated.

VI. SYMPATHETICALLY MAINTAINED PAIN

    A. The exact connection between the sympathetic nervous system (SNS) and the somatic systems is not known.
    B. The current thinking is that in response to injury, the SNS sensitizes the nociceptors and lowers their threshold for activation. The nociceptors happen to transmit pain information through nerves (wide dynamic range

Table 3-3 Adverse effects of acute pain

Cardiovascular	Tachycardia, hypertension, increased SVR, increased cardiac work, increased myocardial O_2 demand
Pulmonary	Hypoxia, hypercarbia, atelectasis, decreased cough, decreased vital capacity and functional residual capacity, V/Q mismatch
Gastrointestinal	Nausea, vomiting, ileus, intolerance for oral intake
Renal	Oliguria, urinary retention
Extremities	Skeletal muscle spasm, limited mobility, thromboembolism
Endocrine	Excessive adrenergic activity, vagal inhibition, catabolic metabolism, increased O_2 consumption
CNS	Sedation, fatigue, anxiety, and fear cause central sympathetic stimulation
Immunologic	Inhibited cellular immunity, increased risk of infection, ?? impaired wound healing ??

[WDR] neurons) that also have their function facilitated by the influence of the SNS. The effect of a lowered threshold for receptor activation means that a higher rate of transmitted neural activity occurs for a given stimulus, even a previously benign one (i.e., light touch).

    C. The alpha-adrenergic receptor may be an important link in the periphery.

    D. Mechanical hyperalgesia in sympathetically maintained pain (SMP) may be the result of the activation of A-beta mechanoreceptors that results in central sensitization and abnormal central processing of noxious afferent input.

VII. MYOFASCIAL PAIN

    A. Myofascial pain (MFP) may be the primary result of a direct injury to muscles or their supporting tissues.

    B. Or it may be the consequence of improper posture and subsequent strain/sprain of muscles and joints that are distant from the original injury.

    C. The tender **trigger points** in muscles and the supporting tissues are *not* areas of chronic inflammation.

    D. There is a localized energy crisis due to muscle spasm and vasoconstriction that results in findings of the biochemical changes of anaerobic metabolism and hypoxia.

    E. A relationship has been found between poor sleep and subsequent inadequate muscle rest that contributes to myofascial pain.

    F. Processing by the CNS of noxious input using such substances as serotonin, catecholamines, endorphins, and neuropeptides also may play a role.

VIII. NEURALGIC PAIN

   A. Neuralgic pain is caused by damage to the nervous system by trauma, infection, metabolic insult, systemic disease, neurologic disease, or exposure to toxins.
   B. The injury to and the repair process in the nervous system can cause pain by the disruption of receptors, altered responses to algesic mediators surrounding the receptors, faulty transmission in the nerve cables that carry the impulses to the CNS, induced changes in the dorsal horn pharmacology, or changes in the central processing of neural input.
   C. The chronicity of the pain may evoke an emotional component that enhances the agony of the pain.

IX. CANCER PAIN

   A. Cancer pain can involve the causes of pain as above under VIII B.
   B. The diagnosis of cancer intensifies the emotional component of "pain" and the patient's perception of the severity of the pain.
   C. Cancer pain often presents as a combination of features of acute and chronic pain.
      1. Pain due to the oncologic process may have features of acute pain (e.g., due to bone metastasis, nerve compression).
      2. Pain related to therapy (e.g., surgery, radiation treatments) may have more characteristics of chronic pain.
      3. Many complaints not directly related to the disease or its therapy can be presented by the patient as "pain" (e.g., fatigue, worry, fear, constipation, mucositis). These will add to the patient's distress and discomfort.

X. CONCLUSIONS

   A. There are different kinds of pain, but all involve *both* physical and non-physical factors.
   B. Pain is more than tissue damage—just taking the pain away does not solve all of the patient's problems. This is especially true in chronic pain.
   C. The purpose of evaluating the patient is to establish the etiology for the pain and from that to generate mechanism-specific therapy.
   D. Pain can be rapidly reduced with medications, surgery, nerve blocks, and stimulation techniques.

E. Effectively treating the side effects of pain therapy, such as nausea, pruritus, and constipation, further improves the patient's sense of well-being.

F. Physical and emotional rehabilitation should follow pain reduction, and restoration of social functioning is reasonable thereafter.

SUGGESTED READINGS

Balter K: A review of pain anatomy and physiology. *Pain Digest* 2:306–330, 1992.

Boissevain MD, McCain GA: Toward an integrated understanding of fibromyalgia syndrome. I. Medical and pathophysiological aspects. *Pain* 45:227–238, 1991.

Fine PG, Hare BD: The pathways and mechanisms of pain and analgesia: a review and clinical perspective. *Hosp Formul* 20:972–985, 1985.

Maze M, Tranquilli W: Alpha-2 adrenoceptor agonists: defining the role in clinical anesthesia. *Anesthesiology* 74:581–605, 1991.

Pasternak GW: Multiple morphine and enkephalin receptors and the relief of pain. *JAMA* 259:1362–1367, 1988.

Raja SN: Reflex sympathetic dystrophy: pathophysiological basis for therapy. *Pain Digest* 2:274–280, 1992.

Raja SN, Meyer RA, Campbell JN: Peripheral mechanisms of somatic pain. *Anesthesiology* 68:571–590, 1988.

Roberts WJ: A hypothesis on the physiological basis for causalgia and related pains. *Pain* 24:297–311, 1986.

Rowlingson JC, Toomey TC: Multidisciplinary approaches to the management of chronic pain, in: Ghia JN (ed) *The Multidisciplinary Pain Center.* Boston, Kluwer Academic Publishers, 1988, pp 45–73.

Whipple B: Neurophysiology of pain. *Orthopaedic Nurs* 9:21–32, 1990.

Woolf CJ: Recent advances in the pathophysiology of acute pain. *Br J Anaesth* 63:139–147, 1989.

CHAPTER 4

THE PHYSIOLOGIC AND METABOLIC RESPONSE TO PAIN AND STRESS

Robin J. Hamill

 I. Metabolic Stress Response
    A. Definition
    B. Precipitating Factors
    C. Pain as an Initiator
 II. Endocrine and Immune Components
    A. Neuroendocrine Axis
    B. Immunologic Effects
III. Pathophysiology
    A. Cardiovascular Effects
    B. Respiratory Effects
    C. Fluid and Electrolyte Homeostasis
    D. Gastrointestinal Alterations
    E. Metabolic Manifestations
    F. Emotional Effects
 IV. Impact of Adequate Pain and Anxiety Management
    A. Cardiovascular Effects
    B. Respiratory Effects
    C. Fluid and Electrolyte Balance
    D. Gastrointestinal Effects
    E. Metabolic Alterations
    F. Emotional Effects
  V. Conclusions
Suggested Readings

I. METABOLIC STRESS RESPONSE

A. Definition

The metabolic stress response (MSR) (Fig. 4-1) is a **complex and multifaceted behavioral, physiologic, and metabolic reaction** that is triggered by a long list of stimuli. This response is characterized by increased adrenergic activity, energy expenditure, and substrate turnover, as well as by sodium and water retention.

B. Precipitating Factors

Factors precipitating the MSR are multiple (see Table 4-1), but have in common the fact that they all represent a potential and/or perceived risk to the integrity and survival of the organism. It should be noted that many activities which are a routine part of care in the intensive care unit (ICU), such as the physical exam, weighing the patient, and chest physiotherapy, have all been shown significantly to increase metabolic rate and energy expenditure.

C. Pain as an Initiator

As an initiator of the MSR, pain is well documented. The degree of response to an injury or operation depends on the extent of tissue damage, the duration of the stimulus, and the degree to which it disrupts normal homeostasis. For example, significant hemorrhage and hypotension from a vascular injury would potentiate the severity of the stress response initiated by a penetrating thigh wound, as compared with the same injury with only soft tissue involvement.

    1. Painful afferent impulses into the spinal cord give rise to the **segmental response,** which includes spinal cord reflex mediated increases in:

        a. **Muscle spasm** (contributing to decreased activity, splinting, hypoventilation).

        b. **Vasospasm** (causing hypertension).

        c. **Inhibition of visceral function** (aggravating hypoventilation, gastric and intestinal distension, impaired digestion).

    2. The **suprasegmental response** refers to the widespread complex of hormonal, metabolic, and immunologic reactions and interactions that

Table 4-1   **Factors activating the metabolic stress response**

Pain	Hypoxia, ischemia
Acidosis	Starvation
Exposure to extreme temperatures	Fear, anxiety
Hypo- or hyperthermia	Hypovolemia, dehydration

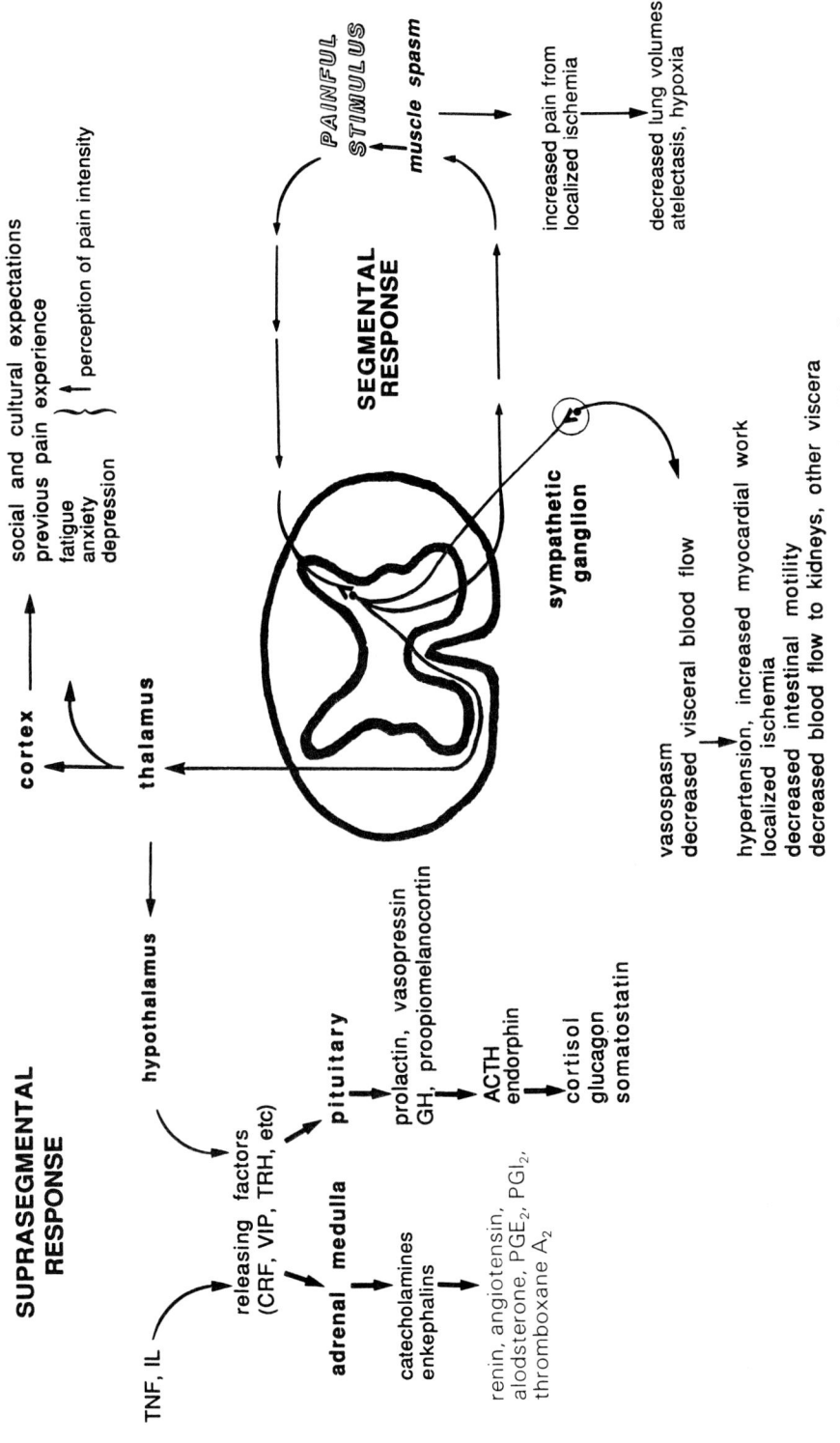

Figure 4-1 The metabolic stress response to a painful stimulus is composed of the segmental, suprasegmental, and integrative components.

result from a painful injury or a host of other noxious stimuli. Afferent impulses stimulate the secretion of releasing factors (e.g., corticotropin-releasing factor, CRF) from the hypothalamus and set off a cascade of teleologically useful alterations in physiology. In the hospital setting, however, where many environmental factors can be controlled, aspects of the MSR may be unnecessary physiologically, and potentially can be detrimental to a patient with impaired organ systems and a limited functional reserve.

3. The **integrative response** reflects the individual's interpretation of the painful experience and is a product of the significance of the pain, the patient's pain experience, his or her emotional state (being angry, afraid, and tired versus being rested and calm), and cultural background. For example, post-laparotomy pain may have very different meanings, depending on the patient's diagnosis. Patients may experience significantly less pain when they learn that their ovarian cyst was benign instead of malignant.

II. ENDOCRINE AND IMMUNE COMPONENTS

A. Neuroendocrine Axis

Stimulation of the **neuroendocrine axis** has effects on water and electrolyte balance and the metabolism of glucose, fat, and protein. This is mediated through a number of hormonal systems.

1. **Afferent neural impulses,** as well as humoral agents such as **interleukin 1 (IL-1)** and **tumor necrosis factor (TNF),** stimulate the hypothalamus, leading to the secretion of **releasing factors,** such as **corticotropin-releasing factor (CRF) and vasoactive intestinal peptide (VIP).** These stimulate the release of hormones from the **pituitary (e.g., prolactin, vasopressin, growth hormone, and proopiomelanocortin).** Proopiomelanocortin is metabolized to adrenocorticotropic hormone **(ACTH) and beta-endorphin.**

2. **ACTH** production is also stimulated by catecholamines, vasopressin, and VIP. ACTH increases the production of cortisol, which, in turn, provides negative feedback and limits the production of ACTH.

3. **Cortisol** stimulates gluconeogenesis and proteolysis, and is, in large part, responsible for the negative nitrogen balance seen in stressed and ill patients. It also increases the adipose tissue's response to growth hormone (GH) and catecholamines, facilitating both lipolysis and further substrate mobilization. Although insulin is also released in response to stress (see below), cellular insulin resistance caused by cortisol and likely due to a post-insulin receptor blockade leads to glucose intolerance and hyperglycemia. The result is increased glucose availability to the brain.

4. The **anti-inflammatory actions of cortisol** act as a brake, controlling the extent of the immune system's response to injury. An uncontrolled immunologic reaction can lead to cellular damage as seen in such syndromes as the Adult Respiratory Distress Syndrome (ARDS), Systemic

Inflammatory Response Syndrome (SIRS), and Multiple System Organ Failure (MSOF). (Refer to Chapters 18 and 22.)

5. In addition, CRF stimulates the **adrenal medulla,** leading to the release of catecholamines and enkephalins. Thus, there is an intimate relationship between the hypothalamic–pituitary–adrenal axis and endogenous opioid production.

6. Stress of many kinds increases serum levels of the **catecholamines** epinephrine, norepinephrine, and dopamine. As messengers of the sympathetic nervous system, catecholamines increase vascular resistance and cardiac output in states of hypoperfusion, redistribute blood to the skeletal muscles and vital organs to prime the organism for fight or flight, facilitate the retention of sodium and water by the kidney, and contribute to the creation of a catabolic state. Catecholamines act synergistically with glucagon and cortisol to increase glucose availability through increased production as well as decreased clearance.

   a. In response to sympathetic stimulation, **epinephrine** is released from the adrenal medulla. It increases glucose availability by stimulating glycogenolysis, gluconeogenesis, and lipolysis, inhibiting insulin release and decreasing peripheral insulin sensitivity. Epinephrine levels remain elevated for approximately 2 days after surgical trauma.

   b. **Norepinephrine (NE)** is released from the sympathetic ganglia, and as such, is an indicator of sympathetic nervous system activity. Most of the NE is taken up at the nerve ending. Thus plasma levels reflect the excess NE that overflows into the bloodstream. The NE levels may be increased for up to 10 days after a surgical procedure.

   c. Dopamine is the immediate precursor of NE. It acts both centrally and peripherally. Peripherally, it modulates the involuntary activity of the sympathetic ganglia, directly decreasing aldosterone production and release, as well as dilating renal vascular beds. Its hemodynamic effects reflect its ability to release NE from sympathetic nerve endings, as well as to exert direct effects on dopaminergic, alpha-, and beta-adrenergic receptors.

7. **Endogenous opioids, beta-endorphin, dynorphin, and the enkephalins,** are produced and stored in the brain, hypothalamus, pituitary, and adrenal medulla. As noted above, their production is closely linked to the synthesis of other stress hormones such as ACTH. Although not well understood, studies using naloxone have suggested that endogenous opioids are involved in the hypotension and myocardial depression associated with septic shock. There is evidence to suggest that endorphins also have immunologic effects, such as enhancing killer cell activity and decreasing neutrophil chemotaxis.

8. **Glucagon, insulin, and somatostatin** are produced in the pancreas and secreted into the portal vein, exposing the liver to high concentrations of the hormones. The balance between the glucagon and insulin levels controls the extent of gluconeogenesis.

a. **Glucagon** increases gluconeogenesis, glycogenolysis, lipolysis, and ketogenesis, through a nonadrenergic receptor mechanism. Secretion is stimulated by hypoglycemia, endorphins, exercise, GH, epinephrine, and glucocorticoids. Levels are increased after surgery or trauma. Glucagon appears to act synergistically with the catecholamines to increase glucose mobilization and availability.

b. **Insulin** secretion is suppressed during stress by an alpha-adrenergic receptor mechanism, further encouraging gluconeogenesis. Although insulin levels are increased after surgery, the levels are inappropriately low given the degree of hyperglycemia. In addition, peripheral sensitivity to insulin is decreased as mentioned above.

c. **Somatostatin** acts as a modulator of the stress reaction and glucose metabolism by inhibiting the release of insulin, as well as of glucagon and GH.

9. Secreted by the anterior pituitary in response to hypothalamic GH-releasing factor, GH causes insulin resistance, increases lipolysis, and promotes the incorporation of amino acids into protein. Many of its actions are mediated by **somatomedins or insulinlike growth factors (IGF)**. A more positive nitrogen balance correlates with increased somatomedin C to IGF-I ratio and GH levels.

10. **Renin, angiotensin II, aldosterone, and antidiuretic hormone (ADH)** are involved in regulating the body's water composition. Increased levels in response to stress lead to water and sodium retention, as well as elevated blood pressure and altered renal perfusion.

a. Decreases in circulating blood volume, blood pressure, renal artery sodium concentration, or beta-adrenergic stimulation provoke the release of **renin** from the juxtaglomerular apparatus in the kidney. Renin is required for the production of angiotensin I, which is subsequently converted to angiotensin II in the lungs.

b. **Angiotensin II** is a very potent vasoconstrictor. It also stimulates the secretion of aldosterone from the adrenal cortex.

c. **Aldosterone** augments sodium reabsorption by exchanging sodium for potassium at the level of the distal tubule in the kidney.

d. **Prostaglandin synthesis** in the medullary interstitial cells of the kidney is also stimulated by stress and hypoperfusion. **PGE_2 and PGI_2 (prostacyclin)** are vasodilators, whose levels parallel those of renin. They appear to modulate the vasoconstrictive effects of angiotensin II and the catecholamines, thereby redistributing renal blood flow from the cortex to the medulla. **Thromboxane A_2** is also produced in the kidney in response to severe stress and decreases renal blood flow by causing vasoconstriction.

11. **Thyroid hormone** metabolism is altered by critical illness, often leading to the **"sick euthyroid syndrome."** This syndrome is manifested by normal levels of thyroid stimulating hormone (TSH), but decreased T_3 levels, low to normal T_4 levels, normal free T_4 levels, and elevated reverse T_3 (rT_3) levels and T_3 resin uptake (T_3RU). Immediately after surgery, TSH

response to thyrotropin releasing hormone (TRH) stimulation is depressed. Furthermore, in severe illness, TSH production seems to be altered such that a less potent TSH is synthesized. Increased dopamine levels, whether endogenous or exogenous, appear to potentiate these changes.

B. Immunologic Effects

1. **Tumor necrosis factor (cachectin)** is a polypeptide released by activated macrophages on exposure to endotoxin. It is responsible for many of the manifestations of septic shock, including the hyperdynamic state, hypermetabolism, fever, hypotension, metabolic acidosis, and acute tubular necrosis. It can cause direct vascular endothelial damage through the production of oxygen-free radicals, as well as stimulate intravascular thrombosis through induction of procoagulant activity. Further, TNF increases IL-1 secretion.

2. **Interleukins** are also mediators of the inflammatory response. IL-1 (endogenous pyrogen or leukocyte endogenous factor) is released from many cell types, but primarily from monocytes and macrophages after exposure to an antigenic stimulus. The beneficial effects include activation of the immune system and fever production, a direct hypothalamic effect. The liver is stimulated by IL-1 to release acute-phase reactants. Other effects include increased endothelial adhesiveness to monocytes, promotion of fibroblast activity, increased protein breakdown, and stimulation of the secretion of ACTH, CRF, endorphins, and TRH.

3. **Bradykinin,** one of the many other substances active in the stress response, is released in response to tissue hypoxia and ischemia. It has been postulated that, through stimulation of intracellular prostaglandin synthesis, bradykinin inhibits hepatic gluconeogenesis, which modulates the effect of glucagon on the hepatocytes. Other factors active in the response to tissue injury and pain include **serotonin, histamine,** and **substance P.**

III. PATHOPHYSIOLOGY

A. Cardiovascular Effects

1. The **cardiovascular effects** of the MSR (without associated sepsis) are primarily the result of increased catecholamine levels. Angiotensin II and ADH also contribute to the hemodynamic manifestations of stress, which include:

    a. **Arteriolar constriction,** which is manifest clinically as hypertension and increased systemic vascular resistance.

    b. **Venoconstriction and decreased venous capacitance.**

    c. **Increased inotropy and chronotropy,** resulting in tachycardia and perhaps dysrhythmias.

2. The net effect of these alterations is an **increased myocardial oxygen consumption ($M\dot{V}O_2$)**. Although not necessarily desirable in the healthier patient, the associated increase in $M\dot{V}O_2$ may be well tolerated. Since oxygen extraction in the myocardium is nearly maximal in the normal setting, increased extraction offers little compensation for increased demands. In the patient with myocardial perfusion limited by critical coronary artery lesions, increased oxygen delivery may not be possible, predisposing the patient to ischemia, arrhythmias, and even myocardial infarction. Attention should be paid to maximizing oxygen delivery by increasing oxygen carrying capacity (hemoglobin) and controlling oxygen demand whenever possible.

B. Respiratory Effects

1. Respiratory effects are a result of increased metabolic rate and alterations in pulmonary vasculature (due to the effects of prostaglandin, bradykinin, etc.), as well as the influence of segmental reflexes. The additional compromise of pulmonary mechanics and lung volumes associated with the supine position and chest or abdominal injury further impairs respiratory function. The clinical results include:
   a. **Increased carbon dioxide production (V_{CO_2})**.
   b. **Increased oxygen consumption (V_{O_2})**.
   c. **Increased V/Q mismatch,** atelectasis, and shunting, all of which predispose to hypoxemia.
2. Also, **muscle spasm, splinting of the chest wall,** and **altered pulmonary volumes** (see Fig. 4-2), limit the ability to cough effectively, impair clearance of secretions, and put the patient at risk of developing atelectasis, progressive hypoxemia, and pneumonia.
3. The net result is an **increased work of breathing,** which further increases metabolic demand.

C. Fluid and Electrolyte Homeostasis

1. Increased **sodium retention** is a result of elevated aldosterone secretion. Catecholamines and cortisol also contribute to the **wasting of potassium, magnesium,** and other electrolytes.
2. **Water retention** and decreased urine output are seen in the face of elevated ADH levels. In patients with marginally compensated congestive heart failure, this effect can be instrumental in complicating their postoperative or postinjury management. In predisposed patients, fluid overload frequently becomes obvious 48 to 72 h after the stressful event as the patient begins to mobilize fluid.

D. Gastrointestinal Alterations

1. Sympathetic stimulation **decreases bowel motility** and shunts blood away from the viscera.

A.

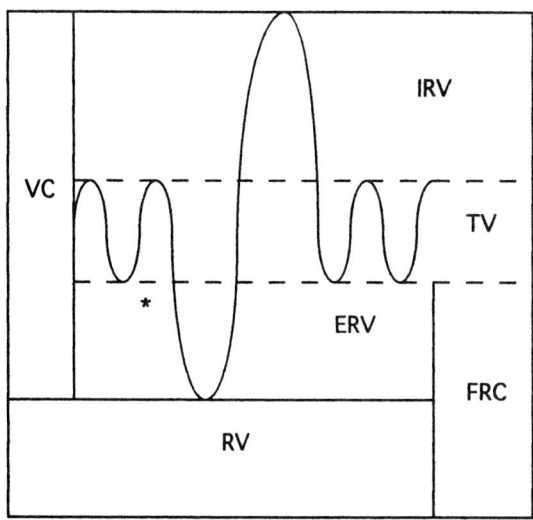

B.

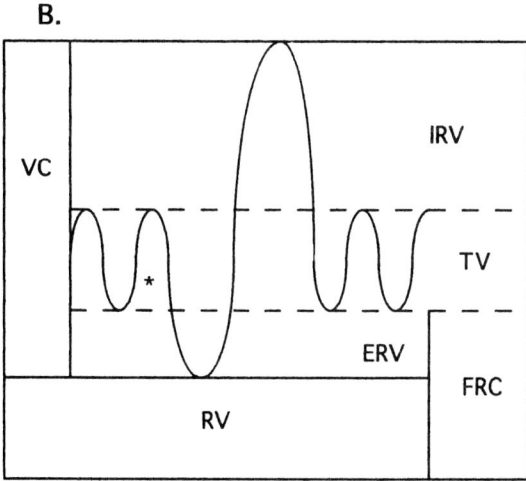

Figure 4-2 Most pulmonary volumes diminish after thoracic or abdominal injury, or simply from maintaining the supine position for an extended period of time. Under these circumstances, the closing volume (*), which normally occurs at a lung volume below normal tidal breathing (*A*), moves into the tidal range (*B*). Consequently, alveoli are closed during tidal breathing, which leads to atelectasis. Obesity and increased secretions further exacerbate this problem. (VC = vital capacity, IRV = inspiratory reserve volume, TV = tidal volume, ERV = expiratory reserve volume, FRC = functional residual capacity, RV = residual volume)

2. **Increased interstitial fluid and bowel edema** further impede motility.

3. Clinically, these effects are made manifest as **nausea, vomiting, and compromised absorption.** In severe stress or illness, **bacterial overgrowth and bowel ischemia** can lead to loss of mucosal integrity, villous atrophy and sloughing, and transudation of bacterial products across the intestinal wall.

4. These changes result in an increased risk of developing **nosocomial pneumonia** and/or the **sepsis syndrome.** In addition, **malabsorption** and increased gastrointestinal losses of fluid and electrolytes occur.

E. Metabolic Manifestations

1. **Carbohydrate metabolism,** under the influence of catecholamines, glucagon, insulin, somatostatin, cortisol, and GH, is altered significantly under stress. The result is increased glucose availability to the brain, skeletal muscles, and vital organs.

2. **Lipolysis** increases in response to epinephrine, GH, glucagon, and cortisol, providing an additional, readily available energy source—free fatty acids.

3. Under stress, protein metabolism is characterized by **proteolysis** and a **negative nitrogen balance.** This can be very resistant to treatment in the critically ill patient despite adequate nutritional intake. Cortisol, TNF, IL-1, and other hormones contribute to the establishment and maintenance of the catabolic state, while GH facilitates the incorporation of amino acids into proteins.

4. **Energy metabolism** is altered such that energy stores are depleted. Hyperglycemia results from the combination of increased insulin resistance, gluconeogenesis, and glycogenolysis. Muscle and hepatic glycogen stores are depleted readily. Lypolysis and proteolysis further aid glucose availability to the brain and other tissues.

F. Emotional Effects

Fear, anxiety, and agitation are frequently seen in critically ill or traumatized patients. These emotions can cause substantial increases in their metabolic rates. If the patient has increased metabolic demands because of a critical illness, particularly in the face of compromised cardiac and/or pulmonary reserve, the increased physiologic demand of these emotions may have a crucial impact because they stress the patient beyond his or her ability to compensate.

IV. IMPACT OF ADEQUATE PAIN AND ANXIETY MANAGEMENT

The effect of adequate management on the stress response has been well demonstrated in the literature over the past 20 years. There are many sites where the physiologic responses to pain can be altered. These are elucidated in Fig. 4-3. The effects of some of these interventions are discussed below.

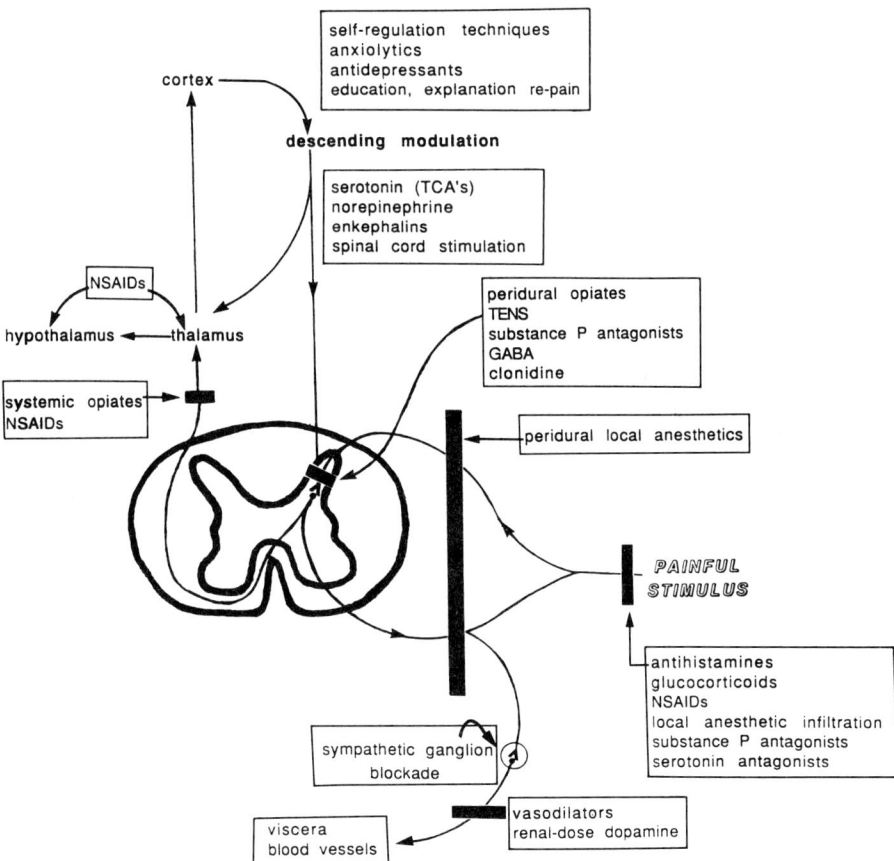

Figure 4-3 Known sites for the modulation and treatment of painful stimuli which can alter the magnitude of the metabolic stress response. (TCA = tricyclic antidepressant, NSAID = nonsteroidal antiinflammatory agent)

A. Cardiovascular Effects

1. As noted above, pain and stress increase myocardial oxygen consumption. If follows that **adequate analgesia** and anxiolysis should decrease or blunt the body's response to stress.

2. Changes in $\dot{V}o_2$ and $\dot{V}co_2$ that result from daily activities in the ICU decrease in the face of parenteral narcotics. **Systemic narcotics** may also have some effect on the endocrine aspects of the MSR.

3. Thromboembolic events are common in the critically ill or traumatized patient despite the use of subcutaneous heparin, elastic wraps or stockings, or intermittent compression boots. Pulmonary emboli are frequent findings at autopsy of ICU patients. **Peridural local anesthetics** increase the rate of arterial inflow, as well as that of venous outflow. Epidural analgesia appears to be associated with a lower incidence of thromboembolic phenomena. Whether this is due to the sympatholytic, vasodilatory effect of the local anesthetic, a direct effect of the local anesthetic on platelet adhesiveness, a neurally mediated alteration in platelet function, or a combination of these effects is not entirely clear.

4. Multiple System Organ Failure (MOSF) can develop as a result of cellular ischemia due to hypoperfusion, whether from hypotension or vasoconstriction and shunting mediated by catecholamines. Cellular ischemia further increases the neuroendocrine stress response, leads to the release of immunosuppressive factors in the blood, and increases the likelihood of sepsis. **Sympathetic blockade with peridural local anesthetics** causes vasodilation in the viscera, depending on the level of the block (liver, T6–T9; pancreas, T5–T11; bowel, T6–T12; kidney, T10–L1). As long as adequate blood pressures are maintained, organ perfusion is maximized.

B. Respiratory Effects

1. Although there is little in the literature evaluating the effects of analgesia and sedation on pulmonary function in the critically ill population, much attention has been focused on postoperative patients.

2. **Parenteral and epidural opioids and epidural local anesthetics** increase forced expiratory volume (FEV_1), vital capacity, and functional residual capacity after thoracic and upper abdominal surgery. The peridurally administered drugs exhibit a more profound improvement as compared with intravenous narcotics. Presumably, decreased pain sensation prevents or blunts the spasm and guarding that would otherwise occur. In *anesthetic* concentrations (e.g., 1.5% to 2.0% lidocaine), peridural local anesthetics cause motor blockade. Most *analgesic* concentrations (e.g., 0.6% to 1.2% bupivacaine) do not cause profound motor blockade.

3. The chance of respiratory failure and/or prolonged intubation is decreased in high-risk patients receiving **peridural analgesia** as compared

with those receiving parenteral narcotics. Similarly, peridural analgesia lessens the likelihood of patients with flail chests requiring intubation and mechanical ventilation.

C. Fluid and Electrolyte Balance

1. Peridural local anesthetics and/or narcotics significantly blunt increases in ADH, aldosterone, and renin after a surgical stimulus, and instead maintain levels near normal. Hormone levels can reach up to five times baseline if only parenteral narcotics are used. The impact of peridural analgesia is more profound in upper abdominal incisions than with lower incisions.

2. A number of studies suggest that perioperative **epidural local anesthetics** decrease the risk of postoperative renal insufficiency or failure.

D. Gastrointestinal Effects

1. Narcotics and **pain** both decrease intestinal motility. Patients receiving effective postoperative peridural analgesia have a more rapid return of bowel function than do those receiving parenteral narcotics.

2. Peridural local anesthetics block sympathetic input to the bowel and viscera, as noted above. Unopposed parasympathetic stimulation should improve peristalsis and organ perfusion however, the effect of adequate analgesia on postoperative or posttraumatic liver dysfunction, pancreatitis, and bowel ischemia has not been well studied.

E. Metabolic Alterations

1. Many daily interventions, such as baths, chest films, and chest physical therapy, increase $\dot{V}o_2$ and $\dot{V}co_2$ significantly above baseline levels. On the other hand, sedatives and analgesics have been shown to decrease metabolic rate.

2. Epidural local anesthetics blunt perioperative increases in cortisol, glucose, lactate, pyruvate, and free fatty acids.

3. Epidural narcotics are less effective than local anesthetics but more effective than parenteral opioids in limiting the metabolic response to stress.

F. Emotional Effects

Education about one's disease and treatment, preservation of normal wake–sleep cycles through the appropriate use of sedatives, and efficacious pain management clearly influence the patient's level of distress and anxiety. The agitated, combative, uncooperative patient uses more energy, compounding the struggle to achieve positive nitrogen balance. He or she is also more difficult to care for (mechanical ventilation, procedures, etc.) and sometimes poses a risk to the self as well as to caretakers. The judicious use of medications improves the patient's actual as well as perceived well-being. A comfortable, rested patient is less likely to be confused or to develop ICU psychosis.

V. CONCLUSIONS

A. The stress response is initiated by a multiplicity of factors, many of which can be influenced by adequate pain management, sedation, and emotional support.

B. Neural blockade with local anesthetics prevents a large part of the stress response initiated by trauma or surgery.

C. Systemic and epidural opiates may lessen the endocrine response to surgery (and trauma), but the effect is less dramatic than that seen with local anesthetics.

D. Epidural narcotics do have a significant impact on the pulmonary, cardiovascular, and psychological response to pain, surgery, and trauma.

SUGGESTED READINGS

Abraham E: Physiologic stress and cellular ischemia: relationship to immunosuppression and susceptibility to sepsis. *Crit Care Med* 19(5):613–618, 1991.

Breslow MJ, Ligier B: Hyperadrenergic states. *Crit Care Med* 19(12):1566–1579, 1991.

Cheung AT, Chernow B: The stress responses to critical illness. *Prob Anesth* 3(2):169–179, April–June 1989.

Hoyt DB, Ozkan AN: Immunosuppression in trauma patients. *J Intensive Care Med* 6(2):71–90, 1991.

Jorgensen BC, Andersen HB, Engquist A: Influence of epidural morphine on postoperative pain, endocrine-metabolic and renal responses to surgery. A controlled study. *Acta Anaesth Scand* 26:63–68, 1982.

Kehlet H: Pain relief and modification of the stress response, in Cousins (ed.): *Acute Pain Management.* New York, Churchill Livingstone, 1986, pp 49–75.

Swinamer DL, Phang PT, Jones RL et al: Effect of routine administration of analgesia on energy expenditure in critically ill patients. *Chest* 92:4–10, 1988.

Tuman KJ, McCarthy RJ, March RJ, et al: Effects of epidural anesthesia and analgesia on coagulation and outcome after major vascular surgery. *Anesth Analg* 73:696–704, 1991.

Yeager MP, Glass DD, Neff RK, et al: Epidural anesthesia and analgesia in high-risk surgical patients. *Anesthesiology* 66:729–736, 1987.

Weissman C: The metabolic response to stress: an overview and update. *Anesthesiology* 73:308–327, 1990.

CHAPTER
5

A MATRIX MODEL FOR THE PSYCHOLOGICAL ASSESSMENT AND TREATMENT OF ACUTE PAIN

Joseph R. Dane
Rodger S. Kessler

I. Background Factors
   A. Primary Background Factors
   B. Patient and Caregiver Attitudes Toward Pain
   C. Corrective Information About Pain
II. Process Factors
   A. Affective and Cognitive Principles
   B. Perceived Control
   C. Patient Status Along the "Recovery" Continuum
III. Individual Difference Factors
   A. Internal Factors
   B. Meaning of Pain
   C. Preexisting Levels of Problem-Solving Skills
   D. Coping Style
   E. Emotional Age
   F. Hypnotic Capacity
IV. Treatment Factors
   A. Goals and Objectives
   B. Models and Psychological Intervention
   C. Levels and Types of Psychological Intervention
   D. Natural Stages of Psychological Treatment
   E. Application of the Matrix Model
V. Case Examples
Suggested Readings

What is psychological about pain?

Pain is a highly complex and multidimensional psychophysiologic experience. This chapter attempts to organize the caregiver's thinking about the psychological dimensions of the pain experience and to assist caregivers in assessing themselves, their patients, and their patients' specific circumstances along these interacting dimensions in order to develop strategies for appropriate psychological intervention. Specific aspects include background factors, process factors, individual difference factors, and treatment factors. These constitute a multidimensional matrix within which patients and caregivers can be placed in a way that allows the development of rational treatment decisions which are specific to the individual patient.

The differences between the emergent and posttriage phases of acute medical care are highlighted, along with the differences in types of psychological strategies appropriate to each phase. However, the psychological dimensions relevant to each phase remain the same. Background factors, process factors, and individual differences factors are discussed as a general context for application of the resulting multidimensional matrix (including treatment factors) to specific patients. Case examples illuminate specific points. For discussion of specific techniques of coping skills training (as distinct from the more general topic of psychological intervention covered in this chapter), see "Self-Regulation Techniques" in Chapter 14.

I. BACKGROUND FACTORS

A. Primary Background Factors

There are two **primary background factors** that influence the psychology of pain:

1. problematic attitudes toward pain among patients and caregivers, including basic misconceptions about pain; and
2. information about pain which helps to rectify these interactions and misconceptions.

B. Patient and Caregiver Attitudes Toward Pain

1. Pain is frequently oversimplified as either imaginary (mind), real (body), or faked (malingering). The reality is that most pain involves variable levels of pathophysiology which interact with varying personality styles that inhibit or facilitate management of the pain experience. Instances of purely "psychogenic" or imaginary pain are *extremely* rare.

2. Both patient and caregiver attitudes toward pain are affected by prior learning, as well as by external pressures and demands of the immediate environment which have nothing to do with the pain itself.

3. Due to unrealistic cultural expectations that medicine and science can do "anything," the lack of adequate pain control is usually interpreted by patients as the deliberate withholding of available relief.

C. Corrective Information About Pain

1. Pain is defined by the International Association for the Study of Pain as an unpleasant sensory *and* emotional experience associated with tissue damage (actual *or* potential) or described in terms of such experience.

Noxious stimulation simultaneously activates both sensory and limbic components of the brain. Any reduction in negative states, whether achieved pharmacologically or psychologically, helps reduce the neurophysiologic experience of pain. The report of pain relief after "merely" talking with someone and feeling cared about does *not* mean that the pain being relieved was imaginary.

There is no single or clear physiologic index of pain. In the early stages of acute pain, cardiovascular and behavioral signs of pain are likely to be present. **Physiologic responses** include increased blood pressure, pulse rate, and respiratory rate, as well as dilated pupils and perspiration, whereas behavioral responses include that the patient focuses on and reports pain, cries and moans, rubs the painful part, exhibits increased muscle tension, or frowns and grimaces. However, a significant degree of physiologic and behavioral accommodation occurs in response to pain which continues over time. **Physiologic accommodation** includes normalization of blood pressure, pulse, respiratory rates, and pupil size, and the presence of dry skin, while **behavioral accommodation** includes that patients may not report pain unless questioned, may remain quiet, may sleep or rest, may turn their attention to things other than pain, may exhibit physical inactivity or immobility, or may have blank or normal facial expressions. *The only valid measure of pain is the patient's subjective report of or communication about the pain experience.*

2. Pain behavior is a form of communication about overlapping sensory and affective events. Pain behavior, therefore, is modified not only by the intensity of the pain, but by everything which influences communication.

3. The sudden appearance of pain behaviors in a previously calm patient when someone enters the room does not necessarily mean that the patient is malingering or manipulative. It *may* indicate the spontaneous but unrecognized use of **pain coping strategies** (e.g., a variant of self-hypnosis through focusing on internal thoughts or external distractions, such as television) and that the patient is a candidate for training in techniques which can build on his or her previously unrecognized skills.

4. The effective **treatment of pain** attempts to have an impact on sensation, suffering, and communication simultaneously, or on as many of these components as possible at a given time, and considers alteration in *any*

Table 5-1 Characteristics of acute versus chronic pain

Acute pain	Chronic pain
Meaning	
Pain as symptom	Pain as disease
Biologically useful	No biologic usefulness
Pathology recognized	Complex physical/psychological interaction
Cure and relief likely	Cure and relief not possible?
Ongoing damage	(Broken fire alarm?)
When will it heal?	It already has healed
"Sorry you're hurting"	"It must all be in your head"
Behavioral impact	
Anxiety	Depression
Temporary adjustments	Major lifestyle changes
Anger	Arrested grief response?
Treatment	
Narcotics useful	Narcotics contraindicated
Little addiction potential	Polyaddiction
Stop!	Keep going!

combination of these as a legitimate target for intervention and a valid index of pain relief.

    5. There is a **crucial difference between acute and chronic pain** which must be communicated to patients and caregivers alike.

        a. Acute pain is the antithesis of chronic pain in three critical domains:

            1. The meaning ascribed to the pain.
            2. The behavioral impact of the pain.
            3. Treatment strategies appropriate for dealing with the pain.

Table 5-1 details the differences in each of these domains.

        b. A useful model for discussing this concept with patients, particularly with respect to neuropathic pain, is that of the "broken fire alarm." Pain is normally taken as an alarm signal for ongoing tissue damage ("fire!"). Most patients have experienced such false alarms, and can understand learning to tolerate the annoyance of recurrent false alarms caused by faulty or hypersensitive wiring, especially when the alarm bell is located close by. One can complain to the maintenance crew, but adapting to the situation and getting on with daily living are up to the individual.

II. PROCESS FACTORS

Process factors in the psychology of pain involve affective and cognitive principles governing the awareness of pain, the importance of perceived control and its relation to coping style, and the patient's status along the recovery continuum.

A. Affective and Cognitive Principles

1. **Negative emotional arousal** leads to increased awareness of pain, while **positive emotional arousal** leads to decreased awareness.

2. The degree of tolerance for pain is directly proportional to the **degree of perceived suffering** (negative emotional arousal) associated with that pain (e.g., childbirth pain is generally perceived as more tolerable than is cancer pain).

3. The **"meaning" attributed to pain** is a major determinant of the response to pain.

   a. Perceived suffering due to pain is largely a function of the meaning attributed to that pain. Further, pain is an information-bearing signal, usually connoting tissue damage and a threat to survival. Since the human mind pays most attention to information which is relevant to survival and can accommodate to or ignore what is informationally neutral (e.g., the sound of a noisy fan), the meaning attributed to the pain is crucial in determining a patient's ability to ignore or accommodate to the pain.

   b. Alterations in meaning and suffering provide a major avenue of treatment for otherwise "refractory" pain by helping patients distinguish and appropriately manage their suffering versus their physical discomfort.

   c. Patients who are not satisfied that the physiologic meaning (i.e., source) of their pain has been identified are particularly likely to resist overt psychological measures for pain relief (e.g., hypnosis or relaxation training) due to a fear of masking the true etiology of their pain and/or a fear that if such techniques are effective, the pain will be discounted as purely psychological. With such patients, effective education about pain is crucial.

4. The influence of classical primary and secondary gain factors can best be understood as altering the meaning of pain and interfering with training in pain management.

B. Perceived Control

1. The absence of perceived control tremendously increases anxiety and reduces the degree to which patients see themselves as able or competent to contribute to their own comfort independently of caregivers' efforts.

2. As patients experience an increase in perceived control, they are more likely to exhibit self-initiated pain management (e.g., heightened pain tolerance and use of self-regulation skills) and increased cooperation with treatment.

3. Exactly what constitutes an increase in perceived control, however, depends on the patient's individual coping style.

C. Patient Status Along the "Recovery" Continuum

1. The **amount of energy and motivation available** for coping effectively with pain is related to the patient's location on the continuum of effective recovery. This continuum is as much psychological as it is physiologic, and consists of two major components: (1) patient movement from "victim of injury" to "manager of recovery" stance, and (2) patient movement through the grief process.

2. "Victim of injury" to "manager of recovery"

   a. The healthy recovery process may begin with patients' feeling victimized by their circumstances and/or blaming those perceived as responsible. For recovery to be successful, such an initial posture, even when justified, must shift to one of effectively managing one's situation and one's personal responses to pain.

   b. Only a management stance is consistent with the initiative and stamina necessary for the effective use of self-regulation training over time.

3. The grieving process

   a. Acute pain can be accompanied by loss of life (e.g., friends, family members), property (e.g., home, car), or function (e.g., spinal cord injury, severe fractures), which precipitates a predictable grief response. Patients' internal management of this response can unwittingly overlap with and complicate the internal management of their pain experience. Further, when the meaning of pain includes chronic pain, permanent physical disfigurement or disability, or terminal illness, resulting changes in lifestyle constitute a psychological "death" as real as the loss of a spouse. The **grief response** to any such death or loss follows the same course as that popularized by Elizabeth Kubler-Ross: **shock, denial, anger, bargaining, mourning, and acceptance.**

   b. Patients can become fixed or arrested in any one or a combination of the stages. Without appropriate psychological intervention, such an arrest can seriously impede effective pain management and recovery. For example, denial and anger may be manifest as an undue focus on physical pain and blame for failures to relieve it, both of which serve to avoid the emotional pain over the loss of physical functioning. Table 5-2 lists indications of a possible **arrested grief response** which may need treatment before pain coping can improve. See "Grief Work" for details of treatment.

III. INDIVIDUAL DIFFERENCE FACTORS

A. Internal Factors

A third major vector in the psychology of pain involves **internal factors** specific to individual patients. These include the specific meaning attributed to

Table 5-2 Patient characteristics indicating possible arrested grief response

1. Is unresponsive to reasonable reassurance about his or her condition.
2. Continues to insist on the need for a clear diagnostic label for the etiology of the pain, even when one is not reasonably available, especially when potentially lethal or occult processes (e.g., cancer) have been ruled out (this may take the form of "doctor shopping" in the outpatient setting).
3. Exhibits unreasonable and unrelenting anger or hostility toward family, caregivers, and others who are supportive.
4. Is obsessively preoccupied with the details of a particular medication or exercise regimen.
5. Persists in focusing on the history and unfairness of the injury, pain, or illness rather than on the recovery process.

---

the pain, based on current circumstances and prior learning about pain; the preexisting level of problem-solving skills; the prevalent coping style and its relation to the perceived locus of control; the prevalent "emotional age"; and the level of hypnotic capacity.

B. Meaning of Pain

1. The exact meaning attributed to pain will vary according to the individual's personal history and prior learning about pain, the character of the illness or injury, and the circumstances surrounding these. Whatever the meaning, it will significantly influence the type and extent of pain behavior displayed.

2. Basic relevant information includes:

   a. How and under what circumstances the pain began (i.e., who is perceived as responsible for the pain, what losses were incurred, etc.).

   b. The patient's understanding of the medical diagnosis and etiology of the pain, especially if dealing with chronic pain.

   c. Environmental factors such as secondary gain, dysfunctional family support of pain behavior, or interpersonal conflict with the caregivers.

   d. Historically based intrapsychic factors (e.g., a history of physical or sexual abuse, where current pain may reactivate disruptive but previously repressed memories and affect, or the pain may be perceived as punishment of the self or others).

   e. Current intrapsychic factors (e.g., perception of the pain as a signal that at least one is still alive; or more typically, pain is a reminder of the frustration, discouragement, anxiety, and depression over the current situation).

C. Preexisting Levels of Problem-Solving Skills

1. The best predictor of future behavior is past behavior. Preexisting levels of problem-solving skills are roughly indicated by how effectively an individual has performed in the major arenas of life: education, work, family, and social interaction. The more positive these indicators, the greater is the likelihood of productive problem-solving behaviors and attitudes toward pain.

D. Coping Style

1. How patients cope can be understood as an internalized way of balancing personal emotional reactions with externally oriented, problem-solving behavior.
2. Whatever the patient is doing (whether we like it or not) *is* his or her way of coping. The issue for caregivers is to understand the patient's way of coping and to interact with it appropriately.
3. **Differences in coping styles** can be broadly characterized by differences between *repressing avoiders* and *coping sensitizers.* Both styles are valid and effective, but are quite different from each other and elicit different responses from caregivers.
    a. **Repressing avoiders** cope by minimizing the seriousness of their condition and maintaining a generally positive attitude (e.g., hoping for the best). They may become anxious when given too much information or too much emphasis is placed directly on their problems. They give the appearance of trusting their caregiver's judgment, and are often described by caregivers as quiet, undemanding, and easy to work with.
    b. **Coping sensitizers** manage their anxiety and emotional discomfort by seeking information and reassurance, and by taking specific action. However, this means that they often ask difficult questions, and insist on talking with people whom they perceive as able to do something about their situation. They are often seen by busy caretakers as troublesome and demanding.
4. Related to the concept of perceived control is that of **locus of control** (LOC). This refers to whether one perceives that the power to effect relevant change lies within oneself or with powerful others. **Internal LOC** is more likely to occur in coping sensitizers, while **external LOC** is more common in repressing avoiders, but this can vary with individuals.
5. Differences in coping style do not preclude the use of self-regulation training. However, rationales offered to encourage their use should remain consistent with the patient's coping style.
    a. For example, patients who cope through the use of repression and avoidance may perceive efforts to teach active involvement in self-regulation techniques as a *loss* of control, since it focuses attention on their condition and on something they must do about it. With such patients, one

should emphasize a more passive and receptive stance, pointing out that their bodies will be able to respond much more effectively to the medications being used, and that they may be surprised at just how little medication it takes to make them feel better as their facility with self-regulation techniques becomes more effective.

   b. Conversely, patients who cope through active involvement in the details of their care manage their anxiety by obtaining information and reassurance and by actively confronting their difficulties. They thus are more likely to perceive active involvement in self-regulation techniques as desirable and as increasing their sense of control. With such patients, one should emphasize an active stance by pointing out the benefits of their being more in charge of their own comfort, and suggest that the occurrence of the pain can become a reminder to use the techniques they are learning.

E. Emotional Age

   1. The concept of emotional age reflects the emotional fluctuations (i.e., **regression**) often generated by the stress of acute pain. Statements such as, "My patient is acting like a 3-year-old," reflect valid and useful intuitive assessments of current personality functioning. The point is that although regressed patients (or staff members) will respond in a manner consistent with the emotional age being exhibited, they also can react either positively or negatively, depending on how one responds to them.

   2. When faced with regression, the goals for caregivers are to (1) distinguish the behavioral and emotional dilemmas being presented by both the patient and staff from the developmental age and particular emotions through which these dilemmas are expressed (see Table 5-3 for example),

Table 5-3 Example of factors to distinguish when faced with regression

Factor	Patient	Staff
Behavioral dilemma	Wants pain relief (= more medication)	Want pain relief, but concerned about addiction, respiratory depression
Emotional dilemma	Can't get what he or she needs, so demands and manipulates via noncompliance	How to avoid being and feeling manipulated
Developmental age	Rebellious adolescent	Appropriately supportive neutral adult, or punitive parent?
Particular emotions	Anger, ambivalence at showing dependency on others	Empathetic, yet angry, frustrated, resent lack of cooperation

and (2) respond to these dilemmas in a manner consistent with therapeutic principles appropriate to the developmental age and type of emotions being exhibited.

3. General **principles for responding to emotional age** include:

   a. Expecting an upset 3-year-old (or a regressed adult) to quit "acting like a child"—this will only generate more upset.

   b. Children (and people in general) will usually calm down once they feel they have been heard (i.e., have experienced an accepting stance which acknowledges the emotions being expressed and avoids judgment, defensiveness, and retaliation, such as guilt-tripping for "bad" behavior).

   c. Emotions demand expression, and identifying emotions through words (i.e., talking with regressed or upset patients about their feelings) can help dilute the regressive need for physical action (e.g., withdrawal and noncompliance) as an expression of these emotions.

   d. Emotional support should be appropriate to the patient's emotional age (e.g., overt caring and nurturance for toddlers and youngsters versus "tough love" for teenagers).

   e. Most children will respond positively to accepting nurturance, and they will react to criticism with temporary compliance, only to express resentment and revenge through longer-term patterns of noncompliance.

   f. Adolescents are desperate to look as though they do not care about the support they so desperately crave, are often suspicious of openly caring responses, respond best to attitudes of respectful neutrality laced with caring, and generally both need and respect clear limits.

   g. Adolescents tend to "hand off" intolerable emotions by attempting to generate these emotions in others (ever notice how a teenager begins to calm down once you have become upset?); acknowledging emotions from a position of neutral respect and offering viable choices within clear limits will go much further toward emotional resolution than will simply acting out such patients' emotions for them.

4. Some children and adolescents need to be upset on occasion, and are unlikely to calm down without time to ventilate, free from constraints.

5. Other children cannot be calmed, and to expect otherwise is a setup for ongoing frustration. In such cases, one should avoid taking the patient's behavior personally, allow the behavior to run its course without recrimination, and isolate the behavior (e.g., close the door, remove roommate, etc.) if it is disruptive to others in the setting.

6. Pervasive or consistent regression in the face of stress (e.g., "My patient *always* acts like an angry adolescent") *may* represent a **character-disordered** patient rather than mere regression. These patients are often accused of manipulative drug seeking by pitting one staff member against another to obtain medications. Such behavior appears naïvely obvious, generating staff comments to the effect that: "This patient must think we're dumb if she thinks we can't see what she's doing." However, such behavior

is *not* consciously manipulative. Rather, due to a delay in emotional development, such individuals cannot tolerate ambivalance in their feelings toward others, and literally perceive and interact with the same person as two separate people, depending on whether the person is perceived as gratifying (good) or frustrating and depriving (bad). Thus the previously nurturing caretaker who, due to the normal demands of the job, must temporarily frustrate such a patient, becomes, in the patient's internal experience, a "bad" person who must be rejected and replaced by alliance with another, "good" caretaker. In sum, it is not simply drugs, but appropriate (i.e., gratifying) caretaking which is being sought. The only effective antidote to such behavior is to:

    a. Recognize what is happening.

    b. Avoid both taking the patient's reactions personally and responding punitively.

    c. Maintain effective rapport.

    d. Develop a clear set of limits which are mutually agreed upon by staff members and clearly communicated to staff members on all shifts.

    7. In dealing with regression, and particularly when dealing with regression in the form of character disorders, it is especially important to avoid personalizing a patient's responses, whether these be positive or negative. The goal is to establish and maintain the rapport so crucial to effective pain management by maintaining a professional stance of empathic neutrality as the patient shifts from one emotional stance or interpersonal alliance to another.

F. Hypnotic Capacity

    1. The profound medical implications of an individual's capacity to experience hypnotic phenomena are not yet appreciated by most caregivers. Hypnosis is a natural state of focused attention similar to that of daydreaming. The purpose of a hypnotic induction is simply to help elicit a similar type of focused attention more reliably and predictably than waiting for it to happen spontaneously. It is crucial to recognize that the attentional focus generated by trauma and emotional arousal also constitutes a type of spontaneous hypnotic induction.

    2. The importance of the hypnotic state is **increased responsiveness to suggestion,** from either the self or others. Such suggestions can produce a range of psychological and psychophysiologic alterations which are distinct from simple relaxation and distraction, with which hypnosis is often confused. In the extreme, this includes such things as surgical levels of anesthesia in the absence of medication, but also includes profound changes in motivation, memory, affect, and sense of time, as well as alterations in blood flow, appetite, gastric secretions, and respiratory functioning.

    3. Hypnotic phenomena can be an asset or a liability, depending on whether they occur spontaneously and unwittingly or are purposefully elicited. For example, patients with significant hypnotic capacity and who are prone to negativity and catastrophizing are likely to alter their pain experience through negative self-suggestion. The resulting alterations in their experience are very real subjectively and may help account for perceived exaggerations in pain reports. These variations can also be quite real physiologically and take such forms as nausea, vomiting, gastric distress, and decreased food intake. When purposefully elicited and directed, either through the assistance of a caregiver or as a result of training patients in specific skills, this same ability to alter psychophysiology through suggestion can contribute enormously to successful medical management, and in particular to the management of pain.

4. The capacity to experience hypnotic phenomena (**hypnotic susceptibility**) is normally distributed, and its measured stability over time (as many as 20 years) is similar to that of IQ measures. This suggests that from 60 to 70 percent of the population can benefit to some extent from the appropriate use of hypnotic strategies. A rough clinical index of hypnotic capacity is the degree to which an individual can become absorbed internally in fantasy (daydreaming) or externally in distraction (television, books).

5. The appropriate use of hypnotic phenomena and strategies requires specialized training, which is well worth obtaining (see section on hypnosis in Chapter 14). Staff members and patients who are unaware of the validity of hypnotic phenomena and do not appreciate their spontaneous occurrence are powerless to recognize, counter, alter, or utilize their presence.

IV. TREATMENT FACTORS

Treatment factors in the psychology of acute pain include goals and objectives consistent with the phase of medical treatment, models, levels and methodologies of psychological intervention, stages of psychological treatment, and application of the matrix model.

A. Goals and Objectives

1. A successful outcome in the psychological management of acute pain is characterized by:

a. achieving **sufficient comfort** (i.e., varying levels of reduction in sensory and/or affective pain components) as opposed to total absence of pain; and

b. increasing the partnership between the caregiver and patient in managing the pain.

2. The specific objectives of psychological intervention differ somewhat according to the **phase of medical care involved.**

   a. During the **emergent/triage phase,** one attempts to establish rapid patient–caregiver interaction, immediate patient compliance and enhanced self-control, and cursory psychological assessment of the patient's behavior. The initiative for the use of psychological strategies during this phase rests primarily with the caregiver.

   b. During the **posttriage/stabilization phase,** one seeks greater psychological understanding of the patient's behavior in ways that help determine how to interact with the patient most effectively. On the patient's part, there are increased understanding of the physical and psychological dimensions of the injury and recovery process, acquisition and practice of psychological strategies that enhance recovery, and enhanced participation in treatment activities. The initiative for the independent use of psychological strategies rests increasingly with the patient during this phase.

3. It is important to understand that the use of psychological strategies can do more than simply facilitate care delivery via increased patient compliance. In particular, the use of self-regulation techniques (see "Models of Psychological Intervention," below) can also have an **impact on the physiology of healing** via alterations in blood flow and reductions in biochemical stress factors.

B. Models of Psychological Intervention

Two basic **models of psychological intervention** are available.

   1. Interpersonal influence model

   a. This model refers to what can be accomplished by the willingness to simply "be" with a patient in the face of powerlessness to "do" anything. The potency of this model for relief of suffering is typically underestimated in busy medical settings. It remains the **primary treatment for regression** due to pain and a sense of powerlessness.

   b. Its impact is achieved through:

   (1) Modeling caregiver tolerance of uncomfortable emotions by a willingness to be present with them.

   (2) Serving as a container for a patient's emotions by recognizing and, when appropriate, addressing displacement of affect onto others, and recognizing persistent anger and other strong affects as a possible avoidance of mourning.

   (3) Avoiding the personalization of a patient's emotional reactions.

   (4) Assessing and providing interactions appropriate to the patient's emotional age at any given time.

Case example An oncology nurse approached the Pain Service psychologist with a sense of urgency concerning a female patient who was requesting inordinate amounts of pain medication because of inadequate relief. A brief discussion indicated that the patient had just been told that her cancer was terminal. Since the psychologist was obligated to see another patient at that time, he encouraged the nurse to ask the patient, "Which pain hurts worse, your cancer or what you have just been told?" The nurse subsequently reported that in response to her question, the patient had burst out crying, and when provided further opportunity to ventilate, had no further requests for additional pain medication.

The point of this example is that when staff members find themselves unwilling to talk with patients about blatantly obvious but emotionally uncomfortable issues, the inhibition to speak is more likely due to the staff members' discomfort with their own emotions than to the patient's discomfort. It is precisely a caretaker's willingness to broach seemingly taboo subjects at an interpersonal level that can alleviate the emotional pressure that complicates and inhibits pain relief.

2. Self-regulation training model

    a. This model seeks to generate and enhance a patient's spontaneous self-regulation of the various cognitive, affective, and physiologic components of pain perception and response to pain (see Chapter 14 for a discussion of specific techniques). The level and type of staff involvement dictated by this model for any given situation are determined through application of the matrix model.

    b. The **basic types of staff involvement** are (1) provision of information and education, (2) training patients in specific coping skills, (3) facilitating a gradual shift from staff-initiated to patient-initiated use of specific coping skills, and (4) follow-up for reinforcement of acquired skills when use of the skill no longer appears to be as effective as previously.

    c. Patients clearly benefit from information about what is to be done during a procedure, and even more powerfully, from information about the kind of sensory experience they can expect during the procedure. However, information must be supplemented by a broader educational approach which addresses gaps in the patient's understanding of and expectations for effective pain management.

    3. These models necessarily overlap in that effective self-regulation training requires a degree of interpersonal relationship which is characterized by traits of the interpersonal influence model.

    4. **Environmental support** for the use of self-regulation techniques is crucial to their success. This support includes educating medical and ancillary staff as to the important benefits of self-regulation training, discouraging and counteracting negative comments (e.g., "You don't really believe in that stuff, do you?"—referring to medical hypnosis) by uninformed staff mem-

bers or personnel, and ensuring protected time in a patient's schedule for the practice of self-regulation techniques (e.g., listening to prescribed audio tapes).

C. Levels and Types of Psychological Intervention

1. It should be remembered that *all* interventions are "psychological" in so far as they affect the patient's attitudes, hopes, beliefs, understandings, motivations, and expectations. Table 5-4 identifies various levels of psychological input from staff and the range of interventions most readily available to each. The content of intervention may differ for each level of input. Where overlap occurs, it is crucial that input be coordinated and consistent so that the patient receives the same basic message with regard to what is being said and done by all levels of staff involved.

2. Table 5-4 further organizes available types of acute interventions and teachable coping skills into categories of "brief/rudimentary" and "extended/complex," based roughly on the time required for the delivery of the intervention and the amount of specialized training necessary for the staff to utilize the intervention. Variants of some interventions apply equally to both categories. (See section on self-regulation techniques in Chapter 14.)

3. Specialized pain consultants

a. Far more psychological interventions and greater benefits are possible with regard to the management of acute pain than are likely to be available in most acute care settings. At best, existing demands on staff time and energy are likely to limit psychological intervention to its most rudimentary levels. The information provided in this text should improve the quality of such interventions.

b. Effective psychological intervention with truly complex pain problems, however, is likely to require a level of expertise and the availability and continuity of care that simply are not possible other than by use of specialized pain consultants.

c. One very effective model for such consultants has been the development of an **Acute Pain Service Psychology Division** as part of an Acute Pain Service run by an Anesthesiology Department. Alternatively, appropriately trained consultants in the department of Behavioral Medicine or Consult/Liaison Psychiatry might be called in, as is typically done in most hospital settings. The distinct advantage of having consultants specifically identified as part of the Acute Pain Service is the implicit validation of psychological intervention as coequal with medical intervention. We have found that this identification does much to forestall patient objections to "talking with a shrink," particularly when the idea of a referral is introduced by an anesthesiologist who obviously considers psychological input to be as important as medical input in the treatment of pain.

Table 5-4 Levels and types of psychological intervention available

I. Levels of intervention
   1. Physician's input
      a. Rapport and interpersonal influence
      b. Information about:
         (1) Procedures and medications
         (2) General medical condition
         (3) Prognosis
      c. Sense of humor
      d. Encouragement
      e. (Rarely, but ideally) use of hypnotic strategies
   2. Nursing/ancillary staff
      a. Same as above, plus
      b. Rudimentary coping skills training
      c. Rudimentary counseling
   3. Specialists in psychological treatment of pain
      a. Same as (2) above, plus
      b. (Ideally) use of hypnotic strategies
      c. Coping skills training, rudimentary and complex
      d. Counseling, ranging from rudimentary to brief psychotherapy
      e. Formal assessment of cognitive and emotional functioning
      f. Complex acute interventions (e.g., psychological preparation for surgery, or use of hypnoanalgesia as sole anesthetic for surgery if indicated)

II. Categories of acute interventions and teachable coping skills
   1. Brief/rudimentary
      a. Distraction
      b. Humor
      c. Music
      d. Reading
      e. Deep breathing and relaxation
      f. Imagery
   2. Extended/complex
      a. Distraction
      b. Deep breathing and relaxation
      c. Imagery
      d. Meditation
      e. Biofeedback
      f. Cutaneous stimulation (massage)
      g. Stress inoculation training
      h. Hetero- and self-hypnosis utilizing complex hypnotic phenomena (e.g., dissociation, sensory alteration, time distortion)
      i. Brief psychotherapy

D. Natural Stages of Psychological Treatment

Just as there are stages of medical treatment which build successively, there are **natural stages of psychological treatment** in acute medical care which must be respected if treatment is to be effective. Further, stages of psychological treatment interact with phases of acute medical care. During the emergent and triage phases of acute care, only the first three stages of psychological treatment (initial rapport, building trust and alliance, and personality assessment) are relevant. During the post-triage/stabilization phase, the later stages of psychological treatment (patient education about pain management, grief work, facilitation of the patient's shift from a victim-of-injury to a manager-of-recovery stance, and patient skill acquisition) gain primary importance. Failure to appreciate the patient's changing psychological needs and phases of treatment becomes increasingly detrimental the longer a patient remains in the acute care setting.

Specific stages of psychological treatment include the following:

1. Establishing initial rapport   At this stage, the patient's basic question concerning pain is, "Will they listen to me?" Since patients are likely to interpret the staff members' interpersonal availability and sensitivity as an index of their willingness to listen to concerns about pain, a crucial step in pain management is taking the time simply to become acquainted with patients interpersonally (e.g., saying "hello," introducing oneself, asking questions about the person's life not directly related to his or her medical care).

2. Building a sense of trust   The patient's next question is "Can I trust them (doctors and staff) to believe me about my pain?" *The reality of the patient's pain should never be questioned. Focus instead on maintaining a partnership in determining how best to manage the pain.*

3. Building a sense of alliance   Like trust, a sense of alliance develops over time. Alliance is consolidated by encouraging patients to tell their story, and by expression of the caregiver's interest in clarifying exactly who did or did not do what, and what did or did not happen that should have happened relative to the patient's condition. As the patient's story becomes clear, it becomes possible to help establish specific priorities and goals in the patient's personal situation, as well as in his or her medical care, thereby freeing the patient's energy for effective management of the pain experience.

4. Personality assessment   This process is not restricted to formal psychological testing. It is an intuitive process engaged in by caretakers and patients alike, and refers to how we generate expectations as to how another person is likely to act. Major pertinent factors include problem-solving history, coping style, and emotional age.

5. Patient education about pain management   In order to offset the typical misconceptions about pain, it is important to provide basic education about pain in a manner which is consistent with the patient's coping style and level of cognitive ability. This education should be a standard part of each patient's care as early as possible in treatment, since efforts to educate which begin after pain control has become a problem are likely to be per-

Table 5-5 What to teach about pain

I. Dispel myths
1. That mind and body are separate
2. That medicine and science can do anything

II. Clarify important distinctions
1. Sensation versus suffering
2. Significance of the "meaning" of pain
3. Acute versus chronic pain
4. Sufficient comfort versus total absence of pain

III. Provide useful models
1. Gate control theory of pain as rationale for psychological impact on pain perception
2. Broken-fire-alarm model for neuropathic pain or pain not associated with identifiable tissue damage
3. Arrested grief response to physical and emotional losses

---

ceived by patients as discounting the reality of their pain. If the pain management has already become problematic, a useful way to begin the education process might be to say, "We know you have real pain, and we know that real pain has serious effects on a person's life that we've only begun to understand. That's why I want to explain to you some basic facts about how pain works, and how we are trying to help you manage it." The focus should be on the provision of sufficient comfort, specifically countering the expectation of total relief at all times, and emphasizing the importance of the patient's management of his or her condition. For a summary of **what to teach,** see Table 5-5.

    6. Grief work

       a. The treatment goal in grief work is facilitation of the acceptance phase and the shift from victim to manager stance. This is achieved by educating the patient about the existence of the normal grief response and its predictable stages, identifying associated losses, recognizing and ventilating related affect (especially anger), and mourning the losses.

       b. It is important that caregivers' expectations and strategies for interacting with patients about their pain correspond with the stage of grief and the phase of treatment involved.

Patients who are stuck in denial or anger, for example, often present with anger about inadequate pain medication. Caregivers miss the point if they merely respond with explanations about potential addiction and respiratory failure. Rather, additional ventilation of anger must be allowed, with the goal of helping patients identify (previously unrecognized) losses which underlie their anger. Simultaneously, caregivers must maintain a professional stance and not take personally the unreasonable expressions of affect which characterize the early phases of grief (e.g., denial, anger, frustration, hopelessness, and helplessness). Instead, they must remain compassionately neutral so as to maintain the rapport necessary for later stages of treatment.

7. **Facilitating the patient's shift from a victim-of-injury to a manager-of-recovery stance** This is less a stage of treatment than it is an ongoing process and goal of treatment. However, caregiver expectations and strategies for specific intervention should be consistent with the patient's location on this continuum at any given time.

8. **Coping skills training**

a. Training in self-regulation skills is a major part of shaping the manager-of-recovery stance, and consists of five phases:

1. **Initial introduction** to the concept of self-regulation. In truly emergent settings, this may consist of experiencing the effective use of techniques which are initiated and sustained by the caregiver, such as a hypnotic induction with suggestions for relaxation and improved comfort. More commonly, this introduction consists of a discussion which includes basic information about pain management (see Table 5-5) followed by the demonstration of a specific technique which the patient eventually can utilize independently.

2. **Provision of specific instructions,** with gradual shaping of the patient's responses.

3. **Supervised and independent practice** of the techniques.

4. **Gradual fading** of caregiver-initiated activities as the patient assumes responsibility for the self-regulation process.

5. **Monitoring** of the patient's progress and possible need for booster interventions or retraining, particularly following setbacks or alterations in the patient's medical or psychological condition.

b. It is important that the patient experience success in the early phases of training, so training should begin with simple techniques that have a high probability of initial success (e.g., simple relaxation through deep-breathing exercises), even if the relative benefit is limited by comparison with more complex phenomena, such as dissociation and sensory alteration.

c. Patients should not be expected to utilize acquired psychological skills effectively 100 percent of the time. Psychological techniques of pain management are not 100 percent reliable, and psychological skills are intended as a supplement to, and not a replacement for, appropriate medication and treatment. Further, it is important to monitor the need for either additional detailed training or a simple booster session following periods of disuse.

d. Ideally, one should avoid openly challenging the patient's use of self-regulation procedures as a way to reduce medications, especially in the early phases of training. When self-regulation training is used to assist in forced reductions of pain medication, it is important that (1) the reduction be gradual and allow reasonable time for skill acquisition; (2) the reduction schedule be discussed and clarified with the patient well ahead of time; (3) the trainer be perceived by the patient as separate from the decision process of how much medication is to be allowed (i.e., that the trainer not be expected to police medication consumption, and, when possible, be separate from regular nursing staff, such as a part of the psychology division of the hospital's Acute Pain Service); and (4) the trainer maintain ongoing contact with the patient throughout the reduction process.

E. Application of the Matrix Model
1. Assessment and positioning of factors within the matrix
  a. Assess and locate relevant staff, setting, and patient characteristics as identified within the matrix model (see Table 5-6 for summary listing of these characteristics).
  b. Identify factors which interfere with the patient's effective management of pain and are in need of treatment. These factors may be related to:

  1. Pharmacologic needs.
  2. Problematic pain perception.
  3. Characterologic issues.
  4. Grief work.
  5. Environmental impediments.
  6. Financial impediments.
  7. Safety issues (e.g., providing aliases for victims of violence).
  8. A need for information, social support, attention, limit setting, specific coping skills (either staff-initiated and sustained, or longer-term patient training), or brief psychotherapy for resolution of specific psychological issues.

  c. Based on the relative locations of staff, setting, and patient variables within the matrix, determine which of the above factors are best treatable (1) by whom, (2) with what sequence of strategies, and (3) in what order.
  d. In determining how best to approach the patient interpersonally at any given time with any given strategy, give particular attention to:

  1. Meaning of the pain for the patient.
  2. The patient's current emotional age.
  3. The patient's position within the grief process.
  4. Matching of staff and patient coping styles.

CHAPTER 5 PSYCHOLOGICAL ASSESSMENT AND TREATMENT 73

Table 5-6 Relevant staff, setting, and patient characteristics for matrix assessment

I. Relevant staff and setting characteristics include:
  A. Potential staff misconceptions about pain
  B. Individual staff coping styles
  C. Ability to avoid personalizing patients' responses
  D. Sensitivity to interpersonal issues
  E. Willingness to "be with" versus insistence on "doing"
  F. Staff attitudes toward role of self-regulation training in pain management
  G. Willingness to identify specific individual as responsible for pain assessment and oversight of pain management

II. Relevant patient characteristics include:
  A. Evidence of previous problem-solving behavior:
    1. Family of origin
    2. Educational
    3. Marital
    4. Vocational
  B. Dominant coping style pattern and sense of self-efficacy
    1. Coping sensitizer
    2. Avoidant repressor
  C. Meaning attributed to the pain
    1. How pain began (e.g., who is perceived as responsible; losses incurred)
    2. Patient's understanding of current and previous medical diagnosis and etiology of the pain (especially important if dealing with chronic pain)
  D. Environmental factors (e.g., secondary gain, dysfunctional family support, interpersonal conflict with staff)
  E. Historically based intrapsychic factors (e.g., physical or sexual abuse)
  F. Current intrapsychic factors (e.g., pain as signal that one is still alive; pain as reminder of discouragement, anxiety, depression over current situation)
  G. Predominant emotional age (distinguish transient shifts versus character disorder)
  H. Level of hypnotic capacity
  I. Position within the grief process
  J. Position on the continuum from a victim-of-injury to a manager-of-recovery stance
  K. Phase of recovery
  L. Phase of medical treatment

e. The process of assessment and strategy selection is necessarily somewhat fluid, and must be adjusted as information and experience accrue with a given patient.

2. Prognostic indicators

a. Within the matrix application process, one can identify both optimum and minimally positive prognostic indicators for the successful use of psychological strategies in acute pain management (see Table 5-7 for summary). The more that patient prognostic indicators deviate from optimum, the more important it becomes to tease out available indicators of patient

Table 5-7 Prognostic indicators

I. Setting
   A. Optimal
      1. All unit staff members are specifically trained in use and teaching of self-regulation techniques
      2. All unit staff members are committed to use these strategies
      3. Formal training in the use of these strategies is available for new staff
      4. Pain specialist consultants are available
   B. Minimal
      1. Availability of at least some trained staff members (e.g., pain specialist consultants)
      2. Commitment of at least one staff person to use of the techniques
      3. Sufficient unit support for and cooperation in the use of the strategies
II. Patient
   A. Optimal
      1. Coping style of "coping sensitizer"
      2. Nonregressed
      3. Minimally depressed
      4. Psychologically minded
      5. High hypnotic capacity
      6. Motivated
         a. Energy available
         b. Positive social support system
   B. Minimal (look for the presence of at least one characterstic in each major category)
      1. Some indication of positive coping history, such as:
         a. Sense of "decent metal" beneath surface appearance (i.e., may look bad now, but there's something there to build on)
         b. *Something* is going or has gone OK in life
      2. Patient shows at least minimal indication of progress with one to three concerted efforts at use of psychological strategies, such as:
         a. Reported sense of improvement
         b. Sense of initiative
         c. Spontaneous insight into own behavior
         d. Compliance with behavioral "hoops" (e.g., increase in pain medication if accompanied by increased activity level)
      3. Patient exhibits capacity for:
         a. Interpersonal relatedness versus constant blaming and distancing
         b. Self-observation
         c. Sense of humor
         d. Cognitive flexibility
         e. Psychological mindedness
      4. Staff experiences some sense of diagnostic clarity about the patient's operative psychological dynamics

and staff resources and to match these as determined from application of the matrix model.

    b. If at least minimal prognostic indicators are not present, there is a clear need for consultation with a pain specialist.

3. Selection of intervention strategy

a. The basic criteria for the selection of an effective intervention strategy include:

1. Can the setting provide the desired intervention(s)?
2. Is the patient capable of participating in and effectively using the intervention?
3. Does the strategy build on existing skills and circumstances?
4. Will the strategy chosen now be useful later?
5. Who can best provide the intervention (i.e., who already has established a relationship with the patient, and is this person equipped to provide the desired intervention)?

b. Since a lack of continuity and a lack of consistency in approach are the first likely sources of difficulty in pain management, it is crucial to identify a specific individual as responsible for the assessment and oversight of pain management for a given patient.

c. Since choosing an intervention without doing an assessment is likely to perpetuate or exacerbate the existing problem, it is important to determine whether a matrix assessment has been done. If assessment is needed, identify individuals having a sufficient relationship with and knowledge of the patient to provide data for the assessment, and carry out the assessment.

d. Identify factors in need of treatment, consider the staff level and type of interventions to be used, and identify who should be involved in and/or informed about the choice of the intervention, and how soon. If needed, arrange a team meeting to discuss the assessment and to evolve a coordinated plan of designated activities.

e. Choose the intervention based on the principle of doing the simplest things first. Begin with interpersonal influence, move to self-regulation training as indicated, and build toward a model of having the patient psychologically equipped for managing the pain of upcoming procedures and conditions. Request a consultation with pain specialists when indicated, and provide access to in-depth psychological preparation prior to major procedures (e.g., surgery) whenever indicated and possible.

V. CASE EXAMPLES

A. Case I

1. Problem A 27-year-old black male presented with second- and third-degree partial-thickness scald burns to 36 percent of his body (primarily his legs). The injury had occurred when the patient fell into a vat of 200°F water at a plastics factory while attempting to rescue a coworker who had just fallen into the same vat. He is now facing a third grafting attempt 3 months after the original injury and following two successive failures exacerbated by the conversion of all donor sites to third-degree-burn equivalents. His graft and donor sites are healing poorly, with no identifiable medical explanation. The patient is anxious and oppositional about the upcoming surgery, depressed, regressively dependent, phobically anxious, very disruptive to nursing staff efforts in anticipation of daily procedures, and oppositionally out of control during these procedures despite heavy medication.

2. Matrix assessment

a. **Setting characteristics** The setting is the burn unit in a tertiary-care teaching hospital. Earlier consultation with Consult/Liaison Psychiatry had identified posttraumatic stress response, but afforded no improvement in his problem behavior. Internal caregivers were frustrated, angry, and impatient with the patient's behavior. Based on a recommendation from the nursing staff, the attending physician made a referral to the Anesthesia Department–based Acute Pain Service Psychology Division.

b. **Patient characteristics**
1. **Environmental factors.** None evident.
2. **Problem-solving behavior.** Previously healthy, verbally interactive married male with a college education, good job, strong religious ties, and family support.
3. **Coping style and behavior.** Coping sensitizer with external LOC exacerbated by regressive catastrophizing tendencies, resulting in obsessive anticipatory rumination prior to each debridement session and disruptive calls and questions to staff before each procedure.
4. **Meaning of the pain**
   a. Punishment for clumsiness and willingness to help others.
   b. Suspiciousness and attribution of malicious intent to staff (based on ketamine-induced interpretation of debridement immediately following initial hospitalization: "The doctors were taking turns at torturing me by cutting off my skin"). The patient was consciously aware of the basis for his fears, but his fears were unrelieved by rational discussion and reassurance.
   c. "Will I live?", based on: (i) a nearly lethal renal failure (from which he had recovered by the time of the consultation request); (ii) progressive conversion of donor sites to third-degree-burn equivalents and projected use of his entire back and buttocks as donor sites for the next grafting attempt; (iii) an impression that his transfer from a smaller local hospital to the tertiary care hospital must mean the

injury was more serious than he had been told; and (iv) statements the patient had made to himself when he had slipped and gone under the water for a second time (e.g., "I'm going to die!").
  5. **Intrapsychic factors**
     a. Historical: None evident
     b. Current: Going to "tanking" room as an unconscious reminder of falling into the vat, which precipitated his injury.
  6. **Predominant emotional age.** Chronologically age-appropriate mixed with intermittent, transient episodes of 6- to 8-year-old attitudes and behavior, mostly around times of debridement or other painful procedures.
  7. **Hypnotic capacity.** Moderate to high (assessed informally by administration of hypnotic induction with suggestions for comfort, relaxation, and pleasant dissociative experiences).
  8. *Phase of* **grief process.** Anger and bargaining (blaming physicians for not caring, attempting to put off necessary procedures).
  9. **Victim-of-injury versus manager-of-recovery stance.** Passive victim whose efforts at self-help were focused on activating assistance from others.
  10. **Phase of recovery**
      a. **Attitudes and beliefs** about etiology of pain: See "meaning of pain" below.
      b. **Distinguishing acute versus chronic pain:** Need to distinguish acute (procedural) pain from chronic pain of deconditioning and disrupted healing process.
  11. **Stage of psychological treatment**
      a. For consultant: Initial rapport and trust/alliance building.
      b. For Burn Unit caregivers and ancillary staff: Patient education, facilitating shift to manager-of-recovery stance.

3. Factors in need of treatment Brief psychotherapy for resolution of specific issues:
  1. Grief work.
  2. Resolution of residual posttraumatic stress disorder and corrective work on preconscious attributions to the meaning of the pain.

Coping skills training:
  1. Initially provided by consultant.
  2. Goal is to have this be patient-initiated.

4. Prognostic indicators
  a. Had a positive coping history.

b. Evidenced sense of humor and ability to comment on own dysfunctional behavior during initial interview.

c. Responded well and rapidly to initial hypnotic induction.

5. Intervention strategy

a. The specialized pain consultant was identified as responsible for matrix assessment and coordination of intervention strategies.

b. Following an explanation and discussion of potential benefits with patient, the consultant provided an initial hypnotic induction with the immediate goal of relaxation and assessment of his capacity for pleasant dissociative experiences. The patient's response was excellent.

c. Hypnotic preparation for increased tolerance of the debridement procedures was accomplished by suggesting amnesia for previous debridement experiences, then sustaining a hypnotic sense of calm and comfort as the patient imagined going through the treatment process with much greater comfort than he had thought possible. Time progression techniques were used for the patient to imagine himself as comfortable and proud of his success following the procedure.

d. The consultant then accompanied the patient through the debridement process, providing a hypnotic induction in the tanking room just prior to beginning the procedure, reinforcing suggestions for analgesia (sensory alteration), dissociation, and distraction (reliving a previous experience of being home with his family at Christmastime).

e. The patient then acquired and perfected the skill of self-hypnosis through independent use of audio tapes prior to and during subsequent therapy procedures.

f. In preparation for upcoming surgery, the consultant performed a hypnotic review of the patient's experience at the time of injury in order to determine his conscious and unconscious attitudes, expectations, and beliefs which might affect his current behavior and difficulties with healing (e.g., inappropriately sustained physiologic stress response producing a disruptive biochemical substrate for healing). With the patient under hypnosis, the consultant provided corrective understandings and ameliorative suggestions consistent with the patient's regressive emotional age in order to counter and reframe feelings of guilt, self-blame, and religious doubt, along with obsessive, ketamine-induced delusions of purposeful mistreatment by the medical staff. Future progression techniques were used for him to imagine and create expectations of a postitive outcome to surgery, including the rapid growth of healthy tissue, effective participation in wound care and the rehabilitation process, good appetite and renal function, a rapid improvement in the ability to ambulate, and a minimal need for pain medications.

6. Outcome

a. An immediate improvement was seen in his ability to tolerate debridement, including a dramatically increased tolerance for range-of-motion exercises, a decrease in the time required for procedures, decreased medication requirements, a nearly total reduction in anticipatory anxiety and associated disruptive behavior, and a significant increase in independent functioning.

b. Following surgery, the graft take was 95 percent, and donor sites healed rapidly. Hetero- and self-hypnosis were continued for pain control and enhanced ambulation, with minimal use of pain medication. The patient was discharged in good condition 15 days after surgery, with complete healing and therapeutic amnesia for significant medical trauma at 4 months. Throughout treatment, nothing had been altered with regard to previous medical procedures or medication regimens, other than a reduction in pain medications. It is argued that in addition to providing anxiety and pain control, hypnosis and suggestion facilitated the healing processes in this patient, presumably via psychoneuroimmunologic pathways.

B. Case II

1. Problem A 34-year-old white male presented with second-degree burns which were at risk of becoming third-degree burns. The patient had been a passenger in a motor vehicle which went out of control. The driver (the patient's best friend from work) was killed, leaving behind a young wife and an infant child. The patient had been progressing well physically, tolerating whirlpool treatment and debridement, with healing occurring during the hospital stay. He was discharged to outpatient treatment, and during one outpatient contact for debridement treatment, complained more of pain than he had during inpatient treatment. He refused tanking and debridement at his second and third outpatient visits, complaining about pain severity without any observed pathophysiology. On the third visit, he was seen in the emergency room by his surgeon, who requested a consultation with the psychology pain specialist.

2. Matrix assessment

a. Setting characteristics The setting was the emergency room in a rural primary care hospital. Prior treatment had been provided by the surgeon and the rehabilitation service, with appreciation for the value of psychological interventions.

b. Patient characteristics

1. **Environmental factors.** None evident.
2. **Problem-solving behavior.** Working-class background with a reasonable work history; a high school graduate; single, with no previous marriages; mother available as support.
3. **Coping style.** Minimally verbal. Reported difficulty in discussing feelings and strategizing about what to do. Mixed avoidant-

repressor and coping sensitizer, with internal LOC and difficulty in relationships. Reported no discussion of the accident or feelings about the accident up to the point of consulting with the psychologist.
  4. **Meaning of pain**
     a. Punishment for the accident and the patient's inability to do anything about it.
     b. Unrecognized reminder of his friend's death, and resulting difficulties for the friend's wife and child.
     c. A way of grieving.
  5. **Intrapsychic factors**
     a. Historically based: None apparent.
     b. Current: Arrested grief response.
  6. **Emotional age.** Congruent with chronological age.
  7. **Hypnotic capacity.** Moderate (assessed by clinical interview with a focus on the history of his ability to become absorbed in imaginative involvement and his degree of fantasy proneness).
  8. **Phase of grief process.** Anger and denial.
  9. **Victim-of-injury versus manager-of-recovery stance.** Victim of injury.
  10. **Phase of recovery**
      a. **Attitudes and beliefs** toward etiology of pain: "There's something wrong. It just hurts more now."
      b. **Distinguishing acute versus chronic:** At risk for the development of a chronic pain syndrome.
  11. **Stage of psychological treatment**
      a. For consultant: Initial rapport and trust/alliance building.
      b. For internal/external caregivers: Patient education, facilitating a shift to the manager-of-recovery stance.

3. **Factors in need of treatment**
   a. Need for an explanation of the necessity for tanking and debridement.
   b. Education about psychological factors in recovering from an accident.
   c. Identification and emotional ventilation of sadness over the loss of his friend and the plight of the friend's young family.
   d. Coping skills training.

4. **Prognostic indicators**
   a. Previous healing and participation in treatment.
   b. Family support.
   c. Willingness to discuss the psychological dimensions of treatment.
   d. Rapid involvement in hypnotic treatment.

5. Intervention strategy

    a. A specialized consultant was called in, who replaced the focus on getting into the whirlpool with a discussion about the accident which had caused the patient's pain. He identified the pain as including an emotional response to the friend's death while in the car with the patient, and with what would happen to the friend's wife and child.

    b. The patient now recognized that coming to the hospital was a painful reminder of the accident. The consultant continued to support the grieving and to make a distinction between grieving and the pain of debridement.

    c. Simple rapid hypnotic induction was used with dissociative focus, allowing the body to do its healing as the patient developed an interpersonal context for emotional healing.

6. Outcome

    a. The consultant met the patient at the rehabilitation center the following day rather than at the emergency room.

    b. He repeated hypnosis with suggestions for dissociation for comfort.

    c. There were no further problems with the tanking procedure.

    d. He followed up with six psychotherapy sessions for further facilitation of the grieving.

SUGGESTED READINGS

Barber TX: Changing "unchangeable" bodily processes by (hypnotic) suggestions: a new look at hypnosis, cognitions, imagining and the mind-body problem, in Sheikh AA (ed): *Imagery and Healing* (Imagery and Human Development Series). Farmingdale, New York, Baywood, 1984.

Bennett HL: Behavioral anesthesia. *Advances* 2:11–21, 1985.

Blankenfield R: Suggestion, relaxation and hypnosis as adjuncts in the care of surgery patients. *Am J Clin Hypn* 33:172–186, 1991.

DeGood D: Reducing medical patients' reluctance to participate in psychological therapies: the initial session. *Prof Psychol Res Prac* 14:570–579, 1983.

Hilgard ER, Hilgard JR: *Hypnosis in the Relief of Pain* Los Altos, California, Kaufmann, 1975.

McCaffery M, Vourakis C: Assessment and relief of pain in chemically dependent patients. *Orthopaed Nurs* 11:13–27, 1992.

Spiegel D: Hypnosis with medical and surgical patients. *Gen Hosp Psychiatry* 5:265–277, 1983.

Turk DC, Michenbaum DM, Gemest M: *Pain and Behavioral Medicine: A Cognitive-Behavioral Perspective.* New York, Guilford, 1983.

Van Dalfsen T, Syrjala K: Psychological strategies in acute pain management, in Hoyt J (ed): *Pain management in the ICU. Crit Care Clinics* 6:421–432, 1990.

PART THREE

PHARMACOLOGIC AGENTS

CHAPTER 6

PHARMACOKINETIC AND PHARMACODYNAMIC CONCERNS IN THE CRITICALLY ILL

Robb McGory

I. Goal of Therapeutic Drug Monitoring
   A. Components of Therapeutic Drug Monitoring
   B. Assumptions for Therapeutic Drug Monitoring
II. Influences on Serum Drug Concentrations
   A. Pharmacokinetics
   B. Disease-Related Alterations in Biopharmaceutics
III. Pharmacokinetic Models
   A. Compartments
   B. Linearity of Elimination
   C. Model of Drug Administration
   D. Individualized Pharmacokinetic Parameters
   E. Mathematical Equations
IV. Pharmacodynamics
   A. Altered Dynamic Responsiveness
   B. Pathophysiologic Influences
   C. Iatrogenic Interventions
V. Summary
Suggested Readings

I. GOAL OF THERAPEUTIC DRUG MONITORING

The goal of monitoring is to provide the most effective drug regimen with the least amount of toxicity. The risk/benefit ratio of the dose, duration of therapy, and potential for toxicity must be assessed for each drug in order to define the limits of therapy.

A. Components of Therapeutic Drug Monitoring
1. **Individualized dosing regimens** are calculated for patients in order to achieve therapeutic serum drug concentrations.
2. **Assessment of drug effectiveness** is performed frequently to correlate patient outcome with assumed/measured serum drug concentrations.
3. **Adjustment of acceptable dosing limits** may be necessary if the patient does not respond to normal patterns of drug use.

B. Assumptions for Therapeutic Drug Monitoring
The following assumptions are made to justify the existence of individualized drug dosing.
    1. Serum drug concentrations correlate directly with tissue levels. Drug molecules follow a gradient from high serum concentration to a lower tissue concentration. Drug will reenter the circulation once the serum concentration falls below the tissue concentration. Serum and tissue levels are therefore related, but never equal. Serum concentrations are monitored as an approximation of tissue levels.
    2. Changes in serum drug concentrations correlate with increased or decreased tissue responsiveness. Disease processes, such as liver failure, renal failure, and malnutrition, may blunt the response to receptor stimulation due to changes in the amount and strength of drug binding to the receptors. Disease may result in an altered chemical composition of the membrane structure, physical distortion of the membrane due to edema, or blocking of receptors by waste products that accumulate in disease states.
    3. Pharmacologic data from noncritical patients are applicable to intensive-care-unit (ICU) patients. The evaluation of drug therapy normally is performed on volunteers or minimally ill patients. The validity of extrapolating this experience to the critically ill patient with multiple-organ dysfunction is suspect, but necessary.

II. INFLUENCES ON SERUM DRUG CONCENTRATIONS

A. Pharmacokinetics

Pharmacokinetics is the study of the time course of drug presence in the body, encompassing the absorption, distribution, metabolism, and elimination of the drug.

   1. The absorption of the drug across cell membranes must occur at several sites. Drug deposited into the gastrointestinal (GI) tract must pass through the cells lining the mucosal surface and the cells of the blood vessels in order to enter the circulation and travel to the target organ. In like manner, drug deposited by subcutaneous, intradermal, or intramuscular injection must pass through cell membranes to enter the blood. The prevalence of direct intravenous (IV) infusion of drugs in critical care is necessary because of disruptions in tissue absorption.

   2. Distribution of the drug describes the transportation and deposition of the drug throughout the body. Very few drugs can be directly administered at the site of need. Drug molecules will vary in their ability to enter fluid compartments and fat tissue, to pass through the blood–brain barrier, and to bind to tissue receptors and carrier proteins such as albumin and alpha-1-acid glycoprotein (Table 6-1).

   3. Metabolism of the drug is the physical alteration of drug molecules. The body reacts to drugs as if they were harmful. Many tissues, primarily the liver, will detoxify the molecule by changing the chemical structure. This

Table 6-1 Protein binding of drugs

Drugs that bind to albumin	Drugs that bind to alpha-1-acid glycoprotein
Carbamazepine	Bupivacaine
Diazepam	Diltiazem
Diltiazem	Dipyridamole
Etoposide	Disopyramide
Ibuprofen	Lidocaine
Indomethacin	Meperidine
Lidocaine	Methadone
Meperidine	Propranolol
Naproxen	Quinidine
Phenytoin	Verapamil
Propranolol	
Quinidine	
Valproic acid	
Verapamil	
Warfarin	

physical change will decrease the ability of the parent drug to stimulate tissue receptors and will increase the water solubility of the metabolite to improve the elimination of the drug.

4. **Elimination** is the final pathway by which a drug or its metabolite is removed from the body. The kidney is the main organ of elimination, while the liver can concentrate drug in bile. Minor routes of drug loss are through secretions, tears, and pulmonary gas exchange.

B. Disease-Related Alterations in Biopharmaceutics

1. Absorption

   a. **Oral absorption** of drugs is reduced in critical care patients due to physical removal by **continuous or intermittent nasogastric suctioning,** reduced passage of the drug through the GI tract secondary to **altered peristalsis,** reduced absorptive surface caused by **villous atrophy,** altered passage through mucosal endothelial cells due to **edematous bowel wall** and **reduced active transport,** and limited passage into the circulatory system because of **poor blood flow** to the microvilli. In addition, **physical drug interactions,** such as magnesium or aluminum with ciprofloxacin or phenytoin with tube feeding, occur in the bowel lumen, hindering movement of the drug through endothelial cell linings owing to its physical size.

   b. **Intramuscular and subcutaneous injections** are prone to limited drug absorption due to **decreased tissue perfusion** during periods of high catecholamine release and to decreased movement of the drug through **altered tissue** that either is edematous or has abnormal contents of fat and protein.

   c. **Intravenous infusions** deposit the drug directly into the bloodstream. However, the drug may become trapped in tissue after **IV infiltration** or in the **dead space of IV tubing,** which is distinct from drug that is **adsorbed onto IV tubing** during infusion, such as occurs with nitroglycerin, insulin, or cyclosporine. The drug may be physically altered by in-line **drug interactions** or by **physical decomposition** while in solution, as with nitroprusside and cyclosporine.

2. Distribution

   a. **Poor perfusion** of target tissue will limit the number of cells that are exposed to the drug.

   b. **Altered receptor binding** will change the amount of drug attached to tissue. Receptors may be physically altered owing to **edema, malnutrition, and down-regulation,** or the binding of drugs to receptors may be blocked by **interacting drugs or uremic toxins.** Decreases in binding will elevate free serum concentrations, allowing tissues with functional receptors to bind more drug, resulting in toxicity.

   c. **Third spacing of fluid** such as ascites or massive edema may result in an additional volume into which the drug can diffuse.

d. **Loss of barrier integrity** may allow the drug to pass into otherwise virgin tissue, such as cerebral spinal fluid or the peritoneal cavity.

3. **Metabolism**

a. **Flow-dependent metabolism** describes the ability of the liver to clear the blood of toxin so rapidly that the amount of drug metabolized is determined principally by the rate of blood flow (Table 6-2). Flow-dependent metabolism is synonymous with the **first-pass effect;** that is, drug enters the circulation of the GI tract and immediately passes through the liver where most of it is metabolized. Diseases and medications that reduce cardiac output or shunt blood to other organs, and surgical revascularization that disrupts blood flow to the liver, will result in accumulation of the drug despite unaltered hepatic cell function. Reduced protein binding may increase the clearance of the drug because the liver primarily extracts unbound drug. Hence the patient may be at higher risk for toxicity due to elevated free concentration of the drug, but the liver will also detoxify the drug more rapidly. Diseases that affect hepatocyte function will also result in drug accumulation, as the inherent ability to metabolize may change the relationship to one of flow-independent metabolism.

b. **Flow-independent metabolism** is not influenced by blood flow. The amount of drug metabolized is limited by the inherent ability of hepatocyte detoxification (Table 6-2). The amount of drug that can be cleared from blood will always be less than the amount of drug that is presented to the liver via blood flow. Diseases that alter hepatocyte function are the primary cause of drug accumulation.

c. **Active metabolites** may appear upon detoxification of the parent compound. This may lead to prolonged therapeutic/toxic presence of drugs such as the benzodiazepines, or it may be beneficial as with the oral angiotensin enzyme inhibitors such as enalapril, which has an inactive parent compound, but an active metabolite (enalaprilat).

Table 6-2 Relation of drug metabolism to hepatic blood flow

Flow-dependent metabolism	Flow-independent metabolism
Isoproterenol	Cyclosporine
Lidocaine	Diazepam
Hydrocortisone	Erythromycin
Morphine	Phenytoin
Meperidine	Theophylline
Metoprolol	Warfarin
Nitroglycerin	
Propranolol	
Propoxyphene	
Verapamil	

Table 6-3 Drug elimination through artificial clearance

Dialysis	Plasmapheresis
Acyclovir	Digitoxin
Atenolol	L-thyroxine
Ceftazidime	Phenytoin
Gallamine	Propranolol
Gentamicin	Salicylate
Nadolol	Tobramycin
Penicillin	
Pentazocine	
Prednisone	
Procainamide	

4. Elimination

a. **Renal disease** will limit the amount of water-soluble parent compound and metabolite that is removed from the blood. Diseases that affect **glomerular filtration, tubular secretion,** and **tubular reabsorption** may decrease the amount of drug that reaches the urine. **Reduction of renal perfusion** will also limit the filtration of the drug.

b. **Extracorporeal dialysis** may remove drug from the blood (Table 6-3). The extent of removal depends upon the **type of dialysis,** the **length of dialysis,** and the **type of filter used.** The size of the drug molecule and the extent of tissue binding determine the potential for drug removal, while the efficiency of dialysis will determine the extent of removal.

c. **Secretions of body fluids** through wounds, burns, or drainage of compartmentalized collections (ascites) may result in enhanced clearance of drug from the body. Patients with reduced renal or hepatic function may need full or greater doses of the drug to maintain therapeutic levels.

III. PHARMACOKINETIC MODELS

Models have been mathematically constructed to describe the behavior of drug molecules once they enter the body. Knowledge of a drug's general behavior improves the ability to optimize dosage changes, as well as to schedule serum samples for the most accurate measurement.

A. Compartments

Compartments are used to equate the mathematical and physiologic distribution of the drug. The drug is administered into the **central compartment,** consisting primarily of the cardiovascular system. It then circulates throughout the body and diffuses into the **peripheral compartment,** which is composed of various tissues, be they specific organs, such as the brain, or a type of tissue, such as fat deposits. Different compartments exist because of large differences in the rate of drug entry into tissue. Most tissues rapidly equilibrate with the bloodstream and are very difficult to distinguish mathematically from the central compartment. The central compartment is the sampling compartment because blood is the most convenient tissue to obtain. Drug levels drawn from the central compartment must be used to predict the effectiveness of the drug in the peripheral compartment.

1. The **one-compartment model** (Fig. 6-1) is the simplest form of drug distribution. Serum and tissue equilibrate so rapidly that the drug appears to diffuse instantaneously throughout the body. Although not completely accurate, this model is the simplest to apply to patient care. Most of the drug distribution into peripheral compartments has occurred by the time a dose has finished infusing. Unless the drug is administered by rapid IV push, drug movement into peripheral tissue is nearly completed by the time required for infusion/absorption. The decrease of serum drug levels throughout the dosage interval reflects only the elimination of drug from the body. Most clinically relevant drugs are described by a one-compartment model.

2. The **multiple-compartment model** (Fig. 6-1) describes delayed drug movement into peripheral tissue compartments, as well as the elimination of drug via the kidneys and liver. Each tissue has an inherent rate at which the drug may attach onto and/or pass through cell surfaces. The serum elim-

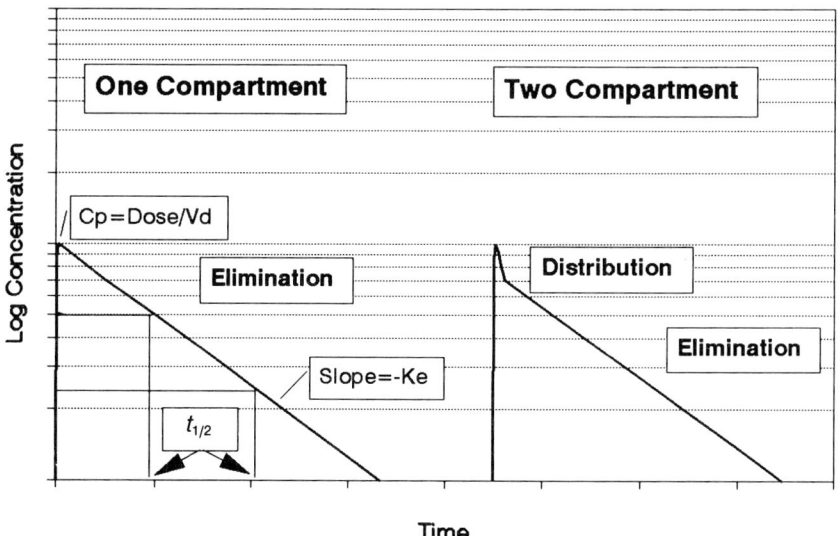

Figure 6-1 One- versus two-compartment model

ination–time curve will indicate a loss of drug from the central compartment at different rates. The initial rapid loss of drug is by distribution into the slowly equilibrating tissue, while the slowest loss reflects elimination of the drug from the body. Recognition of multiple compartments is necessary in order to obtain accurate serum samples for drug measurement. Sampling before the equilibration of compartments will give falsely elevated serum drug levels, and will not correlate with the drug's effect on tissue. Certain drugs, such as vancomycin and digoxin, are large molecules that take a long time to equilibrate. Serum samples drawn prior to 2 h and 6 h after the end of infusion, respectively, will poorly predict patient response to these drugs.

B. Linearity of Elimination

Elimination linearity describes the mathematical pattern of drug elimination from the body.

   1. Linear elimination results when the body eliminates the same percentage of drug per unit time. The percent of drug removed is independent of the starting concentration. The amount of drug removed per unit of time will decrease as the serum concentration decreases. If plotted on a log–linear graph (Fig. 6-1), the serum concentration–time curve will be a straight line throughout the dosing interval. Linear kinetics yield constant drug loss throughout the range of serum concentrations, as well as the entire dosage interval. A percentage change in dose will yield an equivalent desired percentage change in serum concentration. Linear kinetics is also called **first-order kinetics**.

   2. Nonlinear elimination results when the body eliminates the same amount of drug per unit time, while the percentage of drug removed changes. This pattern is due to a saturated elimination process, usually involving an enzyme that transforms the drug molecule. A saturated enzyme is always functioning at its maximum ability. Eventually, enough drug is eliminated to desaturate the enzymes, allowing a shift to linear kinetics as previously described. Dosage adjustments are not made according to a ratio and proportion relationship as with linear kinetics. Because most of the dosage interval is spent in the nonlinear portion of the time curve, small amounts of drug will result in larger than expected changes in serum levels. Nonlinear kinetics is also called **zero-order kinetics**.

C. Model of Drug Administration

The model of drug administration relates serum concentrations to the technique of drug delivery. Variations occur due to the access of IV lines, the ability to take medication orally, and the importance of maintaining tight control of serum concentrations. Each method of administration has a characteristic serum concentration–time profile (Fig. 6-2). **Steady state** occurs

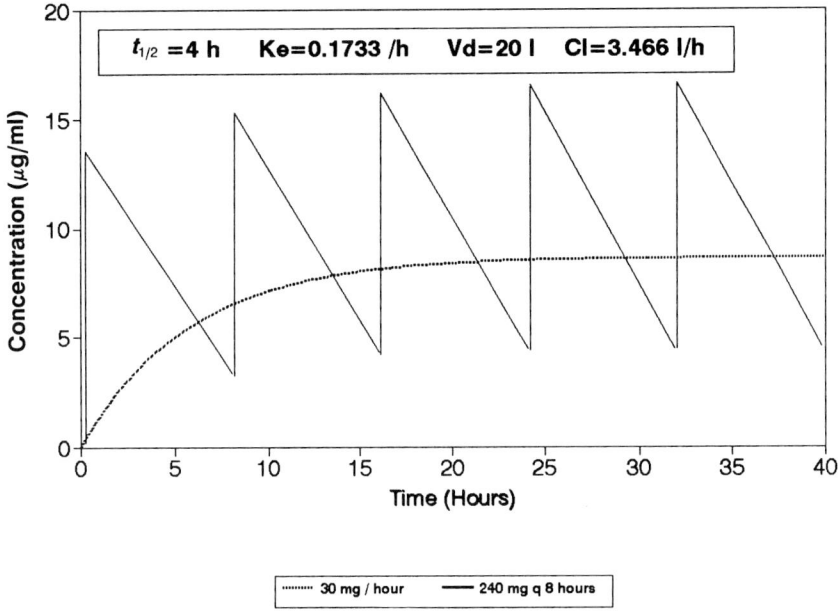

Figure 6-2 Continuous versus intermittent infusion model

when the rate of drug intake equals the rate of drug elimination. Mathematically, the time required to reach steady state is five half-lives. A drug with a short half-life will reach steady state much sooner than will a drug with a long half-life. A **loading dose** may be administered to attain therapeutic concentration quickly and to maintain the patient until the **maintenance dose** reaches steady state.

1. The **continuous infusion** of a drug causes the serum concentration to increase consistently until an invariable level is achieved at steady state. Continuous infusions are useful if a small difference exists between toxic and subtherapeutic serum levels (theophylline, procainamide), and the goal is to maintain a patient at a distinct concentration or the target tissue at a constant level of function (dopamine, dobutamine).

2. **Intermittent infusions** of drugs will result in high **(peak)** concentrations immediately after the end of the infusion and low **(trough)** concentrations just before the next dose. As with continuous infusions, peak and trough levels will increase until steady state is attained. At steady state, the concentration of drug at any time during the dosing interval will be identical to any corresponding time of any subsequent dose. Intermittent infusions are useful when an IV line cannot be dedicated for a continuous infusion or a high peak concentration may be beneficial for tissue penetration (antibiotics). In addition, lowering the serum concentrations to minimum thera-

peutic values at the end of the dosing interval may occasionally be helpful to avoid drug toxicity (gentamicin, amikacin, tobramycin).

3. The **oral administration** of drugs is similar to intermittent infusion. The highest serum concentrations occur soon after drug administration, and decrease throughout the dosing interval. Peak concentrations are affected by the **delay in absorption,** the **extent of absorption (bioavailability),** and the drug lost to the **first-pass effect.** Drugs that are susceptible to the first-pass effect may be administered sublingually to avoid the immediate presentation of drug to the liver after absorption. **Sustained-release dosage forms** of oral drugs have been developed that either mimic the continuous infusion of drug into the circulation, or maintain a drug presence when a short half-life requires frequent redosing of the drug.

D. Individualized Pharmacokinetic Parameters

Parameters (Fig. 6-1) are calculated to assess mathematically each patient's specific dosage needs to meet desired serum concentrations. Once the parameter is known and the appropriate pharmacokinetic model is determined, a dose can be derived.

1. Clearance (Cl) is the volume of blood from which drug will be totally removed over a unit of time (i.e., 1/h). Clearance is dependent on the physiologic function of the organs of metabolism/elimination. If function decreases, the clearance will decrease as well.

2. Volume of distribution (Vd) is the apparent size of the compartment into which a drug disperses. As previously mentioned, drug distribution is influenced by the fluid compartments, protein binding, and fat content of the body.

3. Half-life ($t_{1/2}$) is the time required to decrease the serum concentration by 50 percent. Linear kinetics require the half-life to remain constant at all concentrations, while nonlinear kinetics allow the half-life to decrease as the concentration decreases.

4. Elimination rate constant (Ke) is the fraction of drug removed from the body per unit time (i.e., Ke = 0.15/h = 15% of drug eliminated each hour). The elimination rate constant is a mathematical variation of half-life, that is:

$$t_{1/2} = 0.693/\text{Ke}$$

E. Mathematical Equations

Equations have been derived to individualize dosing to achieve optimal concentrations. Simplified equations are presented here. Refer to the bibliography for a more detailed explanation.

CHAPTER 6 PHARMACOKINETIC AND PHARMACODYNAMIC CONCERNS

1. **Kinetic parameters**
   a. **Volume of distribution:**

   $$Vd = \text{dose/concentration}$$

   where
   - dose = amount of drug administered
   - concentration = peak concentration

   b. **Elimination rate constant:**

   $$Ke = (\ln \text{conc } 1 - \ln \text{conc } 2)/t$$

   where ln = the natural log
   - conc 1 = peak concentration
   - conc 2 = trough concentration
   - t = time between conc 1 and conc 2

   c. **Clearance:**

   $$Cl = Ke \times Vd$$

   $$Cl = 0.693 \times Vd/t_{1/2}$$

Half-life and elimination rate constant are the mathematical correlation between clearance and volume of distribution. Because clearance and volume are only influenced by physiologic function, they are mathematically termed **model-independent parameters.** Half-life and elimination rate constant are influenced only by clearance and volume, and are termed **model-dependent parameters.** The half-life does not increase because a kidney or liver fails, but because the clearance of drug by the kidney or liver decreases. Drug effects may be prolonged or shortened due to changes in the volume of distribution (i.e., fluid shifts, protein binding, fat stores), as well as in the organ of elimination.

2. **Dose adjustment (steady state)**
   a. **Continuous infusion:**

   $$\text{concentration} = \text{rate in/rate out}$$

   where
   - rate in = rate of drug infusion
   - rate out = clearance

The serum concentration at steady state is constant and is the point of equilibrium between the drug's entering the body and the drug's leaving the body.

$$\text{dose } 2 = \text{dose } 1 \times \text{conc } 2/\text{conc } 1$$

where dose 1 = initial rate of infusion
conc 1 = steady-state level after infusion of dose 1
conc 2 = desired serum level
dose 2 = dose to achieve conc 2

Dosage adjustment is simply a ratio and proportion. The amount of change in serum concentration is the same amount of change that must be made in the infusion rate.

b. Intermittent infusion:

$$\text{dose} = \text{conc} \times V_d$$

where concentration is the desired change from the trough to the peak concentration

The magnitude of dose is determined by assuming that the patient is a bag of a given volume, and that you need to place only enough drug in the bag to reach the peak concentration. This concept works for loading doses where the trough is initially zero, and for maintenance doses where drug already exists in the body and the change in serum concentration from trough to peak is therefore less.

$$\text{interval} = \{[\ln(\text{peak}/\text{trough})]/K_e\} + t$$

where peak = desired peak
trough = desired trough
t = time required for infusion

The frequency of drug administration is determined by the time required for the drug to travel from the peak concentration to the trough. This parameter is related to the half-life, or elimination rate concentration. The longer or shorter the half-life, the longer or shorter, respectively, will be the time required to eliminate the drug.

c. Oral administration:

$$\text{dose} = \text{conc} \times K_d \times V_d \times \text{interval}/f$$

where conc = desired average concentration
f = fraction of dose absorbed

Oral dosing of drugs is similar to intermittent infusion. The only mathematical difference is the need to take into account the bioavailability of the drug. Because the absorption of drugs varies among doses, diseases, and patients, the concentration is an average concentration rather than peak or trough.

IV. PHARMACODYNAMICS

Pharmacodynamics describes the relationship between drug concentration at the site of the drug action and the pharmacologic response by the target tissue. Drug effect occurs due to an interaction between the drug and a three-dimensional physical receptor on the cell surface. A change in the structure of the cell surface occurs after the drug has bound to the receptor. This change may open channels in the cell membrane through which electrolytes, or other molecules, can pass, or it may activate intracellular enzymes that catalyze the desired physiologic response. For most drugs, the concentration at the receptor site determines the intensity of the pharmacologic outcome.

A. Altered Dynamic Responsiveness

This is a poorly understood phenomenon. Not all patients react in the same way to equivalent doses or serum concentrations of the same drug. Differences in **receptor structures, intracellular messengers,** and **feedback mechanisms** have been proposed to account for individual differences.

    1. Hypersensitivity is the exaggerated response to receptor stimulation in an otherwise normal situation. Reduced doses may be required if toxic effects of the drug are observed. Although sometimes confused with hypersensitivity of an allergic response, immunity has no known role in receptor hypersensitivity.

    2. Hyposensitivity is the reduced reactivity exhibited by the target organ after receptor stimulation. Although increased doses of drug may be beneficial, toxicity may occur if other organs retain their normal responsiveness to the presence of the drug. A change of agents or supplementation in drugs is usually necessary to overcome hyposensitivity.

    3. Tachyphylaxis/tolerance is the reduced response to receptor stimulation, or the decreased number of receptors that develop during drug administration. In general, larger doses of drug are necessary to maintain therapeutic response. Drugs may be exchanged once tachyphylaxis has occurred (i.e., morphine used after reduced fentanyl effect), or rest periods may be helpful (nitrate-free period when using topical nitroglycerin).

B. Pathophysiologic Influences

Pathophysiologic influences on the cell may change the efficiency of receptor stimulation, as well as the cellular response to receptor signals.

    1. Altered receptor binding is common with disease states. Because the three-dimensional proximity of membrane structures defines the receptor site, changes in membrane continuity and chemical composition can change the receptor. Cell membranes can be physically distorted by **mal-**

nourishment, edema, and **inflammation. Age** can also affect the chemical composition of the membrane, as dietary habits, as well as the fat and protein content of tissues, change with advancing years. The local chemical environment of the receptor may also play a role, as weak acids and bases may be either ionized or nonionized, depending on local pH. The degree of ionization of the drug will affect the amount and strength of chemical binding between the drug and receptor. Catecholamine dysfunction in acidic patients may reflect a lack of receptor affinity.

2. Down-regulation of receptors appears to be a feedback mechanism that occurs after exposure to a drug. Receptor stimulation is reduced by decreasing the **density of receptors** on the cell membrane, such as seen with adrenergic receptors in congestive heart failure or myocardial ischemia. In addition, mechanisms of **enhanced drug removal** may exist that free the receptor site of drug, similar to cholinesterase enzymes in the neuromuscular junction.

3. Antibodies to receptor sites can develop in select disease states. The antibody can either destroy the cell or the receptor site, or bind to the receptor site to block drug entry and stimulation. This may occur with diabetics who possess antibody to insulin receptors. The principle is exploited in transplantation as the monoclonal antibody OKT3 is used to block the antigen-recognition sites on T cells.

4. Altered responsiveness to receptor stimulation is common, as disease may disrupt the intracellular chemical messenger system that is activated by the receptor. Stimulation of a cell surface receptor by a drug begins a cascade of chemical events that results in the anticipated outcome. Intracellular chemicals such as electrolytes and cyclic adenosine monophosphate (cAMP) may be depleted or functionally blocked by other molecules competing for binding sites. The incidence of digoxin toxicity increases when intracellular potassium concentrations fall.

5. Failing physiologic reflexes may account for exaggerated or reduced pharmacologic effects, especially in the elderly. The inability of an organ system to detect or attenuate drug-induced changes could result in an overwhelming drug effect and patient harm. Antihypertensive medications may produce profound effects, as limited vascular responsiveness may not temper the pressure-lowering drug actions. Sedative effects of medication may be intensified by poor cerebral perfusion or disease-related neuronal dysfunction.

6. Discrepant enantiomeric processing is an active area of research that may further define pharmacologic treatments in the future. All chemicals exist as mirror images called enantiomers. Pharmaceutic production cannot easily separate the active component from the inactive mirror image. Different pharmacologic responses and side effects are commonly seen with the enantiomeric molecules. Disease states may influence the pharmacokinetics of the molecules differently, causing side effects to linger long after the desired effect has gone. Currently used assays cannot differentiate these molecules, further confusing the association of desired effects with serum drug levels. Propoxyphene is composed of dextropropoxyphene and levoproxyphene, which have independent outcomes. The dextro form is a pain reliever, while the mirror-image levo molecule is a cough suppressant.

C. Iatrogenic Interventions

Iatrogenic interventions can disrupt the normal role of the body in responding to and clearing the drug. Improved responses can be seen, as well as abnormal results.

1. Drug interactions are often misinterpreted as solely a chemical binding by two agents in physical contact, resulting in inactivation of the molecules. However, the most important interactions are those that affect the physiology of the patient by different mechanisms. Two drugs may have the same or opposite physiologic effect, or may compete for the same cell receptor binding site.

a. Additive interactions are those that give a resulting physiologic effect equal to the sum of the individual effects of each drug. Vasoactive drugs are often additive in their effects of changing blood pressure or cardiac output.

b. Synergism is a resulting effect that is greater than the sum of the individual effects of the drugs. Antibiotics are commonly prescribed in combinations that have different mechanisms of actions in order to increase antibacterial killing power.

c. Antagonism between drugs results in complete reversal or reduction of drug effect. Narcotic and benzodiazepine antagonists are commonly used to block drug effects. Partial agonist/antagonist drugs may exhibit strong affinity to a cell receptor, but result in a weak stimulation of the receptor.

2. Altered drug clearance is common in ICU patients. Physiologic changes induced through mechanical or pharmacologic means may improve or hinder the removal of a drug from the body. Drugs may suddenly lose their effectiveness or cause toxicity, depending on the situation.

a. Altered blood flow to organs can affect the amount of drug reaching the target tissue or reaching the organ of elimination. Vasopressor drugs used in alpha-adrenergic doses will shunt blood to and from select tissues, causing altered presentation of drug to these sites. Renal blood flow will be lowered, reducing the elimination of drugs and metabolites through the kidney. Inotropic agents can improve drug delivery to tissue, but will also increase renal and hepatic perfusion, causing increased clearance of the drug. The clearance of potent anesthetic gases may be reduced if perfusion

Table 6-4 Drugs that affect liver P450 enzyme function

Inducers of drug metabolism	Inhibitors of drug metabolism
Carbamazepine	Cimetidine
Chloral hydrate	Ciprofloxacin
Ethanol	Erythromycin
Phenobarbital	Ketoconazole
Phenylbutazone	Metoprolol
Phenytoin	Omeprazole
Rifampin	Propranolol

of the lungs is altered during surgery, and presumably through aerators used in cardiopulmonary bypass procedures.

    b. Damage to the organ of elimination is common in the critically ill patient. **Prolonged oxygen deprivation** to tissue, **direct cytotoxic agents,** and **physical damage** to an organ through invasive procedures can affect the ability of an organ to clear a drug.

    c. Changes in drug metabolism are commonly seen in patients that are caused by drug interactions (Table 6-4). Overproduction of metabolic enzymes, called **enzyme induction,** and decrease of enzyme function, or **enzyme inhibition,** are best described for the P450 enzyme system of the liver. Many drugs are metabolized by this pathway, including theophylline, benzodiazepines, and cyclosporine. Induction is caused by phenobarbital and rifampin, the hydrocarbons of cigarette smoke, and other chemicals. Conversely, erythromycin, cimetidine, and other agents can inhibit enzymes and cause drug accumulation.

    d. Artificial drug clearance through extracorporeal devices may increase the elimination of a drug, either through dialysis procedures or through plasmapheresis. Dialysis techniques will remove drug only from the serum that is free and unbound. Dialysis of a drug is ineffectual if the drug is a **large molecule** that cannot pass through pores in the dialysis membrane, or if the drug is highly **tissue bound.** Plasmapheresis conversely will remove drug that is bound to serum proteins, but the significance of this is poorly understood as most drugs in this category will be highly tissue bound as well.

V. SUMMARY

Critically ill patients are exposed to many pharmacologic agents. Due to the nature of critical care, the risk of using toxic drugs is more acceptable if a positive outcome can be reasonably expected. The monitoring of clinical outcome and of the toxicity of these drugs is essential because of the altered physiologic responses and increased susceptibility to side effects of this patient population.

SUGGESTED READINGS

Applied Pharmacokinetics: Principles of Therapeutic Drug Monitoring. Spokane, Applied Therapeutics, Inc., 1992.
Friedman H, Greenblatt D: Rational therapeutic drug monitoring. *JAMA* 256(16):2227, 1986.
Levy R, Bauer L: Basic pharmacokinetics. *Ther Drug Monit* 8(1):47, 1986.
Matzke G, St Peter W: Clinical pharmacokinetics 1990. *Clin Pharmacokin* 18(1):1, 1990.
McLean A, Moran D: Clinical pharmacokinetics in patients with liver disease. *Clin Pharmacokin* 21(1):42, 1991.
Welling P: Graphic methods in pharmacokinetics: the basics. *J Clin Pharmacol* 26:510, 1986.

CHAPTER 7

NONSTEROIDAL ANALGESIC AND ANTI-INFLAMMATORY AGENTS

Victor C. Lee
John C. Rowlingson
Robin J. Hamill

I. General Considerations
II. Overview of the Agents
   A. Classes of Agents
   B. Available NSAIDs
   C. Prostaglandins and Pain
   D. Central and Peripheral Analgesic Effects
III. Therapeutic Use of NSAID Agents
   A. Rationale for Use of NSAIDs
IV. Adverse Reactions and Other Concerns Regarding Clinical Therapy
   A. Gastric and Duodenal Ulcers
   B. Renal Toxicity
   C. NSAIDs and Platelet Function
   D. Other Clinical Concerns
V. Summary
Suggested Readings

I. GENERAL CONSIDERATIONS

A. Until recent times, nonsteroidal anti-inflammatory drugs (NSAIDs) were mostly regarded as mild analgesics for the treatment of minor to moderate **chronic pain** conditions in nonhospitalized patients. Typical indications for such use include: inflammatory and degenerative joint disease, myalgias, headache pain, dysmenorrhea, and minor trauma.

B. NSAIDs possess specific **advantages over narcotics,** including:

1. Ease of prescription and administration.
2. Low abuse potential.
3. Absence of controlled substance restrictions.
4. Multiple over-the-counter preparations.

C. Previously, their use in the treatment of acute pain was limited by:

1. A ceiling effect on analgesia.
2. The lack of parenteral forms of NSAIDs.
3. Potential gastrointestinal (GI), hepatic, hematologic, and renal side effects in patients who may already be critically ill.

D. The **rational use of NSAIDs** in **acute pain** conditions is on the rise, based on an improved understanding of pain mechanisms and pain therapy:

1. Pain often involves multiple mechanisms and neuroanatomic substrates.
2. Prostaglandin-mediated pain may be more specifically and efficaciously treated by NSAIDs than by opioid medication.
3. The use of a combination of therapeutic modalities, including NSAIDs as adjunctive medications, may be more effective than single-drug regimens such as morphine intramuscularly.
4. The use of NSAIDs as adjuncts can decrease narcotic dosage, minimizing opioid side effects (e.g., the ventilator-dependent patient may benefit by a reduction of a narcotic-induced respiratory depression).
5. The increased availability of nonoral dosage forms of NSAIDs (e.g., injectable) expands the options for therapeutic use in a variety of settings.

II. OVERVIEW OF THE AGENTS

A. Classes of Agents

1. Of the classes of agents (see Table 7-1) **acidic agents** comprise the bulk of NSAIDs, and are further categorized as carboxylic acids (e.g., **aspirin**), alkanoic acids (e.g., **indomethacin** [Indocin], **ibuprofen** [Motrin, Advil, etc.]), and enolic acids (e.g., **piroxicam** [Feldene]).
2. **Nonacidic agents** comprise a smaller group of compounds, including **acetaminophen** (Tylenol, etc.) and **nabumetone** (Relafen). **Acetaminophen,** while exerting relatively little peripheral anti-inflammatory effect is nonetheless very useful clinically due to its effect on central nervous system

Table 7-1 Nonsteroidal anti-inflammatory agents, by classes

Acidic agents			Nonacidic agents
Carboxylic acids	Alkanoic acids	Enolic acids	p-Aminophenols
Salicylates	*Propionic acids*	*Oxicams*	Acetaminophen
Aspirin	Ibuprofen	Piroxicam	Phenacetin*
Lysine acetyl	Naproxen	Tenoxicam	*Pyrazoles*
salicylate	Fenoprofen		Dipyrone
Choline magnesium	Indoprofen*		
trisalicylate	Suprofen*		*Naphthylalkanone*
Salsalate	Tiaprofenic acid		Nabumetone
Magnesium salicylate	Protizinic acid		
Lithium salicylate*	Pirprofen		
Imidazole salicylate	Flurbiprofen		
	Carprofen		
	Benoxaprofen*		
	Ketoprofen		
Difluorophenyl		*Pyrazolidinediones*	
derivative			
Diflunisal		Phenylbutazone	
		Oxyphenbutazone*	
		Azapropazone	
Fenamates	*Indoleacetic acids*		
Meclofenamate	Indomethacin		
Mefenamic acid	Sulindac		
Flufenamic acid			
Tolfenamic acid	*Aryl acetic acids*		
Pyranocarboxylic acid	Alclofenac*		
Etodolac	Diclofenac		
	Fenclofenac		
	Heteroaryl acetic acids		
	Tolmetin		
	Zomepirac*		
	Ketorolac		

*Drug withdrawn because of toxicity.

(CNS) prostaglandin activity, which gives this drug analgesic as well as antipyretic properties. It is often used in the patient who poorly tolerates the GI irritation caused by many of the acidic NSAIDs (discussed later). **Nabumetone** is a novel pro-drug which undergoes GI absorption and hepatic metabolism before being converted to an NSAID. It poses a reduced risk to the GI tract in its pro-drug form.

   3. Considerations in selecting a class of NSAIDs:

     a. Combinations of NSAIDs of different classes are sometimes employed clinically in the treatment of chronic conditions such as rheumatoid arthritis, although the advantages and disadvantages of this are not fully understood.

      b. Combinations of NSAIDs may increase the risks of organ toxicity, although the mechanisms and specific risks are unknown.
      c. Clinically, switching the class of NSAID used to treat a particular pain condition may result in improved efficacy. This is done empirically, since there is insufficient pharmacologic information concerning the underlying mechanisms of this phenomenon.

B. Available NSAIDs

Table 7-2 lists NSAIDs available in the United States. Oral forms predominate, but some NSAIDs are available in elixir, suppository, and injectable formulations.

Table 7-2 NSAIDs available in the United States—maximum daily doses and dosage forms

Agents		Maximum Adult dose (24 h)	t_{peak} (h)	$t_{1/2}$ (h)	Dosage interval (h)
Salicylates					
Aspirin	e,rs*	3.6–7.2 g	0.5–2	2–30	4
Choline salicylate (Arthropan)	e	4.8–7.2 g	0.5–2	2–30	4
Choline magnesium trisalicylate (Trilisate)	e	3 g	1–2	9–17	8–24
Sodium salicylate (Pabalate, etc.)	i	3.6–5.4 g	0.5–2	2–30	4
Salsalate (Disalcid)		3–4 g	2–4	16	6–12
Propionic acids					
Ibuprofen (Motrin, etc.)	e	3200 mg	1–2	2–3	6–8
Fenoprofen (Nalfon)		3200 mg	1–2	2–3	4–6
Ketoprofen (Orudis)		300 mg	1–2	2–4	6–8
Flurbiprofen (Ansaid)	o	300 mg	1–5	4–6	6–8
Naproxen (Naprosyn)	e	1500 mg	2–4	12–15	12
Naproxen sodium (Anaprox)		1375 mg	1–2	13	6–8
Fenamates					
Meclofenamate (Meclomen)		400 mg	0.5–1	2–3	6–8
Mefenamic acid (Ponstel)		1000 mg	2–4	2–4	6

Table 7-2 (*Continued*)

Agents		Maximum Adult dose (24 h)	t_{peak} (h)	$t_{1/2}$ (h)	Dosage interval (h)
Oxicams					
Piroxicam (Feldene)		20 mg	3–5	50	24
Acetic acids					
Indomethacin (Indocin)	rs,i	200 mg	1–3	2–5	4–12
Sulindac (Clinoril)		400 mg	2–4	8–18	12
Tolmetin (Tolectin)		2000 mg	0.5–1	1–5	6–8
Etodolac (Lodine)		1200 mg	1–2	7	6–12
Diclofenac (Voltaren)		200 mg	1–3	1–2	6
Ketorolac (Toradol)	i	60 mg (oral) 120–150 mg (IM)	0.5–1	4–9	6
Nonacidic agents					
Acetaminophen	e,rs	4 g	0.5–1	1–4	4
Nabumetone (Relafen)		1000 mg	3–6	24	12–24

*Alternative dose forms available in the United States; **rs** = rectal suppository, **e** = elixir, **o** = ophthalmic, **i** = injectable.

Table 7-3 shows the doses of injectable NSAIDs, two of which—**sodium salicylate** (Pabalate, etc.) and **ketorolac** (Toradol)—are marketed in this country.

C. Prostaglandins and Pain

1. NSAIDs block cyclooxygenase, modifying the inflammatory process by preventing the production of prostaglandins from arachidonic acid at the

Table 7-3 Adult dosage guidelines for injectable NSAIDs (daily dosages indicated, as intramuscular or intravenous injections). Sodium salicylate and ketorolac are marketed in the United States.

Agent	Dose (mg)	Dosage interval (h)	$t_{1/2}$	Maximum adult dose (mg/24 h)
Dipyrone	500–1000	6–12	2–5	2500
Sodium salicylate	500–1000	12–24	2–30	500–1000
Diclofenac	75–150	8–12	1–2	75–150
Ketorolac	15–60	6	4–9	75–150
Tenoxicam	20	24	60–75	20

site of tissue injury, thus eliminating the prostaglandin-induced hyperalgesia (i.e., pain hypersensitization) in peripheral tissues.

2. This is a distinctly different mechanism of analgesia from that of narcotics, which inhibit afferent nociceptive impulses at the dorsal horn of the spinal cord and at supraspinal sites by interacting with opioid receptors.

3. There may be alternate mechanisms of action of NSAIDs, such as inhibition of lipoxygenase activity and leukotriene production or membrane stabilization.

4. There appears to be a supraspinal analgesic effect of NSAIDs (discussed below) which is separate and distinct from their action in inflamed peripheral tissues.

5. The issue of inflammation, pain, and corticosteroids deserves mention.

    a. Oral corticosteroids given at doses that produce an anti-inflammatory effect seem to suggest a correlation of analgesia with a reduction in inflammation and swelling in the dental pain model.

    b. In the same model, NSAIDs produce analgesia which exceeds their anti-inflammatory effects. The analgesia achieved with these agents exceeds that produced by corticosteroids even though the anti-inflammatory effect of corticosteroids is greater.

    c. Hence the reduction of inflammation is *not* the most important factor in NSAID analgesia.

    d. **Corticosteroids** are only useful as analgesic agents if the specific disease can be modified by steroid activity (inhibition of cell-mediated immune processes, stabilization of lysosomal membranes, etc.), such as in the treatment of rheumatoid arthritis (typically treated with 5 to 10 mg doses of prednisone) and other connective tissue disorders, and reduction of tumor growth with steroid-sensitive tumors (doses of dexamethasone up to 100 mg have been used) in order to treat cancer pain. Corticosteroids otherwise have little part to play in the management of acute pain disorders.

Certain chronic pain disorders, such as postherpetic neuralgia, reflex sympathetic dystrophy, and lumbar disk disease, have been suggested indications for corticosteroid therapy, although utilization of such therapy is quite variable in clinical practice.

In a critical care setting, corticosteroids are used therapeutically for a variety of clinical entities, such as adrenocortical insufficiency; cerebral edema; spinal cord injury; a variety of respiratory conditions, ranging from bronchial asthma to postintubation stridor; and myasthenia gravis. The underlying therapeutic considerations, as well as the controversies, are beyond the scope of this discussion.

The clinician should be aware of the consequences of corticosteroid therapy, such as adrenal suppression, alterations in glucose and electrolyte metabolism, increased risks of GI hemorrhage, osteoporosis, skeletal muscle myopathy, affective and mental status changes, and changes in leukocyte and lymphocyte count.

D. Central and Peripheral Analgesic Effects

NSAIDs have both central and peripheral analgesic effects; hence, NSAID analgesia is not due solely to peripheral prostaglandin inhibition.

NSAID selection is based on therapeutic goals and the actual need for peripheral anti-inflammatory effect versus central analgesia; for example, **mefenamic acid** (Ponstel), **ketorolac** (Toradol), and **etodolac** (Lodine) are not indicated in the treatment of rheumatoid arthritis because of insufficient peripheral anti-inflammatory activity. On the other hand, however, they have significant central analgesic properties that are clearly useful in other situations. Similarly, acetaminophen is useful clinically as an analgesic and antipyretic, even though it possesses little peripheral anti-inflammatory activity.

III. THERAPEUTIC USE OF NSAID AGENTS

A. Rationale for Use of NSAIDs

1. If NSAIDs are to be utilized for their anti-inflammatory properties (e.g., therapy for rheumatoid arthritis), this may require many days of regular, repeated dosing of the NSAID in order to establish a prostaglandin-inhibiting effect at the relevant tissue site (e.g., synovial fluid).

2. NSAIDs are *not* prostaglandin antagonists; they inhibit prostaglandin synthesis and release. Thus in the setting of preexisting tissue trauma, the analgesic effect of the NSAID may not become apparent until previously released inflammatory mediators have ceased their activity.

3. Although the anti-inflammatory effect may take several days to achieve, the onset of analgesia of most NSAIDs ranges from 10 to 60 min. The injectable NSAIDs are the most rapid in the onset of their analgesic effect (10 min for ketorolac). Gastrointestinal absorption limits the onset of oral NSAID analgesia, but the data are really not sufficient to indicate which oral agents are any more rapid in onset than any others (generally 30–60 min). Nabumetone (Relafen) must first be metabolized by the liver to its active metabolite, but this metabolism is relatively rapid.

4. **Uses of NSAIDs in acute pain situations**

   a. There are obvious **advantages to the use of NSAIDs** as compared with narcotics: fewer respiratory, cardiovascular, and CNS effects; lack of abuse potential; no controlled substance interference with availability for clinical use.

   b. NSAIDs are often used for postoperative pain. But *pre*operative administration may be a more efficacious means of treating postoperative pain in certain situations because of inhibition of prostaglandin synthesis prior to the actual tissue trauma (preemptive analgesia).

c. There is evidence that smooth muscle spasm is a prostaglandin-mediated phenomenon, which may explain the efficacy of NSAIDs in treating dysmenorrhea (uterine smooth muscle spasm), renal colic (ureteral spasm), and biliary colic (sphincter of Oddi spasm).

IV. ADVERSE REACTIONS AND OTHER CONCERNS REGARDING CLINICAL THERAPY

Administration of prostaglandin-inhibiting agents in the surgical population and critically ill patients is *not* without concern of possible adverse effects, particularly in the presence of intercurrent illness and the patient's already-compromised physiology.

A. Gastric and Duodenal Ulcers

1. The risk of GI complication-related hospitalization in NSAID-users is approximately six times that of nonusers. The hospitalized patient receiving corticosteroids and NSAIDs concomitantly has a fifteen-fold risk of gastrointestinal complications compared to patients not receiving either drug.

2. In the hospitalized patient with intercurrent illness and a variety of physiologic stressors, there is a predisposition to ulcer formation with NSAID use—groups at particularly high risk include elderly patients, burn patients, patients with head injuries and/or massive trauma, and patients with a past history of peptic ulcer disease.

3. The mucosal injury from orally-administered NSAIDs is due to direct toxicity of the acidic drugs in contact with the gastric mucosa *as well as* the deleterious systemic effects of NSAIDs on mucosal prostaglandin production. Hence, non-oral forms (e.g., injectable ketorolac) are not risk free because their systemic prostaglandin-inhibiting effect may still jeopardize the gastric mucosa.

4. Duodenal ulcers may be the result of inhibition of intestinal prostaglandin production by enterohepatic recirculation of non-metabolized drug, with indomethacin and the oxicam drugs being theoretically more prone to this.

5. Protective strategies

    a. **Aspirin** is manufactured in a variety of buffered forms (e.g., Bufferin), may be enteric coated (e.g., Ecotrin), or compounded with antacids (e.g., Ascriptin), to reduce direct gastric irritation. A number of NSAIDs pass unabsorbed through the stomach (i.e., **ibuprofen** (Motrin, etc.), **diflunisal** (Dolobid), diclofenac (Voltaren) due to their lipophilicity, minimizing the risks of direct gastric irritation.

    b. **Sucralfate** (Carafate) can be administered for mucosal protection. It acts at existing mucosal lesions by forming a lesion-adherent proteinaceous complex which covers the eroded area. Its use in ulcer healing is more of an established indication than as a prophylactic agent against NSAID-induced ulcers. However, sucralfate is frequently used in critically ill patients at risk for gastritis and peptic ulcer disease. Unlike the H_2 blocking agents (see below) sucralfate does not alter gastric pH. This preserves the acidity of gastric fluid, reducing its potential as a growth medium for bacteria. This may possibly reduce the risk of nosocomial pulmonary infection related to gastric reflux and aspiration (whether occult or clinically apparent).

    c. Misoprostol (Cytotec) is a synthetic PE_1 analog which reverses the deleterious effects of prostaglandin inhibition on gastric mucosa while exerting antisecretory effects on gastric acid production as well. This agent is more effective in prophylaxis against NSAID gastropathy than is **sucralfate**.

    d. Cimetidine (Tagamet), **ranitidine** (Zantac), and **famotidine** (Pepcid) are antihistaminic H_2 blocking agents which inhibit gastric acid secretion, thereby lowering the potential for acid-induced mucosal injury. The prophylactic use of H_2 blocking agents appears to protect the small bowel mucosa more effectively than the gastric mucosa against NSAID-induced ulcers. These medications are frequently used in the critically ill population for GI prophylaxis. Of note, they can cause mental status changes and thrombocytopenia.

    e. Since GI morbidity appears to be related to doses and duration of therapy, there may be advantages to limiting doses and utilizing short courses of therapy (e.g., 48–72 h) in certain situations, such as in improving analgesia and lowering narcotic doses in conjunction with weaning from mechanical ventilation.

B. Renal Toxicity

    1. Prostaglandins produce vasodilation in the kidney and increased renal blood flow. Prostaglandin inhibition therefore decreases renal blood flow, glomerular filtration rate (GFR), and excretion of Na^+, K^+, and free water. NSAID-induced renal injury can include interstitial nephritis, glomerulonephritis, papillary necrosis, and acute tubular necrosis (ATN). **Salsalate** (Disalcid), **sulindac** (Clinoril), and **piroxicam** (Feldene) have been reported as lower-risk agents for renal toxicity, although they are not completely risk free.

    2. The use of NSAIDs in patients with atherosclerotic vascular disease, diabetes, lupus, or intercurrent renal insufficiency is cautioned due to the presence of preexisting renal dysfunction/damage (see Table 7-4). These patients have an increased risk of complications. Such patients may have lower drug clearance rates and therefore may well need less frequent and/or smaller doses of NSAIDs than patients with normal renal function.

    3. NSAIDs should not be used in patients receiving concomitant angio-

Table 7-4 Risk factors for nonsteroidal anti-inflammatory drug nephrotoxicity

1. Age more than 60 years, atherosclerotic cardiovascular disease, concurrent diuretic therapy
2. Renal insufficiency, serum creatinine > 2.0 mg/dL
3. States of renal hypoperfusion
   a. Sodium depletion
   b. Diuretic use
   c. Hypotension
   d. Sodium avid state, such as:
      i. Hepatic cirrhosis
      ii. Nephrotic syndrome
      iii. Congestive heart failure

Modified from Stillman and Schlesinger (see Suggested Readings) with permission.

tensin converting enzyme (ACE) inhibitor therapy, due to the adverse effects on renal blood flow and GFR produced by the combination of these drugs.

4. Renal hypoperfusion from other causes, such as hypovolemia, congestive heart failure, and hepatic cirrhosis with ascites, will put patients at risk for further deterioration of renal perfusion and possible renal injury by NSAIDs (see Table 7-4).

5. Patients at risk should have their renal function monitored if NSAIDs are administered. It may be desirable to lengthen the dosing interval and/or to reduce NSAID doses in patients with elevated serum creatinine levels. If creatinine levels increase suddenly (e.g., 0.5–1.0 mg/dL/24 h), these agents should be stopped. Creatinine clearance rates provide a more accurate assessment of renal function than do serum creatinine levels, but may not be a very cost-effective means of monitoring drug therapy in this particular situation.

C. NSAIDs and Platelet Function

1. NSAIDs interfere with normal platelet function primarily by inhibiting cyclooxygenase, whose activity is necessary for clotting.

2. The cyclooxygenase in platelets exposed to aspirin is permanently blocked (irreversibly acetylated). The antiplatelet effect of a dose of aspirin lasts 7 to 10 days with termination of the effect depending on platelet life span. Other NSAIDs competitively inhibit platelet cyclooxygenase, and their effect may last only 6 to 24 h. They are probably unlikely to have a *clinically significant* impact on surgical bleeding, and the prolongation of bleeding time has not been associated with increased blood loss at surgery.

3. Because the risk of nonsurgical postoperative bleeding complications, such as GI hemorrhage, may be increased in patients taking NSAIDs

at the time of their surgical admission, the issue of whether to continue or discontinue preoperative NSAID therapy is a controversial one.

4. Ketorolac reportedly increases bleeding time, but does not alter platelet count, prothrombin time (PT) or partial thromboplastin time (PTT). Although the increase in bleeding time is *statistically* significant, ketorolac does *not* cause a *clinically* significant increase in actual bleeding. Ketorolac apparently does not interact with heparin, but the situation with coumadin is less clear.

D. Other Clinical Concerns

1. As most NSAIDs produce a **mild elevation in blood pressure,** their use in patients with a history of high blood pressure or intercurrent hypertension should be carefully considered, particularly in the face of cardiac disease. NSAIDs antagonize a variety of antihypertensives, including thiazide and loop diuretics, alpha- and beta-adrenergic blockers, and ACE inhibitors, but do not affect central alpha-2-adrenergic agonists or calcium channel blocking drugs.

2. **Aspirin-induced asthma** probably is pathologically distinct from classic bronchial asthma. A number of salicylate and nonsalicylate NSAIDs may be cross-reactive with aspirin in inducing this syndrome. Contraindicated drugs include **indomethacin** (Indocin), **ibuprofen** (Motrin, etc.), **mefenamic acid** (Ponstel), **phenylbutazone** (Butazolidin), **salsalate** (Disalcid), **diflunisal** (Dolobid), and others. Safe NSAIDs appear to include **sodium salicylate** (Pabalate, etc.), **choline magnesium trisalicylate** (Trilisate), and **azapropazone.** Acetaminophen is well tolerated in such patients.

3. **Hepatitis** has been a reported complication of virtually every class of NSAID. The exact incidence is not known, but it is probably quite low. Aspirin-induced hepatitis is well recognized and usually occurs in conjunction with high doses (exceeding 50 mg/kg/day, or over 10 tablets a day for a 70-kg patient) and serum concentrations exceeding 200 to 250 μg/ml; hepatotoxicity occurs within four weeks of initiating therapy and is usually reversible.

4. The **antipyretic effects** of NSAIDs may blunt signs of postoperative infection.

5. Isolated cases of fulminant **necrotizing fasciitis** (e.g., Fournier's gangrene) have been reported in association with acute NSAID administration. The syndrome is seen in association with impaired functioning or production of granulocytes and/or lymphocytes, which results in a predisposition to group A beta-hemolytic streptococcal infections. This underscores our poor understanding of how NSAIDs may affect normal immune functioning. The incidence of such complications is unknown, but it is certainly quite rare.

6. Prostaglandin inhibition may interfere with normal tissue healing, granulation, and heterotopic bone formation.

V. SUMMARY

   A. NSAIDs are finding increasing application in the management of pain in the acute care setting, particularly as an important adjunctive medication in an analgesic regimen.
   B. The use of these agents is guided by an understanding of the role of prostaglandins in the production of pain and that certain clinical pain entities (inflammatory pain, renal colic, biliary colic, bone pain) are particularly responsive to NSAIDs.
   C. The analgesic effect of NSAIDs is separate from the anti-inflammatory effect. This analgesia may be a central, as opposed to a peripheral, effect, and it occurs within a much shorter time (minutes) than the clinical anti-inflammatory effect (days).
   D. The severity of clinical pain in many acute care situations would probably obviate the use of NSAIDs as sole analgesics. But when used as an adjunct to a primary analgesic agent such as an opioid, there is an important narcotic-sparing effect, which can lower the total narcotic dose. This effect of NSAIDs may offer a clear benefit to patients who are at increased risk of respiratory depression or sedation from narcotics, such as patients with morbid obesity, sleep apnea, or intrapulmonary shunt, all of whom are at significant risk of hypoxia even with mild to moderate sedation.
   E. The common and potentially lethal side effects of NSAIDs on the GI, renal, and hematologic systems *must* influence their clinical use, particularly in the critically ill patient. Although these side effects are not contraindications to the use of NSAIDs in the critically ill patient, surveillance should be carried out (e.g., checking nasogastric aspirates for blood, routine creatinine levels, etc.). Toxicity can be limited by modifying the dosage and the dosing interval and by limiting the duration of administration. For example, in the acute postoperative or posttraumatic phase, regularly scheduled NSAIDs for only 72 h can significantly decrease narcotic requirements.

SUGGESTED READINGS

Agrawal NM, Roth S, Graham DY, et al: Misoprostol compared with sucralfate in the prevention of nonsteroidal anti-inflammatory drug-induced gastric ulcer. A randomized, controlled trial. *Ann Intern Med* 115:195–200, 1991.

Buckley MM, Brogden RN: Ketorolac, a review of its pharmacodynamic and pharmacokinetic properties, and therapeutic potential. *Drugs* 39:86–109, 1990.

Conelly CS, Panush RS: Should nonsteroidal anti-inflammatory drugs be stopped before elective surgery? *Arch Intern Med* 151:1963–1966, 1991.

Dahl JB, Kehlet H: Non-steroidal anti-inflammatory drugs: rationale for use in severe postoperative pain. *Br J Anaesth* 66:703–712, 1991.

Fleming BM, Coombs D: Bleeding diathesis after perioperative ketorolac. *Anesth Analg* 73:232–239, 1991.

Houston MC: Nonsteroidal anti-inflammatory drugs and antihypertensives. *Am J Med* 90(suppl 5A):42S-47S, 1991.

McCormack K, Brune K: Dissociation between the antinociceptive and anti-inflammatory effects of the nonsteroidal anti-inflammatory drugs, a survey of their analgesic efficacy. *Drugs* 41:533-547, 1991.

Piper JM, Ray WA, Daugherty JR, Griffin MR: Corticosteroid use and peptic ulcer disease: role of nonsteroidal anti-inflammatory drugs. *Ann Intern Med* 114:735-740, 1991.

Raja SN, Meyer RA, Campbell JN: Peripheral mechanisms of somatic pain. *Anesthesiology* 68:571-590, 1988.

Sandler DP, Burr R, Weinberg CR: Nonsteroidal anti-inflammatory drugs and the risk for chronic renal disease. *Ann Intern Med* 115:165-172, 1991.

Stillman MT, Schlesinger PA: Nonsteroidal anti-inflammatory drug nephrotoxicity, should we be concerned? *Arch Intern Med* 150:268-269, 1990.

Troullos ES, Hargreaves KM, Butler DP, Dionne RA: Comparison of nonsteroidal anti-inflammatory drugs, ibuprofen and flurbiprofen, with methylprednisolone and placebo for acute pain, swelling, and trismus. *J Oral Maxillofac Surg* 48:945-952, 1990.

CHAPTER 8

OPIATE PHARMACOLOGY

Richard L. Noren

I. Structure
   A. Naturally Occurring Compounds
   B. Semisynthetic Compounds
   C. Synthetic Compounds
II. Mechanism of Action
   A. Endogenous Opiate Receptors
   B. Prohormones
   C. Enkephalins
   D. Dynorphine
   E. Relative Potency
   F. Location of Opiate Receptors
   G. Opioid Receptor Subtypes
   H. Peridural Narcotics
III. Clinically Useful Narcotics
   A. Morphine
   B. Meperidine
   C. Fentanyl
   D. Sufentanil
   E. Alfentanil
   F. Methadone
   G. Propoxyphene
   H. Hydromorphone
   I. Oxycodone
IV. Agonist–Antagonist Drugs
   A. Pentazocine
   B. Butorphanol

C. Buprenorphine
D. Nalbuphine
E. Dezocine
V. Opioid Antagonists
A. Naloxone
B. Naltrexone
VI. Cardiovascular Effects
VII. Respiratory Effects
VIII. Neurophysiologic Effects
IX. Gastrointestinal Effects
Suggested Readings

Opiates date back to the ancient Greeks, who used the term opium to describe the plant alkaloids derived from poppy plants. The word narcotic also has a Greek derivation meaning numbing. The modern use of these compounds began with the isolation of morphine in 1803. Morphine gained favor as an adjunct to chloroform and ether anesthesia in the late nineteenth century, but the failure at the time to appreciate the respiratory complications of narcotics later was recognized and had led to their disfavor by the early twentieth century. The reintroduction of narcotics is the result of the description and utilization of balanced anesthetic techniques since the 1930s.

Opiates are classified as synthetic, semisynthetic, or natural plant alkaloid compounds.

A. Naturally Occurring Compounds

The poppy plant produces two **naturally occurring classes of compounds,** the **phenanthrenes,** such as morphine and codeine, and the **benzylisoquinoline alkaloids** (papaverine, noscapine), which have no opioid activity. Morphine is the principal and most clinically useful naturally occurring opioid.

B. Semisynthetic Compounds

The **semisynthetic compounds** result from the simple chemical modification of morphine (Fig. 8-1). Codeine is the result of a methyl group substitution of the hydroxyl group of the third carbon. Reduction of a double bond on the benzene ring results in hydromorphone, and esterification at the two hydroxyl groups yields heroin. Thebaine, a natural plant alkaloid opiate, has no significant clinical properties, but is the chemical precursor to oxymorphone and oxycodone.

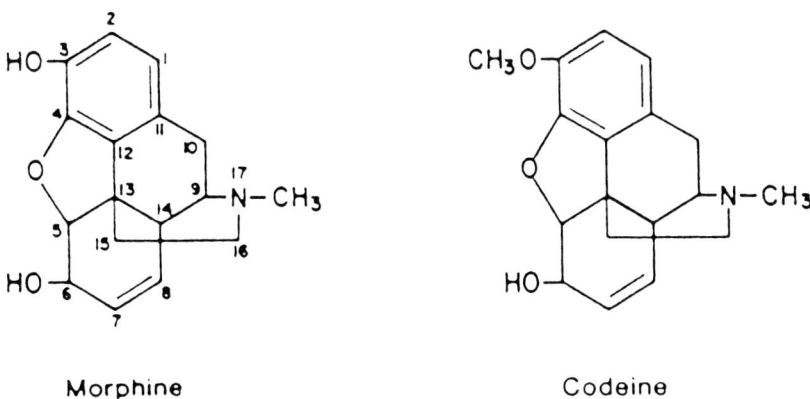

Figure 8-1 Substitution of a methyl group on the naturally occurring morphine molecule results in the semisynthetic compound codeine.

C. Synthetic Compounds

The **synthetic compounds** are structurally similar to morphine but represent completely manufactured compounds and are not chemical derivatives. The synthetic opiates are divided into four groups (Fig. 8-2).

1. Morphinan derivatives (levorphanol [Levo-Dromoran]).
2. Diphenyl derivatives (methadone [Dolophine], *d*-propoxyphene [Darvon]).

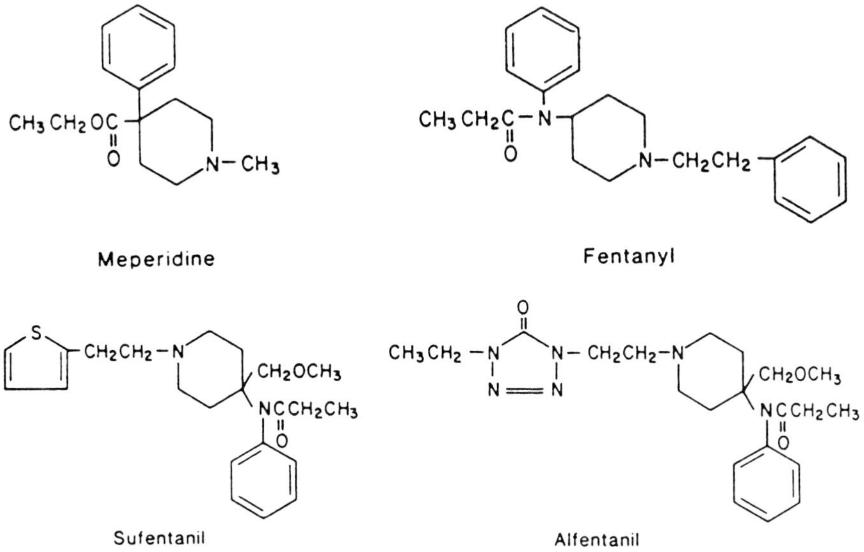

Figure 8-2 Phenylpiperidine derivatives.

3. Benzomorphan derivatives (pentazocine [Talwin]).
4. Phenylpiperidine derivatives (meperidine [Demerol], fentanyl [Sublimaze], alfentanil [Alfenta], sufentanil [Sufenta]).

II. MECHANISM OF ACTION

A. Endogenous Opiate Receptors

Despite the structural dissimilarities, all opiates appear to produce their pharmacodynamic effect by binding reversibly to an **endogenous opiate receptor** located in the central nervous system (CNS). The discovery of opiate receptors resulted in the search for endogenous peptides (**endorphins**) with opiate activity. The peptides are biosynthesized as large polypeptide molecules.

B. Prohormones

Proopiocortin is one example of a **prohormone** which is cleaved to adrenocorticotropic hormone (ACTH) and beta-lipotropin. The latter molecule requires further hydrolysis to produce beta-endorphin, a protein with endogenous opioid activity.

C. Enkephalins

The **enkephalins** are, as a group, pentapeptides which are derived from the precursor proenkephalin. The pentapeptide enkephalins leucine-enkephalin and methionine-enkephalin were the first endorphins described. They were found to contain a common four-amino-acid sequence, Tyr-Gly-Gly-Phe, which is present in all the endorphins despite the differences in their size and biosynthesis. The presence of this sequence in the peptides confers the opioid activity.

D. Dynorphine

Dynorphine, produced in the anterior pituitary like beta-endorphin, is derived from a third precursor, prodynorphin.

E. Relative Potency

The affinity of an opioid for the receptor correlates with its **relative potency.** Only the levorotary form of these stereospecific molecules, when ionized, will bind to the anionic opiate receptor by an opiate agonist or endogenous ligand. Receptor binding has been demonstrated to result in inhibition of adenylate cyclase activity, decreased transport of calcium ions, and inhibition of the release of neurotransmitters like substance P, norepinephrine, acetylcholine, and dopamine. Opioids may also depress sodium channel conductance, resulting in depressed membrane conductance. Serotonin receptors may function to modulate opioid analgesic effects.

F. Location of Opiate Receptors

These **opiate receptors** have been demonstrated in the cerebral cortex, hypothalamus, medial thalamus, amygdala, extrapyramidal regions, the spinal cord (substantia gelatinosa), and sympathetic preganglionic neurons. The receptors modulate afferent and efferent pain stimuli. Electrical stimulation at the midbrain (periaqueductal gray area) or microinjections of morphine result in an antinociceptive transmission down the neuraxis which inhibits the transmission of peripheral nociceptive stimuli to the spinal cord. This stimulation was demonstrated to be inhibited by narcotic antagonists. The substantia gelatinosa within the spinal cord is densely populated with opioid receptors and is the site of direct spinal analgesia.

G. Opioid Receptor Subtypes

Opioid receptors are widely distributed throughout both vertebrate and invertebrate species. In humans, the receptors have been identified and subtyped according to pharmacologic effect and their location (Table 8-1), as in the following.

   1. The **mu receptors** are primarily distributed in the brain and spinal cord. This morphine-binding receptor is associated with supraspinal analgesia. Subclassification of the mu receptors suggests that the mu-1 receptor mediates analgesia and the mu-2 receptor is associated with respiratory depression, bradycardia, euphoria, and dependence.

   2. The **delta receptor** has no selective agonist and modulates mu activity.

   3. Kappa receptors function at the spinal and supraspinal levels, where they have some direct analgesic function in addition to sedation.

   4. Sigma receptors are associated with dysphoria and psychotomimetic effects. They also produce excitatory phenomena, such as tachycardia, tachypnea, mydriasis, and hypertonia.

H. Peridural Narcotics

   1. The presence and identification of **spinal opiate receptors** have led to the application of intrathecal and epidural narcotics. It is presumed that epidurally placed narcotics readily diffuse into the cerebrospinal fluid and bind to opiate receptors within the spinal cord.

Table 8-1 Opioid receptors

Receptor subtype	Effect	Agonist
Mu-1	Supraspinal analgesia; includes periaqueductal nucleus raphe magnus, and locus coeruleus	Beta endorphin
	Prolactin release	Morphine
	Catalepsy	
Mu-2	Respiratory depression	Meperidine
	Cardiovascular effects	Fentanyl
	Decreased GI motility	Sufentanil
	Euphoria	Alfentanil
	Physical dependence	
Delta	Spinal analgesia	Enkephalins
	Modulate mu receptor	
Kappa	Spinal analgesia	Dynorphin
	Sedation	Pentazocine
	Miosis	Butorphanol
	Inhibition of antidiuretic hormone release	Nalorphine
	Respiratory depression	
Sigma	Dysphoria	
	Mydriasis	
	Tachycardia	
	Tachypnea	

2. The analgesia produced is extremely effective for postoperative pain, but will not produce surgical anesthesia. The principal advantages of intraspinal narcotics over parenteral opioids are the complete pain relief achieved with less sedation and improved pulmonary and gastrointestinal (GI) function.

3. The use of intraspinal narcotics is not associated with sympathetic nervous system blockade, and will not produce skeletal motor weakness as seen with local anesthetics. Intraspinal narcotics are associated with variable incidences of pruritus, nausea, respiratory depression, urinary retention, and sedation.

III. CLINICALLY USEFUL NARCOTICS

Narcotics are classified as pure agonists, agonist–antagonists, and antagonists (Table 8-2). Morphine is the **pure opioid agonist** against which all other narcotics are measured. **Agonist–antagonist** drugs such as nalbuphine (Nubain) bind as an agonist at the kappa receptor and as an antagonist at the mu receptors. The agonist–antagonists are not frequently used for surgical anesthesia because their antagonist properties make them less effective.

Table 8-2 Classification of opioid agonists and antagonists

Opioid agonists	Opioid agonist–antagonists	Opioid antagonists
Morphine	Pentazocine (Talwin)	Naloxone (Narcan)
Meperidine (Demerol)	Nalorphine (Nalline)	Naltrexone (Trexan)
Fentanyl (Sublimaze)	Butorphanol (Stadol)	
Sufentanil (Sufenta)	Nalbuphine (Nubain)	
Alfentanil (Alfenta)	Buprenorphine (Buprenex)*	
Codeine	Dezocine (Dalgan)	
Dextromethorphan		
Hydromorphone (Dilaudid)		
Oxymorphone (Numorphan)		
Methadone (Dolophine)		
Heroin		

*Partial agonist.

These drugs may antagonize the analgesia produced by the pure opioid agonists. They offer the distinct advantage of producing analgesia with a limited degree of sedation and respiratory depression. There appears to be a plateau or ceiling effect for these narcotics, after which increasing the dosage does not produce further analgesia. This plateau effect is also present for respiratory depression and sedation. The **opiate antagonists** naloxone (Narcan) and naltrexone (Trexan) are mu, kappa, delta, and sigma receptor antagonists which competitively displace opiate agonists from the receptors.

A. Morphine

1. The intravenous (IV) injection of morphine sulfate (10 mg/70 kg) will produce a plasma concentration in the range of 200 to 700 ng/mL. This concentration will decline rapidly due to the short redistribution half-life. Plasma half-life is 2 to 4 h. The plasma concentration necessary for adequate postoperative analgesia will be achieved or exceeded for only 1 to 3 h. Plasma concentrations following the intravenous (IV) administration do not correlate with the clinical effect. The maximum effect is achieved approximately 20 min following IV injection. The poor lipid solubility, protein binding, and ionization (90 percent) of morphine result in the drug's delayed penetration of the blood–brain barrier and explain this discrepancy. At the time of peak plasma concentration, less than 0.1 percent of the dose has crossed the blood–brain barrier. Morphine is a poorly lipid soluble narcotic and the body distribution is more to muscle than to fat, unlike the phenylpiperidines (meperidine, fentanyl, sufentanil, alfentanil). Morphine is less protein bound than the other opioid agonists. Normally, only 35 percent of the plasma fraction is protein bound, and this may decrease to 20 percent in patients with severe renal or hepatic dysfunction. Albumin is the principal protein. Pathology which alters the normal serum albumin ratios may result in exaggerated responses to the drug.

2. Following **intramuscular (IM) injection, morphine** is rapidly absorbed, with peak plasma concentrations reached in 5 to 45 min. The rate of absorption has been found to be variable; for example, absorption is faster following injection in the deltoid than in the gluteal muscles. After IM injection, 100 percent bioavailability occurs; however, elimination and redistribution will result in maximum plasma concentration of less than 60 ng/mL. The **minimum effective analgesic concentration** of morphine is reported to vary from **6 to 33 ng/mL.** This may explain why single IM doses of morphine sulfate may fail to provide adequate analgesia in some patients with acute pain.

3. The bioavailability of **oral morphine** (20 to 30 percent) is significantly less than with parenteral routes. The short half-life of 4 h requires a frequent dosing interval for effective analgesia. The need to increase the dosing interval has resulted in the creation of sustained-release oral preparations that prolong absorption by limiting the release of the drug from a matrix tablet. These preparations have not increased the bioavailability of the morphine. Peak serum levels after taking the sustained-release preparations of morphine may require as long as 2.5 h to reach as compared with 1 h for morphine sulfate solution. The bioavailability of the sustained-release morphine may be less than for an equivalent dose of morphine solution. The pharmacologic complexities of oral morphine have made it difficult to use any of the preparations for the treatment of postoperative pain. Sustained-release preparations play a significant role in the relief of chronic and malignancy-related pain.

4. Morphine metabolism

   a. Morphine is **biotransformed** into several metabolites. The principal mechanism for metabolism is conjugation with glucuronic acid, which occurs primarily in the liver. The hepatic extraction ratio of morphine is greater than the measured hepatic blood flow. The predominant metabolite is **morphine-3-glucuronide,** which is detectable within 1 min following an IV dose and is present in plasma at concentrations 10 to 20 times that of morphine by 90 min. This metabolite is believed to be inactive secondary to its polarity, which limits the ability to cross the blood–brain barrier. The formation of 3-glucuronide is inhibited by monoamine oxidase inhibitors. Clinically, an exaggerated opiate effect may be seen in some patients on this class of medications who receive morphine.

   b. **Morphine-6-glucuronide** is the second most abundant metabolite. It is found at plasma concentrations similar to that of morphine. Unlike the 3-glucuronide metabolite, **morphine-6-glucuronide is a more potent analgesic than is morphine.** Its increased polarity as compared with morphine results in a decreased ability to cross the blood–brain barrier.

c. The **extrahepatic sites** of morphine metabolism—kidneys, brain, and GI mucosa—have clinical significance. Cirrhotic patients with impaired hepatic clearance of opioid analgesics can have normal clearance of morphine because of these alternative metabolic sites.

d. **Prolonged depression of ventilation** has been noted following the use of morphine sulfate. The relationship of renal function and morphine clearance has been the subject of controversy over the last few years. Morphine clearance is not necessarily decreased in patients with renal dysfunction despite higher plasma concentrations. The **accumulation of morphine-6-glucuronide in patients with renal dysfunction** due to the decreased clearance of this metabolite is the primary cause for the exaggerated respiratory depression and sedation that may be seen.

B. Meperidine (Demerol)

1. Meperidine, 50 to 100 mg IV or IM, produces a variable degree of analgesia. The plasma concentration is described by a biexponential equation. The initial $t_{1/2}$ alpha decay is less than 15 min, with peak serum concentrations reached 10 to 90 min following injection. The $t_{1/2}$ beta elimination is approximately 3 to 4 h. Meperidine is more highly ionized than morphine, but it has a greater lipid solubility. It is highly bound to plasma proteins (70 percent) and primarily to alpha-1 glycoprotein.

2. Generally, a **plasma level of 0.5 to 0.8 μg/mL** is required for **adequate analgesia**. The peak concentration following 100 mg IM meperidine may result in plasma concentrations of 0.2 to 0.8 μg/mL. Thus this dose often results in only brief periods of adequate analgesia. The duration of analgesia may be less than 1 h and depends on the individual's plasma concentration versus the minimal effective analgesic concentration (MEAC) for that individual. Large fluctuations in plasma concentrations result in difficulty titrating meperidine to maintain a steady state. The fluctuations may be overcome by a continuous infusion or by patient-controlled analgesia (PCA) with a frequent dosing interval.

3. **Oral** administration has a **bioavailability of 40 percent**. The plasma concentration achieved by a 100 mg oral dose is subtherapeutic and produces inadequate analgesia. Meperidine's high first-pass hepatic extraction, slow rate of GI absorption, and limited bioavailability result in a plasma concentration of less than 0.2 μg/mL.

4. Meperidine is **primarily metabolized by the liver** and has a high hepatic extraction ratio. Biotransformation therefore is dependent on hepatic blood flow. Approximately 90 percent of the drug undergoes demethylation to normeperidine and hydrolysis to meperidinic acid. Normeperidine is then hydrolyzed to normeperidinic acid. The acidic metabolites are then conjugated and excreted by the kidneys. Renal clearance of

meperidine is normally minimal, with less than 10 percent of a dose excreted unchanged in the urine. Urinary excretion is pH dependent such that with acidification of the urine, 20 to 25 percent of the opioid may be excreted unchanged. In patients with renal impairment, the clearance and half-life may be prolonged, and so smaller than expected doses may be needed.

5. The metabolite **normeperidine** has a renal clearance less than the glomerular filtration rate. The elimination half-life of normeperidine is 15 to 40 h, and the substance can be detected 3 days following the administration of a single dose of meperidine. Patients with **renal disease** are particularly prone to the accumulation of normeperidine, so attention must be given to the size and frequency of the dose. Normeperidine has a direct stimulating effect on the central nervous system (CNS), unlike any other opioid, and at toxic levels may manifest as myoclonus and seizures. The serum level of normeperidine associated with the **CNS irritability syndrome** is variable.

6. The **elderly and the young are more sensitive** to the narcotic effects of meperidine. The decreased plasma protein binding of meperidine in the elderly may result in increased serum concentrations and an apparent exaggerated sensitivity to this narcotic. The **high plasma protein binding of meperidine (60 percent),** principally alpha-1 glycoprotein, will result in an altered narcotic response when any physiologic condition modifies these serum protein levels.

C. Fentanyl (Sublimaze)

1. Fentanyl is a phenylpeperidine synthetic opioid agonist with a potency approximately 100 times that of morphine. Intraoperatively, this drug has great utility because of its pharmacokinetic profile. The **high lipid solubility,** and the ability to cross the blood–brain barrier quickly, accounts for its rapid rate of onset following IV injection (30 s). Following single-dose administration, drug redistribution to inactive tissue sites occurs within 2 min, primarily to fat and skeletal muscle. The CNS levels of fentanyl parallel the plasma level of the drug. Consistent with its high lipid solubility, the volume of distribution is large and the rate of clearance is high. Multiple IV doses or continuous infusion of fentanyl results in gradual accumulation of the drug at inactive tissue sites. Fluctuations in serum concentrations and a prolonged drug effect may result as the drug returns to the plasma from these inactive tissue sites.

2. Fentanyl **metabolism in the liver** is the result of dealkylation and hydroxylation. The inactive metabolites are excreted in the bile and urine. Less than 8 percent of the drug is recovered in the urine as unchanged drug. Hepatic clearance of fentanyl approaches hepatic blood flow and has an extraction ratio close to one. This limits the role of enterohepatic recirculation in secondary plasma peaks. Metabolites are detectable within 2 min following an IV bolus injection.

3. Fentanyl is **80 percent bound to plasma proteins.** The drug is more than 90 percent ionized because of its high pKa (8.4). Clinically, fentanyl appears to have a shorter duration than morphine, and yet the plasma elimination half-life is actually 3 to 4 h. The prolonged elimination time reflects the drug's large volume of distribution (Vd). The large Vd also can account for the variable peak plasma levels and clinical effects in various pharmacokinetic studies.

4. Fentanyl has a **prolonged half-life in elderly patients.** This is due to **decreased clearance** because the drug's Vd does not change with age. Rather, a reduction in hepatic blood flow and decreased plasma protein concentration may account for the age-related changes. Cirrhosis does not prolong the elimination half-life of fentanyl.

5. **Transdermal fentanyl** delivery is an effective, noninvasive route of administration of this narcotic. Blood concentrations can reach the same peaks as with IV administration via the transdermal route. The difficulty with such delivery is the prolonged time between the application of the patch and the achievement of adequate serum levels that produce analgesia. The high lipid solubility results in a subcutaneous reservoir of fentanyl. This deposit is absorbed rapidly into the systemic circulation.

6. The bioavailability of **oral fentanyl** is low because of the drug's high hepatic clearance. Fentanyl has good absorption through the **buccal** mucosa. The fentanyl "lollipop" is a useful premedication technique and route of drug administration in the pediatric population.

D. Sufentanil (Sufenta)

1. Sufentanil is 5 to 10 times as potent as fentanyl. It is twice as **lipid soluble** as fentanyl and has a pKa similar to that of morphine. Eighty percent of the drug is ionized at physiologic pH. The drug is **93 percent protein bound,** with a large fraction bound to alpha-1 glycoprotein. This high degree of protein binding reduces the apparent Vd as compared with fentanyl. Patients with decreased levels of serum proteins, such as the elderly, infants, and those with pathologic conditions which result in decreased serum proteins, may have an exaggerated response to sufentanil. An IV bolus injection of sufentanil results in a rapid effect. Sufentanil's high tissue affinity and lipophilicity result in rapid penetration of the blood–brain barrier and quick onset of opioid effect. Redistribution occurs within 17 min, with 98 percent of the drug out of the plasma by 30 min.

2. **Metabolism** in the liver by N-dealkylation and O-demethylation produces pharmacologically inactive metabolites that depend on the kidneys for elimination. There is extensive reabsorption of sufentanil by the renal tubules, resulting in less than 1 percent of an IV dose being detectable in the urine. A hepatic extraction ratio of 0.8 predicts that any changes in hepatic blood flow should significantly alter elimination. The half-life is

approximately 164 min. The increased protein-bound fraction, smaller Vd, and greater opioid receptor affinity account for the shorter half-life and duration of clinical effect as compared with fentanyl.

E. Alfentanil (Alfenta)

1. Compared with fentanyl, alfentanil has a more rapid onset of action (1 to 2 min) and a shorter duration of effect secondary to drug redistribution (Table 8-3). The **rapid onset** is due to its relatively low pKa of 6.5. Although it is less **lipid soluble** than fentanyl, it readily penetrates the blood–brain barrier due to the low degree of ionization. Ninety percent of the drug is unionized at physiologic pH. The rapid redistribution and hepatic metabolism limit the drug's duration of action. The drug is **90 percent protein bound,** primarily to alpha-1 glycoprotein. The high degree of protein binding and decreased lipid solubility result in a volume of distribution that is one-fourth of that for fentanyl.

2. There is little detectable alfentanil (1 percent) in the urine; this is due to protein binding and renal tubular reabsorption. The drug is metabolized by N-dealkylation to noralfentanil. The metabolites have little opioid activity. The elimination half-life of alfentanil is 70 to 90 min. The apparent Vd is increased in patients with **renal failure,** but the decreased protein binding results in no significant alteration of the clearance or elimination half-life. **Cirrhotic patients** have been shown to have a clearance rate approximately half that of normal controls. Children have a shorter elimination time as compared with adults due to a decreased Vd.

3. The rapid onset and short duration have made alfentanil a useful narcotic for producing rapid anesthesia, and it has been used successfully via IV infusion without causing prolonged or cumulative opioid effects. The short elimination time and small Vd make alfentanil an ideal drug for **continuous IV infusions.**

Table 8-3 Characteristics of commonly used opioids

	% Protein bound	Half-life, h	Equivalent dose to 10 mg IM MSO_4	Onset IV, min
Alfentanil	90	1–1.5	0.3	Rapid
Fentanyl	80	3–4	0.1	Rapid
Sufentanil	93	2.5	0.01	Rapid
Morphine	20–35	2–4	10	10–30
Meperidine	70	3–4	120	1

F. Methadone (Dolophine)

   1. Methadone is a synthetic opioid that is different from most other narcotics. Methadone has a **high oral bioavailability,** approximately 80 percent, and an elimination half-life of 30 to 40 h. Plasma and tissue proteins bind a large fraction of any methadone dose. The drug is **less lipid soluble** than the phenylpiperidines, but redistributes into muscle and fat. The clearance rate for this narcotic is much slower than for the other opioids. The inactive metabolites from the **hepatic metabolism** of methadone are excreted in the bile and urine. Drugs and pathologic states that alter hepatic metabolic functions, such as chemotherapeutic agents and anticonvulsants, will influence the clearance and half-life of methadone.
   2. The **high oral bioavailability** and **prolonged duration** of analgesia make methadone a good choice for patients with chronic intractable pain. These properties have also resulted in methadone's becoming the drug of choice for the suppression of narcotic withdrawal symptoms.
   3. In comparison with morphine, methadone has a similar **side-effects profile.** The incidence of ventilatory depression, miosis, decreased GI motility, and biliary tract spasm at equal analgesic concentrations is equivalent.
   4. Twenty milligrams of methadone following induction of anesthesia will provide postoperative analgesia for at least 24 h.

G. Propoxyphene (Darvon, Wygesic)

   1. Originally prescribed as a nonnarcotic analgesic, propoxyphene is structurally related to methadone (Fig. 8-3). During the 1970s, this drug was prescribed as a nonnarcotic until it was appreciated that tolerance and physical dependence accompanied chronic usage.
   2. The IV administration of propoxyphene results in extensive distribution of the drug because the **Vd is large. Hepatic metabolism** is by N-dealkylation and yields the clinically **active metabolite** norpropoxyphene. The clearance of norpropoxyphene is slower than that of propoxyphene. The half-life of propoxyphene is long, 8 to 24 h, and for norpropoxyphene, the half-life averages 25 h.
   3. The drug is **absorbed completely** after oral administration. Extensive **first-pass hepatic metabolism** results in a bioavailability of only 40 percent. The analgesic efficacy of this narcotic is minimal, with an analgesic potency equivalent to 600 mg of aspirin.
   4. The most common **side effects** following oral administration are nausea, vomiting, vertigo, and sedation. It produces one-third the respiratory depression that codeine does. There is an increased risk of **toxicity** in patients with hepatic disease, who may develop serum concentrations twice those of healthy controls following an oral dose. Seizures and respiratory

depression may occur with high serum concentrations. Propoxyphene and its metabolite norpropoxyphene will accumulate in patients with renal insufficiency. Hemodialysis will not remove either opioid due to the drug's protein binding and large Vd. Clinically, this drug is equivalent to codeine, and may be useful as an analgesic for mild pain that is not responsive to aspirin alone.

H. Hydromorphone (Dilaudid)

Hydromorphone is a derivative of morphine. It has a potency ratio of about 8 to 1 and is more lipophilic than morphine. This narcotic is only 8 percent protein bound and has an oral bioavailability of 50 percent. It has a shorter duration and more sedation but less euphoria than morphine. See Chapter 13 for additional information.

I. Oxycodone (Percocet, Percodan, Tylox)

Oxycodone is available as an oral analgesic in three formulations. Percodan contains oxycodone 5 mg and aspirin 325 mg. Percocet is 5 mg oxycodone and 325 mg acetaminophen, and Tylox has 5 mg oxycodone with 500 mg acetaminophen. Like hydromorphone, this opiate has an oral bioavailability of 50 percent. The half-life is 4 to 5 h.

IV. AGONIST–ANTAGONIST DRUGS

As a group, these drugs are less potent than the pure opiate agonists and lack their efficacy (Fig. 8-4). These drugs have a side-effects profile similar to that of the opiate agonists, but will produce only **limited respiratory depression**. A **maximum or "ceiling" effect of analgesia** is produced, which limits their use for severe pain.

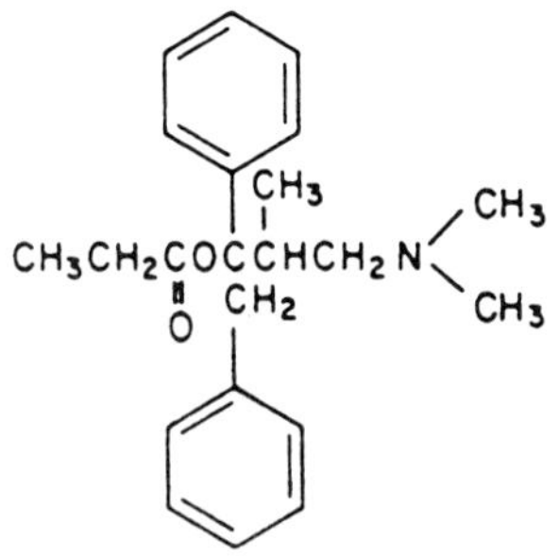

Propoxyphene

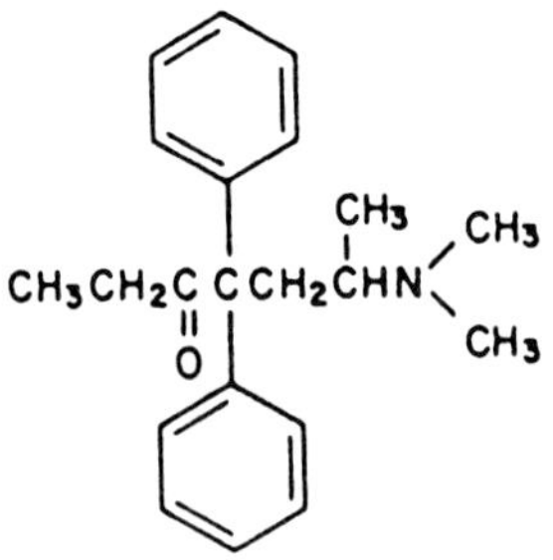

Methadone

Figure 8-3

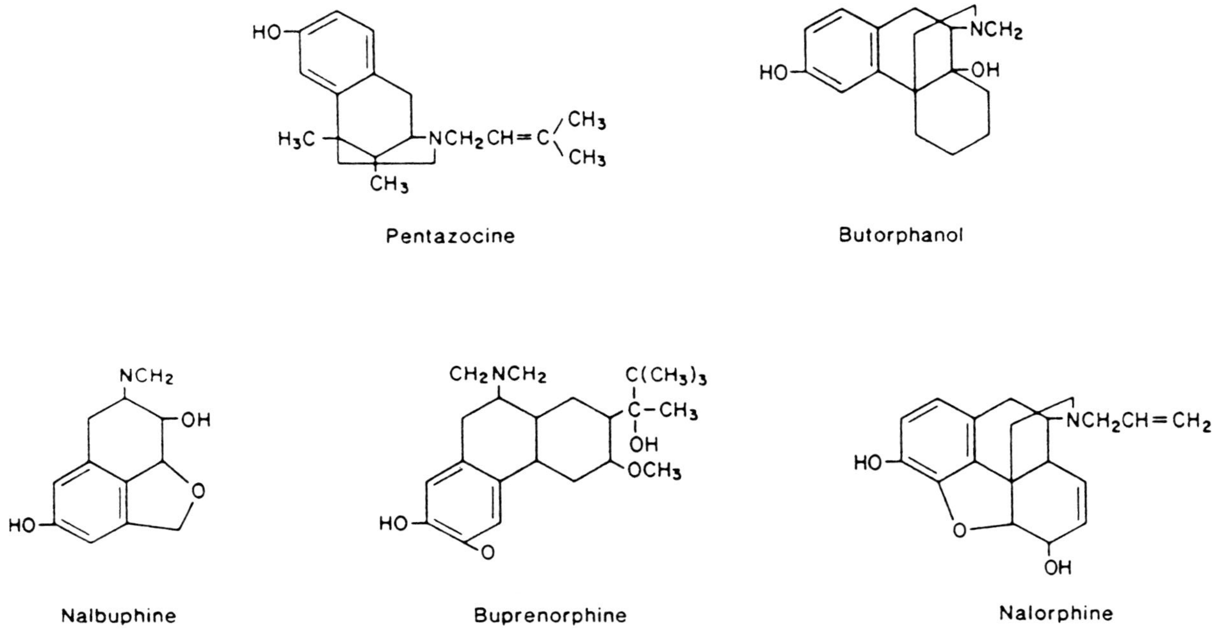

Figure 8-4 Structure of narcotic agonist–antagonist drugs.

A. Pentazocine (Talwin)

1. Pentazocine hydrochloride gained popularity in the 1960s, at a time when there was a strong impetus to develop potent analgesics that lacked any addiction potential. This opioid has agonist properties and some antagonism of opiate effects at different receptors.

2. Abrupt discontinuation following chronic use will result in a **withdrawal syndrome.** The opioid antagonist properties are weak; however, administration of pentazocine to individuals with physical dependence on opioids will precipitate withdrawal symptoms.

3. The drug is frequently prescribed IM or orally. A 50 mg oral dose has an analgesic equivalence equal to 60 mg of codeine. The IM injection of 30 mg produces analgesia and respiratory depression equivalent to 10 mg of morphine sulfate. The bioavailability is low following oral administration (18 percent), due to the drug's high clearance and **first-pass metabolism in the liver.**

4. Pentazocine is metabolized by oxidation into inactive glucuronide conjugates, which are then excreted by the kidneys. The clearance half-time is only 3 to 4 h. The drug's **high lipid solubility** results in minimal amounts of the drug being excreted unchanged in the urine.

5. Despite the label as an agonist–antagonist, when pentazocine is given in analgesic doses equivalent to morphine, an equivalent degree of **respiratory depression** can be expected.

6. Other common **side effects** following administration of pentazocine include sedation and dizziness. Dysphoric reactions have been reported, especially with high doses. There is an **analgesic ceiling effect** above 30 mg.

7. The dose must be decreased by one-third in patients with **hepatic dysfunction.** An oral dose in these patients will result in a serum concentration 300 percent greater than normal due to decreased first-pass hepatic metabolism.

B. Butorphanol (Stadol)

1. Butorphanol is classified as an agonist–antagonist. This drug has **weak antagonist** properties at the mu receptor, and acts primarily as an agonist by producing analgesia at the kappa receptor. The analgesic potency is five times that of morphine.

2. Given IM, 2 mg of butorphanol will produce respiratory depression equivalent to 10 mg of IM morphine. The dose–response curve for **respiratory depression,** however, will plateau, unlike that for the pure opiate agonists (larger doses do not produce increasing ventilatory depressant effects). The **plateau or "ceiling effect"** occurs at doses twice the analgesic dose.

3. The drug is only available in parenteral form. Peak analgesic effect occurs 1 h following an IM injection. The **clearance** half-life is 2 to 3 h. Its

metabolite, hydroxybutorphanol, is inactive, and is excreted primarily in the bile.

   4. Butorphanol's **side effects** include drowsiness, nausea, and diaphoresis. Compared with pentazocine, this drug has a lower incidence of dysphoria and causes fewer cardiovascular changes. Analgesic doses in healthy patients may produce significant increases in cardiac output, pulmonary artery pressure, and left ventricular end diastolic pressures. Increases in biliary pressure and acute biliary spasm are less frequent than with the pure opiate agonists.

   5. The **abuse potential** is less than that associated with the pure agonists; however, withdrawal can occur following abrupt discontinuation after chronic utilization.

   6. The **antagonist properties** may partially reverse the respiratory depression associated with the concurrent use of a pure mu receptor agonist, but not interfere with the agonist's analgesic effect.

C. Buprenorphine (Buprenex)

   1. Buprenorphine is classified as either an **agonist–antagonist or a partial agonist.** The drug is an opiate alkaloid thebaine derivative. It is 33 times as potent as morphine as an analgesic. Given IM, 0.3 mg is equivalent to 10 mg of morphine. This drug is a partial mu receptor agonist, and also binds the delta and kappa receptors. The onset of analgesic effect requires about 30 min following IM injection, and the peak effect may not occur for 3 h. Buprenorphine is lipophilic like fentanyl, but is slow to associate and disassociate from the opiate receptor. Thus the drug has a slow onset of action and plasma levels will not correlate with clinical effect. The analgesic duration is frequently greater than 10 h.

   2. **Metabolism** occurs in the liver and the by-products are excreted in the urine. Two-thirds of the drug is excreted in the bile unchanged. The drug has a high clearance, and after oral administration, would have limited bioavailability. Sublingual administration of buprenorphine has been used successfully to circumvent the first-pass hepatic metabolism.

   3. Nausea and vomiting are the predominant **side effects.** The incidence of euphoria is less than with morphine. Respiratory depression will occur up to a plateau, and increasing doses may improve ventilation due to the narcotic antagonist properties. The **duration of respiratory depression can be prolonged due** to the strong receptor affinity of buprenorphine, and there may be little effect from the opioid antagonists such as naloxone. This resistance is seen with the use of nalbuphine and butorphanol, and the reversal of buprenorphine's effects may require doses of naloxone or doxepram that are much greater than those traditionally used. The hemodynamic effects of buprenorphine are similar to those of morphine. **Withdrawal** can be precipitated in patients with a history of chronic opioid use. Physical

dependence on buprenorphine occurs, and abstinence results in a mild withdrawal syndrome that may take 5 to 10 days to develop.

D. Nalbuphine (Nubain)

1. Nalbuphine is an opioid **agonist–antagonist** that is structurally related to oxymorphone and naloxone. At doses greater than 30 mg, nalbuphine has a **ceiling effect for analgesia and respiratory depression.** Its antagonist properties are about 25 percent as potent as those of nalorphine. The drug acts as an antagonist at the mu receptor and as an agonist at the kappa and delta receptors. Respiratory depression and analgesia are due to kappa-receptor effects. Nalbuphine has an onset of action in less than 10 min and a clinical effect lasting 3 to 6 h.

2. The drug is **metabolized** in the liver and has an elimination half-life equal to its clinical effect.

3. The most common **side effect** is sedation, present in about 33 percent of patients. Unlike other agonist–antagonists, there is a much lower incidence of dysphoria and no significant hemodynamic changes. The drug produces no increase in systolic blood pressure, pulmonary artery pressure, atrial filling pressures, or heart rate. This has led to its use in patients for cardiac catheterization and as a premedication for cardiac surgery. At doses of 0.1 mg/kg, nalbuphine produces sedation, anxiolysis, and respiratory depression equivalent to 0.1 mg/kg of morphine sulfate.

4. The **antagonist properties** of nalbuphine have been used to reverse the respiratory depression of opioid agonists postoperatively while preserving analgesia. The reversal effects of nalbuphine are variable, as reported in several studies. Small doses (2 to 5 mg IV) will **antagonize respiratory depression** following fentanyl, nitrous oxide, and isoflurane anesthesia, and with less decrement of analgesia than naloxone. This effect has not been demonstrated following respiratory depression from morphine. Renarcotization occurs 2 to 3 h after the administration of nalbuphine when it is used postoperatively to reverse the fentanyl-induced respiratory depression in patients following cardiac surgery. Discontinuation following chronic use will produce a mild withdrawal syndrome. Nalbuphine is considered to have a **low abuse potential.**

5. Clinically, small doses of nalbuphine (2 to 5 mg) also reverse narcotic-induced increases in biliary pressure.

E. Dezocine (Dalgan)

1. Dezocine is an opioid agonist–antagonist which is equipotent to morphine at doses of less than 30 mg. Like the other narcotics in this class, there is a **ceiling effect for respiratory depression** and analgesia with repeated

doses. The analgesia is dose dependent at up to 20 mg of dezocine. It is a partial mu and delta receptor agonist. The analgesic and ventilatory depressions are reversible by opioid antagonists such as naloxone.

 2. Administration of dezocine will **potentiate the analgesia produced by pure mu receptor agonists,** unlike other opioid agonist–antagonists.

 3. Hepatic **metabolism** produces glucuronide conjugates, which are excreted in the urine. The drug has a high clearance, with a half-life of 2 to 3 h.

 4. The duration of the clinical effect and the **side-effects** profile are similar to those of morphine. Dezocine has a small incidence of dysphoria following administration, and there is no increased plasma histamine.

 5. There has been interest in the **lack of physical dependence** seen with the use of dezocine in animals. Several studies have failed to demonstrate withdrawal syndromes or the prevention of withdrawal in opioid-dependent primates given dezocine. A human study of the drug in nondependent, former opioid-addicted individuals revealed that these subjects were able to identify dezocine as "dope" as frequently as they did morphine. Dezocine currently is not a scheduled opioid.

V. OPIOID ANTAGONISTS

 A. Naloxone and naltrexone are **pure opioid antagonists.** Structurally, substitution of an alkyl group for a methyl group on an opioid agonist results in the pure antagonists. These drugs have a high affinity for the mu, kappa, and delta receptors. They are able to displace opioid agonists without activating the receptors. Initially, nalorphine and levallorphan were used as antagonists, but had a high incidence of side effects and incomplete reversal. The pure antagonists, naloxone and naltrexone, are frequently used to restore spontaneous ventilation following opioid anesthesia and narcotic overdoses.

B. Naloxone (Narcan)

 1. Naloxone administered IV rapidly (1 to 2 min) **reverses the respiratory depression and analgesia** of opioids. The duration of effect is short (30 to 45 min). An infusion (2 to 10 μg/kg/h) or frequent bolus doses (1 to 4 μg/kg) may be required to prevent renarcotization when used to reverse an opioid that has a longer clearance half-life. The lower doses can be effective in reverse opioid-related pruritus and nausea, whereas the higher dosage may be required for adequate antagonism of respiratory depression.

 2. Naloxone is **metabolized** primarily in the liver by glucuronidation. Bioavailability following oral administration is only 20 percent due to hepatic first-pass metabolism. The reversal of analgesia is the main side effect associated with naloxone.

3. Increased heart rate, blood pressure, nausea, vomiting, pulmonary edema, and cardiac dysrhythmias may accompany the use of naloxone. In the absence of present or impending respiratory arrest, **gentle titration** (0.5 μg/kg incremental doses every 2 to 5 min) for reversal of ventilatory depression will result in a lower incidence of these side effects. The **cardiovascular effects** have been attributed to recurrence of pain, rapid awakening, and increased sympathetic nervous system activity. Opioids decrease central sympathetic stimulation. There is evidence that reversal of this effect can precipitate the cardiovascular response associated with naloxone. It will increase cerebral blood flow and oxygen requirements, and is best avoided in neurosurgical patients. Opioid reversal may be hazardous in patients with pheochromocytoma or chromaffin tumors.

4. Naloxone is able to cross the placenta, and may be used effectively for the reversal of neonatal respiratory depression. Caution must be used with **newborns** of opioid-dependent mothers. Administration of naloxone may produce acute withdrawal in these neonates.

5. There are reports of improved hemodynamics when naloxone is used during **septic and hypovolemic shock.** It is hypothesized that stress-induced release of endorphins and the resultant decreased sympathetic output are reversed by opioid antagonists.

6. There are reports suggesting that naloxone may have a role in the treatment of ischemic or traumatic neurologic injury, Alzheimer's disease, schizophrenia, intractable pruritus, and thalamic pain syndromes.

C. Naltrexone (Trexan)

1. Naltrexone is another pure mu receptor **antagonist.** As compared with naloxone, this drug is effective orally and has a significantly longer half-life (8 to 12 h). Oral administration of a single dose has an antagonist effect that lasts 24 h.

2. Naltrexone undergoes extensive (95 percent) first-pass **hepatic metabolism** and is **excreted primarily by the kidney,** 99 percent in the form of metabolites. Peak serum levels occur approximately 1 h after ingestion.

3. Oral naltrexone has been **used to decrease the incidence of pruritus and nausea associated with epidural morphine,** although it is most frequently used for outpatients with previous histories of narcotic addiction, much in the way that disulfiram (Antabuse) is used for alcoholics.

4. Naltrexone can cause **hepatocellular damage.** It is contraindicated in patients receiving parenteral opioids.

5. **Pupillary constriction** occurs with naltrexone administration. The mechanism is unknown.

VI. CARDIOVASCULAR EFFECTS

A. Opioid use can be associated with hypotension, hypertension, and dysrhythmias. Each narcotic has unique effects on the cardiovascular system. Although morphine is unlikely to cause hypotension in normovolemic, supine, healthy patients, **orthostatic hypotension** may result following the IV administration of morphine. The orthostasis or hypotension associated with morphine may reflect the **reduced sympathetic tone** of peripheral veins. All opioids reduce sympathetic and enhance parasympathetic tone. Thus a patient who is dependent on a high intrinsic sympathetic tone or exogenous catecholamines may have a decrease in blood pressure following opioid administration.

B. Several **mechanisms,** including histamine release, centrally mediated decreased sympathetic tone, vagus-nerve–induced bradycardia, direct venodilation, and splanchnic vessel dilation, may play a role in morphine's hypotensive effects.

1. The **release of histamine** results in an increased stroke volume and a decrease in blood pressure and systemic vascular resistance. Histamine release and the associated cardiovascular changes may be reduced by limiting the rate of morphine infusion to less than 5 mg/min or keeping the patient euvolemic and supine. The use of H_1 (diphenhydramine) and H_2 (cimetidine) blockers will attenuate the cardiovascular effects, with no change in plasma histamine concentration. Fentanyl, sufentanil, and alfentanil do not induce histamine release with IV bolus administration (Fig. 8-5). Meperidine, however, is associated with a higher incidence of histamine release than is morphine.

2. Morphine reduces venous and arterial vascular smooth muscle tone. The venodilation is more significant and of longer duration than the arterial dilation. Intraoperatively, the venodilation may encourage increased fluid replacement. These vascular effects may be due to a **direct effect of morphine on the smooth muscle and a reduction in sympathetic nervous system reflexes.**

3. Morphine-induced hypotension is not related to myocardial depression. All opioids except meperidine cause a decrease in heart rate. Opioid bradycardia is the result of **increased vagal tone** by direct stimulation of the vagal nucleus in the medulla. The degree of induced bradycardia is dose related, although multiple clinical factors appear to attenuate this effect.

4. Morphine may also have a **direct depressant effect** on the **sinoatrial node** and depress **atrioventricular conduction.** Fentanyl-induced bradycardia is attenuated by anticholinergic drugs like atropine. Asystole has been reported following the administration of sufentanil and alfentanil. Direct vagal stimulation, combined with opioid-induced decreases in cen-

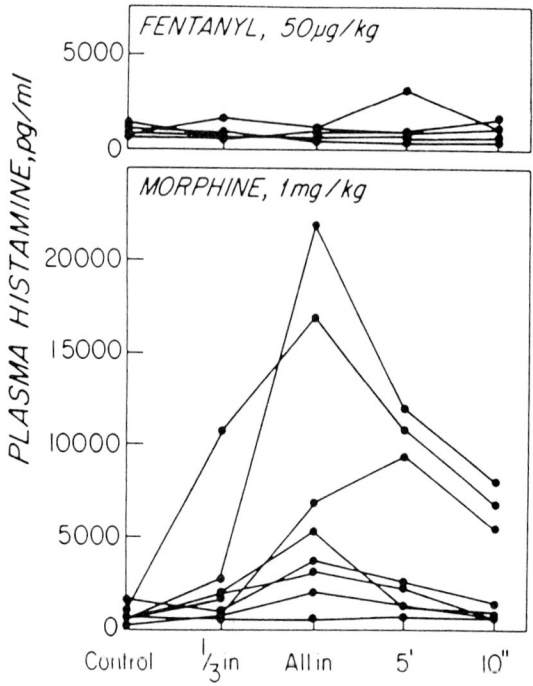

Figure 8-5 Plasma histamine from arterial samples following single bolus injection. (From Rosow CE, Moss J, Philbin DM, Savarese JJ. Histamine release during morphine and fentanyl anesthesia. *Anesthesiology* 56:93, 1982.)

tral sympathetic tone, may explain these episodes of asystole. Fentanyl will prolong the PR interval and atrioventricular node conduction.

C. Meperidine, unlike the other mu receptor agonists, has a **vagolytic effect** and may cause tachycardia. This has been related to the structural similarity of meperidine and atropine. Meperidine decreases the myocardial contractility of cardiac myofibrils in vitro. In comparison with morphine, meperidine will cause a decrease in cardiac output, blood pressure, and peripheral vascular resistance, and an increase in heart rate at low doses.

D. Hypertension and tachycardia during anesthesia with opioids are not direct effects of the opioid. The hypertensive response to intubation or surgical stimulation reflects inadequate anesthesia or inadequate blocking of sympathetic responses to noxious stimuli. The sympathetic and renin-angiotensin system functions remain intact. Fentanyl and sufentanil have a greater capacity to blunt the response to noxious stimulation than does morphine.

VII. RESPIRATORY EFFECTS

A. All mu receptor opiate agonists produce a **dose-dependent depression** of ventilation by directly depressing the brain ventilatory centers. There is a decreased minute ventilatory response to increasing carbon dioxide (CO_2) and the Pa_{CO_2} response curve is shifted to the right. The opioid's effects on the pontine and medullary respiratory centers alter the ventilatory pattern.

B. Patients typically will demonstrate a **decreased respiratory rate** and a compensatory **increased tidal volume.** A delayed expiratory phase, increased pauses, a decreased respiratory rate, and an increase or decrease in tidal volume may result from effects on ventilatory centers. It should be noted that a normal rate with decreased tidal volumes can occur. There is **a decrease in the hypoxic ventilatory drive.** One proposed mechanism for the changes in CO_2 sensitivity is that opioids may decrease the sensitivity of medullary ventilation centers to acetylcholine. The observation that physostigmine may reverse respiratory depression without altering the analgesic properties of opioids by increasing the CNS levels of acetylcholine suggests a cholinergic mechanism.

C. Several factors will alter opioid-induced respiratory depression.

1. **Sleep** seems to potentiate the depressant effects of opioids.
2. **Neonates and elderly** patients are particularly sensitive to the respiratory depressant effects.
3. **Pain and surgical stimulation** will counteract the respiratory depression.

D. The time to peak respiratory depression is shorter with IV fentanyl than with morphine or meperidine, while the length of depression is greater for equipotent doses of morphine and meperidine than for fentanyl. All opioid agonists can produce **delayed respiratory depression,** and several mechanisms may explain this. Sleep, lack of pain, supplemental analgesics, and hypothermia may have a role in this phenomenon. Several studies examining the elimination pharmacokinetics have found that plasma levels frequently have secondary peaks. Secondary fentanyl peaks correlate with the CO_2 response. Sequestration of fentanyl in the stomach secondary to ion trapping may contribute to the secondary serum fentanyl peak.

VIII. NEUROPHYSIOLOGIC EFFECTS

A. Opioids in the absence of hypoventilation produce modest reductions in **intracranial pressure** and **cerebral metabolic rate.** These drugs do not alter the production or absorption of cerebrospinal fluid. **Patients with**

head injury may be more sensitive to opioid effects due to alterations in the integrity of the blood–brain barrier. There are multiple reports of neuroexcitatory phenomena following the administration of large doses of opioids. Focal electroencephalogram (EEG) activity can occur after large doses of the phenylpiperidine derivatives (fentanyl, sufentanil, alfentanil). Meperidine's metabolite, normeperidine, has a long elimination half-life, and has twice the potency to induce seizures as does the parent drug.

    B. Miosis following opioid administration is due to release of cortical inhibition of the Edinger-Westphal nucleus, resulting in pupillary constriction. Atropine can antagonize this opioid effect, as will alterations in sympathetic and parasympathetic tone.

    C. Skeletal muscle rigidity has a variable reported incidence. The rate of injection and the dose may account for this discrepancy. The thoracic and abdominal muscles are primarily sensitive to this opioid effect. Alfentanil in large doses has the highest incidence of muscle rigidity. Extremity movements and tonic–clonic motion may appear as seizurelike movement. The mechanism for muscle rigidity and the relationship of opioid-induced movement to seizures is not clear. Thoracic rigidity alters pulmonary compliance and increases pulmonary artery pressure, centrol venous pressure, and pulmonary artery resistance. Decreased chest wall compliance may interfere with ventilation. Succinylcholine or nondepolarizing muscle relaxants can eliminate this effect. There are reports that thiopental or benzodiazepines may also attenuate or prevent the rigidity.

    D. Unlike general anesthetics which result in generalized CNS depression, opiates block afferent input from peripheral receptors to the CNS. Low doses of fentanyl apparently produce few **EEG changes.** High doses (59 to 70 μg/kg) result in replacement of alpha-wave with slow delta-wave activity, which is consistent with anesthesia and unconsciousness. Sufentanil apparently produces similar EEG patterns at higher dosages. Unlike the volatile anesthetics, burst suppression of EEG activity does not occur with increased dosage.

IX. GASTROINTESTINAL EFFECTS

    A. Gastric emptying is prolonged with opiates. There is a reduction in the peristaltic contractions of the small and large bowels with opiate administration. Peripheral opiate receptors in the myenteric plexus and cholinergic vagal stimulation account for the constipating effect of opioids. The ability to decrease GI motility has resulted in the utilization of opioids for chronic diarrhea. There does not seem to be much tolerance to the constipating effect of opioids.

    B. Biliary tree pressure and sphincter of Oddi tone increase with all opioid agonists. This effect seems to be dose dependent and correlates with plasma levels. Spasm of the biliary smooth muscle can result in biliary colic.

The pain will respond to nitroglycerin, nalbuphine, naloxone, or glucagon. The highest incidence of biliary spasm occurs with fentanyl; morphine and meperidine seem to have a much lower incidence. Mixed agonist–antagonists such as butorphanol can increase biliary pressure, but the effects are less significant when compared with the pure agonists. The incidence of spasm of Oddi's sphincter following fentanyl administration is 3 percent, but there is a 99 percent incidence of increased biliary pressure with fentanyl administration.

C. Opioids increase the incidence of **nausea and vomiting.** Narcotics directly stimulate the chemoreceptor trigger zone in the floor of the fourth ventricle in the area postrema of the medulla oblongata. Increased gastric secretions and delayed gastric emptying times all contribute to opioid-induced nausea. Opiate binding, as a partial dopamine agonist in the chemoreceptor trigger zone, has been proposed as a mechanism for the nausea and vomiting. Apomorphine has the greatest affinity for the dopamine receptor and has a high incidence of nausea associated with its administration. Antagonism of dopaminergic receptors in the medulla will reduce the incidence of nausea and vomiting. Droperidol (Inapsine), a butyrophenone with antidopaminergic properties, is an effective antiemetic. Metoclopromide (Reglan), a dopamine antagonist, acts centrally at the chemoreceptor trigger zone and in the GI tract to increase intestinal motility.

SUGGESTED READINGS

Estafanous FG et al.: *Opioids in Anesthesia.* London, Butterworth's, 1984.
Gourlay GK, Cherry DA, Cousins MJ: A comparative study of the efficacy and pharmacokinetics of oral methadone and morphine in the treatment of severe pain in patients with cancer. *Pain* 25:297, 1986.
Hug CC Jr: *Seminar Anesth* 1:14, 1982.
Jaffe JH, Martin WR: Opioid analgesics and antagonists, in Goodman LS, Gilman AG (eds): *The Pharmacological Basis of Therapeutics,* 7th ed. New York, Macmillan, 1985.
McClain D, Hug CC Jr: Intravenous fentanyl kinetics, *Clin Pharm Ther* 28:106, 1980.
Pasternak G: Multiple morphine and enkephalin receptors and the relief of pain. *JAMA* 259:1362, 1988.
Rosow C, Moss J, Philbin D, Savarese J: Histamine release during morphine and fentanyl anesthesia. *Anesthesiology* 56:93, 1982.
Stanski DR, Greenblatt DJ, Lowenstein E: Kinetics of intravenous and intramuscular morphine. *Clin Pharm Ther* 24:52, 1978.

CHAPTER 9

GENERAL ANESTHETICS IN THE INTENSIVE CARE UNIT

Charles G. Durbin, Jr.

I. Definitions
II. Indications for General Anesthesia in the Critically Ill
III. Inhalation Anesthesia/Analgesia
    A. Nitrous Oxide
    B. Potent Vapors
    C. Halothane
    D. Isoflurane
    E. Enflurane
    F. Methoxyflurane
IV. Hazards of Inhalational Anesthesia
    A. Monitoring
    B. Malignant Hyperthermia
    C. Anesthetic Trace Exposure
V. Intravenous Anesthesia
    A. Barbiturates
    B. Etomidate
    C. Ketamine
    D. Propofol
VI. Specific Conditions and General Anesthesia
    A. Tetanus
    B. Asthma
    C. Control of $CMRO_2$
VII. Summary
Suggested Readings

I. DEFINITIONS

   A. Occasionally, patients in a critical care unit require total insensitivity to environmental stimuli and pain. This total unawareness may be described as **general anesthesia.** Many different, unrelated chemical compounds are capable of producing a state of anesthesia, the exact mechanisms of which are not understood. Three classes of anesthetics are described in this chapter: gaseous anesthetics, volatile (or inhalational) anesthetics, and intravenous (IV) anesthetics. Although used for general anesthesia, the narcotics will not be described in this chapter as they are covered in detail in Chapter 8. Some of these agents may be used in less than anesthetic concentrations and would then be described as sedative, analgesic, or hypnotic in their use.
   B. General anesthesia has several **functional goals:**

   1. Analgesia—absence of pain.
   2. Amnesia—lack of recall of unpleasant events.
   3. Areflexia—not moving in response to stimuli (including reflexes involving the autonomic nervous system).

   C. These components may be provided by a single agent such as a volatile liquid (i.e., halothane), or achieved by the addition of several different classes of drugs, such as muscle relaxants, narcotics, and drugs that produce amnesia. Often the choice of anesthetic technique is determined by the patient's physiology. Each agent or technique has unique side effects which must be taken into account when determining a treatment plan. Some of the major effects and side effects of selected anesthetic agents are listed in Table 9-1 and discussed in greater detail in the text.

II. INDICATIONS FOR GENERAL ANESTHESIA IN THE CRITICALLY ILL

   A. There are several reasons to use general anesthesia in the critically ill:

   1. To abolish pain (and recall) during a surgical procedure.
   2. To treat refractory status epilepticus.
   3. To capitalize on the primary bronchodilatory effects of several of the agents in treating status asthmaticus.

   In addition, whenever a neuromuscular blocking agent is used (such as in treating severe respiratory failure), it is essential to provide adequate sedation and analgesia or to induce general anesthesia (complete unawareness),

Table 9-1 The relative effects of various anesthetic agents on hemodynamic function

Anesthetic agent	Blood pressure	Cardiac output	Heart rate	SVR*	Histamine release	Malignant hyperthermia trigger
Nitrous oxide	↑	0-↑	0-↑	↑↑	0	0
Halothane	↓↓	↓↓	↓	↑	0	++++
Isoflurane	↓	0-↑	↑↑↑	↓	0	+++
Enflurane	↓↓↓	0-↑	↑	↓↓↓	0	+++
Ketamine	↑↑↑	↑	↑↑	↑↑	0	+
Propofol	↓↓	0-↑	0-↑	↓↓↓	+++	0
Barbiturates	↓↓	↓↓	0-↓	↑	0	0
Etomidate	↓	0	0	↓	0	0
Narcotics	0	0	0	↑	+++	0

*SVR = systemic vascular resistance

as the most terrifying human experience is to be paralyzed, awake, and in pain, but be unable to tell anyone.

III. INHALATION ANESTHESIA/ANALGESIA

A. Nitrous Oxide

  1. Nitrous oxide is a common agent used to provide or supplement general anesthesia. It is relatively impotent, and is usually used as an adjuvant with another agent to achieve surgical anesthesia. A more than 100% concentration of nitrous oxide is required to reliably achieve unconsciousness in **healthy** people. However, in subanesthetic concentrations, it is an excellent analgesic agent with rapid onset (several breaths) and offset. Many dentists take advantage of these characteristics in their practice. Popular in the United Kingdom and parts of Europe, a gas mixture consisting of 70 percent nitrous oxide and 30 percent oxygen (Nitrox) is self-administered by patients experiencing intermittent pain. The pain from coronary ischemia, and acute myocardial infarction and that experienced in active labor has been successfully treated this way. A renewed interest in the use of nitrous oxide in this fashion is arising in some areas of the United States.
  2. Concerns about nitrous oxide:
     a. The prolonged use of nitrous oxide causes profound **leukopenia.** At one time, this has been used to advantage to treat leukemia. This fall in

white blood cells (WBCs) is due to inhibition of methionine synthetase, an enzyme important in WBC proliferation. This may be an undesirable side effect in the critically ill, as infection is a common lethal complication. The effects of brief exposures to nitrous oxide on immune system function, such as during a surgical procedure, are not known. Nitrous oxide is a sympathomimetic drug, raising heart rate, cardiac output, and blood pressure slightly. This may be undesirable in patients with increased intracranial pressure (ICP), or hypertension, or in those who are actively or at risk of bleeding. Since nitrous oxide must be used in high concentrations, patients requiring more than 30 percent oxygen are not candidates for its use as a single agent.

  b. Another consideration in using nitrous oxide is its **effect on trapped gas.** Since nitrous oxide is more soluble than nitrogen, air-containing cavities will expand as nitrous oxide equilibrates with the concentration in the blood. This is a particular problem in closed spaces such as the brain (after surgery, lumbar puncture, or pneumoencephalogram), unvented pneumothorax, gaseous abdominal distention, and obstructive sinusitis, and after decompression sickness (for as long as several months). Patients taken to the operating room with any of these conditions should not receive nitrous oxide as part of their anesthetic management. Oxygen, or a mixture of air and oxygen, can be used for ventilation instead of nitrous oxide in these patients.

B. Potent Vapors

  1. The classic volatile anesthetic agent used in the United States, diethyl ether, has been replaced by the more potent, less flammable anesthetic agents halothane, isoflurane, and enflurane.

  2. The concentration necessary to prevent movement from a painful stimulus is called **minimal alveolar concentration** (MAC). This is a convenient way to compare potencies, side effects, and toxicities of inhalation agents.

  3. Specialized equipment is needed to deliver accurate amounts of this and other liquid anesthetic agents. The central component of the anesthesia machine is a calibrated, temperature-compensated vaporizer. A gas-mixing system with calibrated flow meters allows precise delivery of oxygen and other gases to a breathing circuit. The breathing circuit connects the anesthesia machine to the patient, and often includes a carbon dioxide absorbing system to allow conservation of anesthetic gases, moisture, and heat by partial or complete rebreathing.

  4. A scavenging system is required to collect and remove the waste gas. A complete description of the components of the anesthetic delivery system is beyond the scope of this text. For further information and detail, consult Suggested Readings.

C. Halothane

1. The most common agent currently in use is halothane. Halothane is a nonflammable, halogenated hydrocarbon with a high anesthetic potency. An anesthetic concentration of halothane is about 0.7 volume % of the alveolar or exhaled gas mixture (MAC = 0.7%). Halothane has been used in asthmatic patients for operative anesthesia and to treat refractory status asthmaticus. It has a significant **bronchodilating effect.**

2. Halothane is also a potent **myocardial depressant** and must be used carefully in patients with cardiovascular instability. Halothane sensitizes the myocardium to the arrhythmogenic effects of catecholamines. This effect is more profound in the patient with increased pCO_2 or decreased pO_2.

3. By inhibiting **autoregulation of the cerebral vasculature,** halothane increases intracranial blood flow. If ICP is elevated, halothane will increase it further. This is particularly true with cerebral edema from tumors, surgery, or head injury. Potent vapors should be used with caution (if at all) in this patient population. The vasodilation and increased cerebral blood flow (CBF) caused by halothane, enflurane, and isoflurane are partially ameliorated by hyperventilation.

4. Halothane decreases **mesenteric blood flow.** This may cause mild hepatic dysfunction. Elevated liver enzymes (which rapidly return to normal) are commonly seen in healthy patients after halothane anesthesia. Massive hepatic necrosis has rarely been reported after the administration of halothane. **Halothane hepatitis** is believed to have an immunologic basis. The incidence of this condition is rare, less than one occurrence in 50,000 exposures, and may be increased after repeated exposure.

5. Halothane releases bromine when metabolized in the body, and sedation from **bromism** is possible after prolonged exposure.

6. A reversible decrease in urine output with no change in renal function occurs with halothane anesthesia. **Fluoride (F^-), a potential renal toxin,** is released as a result of anaerobic metabolism only.

D. Isoflurane

1. Isoflurane is a halogenated ether about one-half as potent (MAC = 1.2 percent) as halothane. Although isoflurane has a less direct bronchodilatory effect, its successful use in status asthmaticus has been reported. Isoflurane is irritating to the airway. Patients often experience coughing and laryngospasm during anesthetic induction and at light levels of anesthesia.

2. Isoflurane has a less profound direct depressant effect on the heart, and it is a significant **direct vasodilator.** Heart rate often increases with anesthetic levels of isoflurane. The decrease in systemic vascular resistance (SVR) and increase in heart rate act to maintain cardiac output despite decreases in blood pressure.

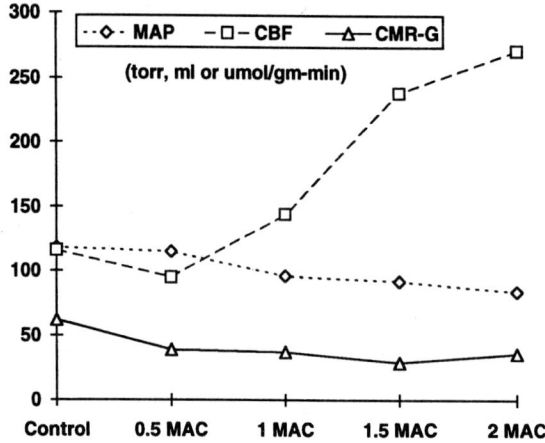

Figure 9-1 Relationship between changes in CMR-g (glucose), MAP, and CBF in rats during isoflurane anesthesia. The reduction in CBF caused by isoflurane occurs below 1 MAC. Above this level, cerebral vasodilation occurs. Matching of metabolism and blood flow occurs at lower anesthetic levels. *(From Maekawa T, Tommasino C, Shapiro HM, et al: Local cerebral blood flow and glucose utilization during isoflurane anesthesia in the rat.* Anesthesiology *65:144–151, 1986.)*

3. At low concentrations of isoflurane (< 0.5 MAC), CBF is decreased in proportion to a decrease in cerebral metabolic rate for oxygen ($CMRO_2$). However, with higher levels of isoflurane (> 1.0 MAC), **cerebral vasodilation** increases CBF in a dose-dependent fashion with little additional decrease in $CMRO_2$ (Fig. 9-1). The matching of CBF and metabolism is better preserved with isoflurane than with halothane or enflurane (Fig. 9-2). Treatment of refractory status epilepticus has been reported with both halothane and isoflurane. Controlled studies demonstrating the superiority of either of these agents over conventional treatment in this condition is lacking.

4. Isoflurane decreases portal blood flow less profoundly than does halothane and hepatic function is unaltered.

5. Normally, only 0.2 percent of the administered isoflurane is metabolized. There is virtually no chance of fluoride nephrotoxicity with isoflurane.

E. Enflurane

1. A stereoisomer of isoflurane, enflurane is less potent (MAC = 1.7%). Like isoflurane, enflurane is irritating to the airway, causing increased secretions.

2. Its potent vasodilating effects are similar to those of isoflurane, but

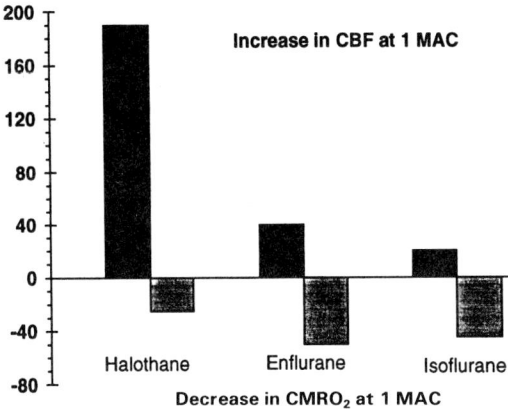

Figure 9-2 The percentage increase of CBF (black bars) and percentage decrease in $CMRO_2$ (shaded bars) for halothane, enflurane, and isoflurane are shown. These effects are demonstrated at anesthetic concentrations (1 MAC). The ratio of $CMRO_2$ to CBF is best preserved with isoflurane. *(From Todd MM, Drummond JC: A comparison of the cerebrovascular and metabolic effects of halothane and isoflurane in the cat.* Anesthesiology *60:276, 1984;* Todd MM, Drummond JC, Shapiro HM: Comparative cerebrovascular and metabolic effects of halothane, enflurane and isoflurane. Anesthesiology *57:A32, 1982;* Murphy FL, Kennell EM, Johnstone RE, et al: The effects of enflurane, isoflurane, and halothane on cerebral blood flow and metabolism in man. Abstracts of Scientific Papers, *1974 ASA Meeting, p 61.)*

enflurane causes less tachycardia. As such, **hypotension** can be a significant problem.

3. Enflurane decreases $CMRO_2$ less profoundly than does isoflurane. In addition, enflurane in high concentrations can cause **seizures,** leading to an increase in $CMRO_2$. It should be used with caution in patients with elevated ICP or a history of seizures.

4. Two percent of the administered enflurane is metabolized, giving rise to F^-. Blood levels of F^- are significantly higher in patients receiving *Isoniazide* (INH), but are unaffected by phenobarbital or ethanol. The free F^- can reach significant levels after as little as 3 MAC hours of enflurane anesthesia (threshold for **renal toxicity** from $F^- = 40$ to $50\ M$). Enflurane should not be used in patients at increased risk of renal impairment or for long periods of time.

5. Like the other potent vapors, enflurane decreases portal blood flow, although this effect is not profound. Liver function abnormalities are rare after enflurane, and no cases of massive hepatic necrosis have been reported.

F. Methoxyflurane

1. Methoxyflurane predates isoflurane and enflurane. Metabolism of this agent is significant because it is very fat soluble and persists in the body for a prolonged period. A significant amount of F^- is released, and **high output renal failure** frequently follows prolonged administration of this agent. It is seldom used today.

A comparison of serum inorganic F^- levels after halothane, enflurane, isoflurane, and methoxyflurane is shown in Fig. 9-3.

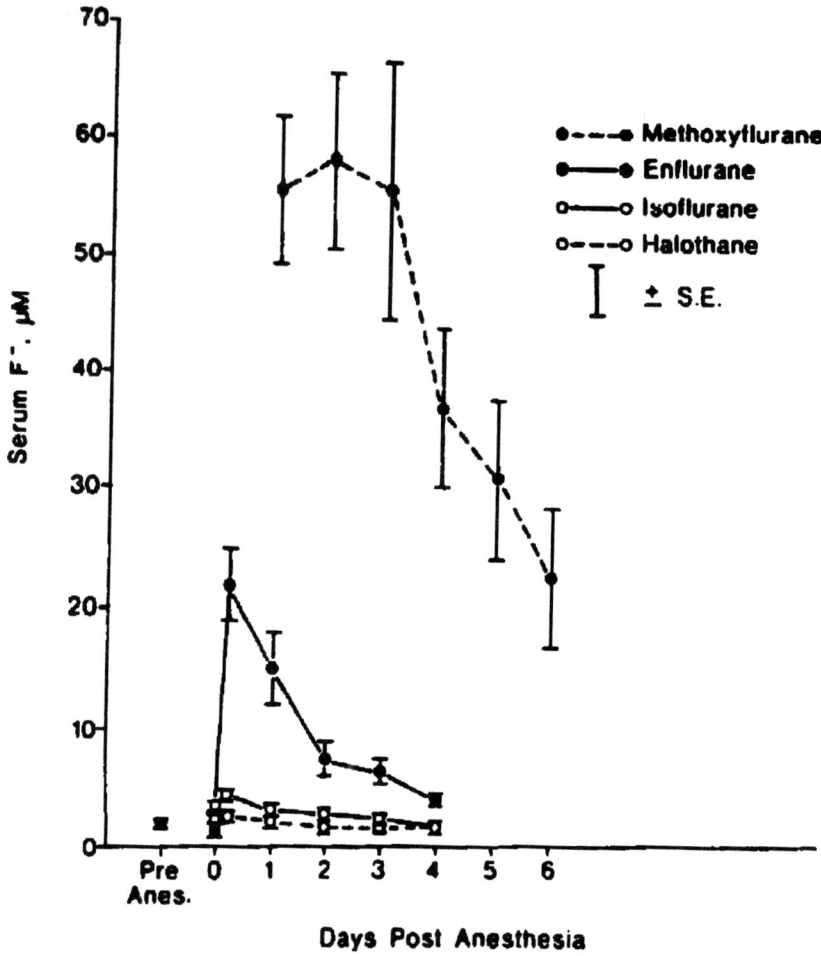

Figure 9-3 Serum inorganic F⁻ levels obtained after halothane, enflurane, isoflurane and methoxyflurane anesthetics. *(From Cousins MJ, et al:* Anesthesiology *44:48, 1974, reproduced with permission.)*

IV. HAZARDS OF INHALATIONAL ANESTHESIA

A. Monitoring

1. Standards (guidelines) have been established for **patient monitoring** during the administration of anesthetic agents in the operating room. This level of monitoring should be provided anywhere that general anesthesia is induced. Patients must have an experienced person administer the anesthetic using safety-checked and monitored equipment. Specific monitors of

the anesthesia machine are needed. Airway pressure, inhaled gas volume, and inspired oxygen concentration must be continuously monitored and alarm systems present and used.

   2. Routine vital signs, including pulse rate, blood pressure, and respiratory rate, must be monitored and recorded frequently (at least every 5 min if they are stable, and more often if they are not). Arterial oxygen saturation must be monitored continuously and recorded and exhaled carbon dioxide and other gases should be measured. The aggressiveness of patient monitoring (i.e., central venous and arterial catheters) should be determined by the severity of illness and stability of the patient.

   3. Anesthesia machines often include mechanical ventilators; however, these ventilators may be unable to provide adequate support of gas exchange if lung compliance is very low or airway resistance is extremely high. Some intensive-care mechanical ventilators (such as the Siemens machines) have provisions for adding anesthetic agents directly to the patient circuit. Familiarity and experience with these devices are necessary for safe patient care.

B. Malignant Hyperthermia

   1. Malignant hyperthermia is a potentially lethal condition arising during anesthetic exposure. It is due to a genetic defect in calcium metabolism in muscle, resulting in runaway metabolism, metabolic and respiratory acidosis, and temperature rise. It is triggered by halothane and all other potent inhalational anesthetics. The incidence is less than one in 30,000 anesthetics, and the diagnosis is made by in vitro muscle biopsy caffeine-contracture testing. There are no symptoms or reliable signs of this inheritable, potentially lethal disorder prior to anesthetic exposure. Patients with a family history of the disease are considered at risk.

   2. Depolarizing neuromuscular blocking agents (succinylcholine) are also trigger agents in this condition, and act synergistically with potent agents to provoke the most rapidly fatal form.

   3. If suspected and treated early, this syndrome can be completely reversed by administration of **dantrolene sodium** IV at a dose of 2.5 mg/kg repeated up to a 10 mg/kg total dose.

C. Anesthetic Trace Exposure

   1. A significant problem in using nitrous oxide or any of the inhalational anesthetics is environmental pollution and its effects on caregivers and patients in the vicinity.

   2. Prolonged exposure to low levels of anesthetic gases may increase spontaneous abortion rates in women.

3. A degenerative neurologic condition with tremors and intellectual changes has also been related to prolonged repeated exposure to nitrous oxide inhalation.

4. The Occupational Safety and Health Administration (OSHA) has endorsed standards for the allowable levels of trace anesthetic gases in locations where they are used. Although there is little evidence to support these limits, nitrous oxide is allowed up to 25 ppm and potent agents up to 0.5 ppm. Elaborate gas-scavenging systems are necessary to achieve these levels. Failure to provide adequate scavenging can result in federal penalties and fines to the institution, as well as lawsuits instituted by affected workers. Short-term effects of exposure to low levels of anesthetic gases are: loss of concentration, sleepiness, giddiness, and headaches. These effects on caregivers must be considered when using inhalational anesthetics without proper scavenging. Environmental pollution is a technical concern that must be addressed if these agents are to be employed safely in the intensive care unit (ICU).

V. INTRAVENOUS ANESTHESIA

Anesthesia with one or several agents is simple to administer by the IV route in the operating room and the ICU, and provides an alternative to the mechanical complexity of general anesthesia. Single complete agents include the barbiturates, ketamine, propofol, and etomidate. High-dose narcotics, discussed in Chapter 8, can also produce profound analgesia and sedation, but do not provide amnesia with any predictability. Narcotics are often used to supplement the analgesia of other anesthetic agents and techniques.

A. Barbiturates

Barbiturates are derivatives of barbituric acid and have various durations of action based on their lipid solubility. Very soluble agents such as thiopental or amytal are used to induce anesthesia because of their rapid action and very short duration of action (minutes). Their effect is terminated by redistribution into fatty tissues. Continuous infusion of these agents results in saturation of fat stores and long duration of coma. After several days of pentothal infusion, for example, consciousness may not return for weeks because the drug's effect is terminated by hepatic metabolism and renal excretion.

1. The barbiturates profoundly **depress global brain function** and are capable of totally, yet reversibly, abolishing electroencephalogram (EEG) activity. A spike and dome or burst suppression pattern is pathognomonic for barbiturate-induced cerebral electrical suppression. Barbiturates

decrease cerebral metabolism and blood flow proportionately, and are useful agents in the treatment of increased ICP of any cause. Barbiturates have been used to treat seizures for many years. Induction of anesthesia with barbiturates often terminates status epilepticus. Other analeptic agents can then be given and barbiturate depression of mental status lightened. Seizures often reemerge when barbiturates are withdrawn.

2. Barbiturates are **profound cardiac depressants.** Because of a direct vascular smooth muscle constrictive effect, blood pressure is often maintained despite a marked decrease in cardiac output. Invasive cardiac monitoring and vasoactive drug infusions are indicated when barbiturates are used to induce coma. Even with brief administration, such as during the induction of anesthesia, cardiovascular collapse may occur. This is most often due to hypovolemia in a patient maintaining normal blood pressure by elevated sympathetic tone. Central nervous system depression from any anesthetic agent can result in a profound fall in blood pressure under these circumstances.

B. Etomidate

A nonbarbiturate induction agent, etomidate has been suggested for use in place of pentothal in patients who are less than hemodynamically stable. Like the barbiturates, etomidate decreases cerebral metabolic rate more than blood flow and reduces ICP. It is less depressing to the heart than the barbiturates, and blood pressure is well maintained. It may be painful on injection, and patient movements commonly occur briefly. Etomidate profoundly **suppresses adrenal function.** This seems to be of little consequence in healthy patients undergoing routine operations. Infusions used for sedation in the critically ill, however, have been associated with increased morbidity. The exact etiology of this is unclear, but it presumably is related to inhibited basal cortisol production and a limited ability to respond to stress.

C. Ketamine

Similar to the psychotropic agent phencyclidine (PCP), ketamine produces analgesia and anesthesia. At low doses, 0.25 to 0.5 mg/kg IV, it produces excellent analgesia without loss of consciousness. At higher doses, a dissociative anesthetic state ensues. Patients report vivid and sometimes unpleasant dreams after ketamine anesthesia. These are less frequent if a narcotic, barbiturate, or benzodiazepine is also given.

1. Ketamine is short in duration of effect (10–15 min), may be repeated for longer needs, and has no direct toxic effects. A direct myocardial depressant, it is also a **sympathomimetic** drug that normally increases blood pressure and heart rate, maintaining cardiac output through the release of epinephrine and norepinephrine even in the critically ill. In active bleeding or

hypertensive conditions, this effect may be undesirable, and with hypovolemia, a profound fall in blood pressure may occur because the direct myocardial depression effect may predominate.

   2. As **ICP can be profoundly increased,** this agent should be used with caution in patients at risk of cerebral herniation.

   3. Ketamine is excellent for patients requiring repeated surgical or painful medical procedures, such as burn debridement or chemotherapy infusions. It is very useful in children, who seem to have a lower incidence of "bad dreams" than do adults.

   4. Ketamine has direct **bronchiolar dilating effects** and has been used to treat status asthmaticus.

   5. It has also been reported to be successful in treating status epilepticus, although the exact mechanism for this effect is not understood.

D. Propofol

Used as an induction agent as well as a complete anesthetic agent, **propofol** has the unique advantage of allowing a rapid emergence from anesthesia after termination of the infusion. This drug has been used in the ICU for periods as long as several days with no delay in emergence. Unlike most other anesthetic agents, nausea and vomiting are rare after its use. Anesthetic induction doses are 1.5 to 2.5 mg/kg in healthy adults, which should be reduced to 0.5 to 1 mg/kg in the ill or elderly. Sedative doses are 10 to 50 μg/kg. The same dose per minute can be used for continuous infusion; however, the effect should be judged by patient response. Reported effective infusion rates are from 20 to 2000 μg/kg/min in the ICU for up to 10 days.

   1. A major issue in using this agent in the ICU is its effect on the cardiovascular system. A profound **fall in blood pressure** often occurs. This is believed to be due to the release of histamine, but also may be due to direct myocardial depression with some vasodilatation. Hypertensive and hypovolemic patients are particularly likely to develop this problem. Continuous infusion rather than bolus administration minimizes these effects.

   2. Propofol is rather insoluble in water and is administered in a lipid emulsion. This is an excellent growth medium for bacteria and, if sepsis is to be avoided, a continuous infusion solution must be changed after 8 hours. The place of propofol in the ICU is not yet known.

VI. SPECIFIC CONDITIONS AND GENERAL ANESTHESIA

A. Tetanus

General anesthesia has been used to support patients with tetanus. Both muscle rigidity and autonomic instability result from this toxin produced by

Botulinum tetanii. Muscle relaxants may be needed to allow mechanical ventilation of these critically ill patients. General anesthesia, inhalation or IV, may improve respiratory and hemodynamic status by decreasing muscle spasms and sympathetic lability in response to noxious stimuli.

B. Asthma

As mentioned above, status asthmaticus has been treated with inhalational anesthesia, and IV ketamine has also been useful. Only case reports support either approach, and no controlled studies have been performed to demonstrate convincingly that either approach is superior to conventional therapy. Propofol is probably contraindicated in asthma due to its release of histamine.

C. Control of $CMRO_2$

Anesthetic depression of brain metabolism is occasionally used for therapeutic reasons.

1. The effect of barbiturates and etomidate on increased ICP is well recognized. These drugs lead to profound alterations in mental status and evaluation of the underlying disease is impossible.

2. They may be lifesaving in the patient with a treatable life-threatening, expanding, intracerebral mass lesion.

3. They may also have effects on the immune system that lead to uncontrolled infection.

4. The use of these cerebroprotective agents (primarily barbiturates) in cardiac arrest (total cerebral ischemia) has not been proved. The profound depression of cardiac function is a factor that limits their use in this situation.

VII. SUMMARY

General anesthesia is occasionally necessary in the critically ill patient. During painful surgical or medical procedures and therapeutic paralysis, abolition of awareness is essential. Control of status asthmaticus and status epilepticus may require general anesthesia. Anesthesia can be provided by inhalation of anesthetic vapors or by the IV route. Anesthetic standards for safety and monitoring must be guaranteed where general anesthesia is provided. Specific patient issues guide the choice of the particular anesthetic technique. Safe and effective patient management requires appropriate experience and skill.

SUGGESTED READINGS

Arnold WP: Environmental safety including chemical dependency, in Miller RD: *Anesthesia,* 3rd ed. New York, Churchill Livingstone, 1990, pp 2407–2420.

Bierman MI, Brown M, Muren O, et al: Prolonged isoflurane anesthesia in status asthmaticus. *Crit Care Med* 14:832, 1986.

Cousins MJ, Greenstein LR, Hitt BA, Mazze RI: Metabolism and renal effects of enflurane in man. *Anesthesiology* 44:44, 1976.

Durbin CG Jr: Neuromuscular blocking agents and sedative drugs: clinical uses and toxic effects in the critical care unit. *Crit Care Clin* 7:489–506, 1991.

Farling PA, Johnston JR, Coppel DL: Propofol infusion for sedation of patients with head injury in intensive care: a preliminary report. *Anaesthesia* 44:222, 1989.

Maekawa T, Tommasino C, Shapiro HM, et al: Local cerebral blood flow and glucose utilization during isoflurane anesthesia in the rat. *Anesthesiology* 65:144–151, 1986.

Mazzi RI, Lecky JH: The health of operating room personnel. *Anesthesiology* 62:226–228, 1985.

Murphy FL, Kennell EM, Johnstone RE, et al: The effects of enflurane, isoflurane and halothane on cerebral blood flow and metabolism in man. *Abstracts of Scientific Papers,* 1974 ASA Meeting, p 61.

National Institute for Occupational Safety and Health: *Criteria for a Recommended Standard: Occupational Exposure to Waste Anesthetic Gases and Vapors.* DHEW (NIOSH) Publication nos. 77-140, 1977.

Orko R, Rosenberg PH, Himberg J-J: Intravenous infusion of midazolam, propofol and vecuronium in a patient with severe tetanus. *Acta Anaesthesiol Scand* 32:590, 1988.

Park GR, Manara AR, Mendel L, Bateman PE: Ketamine infusion: its use as a sedative, inotrope and bronchodilator in a critically ill patient. *Anaesthesia* 42:980, 1987.

Spence AA: Environmental pollution by inhalation anaesthetics. *Br J Anaesth* 59:96–103, 1987.

Strube PJ, Hallam PL: Ketamine by continuous infusion in status asthmaticus. *Anaesthesia* 41:1017, 1986.

Todd MM, Drummond JC: A comparison of the cerebrovascular and metabolic effects of halothane and isoflurane in the cat. *Anesthesiology* 60:276, 1984.

Todd MM, Drummond JC, Shapiro HM: Comparative cerebrovascular and metabolic effects of halothane, enflurane, and isoflurane. *Anesthesiology* 57:A332, 1982.

Watt I, Ledingham I McA: Mortality amongst multiple trauma patients admitted to an intensive therapy unit. *Anaesthesia* 39:973, 1984.

CHAPTER
10

PHARMACOLOGY OF LOCAL ANESTHETICS

Cosmo DiFazio
Andrew M. Woods

I. The How and Where of Local Anesthetic Action
   A. Stimulation of a Nerve
   B. Ionic Currents
   C. Action Potential
   D. Potassium Ion Outflow
   E. Membrane Stabilization
   F. Dose-Related Inhibition
II. Chemical and Physical Properties
   A. Lipid Solubility
   B. Ionization
   C. Protein Binding
   D. Chiral Forms (Stereoisomers)
III. Blood Levels and Toxicity
   A. Peak Blood Levels
   B. Systemic Toxicity
   C. Treatment of LA-Induced Seizures
   D. Cardiac Toxicity
IV. Clinical Applications to Improve Safety
   A. Selecting a Dose
   B. Fractionating the Dose
V. Modification of Onset of Action
   A. pH Changes
   B. Carbonated Solutions
   C. Warming of the Solution
VI. Opiate–LA Combinations
Suggested Readings

I. THE HOW AND WHERE OF LOCAL ANESTHETIC ACTION

A. Stimulation of a sensory nerve results in a **propagated impulse** that passes along the course of the nerve from the peripheral site of stimulation to the central nervous system (CNS), where perception of the stimulus takes place.

B. The electrical signal in excitable nerve tissue is the result of propagated **ionic currents** that are created by a transient alteration in the concentration gradient across the nerve cell membrane for several ionic species. The ionic concentration of sodium (Na+) is high extracellularly and low intracellularly, while that of potassium (K+) is low extracellularly and high intracellularly. The **ionic gradients** for sodium and potassium are maintained across the cell membrane by an ion-translocating, **sodium–potassium–adenosine triphosphate (ATP) pump** mechanism within the nerve.

C. The initial upswing of an **action potential** associated with a nerve impulse is caused by an increase in permeability of the nerve membrane to sodium ions such that they move intracellularly. This results in **depolarization** of the nerve in the area of the open channels. It has been postulated that the action potential causes a conformational change in the nerve membrane lipoprotein and alters the sodium channel.

D. Potassium ion outflow in the area of depolarization commences more slowly and later than the movement of the sodium ions, and peaks after the **inward movement of the sodium ions** subsides. Both ions are subsequently restored to their prestimulation intra- and extracellular concentrations by the **sodium–potassium–ATP-dependent pump** mechanism.

E. Local anesthetic (LA) drugs prevent the development of the action potential in a nerve by preventing sodium ions from moving intracellularly through the sodium channels. This effect has been referred to as **membrane stabilization,** because the resting membrane potential is unaffected by further nerve stimulation.

  1. Present in both cationic (acid) and anionic (base) forms when deposited outside the nerve, LAs are believed to penetrate the lipid bilayer structure of the cell membrane in their lipid-soluble, uncharged base form.

  2. Once in the axoplasm, the LA will reequilibrate into the charged cationic and free-base forms in accordance with the drug pKa and the pH of the axoplasm.

  3. The cationic form of commonly used LA drugs enters the sodium channel from the axoplasmic (intracellular) side of the nerve membrane, binds to an anionic site within the sodium channel, and physically or ionically blocks sodium ion movements in the channel (Fig. 10-1).

F. The LA is in a constant process of binding and releasing from receptors in the sodium channel. As long as there is a critical mass of LA at the sodium channel, that portion of the nerve remains "blocked."

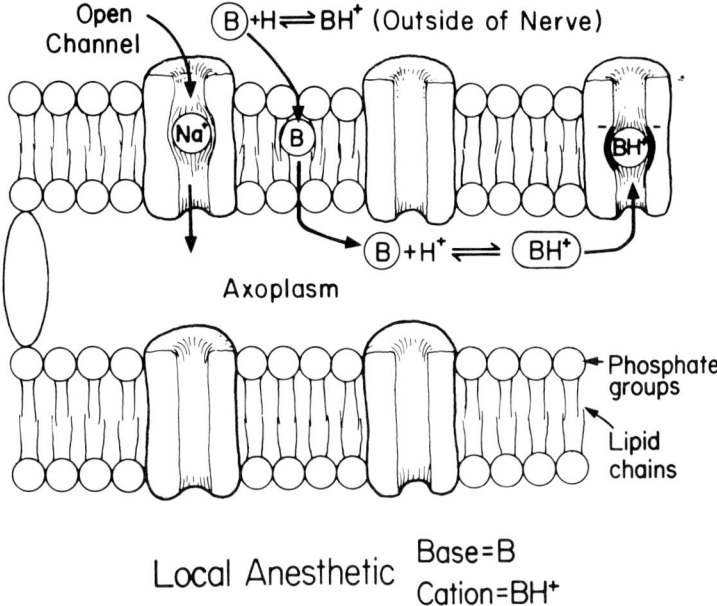

Figure 10-1 The action of LAs at the sodium channel. The base form of the drug passes through the cell membrane. It then enters the channel in the cationic form from the axoplasmic side of the nerve membrane.

II. CHEMICAL AND PHYSICAL PROPERTIES

The **chemical and physical properties** and equipotent concentrations of LA drugs are illustrated in Table 10-1. The physical properties of lipid solubility, pKa (ionization), and protein binding can be directly related to LA potency, onset of action, and duration of action, while the chemical structure determines the metabolism and elimination of these drugs in the body.

A. Lipid Solubility

The aromatic group (benzene ring) present at one end of the LA molecule is the major determinant of the lipid solubility (Fig. 10-2). The significance of this property is that the uncharged base form is lipid soluble and readily passes through the lipid-containing nerve membrane to reach the axoplasm and the LA site of action. Lipid solubility is associated with the **potency** of the LAs: the more lipid-soluble drugs are the more potent LA drugs.

Table 10-1 Physical properties and equipotent concentrations of local anesthetics

	Procaine	Lidocaine	Mepivacaine	Bupivacaine	Etidocaine	Ropivacaine
Molecular weight	236	234	246	288	276	274
pKa	8.9	7.7	7.6	8.1	7.7	8.0
Lipid solubility	1	4	1	30	140	2.8
Partition coefficient	0.02	2.9	0.8	28	141	9*
Protein binding	5	65	75	95	95	90–95
Equipotent concentration, %	2.0	2.0	1.5	0.5	1.0	0.75

*Estimated from data by Rosenberg PH, Kytta J, Alila A, et al: Absorption of bupivacaine, etidocaine, lignocaine and ropivacaine into N-heptane, rat sciatic nerve, and human extradural and subcutaneous fat. Br J Anaesth 58:310–314, 1986.

B. Ionization

1. At the end opposite the benzene ring, the LA molecules contain an amino group, and this group determines the hydrophilic activity and ionization of the molecule. This amino group is capable of accepting a hydrogen

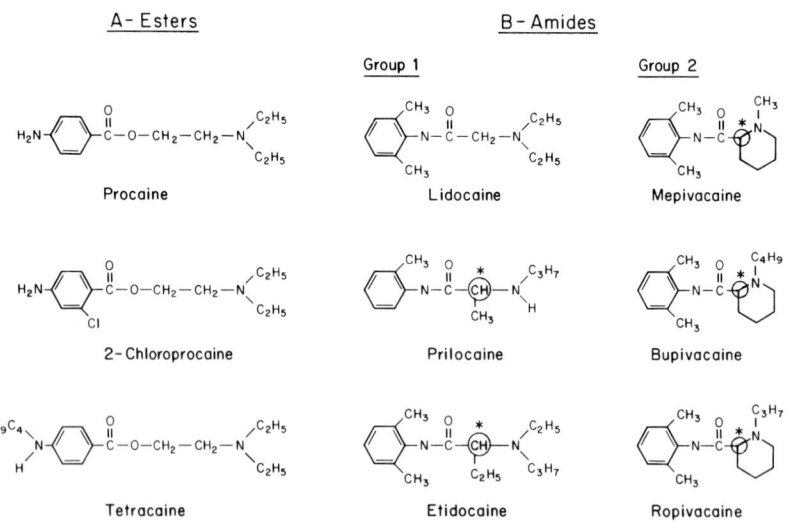

Figure 10-2 The structure of LAs. The benzene ring confers lipid solubility, while the amino group at the other end of the molecule determines hydrophilic activity and ionization of the drug. Only drugs with an asymmetric carbon atom (*) can exist as stereoisomers.

ion (H+), and in so doing, converts the un-ionized base form of the drug into the cationic form of the drug (Fig. 10-3). The proportion of each form (un-ionized base and cation) present is determined by the **pKa** of the drug, the pH of the solution, and the relationship described by the Henderson-Hasselback equation:

$$pKa = pH + \log [cation/base]$$

2. For LAs, the coexistence of the two drug forms, the charged cation and the uncharged base form, is important: it is believed that the unionized (base) form penetrates the nerve membrane and the ionized (cation) form produces blockade of sodium ion movement through the sodium channel. The LAs have a pKa greater than 7.6. The closer the pKa is to body pH, the greater is the fraction of drug present in its base form.

3. With many LAs, the **speed of onset** can be related to the degree of difference between the pKa and normal body pH. As a general rule, the lower the pKa, that is, the closer the pKa is to body pH, the shorter is the onset time for the induction of local anesthesia.

4. The LAs injected into **infected tissues** are much less effective than in normal tissue. The acidic environment of inflamed tissue causes more of the LA to be present in the ionized form, making it unable to penetrate the neuronal membrane and subsequently to block the ion channel. The same nerve may be readily blocked, however, if the LA is administered proximal to the infected area.

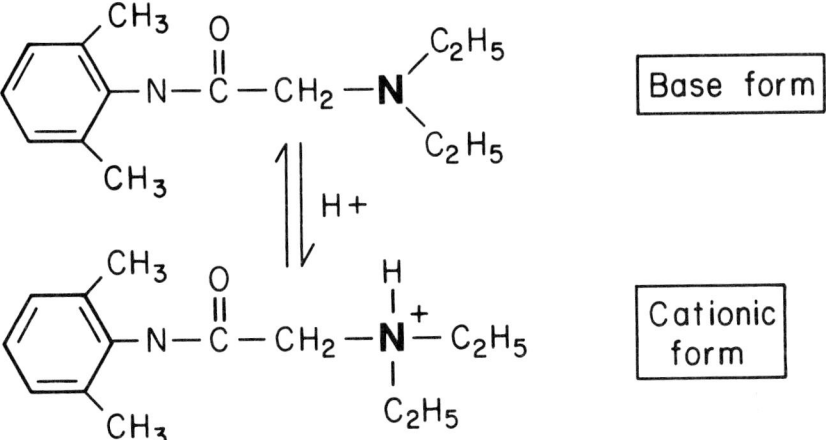

Figure 10-3 Ionization. The amino group is capable of accepting a hydrogen ion (H+), which converts the base form of the drug into the cationic form. It is the cationic form that binds to the sodium channel.

C. Protein Binding

1. Most of the LA in the body is bound to proteins (plasma and tissue). In their bound form, LAs are not pharmacologically active; therefore, the degree of protein binding has implications for the activity, toxicity, and metabolism of these drugs.

2. For LAs, the important binding proteins in plasma are **alpha$_1$-acid glycoprotein** and **albumin**. Alpha$_1$-acid glycoprotein is characterized as a high-affinity, low-capacity binding system, while the binding to albumin is characterized by low affinity and high capacity. Binding to alpha$_1$-acid glycoprotein occurs preferentially. Protein binding of LAs is also influenced by the pH of the medium in that the percentage of bound drug decreases as pH decreases. The practical importance of this is that, with the development of acidosis, the fraction of free drug increases in all compartments, and this can alter LA toxicity.

3. The fraction of drug bound to protein in plasma also correlates with the **duration** of LA activity; that is, **bupivacaine** (Marcaine) and **etidocaine** (Duranest) are 95 percent bound and slightly longer acting than **ropivacaine** (90 percent to 95 percent bound), which in turn is longer lasting than **mepivacaine** (Carbocaine, 75 percent bound), which is longer acting than **lidocaine** (Xylocaine, 65 percent bound), which in turn is longer acting than **procaine** (Novocaine) or **2-chloroprocaine** (Nesacaine), which are 5 percent bound.

D. Chiral Forms (Stereoisomers)

1. Stereoisomers of the LAs etidocaine, mepivacaine, bupivacaine, prilocaine, and ropivacaine have been recognized. For stereoisomerism to be present, an **asymmetric carbon atom** must be present in the molecule, and these asymmetric carbons are indicated in Fig. 10-2.

2. For **etidocaine**, little difference in activity or toxicity has been observed for the two respective isomers (Table 10-2). For **mepivacaine**, a longer duration of infiltration anesthesia was produced with the S isomer than with the R isomer, and little difference in toxicity between the isomers

Table 10-2 Anesthetic duration and toxicity of LA isomers*

Drug	Duration	Toxicity
Etidocaine	S = R	S = R
Mepivacaine	S > R	S = R
Bupivacaine	S > R	S < R
Ropivacaine	S > R	S < R

*S, R = isomeric forms

was observed. With **bupivacaine,** infiltration anesthesia was also of longer duration with the S isomer, and the S isomer had lower systemic toxicity as compared with the R isomer. When the isomers of **ropivacaine** were evaluated, the S isomer of the drug was found to have a longer duration of blockade and lower toxicity than its R form. Additionally, in studies of cardiac electrophysiologic toxicity, ropivacaine in the S form, at equipotent nerve blocking doses, appears to have a safety margin that is almost twice that of bupivacaine, which is a mixture of R and S isomers (i.e., racemic mixture).

III. BLOOD LEVELS AND TOXICITY

After administration, LAs either enter the nerve, get absorbed into the systemic circulation, or enter into fat surrounding the nerves. The resulting blood level is the summation of factors, including the dose of the drug administered and the absorption of the drug from the injection site (site vascularity).

A. Peak Blood Levels

Local anesthetics develop a **peak blood level** that is directly related to the dose administered at a given site. As a general rule of thumb, using lidocaine as an example, a 1 mg/kg dose given as an epidural or caudal results in approximately a 1 μg/mL peak blood level. When this dose (1 mg/kg) is used in less vascular areas, as for an axillary brachial plexus block or when this dose of drug is administered subcutaneously, a peak blood level of approximately 0.5 μg/mL occurs. In contrast, when giving lidocaine (1 mg/kg) into a highly vascular area, such as an intercostal block, approximately a 1.5 μg/mL peak blood level occurs (Fig. 10-4). It should be noted that LAs, like most drugs, can accumulate when administered as an infusion. Further, the amide LAs are almost entirely eliminated through hepatic metabolism. Thus repeated dosing or infusion of LAs should be used with caution in the patient with significant metabolic hepatic dysfunction and the patient monitored closely for early signs of systemic toxicity.

B. Systemic Toxicity

Knowledge of the potential LA blood levels is important, since **systemic toxicity is correlated with blood levels** and how rapidly they are achieved. For example, lidocaine blood levels of 1 to 5 μg/mL are considered therapeutic in the treatment of cardiac arrhythmias and as a supplement to general anesthesia. The effects of lidocaine on the brain are paradoxical. At these low blood levels, it is an anticonvulsant, whereas at elevated blood levels (10 to 12 μg/mL), the drug produces **seizures.** The signs and symptoms that appear

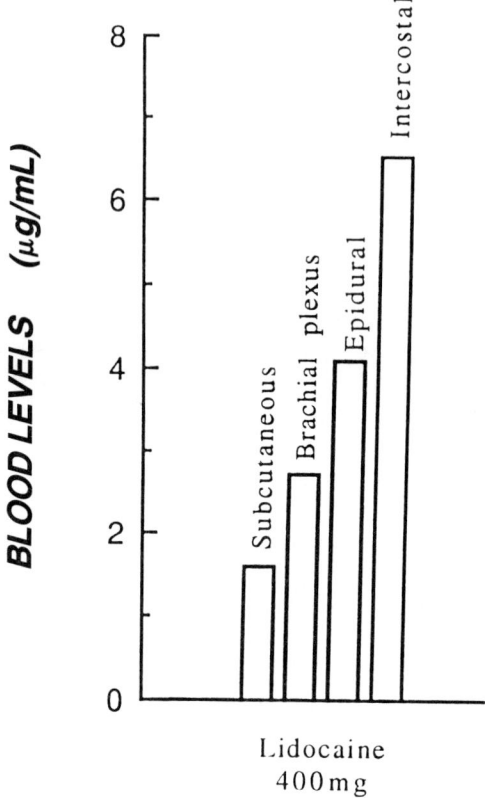

Figure 10-4 The peak blood level of LA is determined by the site of injection, as well as the dose given. The more vascular the region injected, the higher is the blood level that is achieved.

before the onset of seizures with lidocaine usually include **slow speech, jerky movements, tremors, and hallucinations.** As the peak blood level of the LA is further increased, **cardiac toxicity** becomes a concern. Lidocaine levels above 25 μg/mL are necessary for cardiac toxicity. By contrast, for bupivacaine, blood levels of approximately 4 μg/mL are associated with seizures and blood levels of approximately 6 μg/mL are associated with cardiac toxicity.

C. Treatment of LA-Induced Seizures

The treatment of LA-induced seizures consists primarily of preventing aspiration and the detrimental effects of hypoxia. Therefore, the primary concern should be adequate ventilation with 100 percent oxygen. Due to the brief nature of LA-induced seizures, usually oxygen delivered through a mask with positive pressure (e.g., self-inflating bag) suffices, but paralysis and intubation may be required. Secondarily, suppression of seizures can be achieved by raising the seizure threshold of the CNS with an intravenous dose of either thiopental (50 to 100 mg) or a benzodiazepine such as midazolam (1 to 2 mg) or diazepam (2 to 5 mg). Cardiac output and cerebral blood flow are increased during seizure activity, and hence high brain levels of LAs will rapidly dissipate with the redistribution of the drug to other tissue compartments.

D. Cardiac Toxicity

Cardiac toxicity of the long-acting LA drugs such as bupivacaine and etidocaine has been observed. Cardiac arrest with difficult, and often unsuccessful, resuscitations in obstetric patients has been the subject of a number of case reports.

1. Animal studies have provided an insight into the cardiotoxicity of the different LA agents. All LAs have been observed to cause a **dose-dependent depression of the contractility of cardiac muscle.** This cardiodepressant effect on contractility also **parallels the anesthetic potency of the LA** in blocking peripheral nerves. Therefore, bupivacaine, which is four times more potent than lidocaine in blocking peripheral nerves, is also four times more cardiodepressant with respect to contractility. Experimental studies have also shown that all LAs produce a **dose-dependent depression of conduction velocity in cardiac tissue,** including intra-atrial, A-V nodal, His-Purkinje, and intraventricular pathways. In studies that assessed the potential for producing this electrophysiologic toxicity, bupivacaine has been shown to be approximately 16 times more toxic than lidocaine. This effect is out of proportion to the anesthetic potency of the drug in blocking peripheral nerve conduction. Deaths from bupivacaine overdoses have been characterized by a progressive prolongation of ventricular conduction, a widened QRS complex, and the sudden onset of ventricular fibrillation. It has been theorized that the delay in ventricular conduction predisposes to reentrant phenomena and leads to ventricular dysrhythmias. In comparing the new LA ropivacaine with bupivacaine, bupivacaine was found to be approximately twice as toxic as ropivacaine, while bupivacaine's nerve blocking potential was essentially the same as for ropivacaine.

2. **Increased cardiac toxicity of LAs also occurs in the presence of acidosis, hypoxia, hypercarbia, or hyperkalemia.** Cardiotoxicity of the long-acting agents may also be increased in the pregnant patient.

IV. CLINICAL APPLICATIONS TO IMPROVE SAFETY

Since systemic toxicity is directly related to blood levels of LAs, the potential for producing systemic toxicity can be markedly reduced in the clinical situation by the following actions.

A. Selecting a Dose

The dose of LA selected should be associated with clinically safe blood levels based on the site of injection. As a general rule, a safe, maximum drug dose should be selected so that the peak blood concentration does not exceed one-half of the convulsant blood level. Maximum recommended doses of commonly used LA drugs are listed in Table 10-3.

B. Fractionating the Dose

The dose of drug should be administered in a manner that identifies an unintended intravascular injection by adhering to the practice of **fractionating the dose** of LA and **aspirating frequently during injection.** The addition of epinephrine in a 1:200,000 concentration to a small test dose has also been advocated for the more rapid recognition of intravascular injections.

V. MODIFICATION OF ONSET OF ACTION

To achieve neural blockade within an acceptable period, various approaches have been used to facilitate the onset of action. The LA drugs pass through the nerve membrane in the unionized, lipid-soluble base form, and within the nerve axoplasm reequilibrate with the ionic form that is active within the sodium channel. The rate-limiting step in this cascade is penetrating through the nerve membrane.

A. pH Changes

1. Marked decreases in onset time have been achieved with major pH changes in the LA solution being injected. These alterations occur most frequently when commercially available LA solutions containing epinephrine are pH adjusted. The epinephrine in the LA solutions requires a very acidic

Table 10-3 Maximum recommended doses of LAs (in mg/kg)

	Plain solution	With epinephrine	Infusions
Procaine*	7.0	10.0	--
Chloroprocaine*	10.0	15.0	--
Lidocaine†	4.0	7.0	2.0 mg/kg/h
Bupivacaine‡	2.0	2.5	0.5 mg/kg/h
Mepivacaine†	4.0	7.0	1.6 mg/kg/h

Dose may be repeated every *45 min, †1.5 h, or ‡3 h in patients with normal renal and hepatic function and *normal plasmaesterase activity.

solution for stability. Decreases of more than 50 percent in onset time for epidural anesthesia occurred when the pH of commercially available lidocaine with epinephrine with a pH of 4.5 was raised to a pH-adjusted level of 7.2.

  2. Increases in the amount of free base in solution achieved by increases in pH are limited by the solubility of the free base in solution. Attempts to increase the pH of the LA solution beyond this point do not result in a decrease in the onset time of blockade, since the saturation of the base is exceeded and a precipate forms. The amount of bicarbonate that can be added to LA solutions is shown in Table 10-4.

B. Carbonated Solutions

Another approach to shortening onset time for producing surgical anesthesia is the use of **carbonated LA solutions**. Bromage found that the spread of anesthesia was more extensive, and that a better quality of neural blockade resulted when carbonated lidocaine, rather than lidocaine hydrochloride solution, was used.

C. Warming of the Solution

Yet another technique demonstrated to modify latency is the **warming of the LA solution**. Although the exact mechanism for this change is not entirely

Table 10-4 Addition of bicarbonate to adjust pH of LA solutions

	HCO_3 (mEq/10 cc^3 LA)*	pH after HCO_3
2-Chloroprocaine 2%	1.0	7.47
3%	1.0	7.43
Mepivacaine 1%	1.0	7.27
1.5%	0.5	6.98
Bupivacaine 0.25%	0.025	6.97
0.5%	0.012	6.62
0.5% w/ epi	0.075	6.28
Lidocaine 1%	1.0	7.41
1% w/epi	1.0	7.15
1.5%	1.0	7.26
1.5% w/epi	1.0	7.09
2%	1.0	7.21
2% w/epi	1.0	7.02

*8% $NaHCO_3$ has 1 mEq/cc of HCO_3.

Adapted from Peterfreund RA, Datta S, Ostheimer G: pH adjustment of local anesthetic solutions with sodium bicarbonate: laboratory evaluation of alkalinization and precipitation. *Reg Anesth* 14(2S):74, 1989.

clear, it would appear that a major part of it is due to the increase in the pKa of the LA that occurs with increases in temperature of the solution.

VI. OPIATE-LA COMBINATIONS

There has been a great deal of interest in the use of combinations of LAs and opiates to improve the quality and duration of regional anesthesia. Onset is more rapid and anesthesia is more complete and more prolonged when opiates are added to dilute bupivacaine solutions for epidural use. Studies have shown that very dilute solutions of LA combined with an opiate produce anesthesia that is comparable to that produced by a more concentrated solution of the same LA alone. The primary benefit of LA-opiate combinations is that the dose of each drug is substantially lower than that needed if either drug is used alone. As such, the risk of side effects and/or toxicity is decreased.

SUGGESTED READINGS

Bromage PR, Burfoot MF, Crowell DE, et al: Quality of epidural blockade. III: Carbonated local anesthetic solutions. *Br J Anaesth* 39:197-208, 1967.

Carpenter RL, Mackey DC: Local anesthetics, in Barash PG, Cullen BF, Stoelting RK (eds): *Clinical Anesthesia,* 2nd ed. Philadelphia, Lippincott, Chap 20, pp 509-544, 1992.

Clarkson DW, Hondegham LM: Mechanism of bupivacaine depression of cardiac function: fast block of sodium channels during the action potential with slow recovery from block during diastole *Anesthesiology* 62:396-405, 1985.

Covino BG: Pharmacology of local anesthetic agents. *Br J Anaesth* 5:701-716, 1986.

DeJong RH: Local anesthetics, in Raj PP (ed): *Practical Management of Pain.* Chicago, Year Book Medical Publishers, Chap 31, 1986.

Denson DD, Mazoit JX: Physiology, pharmacology, and toxicity of local anesthetics: adult and pediatric considerations, in Raj PP (ed): *Clinical Practice of Regional Anesthesia.* New York, Churchill Livingstone, pp 73-105, 1991.

DiFazio CA, Carron H, Grosslight KR, et al: Comparison of pH-adjusted lidocaine solutions for epidural anesthesia. *Anesth Analg* 65:760, 1986.

Justins DM, Knott C, Luthman J, et al: Epidural versus intramuscular fentanyl: analgesia and pharmacokinetics in labour. *Anaesthesia* 38:937-942, 1982.

Reiz S, Nath S: Cardiotoxicity of local anaesthetic agents. *Br J Anaesth* 58:736-746, 1986.

Tucker GT, Mather LE: Pharmacology of local anesthetic agents. *Br J Anaesth* 47:213, 1975.

CHAPTER 11

SEDATIVES, ANXIOLYTICS, AND OTHER ADJUNCT MEDICATIONS

Marcia L. Buck

I. Benzodiazepines
   A. Indications
   B. Adverse Effects
   C. Contraindications
   D. Pharmacokinetic Parameters
   E. Common Medications
   F. Fumazenil (Mazicon)
II. Barbiturates
   A. Indications
   B. Adverse Effects
   C. Contraindications
   D. Pharmacokinetic Parameters
   E. Common Medications
III. Chloral Hydrate
   A. Indications
   B. Adverse Effects
   C. Contraindications
   D. Pharmacokinetic Parameters
   E. Administration
IV. Antihistamines and Anticholinergics
   A. Indications
   B. Adverse Effects

        C. Contraindications
        D. Common Medications
   V. Butyrophenone Tranquilizers
        A. Indications
        B. Adverse Effects
        C. Contraindications
        D. Pharmacokinetic Parameters
        E. Common Medications
  VI. Phenothiazine Tranquilizers
        A. Indications
        B. Adverse Effects
        C. Contraindications
        D. Phamacokinetic Parameters
        E. Common Medications
 VII. Tricyclic Antidepressants
        A. Indications
        B. Adverse Effects
        C. Contraindications
        D. Pharmacokinetic Parameters
        E. Common Medications
VIII. Anticonvulsants
        A. Indications
        B. Adverse Effects
        C. Common Medications
  IX. Skeletal Muscle Relaxants
        A. Indications
        B. Adverse Effects
        C. Contraindications
        D. Common Medications
Suggested Readings

Pain management often includes measures to improve sleep and relieve agitation. Sedatives, anxiolytics, and other adjunctive medications may be utilized, alone or in combination with opioids, to improve patient comfort in the intensive care unit (ICU).

I. BENZODIAZEPINES

The benzodiazepines provide both sedation and relief from agitation, as well as having anticonvulsant and indirect muscle relaxant properties. In addition, they also induce anterograde amnesia, a potential benefit in the ICU. These agents act at gamma-aminobutyric acid (GABA) receptors throughout the central nervous system (CNS), modulating the effects of this inhibitory neurotransmitter. The most frequently used agents in the acute care setting are diazepam, lorazepam, and midazolam.

A. Indications

1. Sedation for procedures Benzodiazepines are used to provide sedation during imaging procedures such as computed tomography (CT) and magnetic resonance imaging (MRI) as well as endoscopy and other diagnostic procedures.

2. Prolonged sedation Benzodiazepines have also been used to provide prolonged sedation, often during mechanical ventilation, alone or in combination with analgesics. Patients requiring the use of neuromuscular blocking agents to facilitate ventilation *must* receive adequate sedation, and benzodiazepines are often used for this purpose.

B. Adverse Effects

1. Adverse CNS effects include excessive sedation, ataxia, confusion, and dizziness, which typically occur with initial doses and diminish as tolerance develops with continued therapy. The critically ill patient is at greater risk for adverse CNS effects, since a reduction in renal or hepatic function increases the potential for drug accumulation.

2. Paradoxical excitation may occur in some patients, manifesting itself with irritability, agitation, anxiety, auditory and visual hallucinations, or hostility. A decrease in dose or the use of an alternative agent may be necessary. Excitation occurs most frequently in children, elderly patients, and those with reduced elimination capability.

3. Respiratory depression may occur with the rapid administration of large doses of benzodiazepine. These agents cause a decrease in both tidal volume and respiratory rate. Elderly patients and those with chronic pulmonary disorders are at greatest risk. Assurance of adequate ventilatory function or assistance is necessary prior to initiating benzodiazepine therapy.

4. Cardiovascular effects are generally minimal, but may be more pronounced in the critically ill. Hypotension and bradycardia are most commonly reported. Both respiratory and cardiovascular adverse effects may be solely the result of benzodiazepine-induced physiologic depression, but may also be related to the rapid intravenous (IV) administration of products which contain propylene glycol as a vehicle. These products must be given slowly to prevent toxicity (see below).

5. Other adverse effects associated with benzodiazepine use include blurred vision, myalgias, nausea and hiccups, constipation, changes in urination patterns, urticaria, rash, photosensitivity, and thrombophlebitis.

C. Contraindications

Benzodiazepines do *not* provide analgesia, and thus are contraindicated as a single-agent therapy in patients who are experiencing pain. A reduction of dose is needed in elderly patients or in patients with impaired hepatic or renal function due to the potential for reduced serum protein binding and accumulation of drug and active metabolites.

D. Pharmacokinetic Parameters

Benzodiazepines are available in a variety of dosage forms. They are well absorbed after oral administration and quickly distribute into the CNS (Table 11-1). The duration of effect is related to redistribution out of the CNS. All benzodiazepines are metabolized in the liver, with some agents producing pharmacologically active metabolites. Diazepam has the disadvantage of producing several metabolites with long elimination half-lives. Midazolam produces an active metabolite with an elimination half-life of 1 h.

E. Common Medications

1. Diazepam (Valium) Diazepam has a long history of use in the ICU, although it has been replaced by lorazepam and midazolam. It may be administered by a number of routes, but in the ICU, it is most frequently given IV. A dose of 2 to 5 mg may be administered for moderate anxiety and 5 to 10 mg for severe anxiety every 3 or 4 h, depending on patient response. In acute situations, diazepam may be administered every hour. Diazepam products contain propylene glycol and should be administered no faster than 5 mg/min.

2. Lorazepam (Ativan) Lorazepam is frequently utilized in combination with haloperidol for treatment of the severely agitated, delirious patient. Like diazepam, lorazepam may be administered by oral, intramuscular (IM), and IV routes. Dosing requirements depend on the degree of agitation. Doses of 2 to 4 mg (0.05 mg/kg) IM or of 0.5 to 1 mg IV may be administered as frequently as every hour, until adequate sedation is achieved. Maintenance doses are usually required every 4 to 6 h. The recommended maximum for a single dose is 4 mg to avoid respiratory depression, although the

Table 11-1 Benzodiazepine pharmacokinetic characteristics

Medication	Onset, min*	Duration, h	$t_{1/2}$, h
Diazepam	1–2	0.25–1	20–50
Lorazepam	1–5	12–24	10–20
Midazolam	1–2	1–2	1.5–3.5

*IV administration; $t_{1/2}$ = elimination half-life.

safe use of higher doses with appropriate management of ventilation has been reported in the literature. Repeated doses may be increased until sedation has been achieved. In cases of severe agitation, doses as high as 240 mg have been given over a 24-h period. Lorazepam products contain propylene glycol and should be administered at a rate no faster than 2 mg/min.

   3. **Midazolam (Versed)** Although only recently marketed, midazolam has become widely used due to its short duration of action, which allows a rapid titration of dose to patient response. Although midazolam is available only in an injectable form, it has also been administered orally, rectally, and intranasally. The most common route of administration for prolonged sedation is by continuous IV infusion. This method should be used with caution, however, due to the potential for accumulation of drug and metabolite in critically ill patients. Accumulation is observed more frequently in patients with impaired hepatic or renal function, obese patients, and the elderly. A 5 to 10 mg loading dose may be infused over 10 to 20 min, followed by an infusion starting at 0.1 mg/kg/h. The IV midazolam products do not contain propylene glycol.

F. Flumazenil (Mazicon)

   1. Recently, a specific **benzodiazepine antagonist** has become available. However, the role of flumazenil in acute care is still controversial. It may be beneficial in those cases where inadvertent administration of an excessive dose has occurred or when rapid reversal of sedation is necessary. A dose of 0.2 mg may be administered over 15 s to reverse the effects of midazolam.

   2. Flumazenil is a competitive antagonist and must be present for a duration longer than that of the benzodiazepines. Repeated doses of 0.2 mg may be given every 60 s, to a total dose of 1 mg. Flumazenil should be used with caution in patients who are physically dependent on benzodiazepines due to the **potential to induce withdrawal and** in patients who may be prone to **seizures** after the anticonvulsant properties of the benzodiazepine have been reversed.

II. BARBITURATES

The barbiturates provide sedation by inducing a generalized depression of CNS function. The exact mechanism remains unknown. It has been proposed that these agents act by inhibiting oxidative phosphorylation, resulting in a decrease in adenosine triphosphate (ATP) function and a slowing of CNS activity.

A. Indications

1. Sedation Barbiturates no longer are standard therapy for sedation in critically ill patients. Their dose-limiting adverse effects and hyperalgesic properties prevent them from being useful in many patients. They may, however, play a role in combination therapy or in regimens utilizing alternating sedatives.

2. Barbiturate coma This may be used in the patient with severe head injury to avoid unwanted increases in intracranial pressure (ICP). This treatment is reserved for patients refractory to standard therapies, such as hyperventilation and mannitol administration. Barbiturates decrease cerebral oxygen consumption and increase cerebrovascular tone, resulting in a reduction of cerebral blood flow. Agents with a short duration of action, such as pentobarbital and thiopental, allow ease of dose titration.

B. Adverse Effects

1. With regard to **CNS effects,** barbiturates may cause excessive sedation, dizziness, and headache. Paradoxical excitation, similar to that described with benzodiazepines, may occur.

2. Respiratory depression is associated with high-dose therapy and reflects the general CNS depression induced by barbiturates. Depth of respiration is affected, with little change in respiratory rate.

3. With regard to **cardiovascular effects,** barbiturates may induce direct cardiovascular depression, as well as increase venous compliance, resulting in venous stasis. Thiopental may produce profound hypotension and reduce cardiac output from 10 to 35 percent with moderate doses and up to 50 percent with larger doses. Reflex tachycardia and other compensatory mechanisms may minimize the clinical significance of this effect. The IV preparations of some barbiturates contain propylene glycol, and the same cautions discussed with benzodiazepines apply.

4. Other adverse effects may include hypersensitivity reactions, adverse gastrointestinal (GI) effects, elevated serum ammonia concentrations, and thrombocytopenic purpura.

C. Contraindications

Barbiturates increase sensitivity to pain and should not be used as single-agent therapy in patients experiencing pain. These agents are eliminated via hepatic metabolism through the cytochrome P450 enzyme system and should be used with caution in patients with impaired hepatic function. In addition, a number of potential drug interactions with medications also dependent on the hepatic cytochrome P450 enzyme system for elimination are possible. Barbiturates induce this metabolic system and may increase the elimination of other drugs.

D. Pharmacokinetic Parameters

Barbiturates may be administered by oral, rectal, or parenteral routes. Distribution to the brain is rapid and duration is dependent on redistribution from the CNS to other highly vascular tissues, such as the heart and kidneys (Table 11-2). Barbiturates are metabolized to inactive compounds by the liver prior to excretion. The rate of elimination varies considerably within this class of drugs, and may vary depending upon the method of administration. Studies performed during pentobarbital-induced coma have shown an increased clearance rate as compared with single-dose studies, possibly the result of induction of metabolic pathways.

E. Common Medications

1. Phenobarbital (Luminal) Although better known as an anticonvulsant, phenobarbital may also be useful for periodic sedation. A typical oral dose for sedation with phenobarbital is 15 to 30 mg daily. Higher doses may be needed, based on patient response. Phenobarbital may also be administered IV, but the rate of infusion should not exceed 2 mg/kg/min.

2. Secobarbital (Seconal) For preoperative or procedural sedation, the usual oral dose of secobarbital is 100 to 300 mg, administered 1 to 2 h prior to the procedure. For agitation, a dose of 30 to 50 mg may be given IV. Additional doses may be given at 5-min intervals, to a maximum of 500 mg.

Table 11-2 Barbiturate pharmacokinetic characteristics

Medication	Onset*	Duration	$t_{1/2}$
Phenobarbital	IV 5 min PO/PR 20–60 min	10–12 h	2–6 days
Secobarbital	PO/PR 15–30 min IM 7–10 min IV 1–3 min	3–4 h	30 h
Pentobarbital	PO/PR 15–60 min IM 10–20 min IV 1 min	3–4 h	15–50 h
Thiopental	PR 10 min IV 30–40 s	20–30 min	3–8 h
Methohexital	PR 10 min IV 1 min	20 min	3–8 h

*PO/PR oral or rectal routes; IM intramuscular; IV intravenous.

3. Pentobarbital (Nembutal) To treat severely agitated patients, pentobarbital is administered IV at a dose of 100 mg, with supplemental doses given after 1 min to a total of 200 to 500 mg. A concentration of 50 mg/mL may be given, at a rate no faster than 50 mg/min. To induce barbiturate coma, a loading dose of 5 to 35 mg/kg may be given over 10 to 20 min, followed by the infusion of 1 to 4 mg/kg/h or intermittent doses of 3 to 4 mg/kg every 3 to 4 h. Higher loading doses (20 to 35 mg/kg) have been used to produce therapeutic concentrations of 25 to 40 μg/mL within 2 to 3 h.

4. Thiopental (Pentothal) Thiopental may be administered rectally or IV. To provide sedation, 25 mg/kg of the rectal suspension may be used. The maximum dose recommended is 4 g. Doses of 25 to 50 mg IV may be given every 20 to 40 s until adequate sedation or CNS depression is achieved. For the control of an agitated patient, a loading dose of 2 to 5 mg/kg has been recommended, followed by a continuous infusion of 1 to 5 mg/kg/h. Additional bolus doses of 50 to 100 mg may be given if the degree of sedation is inadequate. Serum thiopental concentrations of 10 to 20 μg/mL are associated with adequate sedation. To induce barbiturate coma, a loading dose of 20 mg/kg should be given over one h, followed by an infusion of 3 to 10 mg/kg/h. *Accumulation of thiopental should be anticipated;* a period of 2 to 3 days following discontinuation of therapy may be needed for the patient fully to regain consciousness.

5. Methohexital (Brevital) Another ultrashort-acting barbiturate, methohexital may be used to provide sedation. In children, doses of 0.5 to 5 mg/kg may be administered IV or 20 to 35 mg/kg may be given rectally using a 10% solution. Rectal dosing, although more difficult to administer, is advantageous in patients in whom IV access is limited. Adults usually respond well to incremental doses of 0.25 to 1.0 mg/kg.

III. CHLORAL HYDRATE

Although its specific mechanism of action remains unknown, chloral hydrate (Noctec) appears to induce a general depression of CNS function, similar to barbiturates.

A. Indications

Chloral hydrate is useful for short-term administration. The relative lack of adverse respiratory and cardiovascular effects associated with routine dose administration makes chloral hydrate beneficial in unstable patients who might not tolerate benzodiazepines or barbiturates.

B. Adverse Effects

1. With regard to **CNS effects,** excessive or prolonged sedation may result from the use of high doses or long-term administration. Paradoxical excitation may also occur. Headache, dizziness, ataxia, hallucinations, and malaise have been reported in rare cases.

2. The lack of adverse **cardiovascular effects,** as described above, is an advantage of chloral hydrate use. Both supraventricular and ventricular arrhythmias have been reported, usually following the ingestion of toxic quantities. Lidocaine, phenytoin, or beta-adrenergic blocking agents have proved effective treatment in these cases.

3. Among **GI effects,** nausea and vomiting may be present in up to 5 percent of patients receiving chloral hydrate. Its bitter taste and hyperosmolar concentration may play a role in this regard. More severe adverse effects, including hemorrhage, necrosis, and perforation of the stomach, have also been reported.

4. **Other adverse effects** include rash, leukopenia, eosinophilia, ketonuria, and isolated cases of apnea and laryngospasm.

C. Contraindications

Chloral hydrate should not be used in patients with significant hepatic impairment. Pharmacologic activity depends on conversion of chloral hydrate to trichloroethanol by alcohol dehydrogenase, primarily in the liver. In addition, accumulation may occur in patients with impaired renal function.

D. Pharmacokinetic Parameters

Chloral hydrate is rapidly absorbed following oral or rectal administration. Sedation occurs within 30 min to 1 h and lasts approximately 4 to 8 h in adults. It is believed that the sedative activity of chloral hydrate is due to the **trichloroethanol metabolite,** rather than to the parent compound. Trichloroethanol has an elimination half-life of 8 to 11 h in adults.

E. Administration

When administered orally, the dose should be diluted or given with liquids. Oral administration is not recommended in patients with oral or gastric lesions. The solution may also be given rectally, mixed with olive oil, as a retention enema. Rectal suppositories are also available. The dose by either route is 250 mg to 1 g and may be repeated every 6 to 8 h as needed. Again, the clinician is reminded of the long half-life of trichloroethanol and the potential for drug accumulation with repeated dose administration.

IV. ANTIHISTAMINES AND ANTICHOLINERGICS

Antihistamines act by competitive inhibition at histamine H_1 receptors, blocking histamine release. Many antihistamines also possess anticholinergic activity and may be used to produce sedation in the critically ill. Anticholinergics such as scopolamine may also be utilized. Unlike atropine, scopolamine possesses significant CNS depressant effects.

A. Indications

These agents may be used for periodic sedation. They are low-potency agents and are often used in conjunction with other therapies. Their beneficial effects are frequently outweighed by their adverse effects.

B. Adverse Effects

1. Additional effects on the CNS account for many of the adverse effects of this group. Excessive sedation, dizziness, blurred vision, ataxia, headaches, and muscle weakness may occur with antihistamine use. Repeated use frequently results in tolerance to these adverse effects, as well as the beneficial sedative effects. Paradoxical excitation may occur, resulting in symptoms of restlessness, insomnia, tremors, delirium, and possibly seizures. Respiratory depression secondary to generalized CNS depression may occur with the administration of large doses.

2. **Cardiovascular effects,** including hypotension, hypertension, tachycardia, and other arrhythmias, have been reported with antihistamine use, but the overall incidence is low.

3. **Other adverse effects** include nausea, vomiting, changes in bowel habits, hypersensitivity, flushing, dryness of the mouth, dysuria, urinary retention, impotence, vertigo, blurred vision, and tinnitus.

C. Contraindications

Anticholinergics, as well as antihistamines with pronounced anticholinergic activity, should be used with caution in patients with angle-closure glaucoma, cardiovascular instability, difficulty with urination, or myasthenia gravis.

D. Common Medications

1. **Hydroxyzine (Atarax)** Hydroxyzine has both antihistaminic and anticholinergic properties, producing sedation and an anxiolytic effect, but little, if any, analgesic activity.

a. Pharmacokinetic parameters Hydroxyzine may be administered orally or parenterally. The onset of action following oral administration occurs in 15 to 30 min. Sedative effects last for 4 to 6 h following a single dose. Little is known about the pharmacokinetic characteristics of this agent. Hydroxyzine appears to undergo hepatic metabolism, with excretion of metabolites taking place in the feces and bile.

b. Administration To provide sedation and anxiolytic effects, a dose of 50 to 100 mg may be administered by oral or IM routes every 4 to 6 h. Although not recommended, hydroxyzine may be given IV, diluted to 50 mL and administered over at least 4 to 5 min. Its IV administration has been associated with an increased incidence of hypotension, tachycardia, and hemolysis.

2. Diphenhydramine (Benadryl) When a mild agent is desired, diphenhydramine has also been utilized for sedation.

a. Pharmacokinetic parameters Diphenhydramine is available for both oral and parenteral administration. Although well absorbed following oral administration, it undergoes extensive first-pass metabolism, reducing oral bioavailability to 40 to 60 percent. Peak concentrations occur 1 to 4 h following an oral dose. Diphenhydramine is extensively metabolized; less than 1 percent is excreted as unchanged drug. The elimination half-life in adults has been estimated at 2 to 10 h.

b. Administration Diphenhydramine is typically administered by parenteral routes in the ICU. The usual IM or IV dose is 10 to 50 mg q 2 to 4 h, although doses as high as 100 mg may be required. The recommended maximum daily dose is 400 mg.

3. Scopolamine Like the antihistamines, scopolamine may be useful as a mild sedative or as adjunctive therapy. However, there have been few published reports of its use in the acute care setting.

a. Pharmacokinetic parameters Scopolamine may be administered by a variety of routes. Sedation occurs within 10 min of IV administration and lasts for 1 to 2 h. Scopolamine is metabolized in the liver, with less than 5 percent excreted unchanged in the urine.

b. Administration The usual parenteral dose of scopolamine is 0.3 to 0.65 mg given every 6 to 8 h. Higher doses may be required to achieve adequate sedation in some patients.

V. BUTYROPHENONE TRANQUILIZERS

Haloperidol and droperidol are members of a class commonly referred to as major tranquilizers. The mechanism of action of these agents is still unclear, but involves blockade of dopaminergic receptors, resulting in CNS depression at the subcortical level of the brain. Haloperidol and droperidol also inhibit the chemoreceptor trigger zone in the CNS, providing antiemetic effects.

A. Indications

These agents are indicated for the agitated, delirious patient who fails to respond adequately to nonpharmacologic methods or other sedatives. Butyrophenone use in the ICU has been well documented and offers the advantages of limited respiratory effects and little potential for the development of tolerance or dependence.

B. Adverse Effects

1. **The CNS effects** of drowsiness, lethargy, changes in sleep patterns, and, in some cases, extrapyramidal (Parkinsonian) reactions such as akathesia and dystonia may occur following haloperidol or droperidol use. These effects typically are seen early in therapy and resolve with dose reduction or withdrawal of therapy. Administration of an anticholinergic agent such as diphenhydramine (see above) or benztropine (1 to 2 mg IV or IM) may also be used to relieve symptoms. Extrapyramidal symptoms seldom occur with IV haloperidol. The reason for this is unknown, but it may involve the concurrent use of lorazepam, which possesses a minor degree of anticholinergic activity.

2. **Neuroleptic malignant syndrome (NMS)** may be seen with butyrophenone use and result in hyperthermia, severe extrapyramidal reactions, altered mental status, and autonomic instability. The syndrome is rare, but can be fatal. It is not dose related. Treatment involves supportive care and the administration of dantrolene, a muscle relaxant (see dosing guidelines under "Dantrolene") and bromocriptine, a dopamine antagonist (5 to 10 mg PO every 8 h).

3. **Cardiovascular effects** include hypotension, which may occur with haloperidol use, but is more common with droperidol, due to its greater alpha-adrenergic antagonism. Hypovolemic patients are more susceptible to this adverse effect. In rare cases, arrhythmias have occurred with butyrophenone use.

4. **Other adverse effects** include excessive anticholinergic effects, laryngospasm, bronchospasm, blood dyscrasias, and, in rare cases, endocrine and metabolic effects.

C. Contraindications

These agents should be used with caution in patients with cardiovascular instability. Butyrophenones may also lower the seizure threshold and should be used with caution in those patients with a history of seizures or abnormal electroencephalogram (EEG) activity. These agents are contraindicated in comatose patients and patients with Parkinson's disease.

D. Pharmacokinetic Parameters

Haloperidol may be given by oral or parenteral routes. Droperidol is available only in injectable form. Both agents are well absorbed, although haloperidol undergoes extensive first-pass metabolism, resulting in a bioavailability of 60 percent (Table 11-3). Peak haloperidol concentrations after oral dosing may not result for 2 to 6 h, making this route inappropriate for most acute situations. Both agents are metabolized by the liver and excreted in urine and bile. Haloperidol is converted to hydroxyhaloperidol, which may possess pharmacologic activity.

E. Common Medications

1. Haloperidol (Haldol) Given alone or with a benzodiazepine or opioid, haloperidol is one of the most frequently utilized agents in the ICU to treat the agitated patient. It is frequently administered IV, although this route has not been approved by the Food and Drug Administration. Doses utilized in the ICU are based on the level of delirium: 0.5 to 2 mg for mild agitation, 2 to 5 mg for moderate agitation, and 10 to 20 mg for severe agitation. These doses may be repeated at 20 to 30 min intervals until the desired level of calmness is reached. Frequently the repeated dose is twice the initial amount.

There has been much controversy over the appropriate dosing regimen, with some authors reporting success with extremely high-dose therapy (up to 150 mg as a single dose or 945 mg in 24 h). In severe cases, the use of a continuous infusion has been reported to be successful, beginning at 15 mg/h and titrating to response. After control has been achieved, doses of 0.5 to

Table 11-3 Butyrophenone pharmacokinetic characteristics

Medication	Onset, min*	Duration, h	$t_{1/2}$, h
Haloperidol	10–30	6–12	12–38
Droperidol	3–10	2–4	2–3

*IV administration.

3 mg are given every 6 to 24 h, depending on the recurrence of symptoms. Therapy is usually tapered over 2 to 5 days before being discontinued.

2. Droperidol (Inapsine) Droperidol is used more often as a component of anesthesia or to provide antiemetic effects during the administration of chemotherapy or after surgery. It produces more sedation than haloperidol does, and is associated with a greater incidence of adverse effects. As an adjunct to opioid therapy, droperidol may be administered at a dose of up to .25 mg/kg given IV or IM every 4 h. As a sedative for short procedures, IV doses of 2.5 to 10.0 mg have been given 30 min prior to the procedure.

VI. PHENOTHIAZINE TRANQUILIZERS

Like the butyrophenone tranquilizers, phenothiazines primarily exert their effects by blocking dopamine-mediated nerve transmission, resulting in a reduction in agitation and restlessness. These agents also possess antihistaminic properties.

A. Indications

Phenothiazines are used infrequently in critically ill patients. Their utility as sedative/anxiolytics has been surpassed by newer, shorter-acting agents.

B. Adverse Effects

Hypotension is the most frequent dose-limiting adverse effect seen in the acute care setting. There are numerous adverse effects associated with phenothiazine use, including those described for butyrophenones (see above), as well as agranulocytosis, dermatoses, photosensitivity, ocular changes, adverse GI effects, and hypersensitivity reactions.

C. Contraindications

The cautions associated with butyrophenone use also apply to the phenothiazines, primarily cardiovascular instability and lowering of the seizure threshold. In addition, phenothiazines should be used with caution in patients with impaired hepatic or renal function.

D. Pharmacokinetic Parameters

Although the phenothiazines have been available for many years, little information can be found on their pharmacokinetic characteristics. All are fully absorbed, although somewhat erratically, and are metabolized by the liver. Elimination half-lives range from 10 to 20 h in adults. Some metabolites have pharmacologic activity. The parent drug and metabolites are excreted in urine and bile.

E. Common Medications

1. Chlorpromazine (Thorazine) Although the first widely used medication for the treatment of delirium, chlorpromazine is now only rarely utilized for this purpose. Doses of 25 to 50 mg IM may be given, followed by repeat dosing at 1 h. Severe cases may require doses up to 400 mg every 4–6 h. Doses of 2 mg IV may be given at 2-min intervals, up to 25 mg or until the desired level of sedation is achieved.

2. Prochlorperazine (Compazine) Prochlorperazine bears a great similarity to chlorpromazine. It is effective treatment for agitation and delirium, but is rarely used due to the high incidence of extrapyramidal symptoms associated with it. Prochlorperazine may be administered by oral or IM routes, with the latter method used in the acute care setting. For prompt control of agitation, 10 to 20 mg may be given. Repeat dosing may be necessary within 1 to 4 h. If prolonged therapy is desired, doses of 10 to 20 mg every 4 to 6 h have been recommended.

3. Promethazine (Phenergan) is used for both its sedative and anticholinergic properties. Unlike chlorpromazine and prochlorperazine, it has virtually no antipsychotic properties. When administered for sedation, the standard adult dose of promethazine is 25 to 50 mg. Additional doses may be given at intervals of 4 h, if needed. When administered IV, promethazine should be given at a rate no greater than 25 mg/min to avoid irritation.

VII. TRICYCLIC ANTIDEPRESSANTS

The tricyclic antidepressants act by blocking the reuptake of neurotransmitters at the neuronal membrane, thereby potentiating their activity. Most important, they block the reuptake of serotonin and norepinephrine, key neurotransmitters that may be reduced in depression and chronic pain. Although any agent in this group may be effective, amitriptyline and doxepin have been more widely reported in the medical literature.

A. Indications

Antidepressants may be useful both in those patients who develop depression during a prolonged illness and in some patients with chronic pain. A variety of benign and malignant pain syndromes have been shown to respond to antidepressant therapy, with success rates from 40 to 70 percent. It has been suggested that the mechanism for this improvement is multifactorial, including raising the pain threshold, allowing improved sleep, and altering the perception of pain. When utilized for the treatment of pain, these agents are frequently used in combination with nonsteroidal antiinflammatory agents or opioids. Although these agents have not been studied in the acute pain setting, low doses given at bedtime should provide the same benefits seen with chronic pain: an improved sleep pattern and a higher pain threshold, while avoiding the emotional depression that can be seen with long-term benzodiazepine use.

B. Adverse Effects

1. Anticholinergic effects The most common adverse effects are those related to excessive anticholinergic activity, such as dry mucous membranes, blurred vision, increased intraocular pressure, urinary retention, hyperthermia, and constipation. These agents may reduce esophageal sphincter tone, resulting in gastroesophageal reflux. Amitriptyline possesses more anticholinergic activity than doxepin.

2. Adverse CNS effects may also occur, including excessive sedation, weakness, lethargy, and fatigue. A paradoxical excitation or worsening of depression may take place. Seizures may result from toxic tricyclic antidepressant ingestions. Patients should be closely monitored while receiving therapy. As with tranquilizers, these agents may cause the development of extrapyramidal symptoms or NMS.

3. In the **cardiovascular system,** all of these agents are capable of producing arrhythmias by prolonging ventricular depolarization similar to the effect of quinidine. Hypokalemia and hypomagnesemia may predispose patients to arrhythmias. In addition, the anticholinergic effects of these agents may cause hypotension and reflex tachycardia.

4. Other effects include respiratory depression, which may result with excessive doses. Other, less frequent adverse effects include hematologic disturbances, transient elevation in serum transaminase levels, jaundice, hepatitis, and hypersensitivity reactions, as well as adverse GI and endocrine effects.

C. Contraindications

Tricyclic antidepressants are contraindicated in patients with cardiovascular instability, including patients with recent myocardial infarction. The contraindications to anticholinergic administration also apply to these agents.

D. Pharmacokinetic Parameters

Amitriptyline is available for both oral and parenteral administration. Doxepin is available for oral use only. These agents are well absorbed and widely distributed throughout the tissues (Table 11-4). They are metabolized by the liver, producing active metabolites.

E. Common Medications

1. Amitriptyline (Elavil) Amitriptyline therapy for the treatment of depression or the management of pain must be titrated to individual patient response. Starting doses of 75 to 100 mg PO have been suggested for the treatment of depression. The daily dose can be divided; however, it is often preferable to give a single dose at bedtime to avoid unwanted daytime sedation. Peak antidepressant effects generally are not seen until after 2 weeks or more of therapy; however, improvement in sleep patterns may take place sooner. Lower doses are often used initially in the treatment of pain, starting at 10 to 25 mg at bedtime and titrating to patient response. Doses up to 150 mg have been required in some patients.

2. Doxepin (Adapin) Doxepin is administered orally, in a single daily dose, for either antidepressant or analgesic effects. The initial analgesic dose should be low, 30 to 50 mg/day, and titrated upward based on patient response. The maximum single dose recommended is 150 mg; however, some patients may require up to 300 mg/day given in divided doses.

VIII. ANTICONVULSANTS

Several commonly used anticonvulsants possess analgesic properties. Although the mechanism is not well understood, these agents provide stabilization of neuronal membranes and block pain transmission.

Table 11-4 Tricyclic antidepressant pharmacokinetic characteristics

Medication	Peak, h*	$t_{1/2}$, h
Amitriptyline	2–12	10–50
Doxepin	2	6–8

*Time to peak serum concentration.

A. Indications

Anticonvulsants have proved useful in the management of a number of types of neuralgic pain. These agents have been found to be effective treatment for pain associated with trauma, laminectomy, lancinating pain, and amputation (phantom limb pain syndrome), as well as pain associated with malignant and diabetic neuropathies, trigeminal neuralgia, and scleroderma. Anticonvulsants may also be used to treat thalamic (central) pain, reflex sympathetic dystrophy, and dysesthetic pain following spinal cord injury.

B. Adverse Effects

All agents described in this section may cause adverse GI effects, blood dyscrasias, and CNS effects, such as drowsiness, dizziness, ataxia, and vision difficulties. Phenytoin use has been associated with gingival hyperplasia, hypertrichosis, rash, Stevens-Johnson syndrome, lymphadenopathy, and osteomalacia. The IV products contain propylene glycol (refer to "Benzodiazepines"). Carbamazepine may also cause agranulocytosis, adverse cardiovascular and neurologic effects, hepatic and renal complications, and hypersensitivity reactions. Valproic acid use has been associated with adverse hepatic effects, including rare, idiosyncratic fatal hepatitis. All of these agents rely on hepatic metabolism for elimination. Impairment of hepatic function may allow drug accumulation and lead to toxicity.

C. Common Medications

1. Phenytoin (Dilantin) One study has shown phenytoin to be effective in approximately 20 to 40 percent of patients with neuralgic pain. The limiting factor for phenytoin is its adverse side-effects profile.

a. Pharmacokinetic parameters Phenytoin is available for both IV and oral use. Bioavailability varies with the products used. Phenytoin is highly protein bound; free drug may be increased in patients with reduced serum protein concentrations. Phenytoin is metabolized in the liver to inactive metabolites by a nonlinear process (Michaelis-Menten pharmacokinetics). Elimination "half-life" varies greatly, with an average of 20 to 24 h.

b. Administration Phenytoin dosing is correlated to serum phenytoin concentrations. Serum drug concentrations greater than 20 μg/mL are associated with a higher incidence of adverse effects. Most patients will respond at serum concentrations between 15 and 20 µg/mL. Therapy may be initiated with a dose of 100 mg every 8 to 12 h.

2. Carbamazepine (Tegretol) Carbamazepine is believed to act by inhibiting polysynaptic reflex activity and blocking potentiation of nerve transmission at the spinal cord.

a. Pharmacokinetic parameters Carbamazepine is administered orally; peak serum concentrations occur 2 to 8 h following a dose. Carbamazepine is metabolized through the cytochrome P450 enzyme system and induces its own metabolism. Maximum autoinduction occurs at 17 to 31 days, after which the rate of metabolism is relatively stable. While the initial elimination half-life is typically 25 to 65 h, after repeated dosing, it may be as short as 12 to 17 h. This period of autoinduction must be considered when initiating therapy. One of the metabolites, carbamazepine-10,11-epoxide, appears to possess both anticonvulsant and analgesic activity.

b. Administration Doses for the treatment of pain with tablets generally begin at 100 mg every 8 to 12 h; use of the suspension requires more frequent dosing (i.e., 50 mg every 6 h). Doses are then increased until relief is achieved. A maximum daily dose of 1200 mg has been suggested, since higher doses do not appear to elicit any additional benefit. The effective serum concentration for analgesic effect appears to be similar to the established anticonvulsant therapeutic range of 4 to 12 µg/mL. Drowsiness and ataxia begin at serum concentrations greater than 10 µg/mL.

3. Valproic Acid (Depakene) Although less information is available on its use as an analgesic, valproic acid may also provide relief for some patients, particularly in phantom limb pain syndromes.

a. Pharmacokinetic parameters Valproic acid is available for oral administration as an acid in the sodium salt form. The salt rapidly converts to free acid in the stomach. Peak serum concentrations are reached in 1 to 4 h. Divalproex sodium, a delayed-release formulation which peaks in 3 to 5 h, is also available. Valproic acid is metabolized in the liver to a number of inactive metabolites. The elimination half-life of valproic acid is 5 to 20 h.

b. Administration The initial dose of valproic acid is 15 mg/kg/day, in two or more divided doses. Doses must be titrated to patient response. Patients usually respond at doses lower than those required to achieve therapeutic anticonvulsant serum concentrations of 50 to 150 µg/mL.

IX. SKELETAL MUSCLE RELAXANTS

These relaxants should be used only as adjunctive therapy in the critically ill. They do *not* provide analgesia or adequate sedation for patients. They may, however, lessen the need for high doses of other agents.

A. Indications

Muscle relaxants are indicated for musculoskeletal pain and the treatment of muscle spasms that may result in pain or discomfort, or be counterproductive to physical therapy.

B. Adverse Effects

The adverse effects most commonly seen with these agents include drowsiness, dizziness, ataxia, tremor, headache, and changes in temperament. These effects are usually transient and resolve with continued therapy. In addition, rash, hypotension, dyspnea, chest pain, and syncope may occur. Both baclofen and cyclobenzaprine may have adverse GI effects, including nausea, vomiting, altered taste, constipation or diarrhea, anorexia, and abdominal pain. Dantrolene use has been associated with hepatitis, but this idiosyncratic reaction is rare. Females, patients taking estrogens, and patients more than 35 years of age are at higher risk. An elevation in serum bilirubin may be a beneficial marker for predicting hepatic injury from dantrolene.

C. Contraindications

These agents are contraindicated in patients where spasticity is necessary to maintain function (e.g., some patients with cerebral palsy), or in cases of cardiovascular instability or hypersensitivity to the drugs. Muscle relaxants should be used with caution in patients with seizure disorders, as they may mask or worsen the condition. A reduction in dose is necessary in patients with renal or hepatic dysfunction.

D. Common Medications

  1. **Baclofen (Lioresal)** Baclofen may be useful in patients with a variety of underlying causes of spasticity, including spinal cord and head injuries, multiple sclerosis, and cerebral palsy. In addition, baclofen has been shown to be effective in patients with some types of neurogenic pain. The mechanism of action is not well understood; primary activity occurs at the spinal cord level. Baclofen, a derivative of GABA, blocks afferent nerve pathways and may act as an inhibitory neurotransmitter.

a. Pharmacokinetic parameters Baclofen is well absorbed after oral administration, with peak serum concentrations occurring within 2 to 3 h. Most of the drug is excreted unchanged in the urine; less than 20 percent is metabolized. The elimination half-life of baclofen is 2 to 4 h.

b. Administration An initial dose of 5 mg given every 8 h has been recommended. The daily dose may be increased by 15 mg/day every 3 to 5 days until beneficial effects are seen. Optimal effects may not be observed for several weeks. Most patients will respond to doses of 40 to 80 mg daily. In those patients who fail to respond to oral therapy, an injectable form for intrathecal administration is available under orphan drug status.

2. Cyclobenzaprine (Flexeril) Cyclobenzaprine produces a combination of CNS depressant, skeletal muscle relaxant, and anticholinergic effects. Its precise mechanism of action remains unknown, although it is likely a central effect with little direct effect on muscle. Cyclobenzaprine is chemically related to the tricyclic antidepressants and possesses many of their adverse effects.

a. Pharmacokinetic parameters Cyclobenzaprine is well absorbed orally and undergoes partial first-pass hepatic metabolism. It is extensively metabolized, with the metabolites excreted in urine and bile. The elimination half-life of cyclobenzaprine has been estimated in adults to be as long as 1 to 3 days.

b. Administration The usual adult dose of cyclobenzaprine is 20 to 40 mg/day in two to four divided doses. The suggested maximum daily dose is 60 mg.

3. Dantrolene (Dantrium) Useful not only for its activity as an antispasmodic, dantrolene is also an important therapy for NMS induced by other medications.

a. Pharmacokinetic parameters Dantrolene is available for oral and parenteral use. Oral bioavailability is approximately 30 to 40 percent. Peak concentrations are reached within the first 5 h after oral dosing. Dantrolene is metabolized in the liver to several compounds, including 5-hydroxydantrolene, which is pharmacologically active. The metabolites are excreted in the urine. The elimination half-life of dantrolene is 7 to 9 h.

b. Administration To reduce postoperative muscle pain, doses of 100 to 150 mg may be given orally every 2 h in adults beginning preoperatively. For management of malignant hyperthermia (see Chapter 9) or NMS, an initial dose of 1 to 2 mg/kg IV is recommended. This dose may be repeated until symptoms subside or until a total dose of 10 mg/kg is reached. Oral doses of 4 to 8 mg/kg/day may be given for up to 3 days after a crisis to prevent the recurrence of symptoms.

SUGGESTED READINGS

Adams F: Emergency intravenous sedation of the delirious, medically ill patient. *J Clin Psychiatry* 49(12,Suppl):22–26, 1988.

Amrein R, Hetzel W: Pharmacology of drugs frequently used in ICUs: midazolam and flumazenil. *Intensive Care Med* 17:S1–S10, 1991.

Burns AM, Shelly MP, Park GR: The use of sedative agents in critically ill patients. *Drugs* 43(4):507–515, 1992.

Crippen DW: The role of sedation in the ICU patient with pain and agitation. *Crit Care Clinics* 6(2):369–392, 1990.

Fish DN: Treatment of delirium in the critically ill patient. *Clin Pharmacy* 10(6):456–466, 1991.

Onghena P, Van Houdenhove B: Antidepressant-induced analgesia in chronic non-malignant pain: a meta-analysis of 39 placebo-controlled studies. *Pain* 49:205–219, 1992.

Winer JW, Rosenwasser RH, Jimenez F: Electroencephalographic activity and serum and cerebrospinal fluid pentobarbital levels in determining the therapeutic end point during barbiturate coma. *Neurosurgery* 29(5):739–742, 1991.

Woster PS, LeBlanc KL: Management of elevated intracranial pressure. *Clin Pharmacy* 9(10):762–772, 1990.

CHAPTER
12
NEUROMUSCULAR BLOCKING AGENTS

John Campbell

I. Introduction
II. Uses
   A. General Considerations
   B. Intubation
   C. Ventilation
   D. Surgical Access
   E. Seizures
   F. Shivering
   G. Safety
III. Physiology
IV. Classes
   A. Depolarizing Agents
   B. Nondepolarizing Agents
V. Depolarizing Agents
   A. Succinylcholine
VI. Nondepolarizing Agents
   A. Long-Acting Agents
   B. Intermediate-Acting Agents
   C. Interactions
VII. Monitoring of Neuromuscular Blockade
   A. Clinical Monitoring
   B. Peripheral Nerve Stimulation
VIII. Reversal of Neuromuscular Blockade
   A. Spontaneous Reversal
   B. Use of Anticholinesterases
Suggested Readings

I. INTRODUCTION

A. This chapter provides an overview of the advantages, disadvantages, and problems associated with the use of neuromuscular blocking agents (NMBs) in acutely injured and critically ill patients.

B. These **blocking agents have no sedative, amnestic, anesthetic, or analgesic properties.** An important concept to remember is that the use of NMBs should be as adjunctive therapy only.

C. Patients with acute injuries and/or serious illness are nearly always suffering from pain to varying degrees, as well as emotional and psychological stress, which are as much a priority for treatment as the underlying problems. The NMBs do nothing to alleviate these problems, and by removing the patient's ability to communicate, can only make matters worse. Not only is the patient unable to inform the carers of his or her pain and distress, but the state of paralysis and hopelessness created is itself frightening to an awake, conscious patient. Therefore, it cannot be overemphasized that NMBs must be used in combination with other agents or techniques which ensure the physical and emotional comfort of the patient at all times. This will require a combination of sedation, analgesia, and amnesia throughout the duration of treatment with NMBs. Due to problems with the assessment of pain and anxiety in the paralyzed patient, it is preferable to administer these agents on a regular schedule or as an infusion rather than "as needed." **A still, paralyzed patient is not necessarily a comfortable, happy one.**

II. USES

A. General Considerations

1. An NMB should only be used to obtain, protect, and maintain a safe, secure airway; to assist with artificial ventilation when required; to enable surgical access, if an operation is to be undertaken; and to facilitate a controlled reduction of the metabolic rate in profoundly hypermetabolic patients.

2. The use of an NMB renders the patient paralyzed and unable to maintain his or her own airway or ventilation. Therefore, NMBs must be used only where there are proper facilities and personnel capable of maintaining them. **Oxygen, suction, appropriately sized face masks, and positive-pressure ventilation bags must always be immediately available whenever a patient receives an NMB.**

3. Endotracheal tubes can be passed safely under topical anesthesia alone, and so the addition of the potential risks of NMBs must be considered and their use restricted to those patients for whom they are indicated.

B. Intubation

1. The NMB can be used to assist in the placement of an endotracheal tube into the trachea to obtain, protect, and maintain a safe, secure airway. The purpose of the NMB is to prevent the patient from coughing or developing laryngospasm during instrumentation of the airway and passage of the endotracheal tube. In awake or semiconscious patients, parenteral analgesia and sedation, preferably including an amnestic agent, must be used before the administration of NMBs and/or intubation.

2. Intubation of a patient against his or her will constitutes assault and battery. In an emergency situation, a medical judgment must be made regarding the patient's competence to make such a decision, particularly in the presence of mind-altering states such as hypoxia or severe hypercarbia or after the ingestion of drugs.

3. If the patient is unconscious, an endotracheal tube can often be passed without the use of NMBs, but coughing and/or laryngospasm may still occur.

4. Nearly all patients presenting with an acute injury or serious illness must be assumed to have a full stomach, and therefore they are at increased risk of aspiration. Hence care must be taken to minimize the risk of regurgitation. This may include:

    a. Applying cricoid pressure.

    b. Expeditiously securing the airway after paralysis.

    c. Removing gastric contents by suctioning before sedatives and relaxants are administered.

    d. Raising the head of the bed 30 to 45 degrees (affects passive regurgitation only).

C. Ventilation

1. Another use for NMBs is to maximize the effectiveness of **artificial ventilation** when this cannot be easily achieved with adequate levels of analgesia and sedation. Sufficient analgesia and sedation must be maintained throughout the duration of use of the NMB.

2. Advantages

    a. An NMB may decrease airway pressures by reducing chest and abdominal wall resistance, especially if the patient is coughing, shivering, having seizures, or suffering from significant muscle spasms as with tetanus.

    b. The NMB can lessen the work of breathing, and thereby reduce metabolic rate and oxygen requirements. This is particularly useful in the patient with severe sepsis and/or adult respiratory distress syndrome (ARDS), where high metabolic rate and increased dead space can necessitate the use of extremely high minute ventilations.

3. Disadvantages

a. The patient may be unable to communicate awareness, pain, or distress to the staff.

b. Also, the staff must be able to provide and monitor adequate ventilation since the patient is unable to control and regulate his or her own.

c. Finally, inadvertent extubation is a life-threatening situation and requires the immediate presence of a professional skilled in airway management.

D. Surgical Access

Patients with acute injuries often need emergency surgery, in which case NMBs may be required to **facilitate surgical exposure,** especially for thoracic, abdominal, and airway surgery. This subject is covered in detail in anesthesiology texts.

E. Seizures

In status epilepticus, NMBs can be used to obtain and maintain an airway, to prevent self-injury to the patient, and to reduce oxygen uptake, but only after specific antiepileptic agents have been unsuccessful and the patient has been adequately sedated.

F. Shivering

Metabolic rate and/or fever may need to be aggressively reduced with the use of cooling blankets and/or ice. In a limited number of cases, this need is profound enough to warrant the use of NMBs to prevent the higher metabolic demands and consequently increased oxygen consumption caused by shivering.

G. Safety

Occasionally, NMBs may be used to prevent spontaneous movements or responses to stimuli in sedated patients to prevent injury or to allow the insertion of invasive monitors. This should be considered only after administration of adequate sedation or in cases where the sedative administration is limited by hemodynamic instability.

III. PHYSIOLOGY

A. As their name implies, NMBs act at the **neuromuscular junction** (NMJ) between the nerve terminal and the muscle motor end plate. **Acetylcholine** acts as the neurotransmitter across the NMJ. Nerve action potentials cause the release of acetylcholine from the nerve terminal which crosses the synapse to bind with postjunctional receptors on the muscle end plate. This results in depolarization of the end plate, leading to contraction of the muscle fiber.

   B. Acetylcholine is then rapidly metabolized by acetylcholinesterase within the NMJ and removed from the muscle end plate, thereby permitting the end plate to repolarize, ready for the next depolarization and muscle contraction.

IV. CLASSES

There are two classes of NMBs based on their action at the NMJ.

A. Depolarizing Agents

   1. These agents bind to the receptors and cause a prolonged depolarization of the muscle end-plate membrane. This results in an extended refractory period during which further depolarization of the membrane by acetylcholine cannot occur. This is manifest by a brief muscle contraction, and then fasciculation of the muscle, followed by relaxation. The **duration of effect** is determined by the rate of removal of the depolarizing NMB from the receptors.
   2. Depolarizing agents are also known as **noncompetitive blockers** because, unlike nondepolarizing NMBs, they cannot be overcome by increasing the concentration of acetylcholine at the receptor site.

B. Nondepolarizing Agents

   1. These agents act by occupying the receptor sites on the postjunctional muscle end-plate membrane and blocking the binding of acetylcholine. This prevents depolarization of the membrane and thereby blocks neuromuscular transmission.
   2. They act as a **competitive block** in that when the levels of the NMB at the receptors are low enough, an increase in the levels of acetylcholine, as achieved by the administration of an anticholinesterase (which blocks the breakdown of acetylcholine), can overcome the block.

V. DEPOLARIZING AGENTS

A. Succinylcholine

Succinylcholine remains the only member of this class used clinically. Its structure is two acetylcholine molecules joined together.

1. **Uses**
   a. Succinylcholine is the NMB of choice for rapid intubation of the trachea, and it is used to maintain and protect the airway when required.
   b. It can be used as an infusion for short procedures such as bronchoscopy or diagnostic laryngoscopy.
2. **Actions**
   a. Succinylcholine binds to the postjunctional receptors of the NMJ and initiates a persistent depolarization of the muscle end plate.
   b. Because of its similarity to acetylcholine, it acts at cholinergic receptors throughout the body, which explains many of its side effects (see "Complications" below).
3. **Clearance**
   a. Succinylcholine is metabolized by a plasma cholinesterase, called **pseudocholinesterase**.
   b. Unlike acetylcholine, succinylcholine is not metabolized locally in the NMJ, but in the plasma. This means that the concentration of succinylcholine at the muscle end plate is determined by the rate of breakdown and removal from the plasma, creating a concentration gradient down which the molecules diffuse away from the NMJ. Metabolism will be slower in patients with genetic **pseudocholinesterase deficiency** ($\frac{1}{25}$ of the population is heterozygote, $\frac{1}{2800}$ is homozygote).
4. **Advantages**
   a. Its **rapid onset** provides optimal intubating conditions in 60 to 90 s.
   b. The **short duration of action,** 3 to 5 min, is attributable to the rapid metabolism by plasma cholinesterase. This results in only a small fraction of the administered drug reaching the NMJ, and rapid removal of the fraction that does. Because of the prevalence of pseudocholinesterase deficiency in the general population, succinylcholine should not be assumed to be short acting. The effect is slightly prolonged in heterozygotes, but markedly prolonged in the homozygote (hours).
   c. The **duration of action is not affected by renal failure,** and is only prolonged when hepatic failure is advanced enough to cause a significant decrease in the levels of plasma cholinesterase. Plasma cholinesterase levels can also be reduced in late pregnancy, cancer, burns, and shock hypothyroidism, and after exposure to ecothiopate eye drops, anticholinesterases, phenelzine, or organophosphates.
   d. Succinylcholine **may be given intramuscularly** to children (1–3 mg/kg) when venous access is a problem, but rapid control of the airway is required.

5. **Complications**
   a. **Autonomic complications,** stimulation of cholinergic receptors, including autonomic ganglia, can result in hypertension and tachycardia, as well as decrease the threshold for ventricular arrhythmias. Also, stimulation

of the cardiac muscarinic (vagal) receptors can cause bradycardia, especially with repeated doses, and bronchospasm. The occurrence of these may be dose related.

b. Histamine release is normally mild, but may cause flushing and a fall in blood pressure. This is usually counteracted by the ganglionic effects described above.

c. Hyperkalemia is another possible complication. The administration of succinylcholine causes a rise in extracellular potassium levels, which is normally of little or no consequence, but in certain conditions, in which tissue trauma or prolonged inactivity predominate, it can be large enough to be life threatening due to the ensuing cardiac arrhythmias. Examples include:

   i. Burns.
   ii. Trauma, especially skeletal muscle damage.
   iii. Sepsis, especially peritonitis.
   iv. Paralysis, especially spinal cord damage.
   v. Closed head injury.
   vi. Upper and lower motor neuron disease.
   vii. Neuromuscular diseases, especially if associated with muscle wasting, including some muscular dystrophies, stroke, Guillain-Barré syndrome, and poliomyelitis.
   viii. Prolonged bed rest.

Patients with these conditions are most at risk during the period from 7 days after the onset of the injury or tissue damage until 9 months later; however, problems can occur as early as 24 h after the injury, and may persist for at least a year. The rise in serum potassium level may also be significant when the extracellular potassium level is already elevated, such as in renal failure.

d. Malignant hyperthermia (MH) may be **triggered by succinylcholine** in susceptible individuals, most often children. Other triggers include the potent anesthetic gases **halothane, enflurane, and isoflurane.** It results from decreased calcium reuptake from the sarcoplasmic reticulum within the muscles. A rapid increase in intracellular calcium precipitates severe hypermetabolism and the production of massive quantities of metabolic products, especially heat, lactic acid, and carbon dioxide. Clinically, MH presents as tachycardia, atrial and ventricular dysrhythmias, tachypnea, and cyanosis. Muscle rigidity after administration of succinylcholine is also suspicious for early MH. Fever, a late sign, may be dramatic (42 to 44°C) and worsens prognosis. Arterial blood gases show hypoxemia, respiratory and metabolic acidoses, and hypercarbia. Hyperkalemia also occurs, and later, creatine phosphokinase and myoglobin can reach extremely high levels. The onset of MH usually leads rapidly to death, unless the stimuli are removed and appropriate treatment initiated at once. The **treatment of MH** includes:

   i. Removal of triggering stimuli.
   ii. Hyperventilation with 100% oxygen.

  iii. Dantrolene 1 to 2 mg/kg intravenously (IV) every 5 min as required to a total dose of 10 mg/kg. This slows calcium release from the sarcoplasmic reticulum.
  iv. Sodium bicarbonate 2 to 4 meq/kg IV while awaiting the first arterial blood gas.
  v. Insulin 20 units IV and 50 mL 50% dextrose IV.
  vi. Aggressive body cooling, including cooling blanket, ice packs, and cold IV fluids.
  vii. Maintenance of urine output greater than 2 mL/kg/h to prevent inspissation of myoglobin in the renal tubules. Mannitol is present in the dantrolene preparation, but furosemide may also be needed.
 e. Masseter spasm may or may not be a prelude to MH, but can make intubation and airway management difficult.
 f. Prolonged apnea occurs when there is a decreased rate of metabolism of succinylcholine in the plasma; a hereditary atypical plasma cholinesterase; or a reduced amount of normal plasma cholinesterase due to liver failure, cachexia, malnutrition, etc.; or when a large dose or repeated doses of succinylcholine are administered resulting in a competitive, nondepolarizing type of block, the exact cause of which remains unclear.
 g. Raised pressures in certain body compartments may cause further deterioration of the patient's condition, for example: intracranial pressure in patients with head injury; increased intraocular pressures, which means that patients with penetrating eye injuries are at risk of expelling vitreous humor and further jeopardizing visual integrity; or increased intragastric pressure, which magnifies the risk of reflux and aspiration.
 h. Myoglobinuria may be seen in patients with severe skeletal muscle damage and result in acute renal failure. This may also occur in malignant hyperthermia, as noted above.
 i. Sustained contractions may be experienced by myotonic patients.
 j. Myalgias as a result of random but intense muscle contractions take place, but probably are not a significant problem in this group of patients.
 k. Allergic reactions are seen, but are uncommon.

VI. NONDEPOLARIZING AGENTS

Nondepolarizing agents represent a relatively large group of drugs which competitively block the action of acetylcholine at the muscle end-plate membrane, thereby preventing depolarization. The choice as to which agent to use depends on the patient's condition, as well as the side-effects profile and duration of action of the individual drugs (Table 12-1).

A. Long-Acting Agents

Among long-acting agents are doxacurium (Neuromax), metocurine (Metubine), pancuronium (Pavulon), pipecuronium (Arduan), and *d*-tubocurarine (Curare).

1. Pancuronium, *d*-tubocurarine, and metocurine are the established agents in this group. Of these, **pancuronium** is the most commonly used in this group of patients because of its sympathomimetic actions, which tend to maintain blood pressure and cardiac output.

2. **Metocurine** and ***d*-tubocurarine** must be used with care because of their ganglion-blocking and histamine-releasing effects, which tend to reduce blood pressure.

3. **Doxacurium and pipecuronium** are two recently released drugs which fall into this group, but have not yet been fully assessed for this type of patient, particularly for long-term treatment. Doxacurium would appear to offer the most advantages over the older agents because of its very clean cardiovascular profile.

4. **Clearance** varies according to which drug is used (Table 12-2).

    a. Pancuronium and pipecuronium are partially metabolized in the liver and so their duration of action may be prolonged by severe liver failure.

    b. Most rely heavily on excretion by the kidneys for their removal and their duration would be markedly prolonged in renal failure. Metocurine is almost entirely excreted by the kidneys. *d*-Tubocurarine, on the other hand, is minimally metabolized, but 40 percent is excreted by the liver and 60 percent by the kidney.

5. **Advantages**

    a. Their long, relatively predictable duration of action allows infrequent bolus dosing.

Table 12-1 Suggested doses, onset, expected durations, incremental follow-up doses, and infusion rates

	Bolus (mg/kg)	Onset (min)	Duration (min)	Increments (mg/kg)	Infusion (µg/kg/min)
Succinylcholine	1.0	1–2	3–5	0.25	50–100
Mivacurium	0.2	3–4	15–20	0.1	5–10
Atracurium	0.5	3–4	20–30	0.1	5–10
Vecuronium	0.1	3–4	20–30	0.02	1–2
d-Tubocurarine	0.5	3–4	60–90	0.1	–
Pancuronium	0.06	3–4	60–90	0.02	–
Metocurine	0.3	3–4	60–90	0.05	–
Pipecuronium	0.1	3–4	60–90		–
Doxacurium	0.06	4–5	60–90	0.01	–

Table 12-2 Clearance rates (+ stimulates, − blocks)

	Metabolism		Excretion	
	Plasma	Hepatic	Hepatic	Renal
Succinylcholine	++*	−	−	−
Mivacurium	++*	−	−	−
Atracurium	++†	+	−	−
Vecuronium	−	+	++	+
Pancuronium	−	+	+	++
Pipecuronium	−	+	+	++
d-Tubocurarine	−	−	+	++
Doxacurium	−	−	+	++
Metocurine	−	−	−	++

*Plasma cholinesterase.
†Hoffman elimination.

    b. Also, the choice of agent may be tailored to the clinical situation according to the duration of action, metabolism, excretion, and cardiovascular side effects.

    c. In addition, they are relatively inexpensive, particularly d-tubocurarine and pancuronium.

  6. Disadvantages

    a. Infusions or repeated doses may lead to accumulation and a markedly prolonged duration of action.

    b. Also, because they are slower in onset than succinylcholine, there is an increased risk of aspiration.

    c. Significant hypoxemia is a risk if control of the airway is lost and intubation is impossible. Therefore, it cannot be overemphasized that these agents should be used only with adequate airway equipment and personnel skilled in airway management immediately available.

    d. These agents do not provide any analgesia or sedation, and so an awake, paralyzed patient is a possibility that must be considered and prevented at all times.

    e. In addition, most have some cardiovascular side effects (Table 12-3).

B. Intermediate-Acting Agents

These agents include atracurium (Tracrium), mivacurium (Mivacron), and vecuronium (Norcuron).

  1. Atracurium and **vecuronium** have well-established roles in the management of patients with acute injury and serious illness.

Table 12-3 Histamine release and interaction with other cholinergic autonomic receptors (+ stimulates, − blocks, 0 no effect)

	Histamine	Cardiac	Ganglia
Succinylcholine	+	++	++
Mivacurium	+	0	0
Atracurium	+	0	0
Vecuronium	0	0	0
d-Tubocurarine	++	0	−
Pancuronium	0	−	0
Metocurine	+	0	−
Pipecuronium	0	0	0
Doxacurium	0	0	0

   2. **Mivacurium** is a recently released agent that is still being evaluated and its role remains unclear.
   3. **Clearance** again varies with each drug (Table 12-2).
      a. **Atracurium** is unique in that a large proportion is cleared by **Hoffman elimination,** a pH and temperature-dependent nonenzymatic hydrolysis, as well as by hepatic ester hydrolysis. Hence the half-life of the drug is least affected by impaired renal or hepatic function.
      b. **Vecuronium** offers the advantage of a significant degree of hepatic metabolism compared with the other nondepolarizing agents. As such, it can be used readily in patients with renal failure without the risk of excessively prolonged effect.
      c. **Mivacurium** is unusual in that it is metabolized by plasma cholinesterase, like succinylcholine. Therefore, its clearance is only likely to be prolonged when the amount of plasma cholinesterase produced is reduced, as in severe hepatic failure, cachexia, or very severe malnutrition (see "Depolarizing Agents—Advantages").
   4. **Advantages**
      a. The duration of action is relatively predictable.
      b. Also, there is less risk of accumulation than seen with the long-acting agents, and so they can be given by infusion with less likelihood of having prolonged recovery times.
      c. There is little change in their duration of action in disease states, although the duration of vecuronium may be prolonged in renal failure.
      d. Finally, there are minimal cardiovascular side effects.
   5. **Disadvantages**
      a. Large total doses may be required, and so the drugs can be rather expensive.
      b. Also, atracurium can release histamine if given in large doses as a

bolus. Administration of the dose over several minutes and adequate hydration minimize this effect.

    c. There have been reported incidences of prolonged action with large doses of vecuronium, although the relationship has not yet been confirmed and the etiology remains uncertain.

    d. The metabolism of atracurium by Hoffman elimination produces **laudanosine,** which, in large doses, causes central nervous system stimulation. This has not been reported to be clinically significant to date.

C. Interactions

The effect and duration of nondepolarizing NMBs may be affected by various disease states and physiologic conditions, as well as by other drugs.

  1. Potentiation of the neuromuscular blocking effect occurs with:
    a. Acid-base imbalance.
    b. Hypothermia.
    c. Acute hypokalemia.
    d. Severe hypermagnesemia.
    e. Myasthenia gravis and myasthenic syndrome.
    f. Collagen vascular diseases.
    g. Volatile anesthetics.
    h. Aminoglycoside antibiotics.
    i. Dantrolene.
    j. Calcium channel blockers.
    k. Local anesthetics.
  2. Resistance to neuromuscular blockade can be seen with:
    a. Burns.
    b. Phenytoin.
    c. Theophylline.

VII. MONITORING OF NEUROMUSCULAR BLOCKADE

Monitoring may be needed to assess both the degree of block and the adequacy of reversal. It is important to ensure adequate blockade when required, and also to avoid overdosage, particularly when using infusions or repeated doses over prolonged periods.

A. Clinical Monitoring

Neuromuscular blockade is usually **monitored clinically** in the intensive care setting in order to achieve the desired result with the minimum dose and side effects. Profound blockade is usually required for intubation, when a full dose of the chosen NMB should be given. For more prolonged use, the level of blockade needed should be just enough to allow the desired therapy and remove the unwanted symptoms. The block should be continually reassessed and adjusted.

B. Peripheral Nerve Stimulation

The level of neuromuscular blockade can be assessed by trained personnel using a **peripheral nerve stimulator**. A supramaximal electrical stimulus is delivered to a peripheral nerve, resulting in an evoked response in the muscles supplied by that nerve. Depending on the type of stimulus and the class of NMB, the pattern of response elicited indicates the degree of block present. When monitoring nondepolarizing NMBs, the **train-of-four** stimulus can give a rough estimate of the percentage of receptors blocked. If the fourth twitch is lost, 75 percent of the receptors are blocked; if two twitches are lost, 80 percent are blocked; for three twitches lost, 90 percent are blocked; and no twitches present indicates 100 percent blockade.

VIII. REVERSAL OF NEUROMUSCULAR BLOCKADE

A. Spontaneous Reversal

Spontaneous recovery from neuromuscular blockade occurs when the levels of NMB have been reduced enough by metabolism and/or excretion to allow the action of acetylcholine at the postjunctional receptors.

1. At present, succinylcholine cannot be reversed pharmacologically, but because it is rapidly metabolized by pseudocholinesterase, this is rarely a clinical issue.

2. In the intensive care setting, it is usual to allow spontaneous recovery whenever possible to ensure full reversal and avoid the return of blockade. It is imperative to ensure full return of muscle function and strength before ventilatory assistance is removed. If the neuromuscular blockade needs to be reversed for clinical reasons, such as the need for a more complete neurologic examination, this can be accomplished by using an anticholinesterase.

B. Use of Anticholinesterases

Anticholinesterases such as **neostigmine** (Prostigmine) and **edrophonium** (Tensilon) prevent the breakdown of acetylcholine within the neuromuscular junction and thereby increase the amount of acetylcholine at the receptor site in competition with the NMB.

1. Nondepolarizing agents act competitively with acetylcholine and so,

when their level at the receptors has fallen sufficiently, they can be reversed by the administration of an anticholinesterase drug.

2. There is also an increase in acetylcholine at other cholinergic receptors in the body. In order to avoid the muscarinic side effects, particularly the resultant bradycardia and possible asystole from increased vagal stimulation, an anticholinergic agent (e.g., atropine or glycopyrrolate [Robinul]) should be administered with the anticholinesterase.

SUGGESTED READINGS

Katz RL: *Muscle Relaxants,* Orlando, Florida, Grune & Stratton, 1985.

Miller RD, Savarese JJ: Pharmacology of muscle relaxants and their antagonists, in Miller RD (ed): *Anesthesia,* 3rd ed. New York, Churchill Livingstone, chap 12, pp 390–435.

Stoelting RK, Dierdorf SF, McCammon RL: *Anesthesia and Co-existing Disease,* 2nd ed. New York, Churchill Livingstone, 1988.

Wood M: Cholinergic and parasympathomimetic drugs. Cholinesterases and anticholinesterases, in Wood M, and Wood A (eds): *Drugs and Anesthesia: Pharmacology for Anesthesiologists,* 2nd ed. Baltimore, Williams & Wilkins, 1990, pp 83–110.

Wood M: Neuromuscular blocking agents, in Wood M, and Wood A (eds): *Drugs and Anesthesia: Pharmacology for Anesthesiologists,* 2nd ed. Baltimore, Williams & Wilkins, 1990, pp 271–318.

PART FOUR

APPLICATIONS OF MODALITIES AND TREATMENT OPTIONS

CHAPTER
13

TECHNIQUES OF NARCOTIC AND LOCAL ANESTHETIC ADMINISTRATION

John C. Rowlingson
Robin J. Hamill

I. Introduction
   A. General Issues
   B. Advantages of Regional Analgesia
   C. Potential Disadvantages of Regional Analgesia
   D. Contraindications to Regional Analgesia
   E. Sources of Complications
II. Parenteral Techniques
   A. Intramuscular Injections
   B. Intravenous Injections and Infusions
   C. Subcutaneous Injections and Infusions
   D. Patient-Controlled Analgesia
III. Epidural Analgesia
   A. Description
   B. Anatomy
   C. Indications
   D. Contraindications Unique to Epidural Analgesia
   E. Complications
   F. Technique of Epidural Catheter Placement
   G. Drugs
   H. Epidural Versus Spinal Analgesia
IV. Subarachnoid (Spinal) Analgesia
   A. Description
   B. Anatomy

    C. Indications and Contraindications
    D. Complications
    E. Technique
    F. Drugs
    G. Pros and Cons of Spinal Analgesia
  V. Sympathetic Nerve Blocks
    A. Cervicothoracic (Stellate Ganglion) Block
    B. Lumbar Sympathetic Block
    C. Celiac Plexus Block
    D. Intravenous Regional (Bier) Block
  VI. Plexus Blocks
    A. Brachial Plexus
    B. Cervical Plexus
    C. Lumbar Plexus
  VII. Peripheral Nerve Blocks for Analgesia
    A. Infiltration of Wound Margins or Incision Irrigation
    B. Paravertebral Blocks
    C. Intercostal Nerve Blocks
    D. Intrapleural Administration of LA
    E. Ilioinguinal Nerve Block
    F. Femoral Nerve Block
    G. Suprascapular and Intrabursal Blocks
    H. Occipital Nerve Block
VIII. Trigger Point Injections
Suggested Readings

I. INTRODUCTION

A. General Issues

1. **Assessment** of the patient is crucial to achieving the diagnosis as to what is physically and psychologically wrong with the patient, as well as a database which is the basis upon which decisions about treatment are made.

2. Patients with critical illness and acute injury exhibit **physiologic and metabolic derangements.** These will affect their **morbidity and mortality** and will influence the patient's tolerance of the effects and consequences of therapeutic modalities.

3. All modes of therapy have **risks and benefits.** These will be amplified in the critically ill patient because this patient may have less physiologic reserve.

4. **The judicious application of analgesic techniques** to critically ill patients can accomplish the goals of pain reduction without contributing such perils as nausea, vomiting, sedation, or mental status change, while maximizing comfort and decreasing the emotional reaction to the acute, painful condition and the hectic atmosphere of the intensive care unit

(ICU). Pain, anxiety, and distress can magnify the metabolic stress response to illness or injury and further tax a hypermetabolic patient.

B. Advantages of Regional Analgesia

Regional analgesia techniques offer the following **advantages** (also see Chapter 24).

1. Analgesia without sedation of the central nervous system (CNS) and probably fewer drug-related side effects given the need for less medication.
2. Effective blockade of noxious afferent input to the CNS such that the stress response is diminished and the patient suffers less physiologic compromise.
3. Effective analgesia that boosts the patient's outlook.
4. Quiet awakening from general anesthesia or prolonged sedation.
5. Techniques that involve patient contact and that are repeatable and nonaddicting.
6. Techniques that facilitate the patient's cooperation with rehabilitation regimens, such as cough and deep-breathing routines and physical therapy.

C. Potential Disadvantages of Regional Analgesia

Regional analgesia techniques are associated with the following **potential disadvantages.**

1. Unpredictability as to the clinical result with regard to the onset of relief or the intensity and duration of the block.
2. Expected physiologic effects, such as numbness and weakness with local anesthetic (LA) use.
3. Side effects (which are *not* the same as complications), such as hypotension, LA drug toxicity, headache, and backache.
4. Complications related to the invasive nature of the therapy or the equipment, such as overflow of LA to nontargeted tissue and needle or catheter trauma.
5. The impracticality of blocking some body areas.
6. The need for extra equipment, time to provide the therapy, special monitoring of the patient, and extra personnel to furnish the mandatory follow-up and to address problems expeditiously when they arise.

D. Contraindications to Regional Analgesia

1. It is important to share accurate information about the risks and benefits of a given procedure with the patient, and to set up the work area for

performing regional analgesia so that any and all contingencies can be handled efficiently. Once initiated, it is imperative to discriminate side effects from true complications from events that are not related to the regional analgesia. If these criteria cannot be fulfilled, regional anesthesia should not be undertaken.

   2. **Anticoagulation** to clinically significant levels can cause excessive bleeding from the trauma of the procedure. The most important issue is where in the body the bleeding occurs. For example, a 50 cc hematoma in the groin after a femoral nerve block is uncomfortable, whereas the same volume of blood in the epidural space may cause paraplegia.

   3. **Infection at the site** of necessary needle insertion carries the risk of contaminating the deeper tissues with the causative organism and worsening the extent of the infection.

   4. The **presence of active, untreated blood-borne infection** can lead to seeding of the injection site. This is primarily a concern when a catheter is to be placed for a number of days.

   5. The **patient's refusal** of the procedure is an absolute contraindication to an invasive procedure.

   6. The **lack of appropriately trained personnel** to perform the procedure and monitor the patient or to manage the emergencies created by the intervention (e.g., LA toxicity, epidural hematoma) demands that other, perhaps more conventional, techniques be used.

   7. A **history of allergic reaction** to the narcotic or LA drug proposed for use does not eliminate the option of regional analgesic techniques because alternative drugs may be available, but it may limit the therapeutic value offered by the modality. For example, while narcotic alone may offer reasonable analgesia, larger doses will be required than if an LA were also used. The larger dose of narcotics will magnify the side-effects profile of the drug (e.g., more itching and nausea).

E. Sources of Complications

The **complications of regional analgesia** include the following sources.

   1. Improper patient selection.
   2. An appropriate patient, but an improper technique.
   3. The lack of informed consent.
   4. Local anesthetic or other drug toxicity that is poorly managed.
   5. Expected physiologic effects that are inadequately anticipated (e.g., severe hypotension after peridural LA due to inadequate volume resuscitation).
   6. Problems due to the needle or catheter, including nerve injury, bleeding, infection, and breakage.
   7. Errors in the performance of the technique.

8. Errors in the management of the patient.

9. Inadequate attention to aftercare, that is, dealing with what issues *the patient* feels are important.

II. PARENTERAL TECHNIQUES

A. Intramuscular Injections

1. For many years, intramuscular (IM) injections were the standard of care for pain management. The injections *cause* pain. Further, especially in the critically ill population, absorption is very unpredictable. Given on an as-needed basis, the delay between initial discomfort and the onset of analgesia could be substantial (often hours).

2. This technique tended to provide the patient with intermittent analgesia, but this was frequently associated with high levels of sedation and, possibly, significant respiratory depression. This alternated with periods of pain, frustration, and anxiety, providing marginal analgesic satisfaction.

B. Intravenous Injections and Infusions

1. Intravenous (IV) administration offers more rapid onset of pain relief, but a faster and higher peak concentration than the same dose given IM. The result is even wider swings, ranging from sedation to pain and back, and the need for more frequent, smaller doses, which will require more intensive nursing attention to observe for respiratory depression.

2. Small boluses (**divided dosing**) are appropriate for titrating analgesia prior to beginning patient-controlled analgesia (PCA), or for management of short, painful procedures. **Infusions** minimize the cyclic variations in blood level and provide a more constant drug effect from which to evaluate the patient (e.g., neurologically). The primary concern is the possibility of gradual accumulation of drug. This is of particular concern in the patient with renal insufficiency. See Table 13-1 for suggested bolus dosing ranges. Infusion doses are listed in Table 13-2. The doses and intervals may need to be adjusted for hepatic and renal insufficiency, old age, and diabetes.

C. Subcutaneous Injections and Infusions

Injections and infusions by the subcutaneous (SQ) route are usually reserved for patients with poor venous access or who will need parenteral analgesic medications for a long period. Doses are similar to those administered IV once a blood level has been established. Loading doses may need to be higher for infusions and PCA (see below) administered by the SQ route. Further, the time to onset of the effect will be longer and the peak blood level lower

Table 13-1 Dosing and interval of IM and IV* opioid medications

	Dose	Interval, h
Morphine	0.1–0.25 mg/kg	3–4
Meperidine	1.0–2.0 mg/kg	2–4
Fentanyl	0.001–0.002 µg/kg	2–4
Hydromorphone	0.015–0.03 mg/kg	3–4
Methadone	0.1–0.2 mg/kg	6–8
Codeine	0.75–1.5 mg/kg	3–4
Buprenorphine	0.003–0.004 mg/kg	6–8
Butorphanol	0.02–0.04 mg/kg	3–4
Nalbuphine	0.1–0.25 mg/kg	3–4

*IV administration should be given as divided dose, titrated to effect.

than with IV administration of the same dose. Infusions via the SQ route are not often used in the acute setting or the critically ill population because of variable superficial blood flow.

D. Patient-Controlled Analgesia

A commonly used mode of opioid administration for acute pain management, PCA offers the patient the advantage of control over the administration and titration of the drug to his or her personal requirements, usually with a good margin of safety so that overdosing is very difficult. On the other

Table 13-2 Starting doses* for IV and SQ† infusions

Morphine†	1–3 mg/h
Hydromorphone†	0.2–0.6 mg/h
Fentanyl	100–300 µg/h
Sufentanil†	10–30 µg/h

*For those already taking narcotics, requirements may be substantially higher. To determine an appropriate starting rate:
  1. Calculate the 24-h narcotics need.
  2. Divide this by 24 and set infusion rate accordingly.
  3. Increase or decrease the dose by 25 to 50 percent for inadequate analgesia or excessive side effects.

†Due to the high potency of these drugs and the small volume needed, they are the best choices for SQ infusions (high-potency morphine: up to 100 mg/mL).

hand, its use is limited to those who are capable of comprehending the concept of self-administration.

   1. Patient selection   Children as young as 5 to 6 years of age may be capable of appropriate use. In less mature children, parent-initiated administration can be used, depending on the parent's motivation and sensitivity to the child's needs. Patients who are confused, forgetful, or mentally or physically unable to access the injection button are not good candidates.

   2. Setting the pump

      a. A **loading dose** of narcotic can be administered through the pump, but this is usually reserved for initiation of PCA therapy or for "catching up" when the patient has a subtherapeutic blood level.

      b. Self-administered doses (SADs) are those initiated by the patient. Table 13-3 shows suggested starting doses for healthy patients who are narcotic naïve. If the patient has a history of chronic narcotic use, these doses may be grossly inadequate, and adjustments will need to be made to meet the needs of the patient. For example, the usual postoperative patient may do very well with morphine, basal of 1 mg, SAD of 1 mg, and lockout of 6 min. A cancer patient taking large doses of narcotics at home, on the other hand, may have inadequate relief with a basal of 10 mg, SAD of 4 mg, and lockout of 5 min. Ideally, the dosing (SAD and basal rate) is adjusted in such a way that the patient needs no more than one to two SADs per hour.

      c. Basal rate refers to the constant infusion provided by the pump. The basal rate offers the patient a guaranteed level of analgesia without his or her active participation and provides the "luxury" of waking up from several hours of uninterrupted sleep without excruciating pain. Patients with very low dose requirements or with poor drug clearance may not need a basal rate, and may be at risk of drug accumulation if a significant basal rate is used.

      d. Lockout period (LOP) is the minimum time allowed between SADs. If the LOP is 10 min and the patient pushes the button 20 times in 6 min, he or she will still receive only one dose. The LOP should be set according to the onset of action of the drug. However, shorter LOPs allow patients

Table 13-3   Suggested IV and SQ* PCA doses†

Drug	Dose, µg/kg	Basal, µg/kg	Lockout, min
Morphine*	10–30	10–30	8–10
Hydromorphone*	1.5–4	1.5–4	5–8†
Meperidine	100–300	100–300	8–10
Fentanyl	0.1–0.3	0.1–0.3	5–8
Sufentanil*	0.01–0.03	0.01–0.03	5–8†

*Due to the high potency of these drugs and the small volume needed, they are the best choices for SQ PCA (high-potency morphine: up to 100 mg/mL).
†Doses recommended apply to most healthy, narcotic-naïve patients.

greater freedom in titrating the analgesia to meet their needs for painful interventions such as chest physiotherapy. Thus shorter LOPs will improve patient participation in his or her own care. LOPs of 5 to 10 min are usually desirable.

        e. The **hourly limit** also needs to be set, and should represent the upper limit of the dose that the practitioner would wish the patient to receive. This is usually the total of all available doses plus the basal dose. However, in some circumstances, the physician may choose a lower hourly limit, as for a patient with impaired drug clearance, while providing a more generous SAD and shorter LOP. This gives the patient the ability to cover painful procedures more effectively.

III. EPIDURAL ANALGESIA

A. Description

The epidural space is continuous from the foramen magnum to the tip of the coccyx. The space can be entered with a needle anywhere along this course, or a catheter can be inserted for the continuous infusion of drug.

B. Anatomy

The needle passes through the skin and the supraspinous and interspinous ligaments to the ligamentum flavum (LF). The LF is thickest (5 to 6 mm) in the lumbar area. If the needle penetrates further, the dura and/or the arachnoid membranes can be pierced, and it will ultimately enter the cerebrospinal fluid (CSF). The epidural space has many veins, as well as fatty tissue. Whereas **spinal anesthesia** is given only through the lumbar area at or below the end of the spinal cord to minimize the risk of neural injury, **epidural analgesia can be provided at the cervical, thoracic, lumbar, or caudal level.** Because of the risk of neuronal injury and arachnoiditis associated with indwelling subarachnoid catheters, the following discussion will focus on epidural analgesia.

C. Indications for Epidural Analgesia

        1. The management of **postoperative pain** (see Chapter 24).

        2. The management of **posttraumatic pain** of the thorax, abdomen, or lower extremities.

        3. The management of **vascular insufficiency,** particularly after major vascular reconstructions (trauma), limb reimplantation, or myocutaneous flap grafts.

        4. The treatment (and possibly prevention) of phantom limb pain and sympathetically maintained pain.

D. Contraindications Unique to Epidural Analgesia

1. Use of LAs in a patient with **active bleeding,** uncorrected **hypovolemia,** or **hypotension** of a different etiology, because the associated sympathectomy may cause profound hypotension. Opioid drugs alone can be given epidurally, however, because they do not cause a sympathectomy.

2. The presence of **spinal metastases, active leukemia,** or **septicemia** due to a risk (at least theoretically) of seeding of the CSF.

E. Complications

1. There may be **systemic toxicity** to the LA drug given because of the large dose required as a bolus or due to accumulation from an infusion. Tinnitus and circumoral numbness are early signs of toxicity. At higher levels, seizures and cardiovascular collapse can occur. (See Chapter 10.)

2. Dural puncture with subsequent spinal anesthesia to high levels **(total spinal)** can occur when the dose was intended for the epidural space. The analgesic dose for the epidural space is 10 times that required in the subarachnoid space. **Post–dural-puncture headache** can also occur. The incidence of headache is up to 80 percent after puncture with a 17-gauge epidural needle versus less than 1 percent with a 24-gauge Sprotte needle. Management is discussed in Chapter 16.

3. Symptoms of **epidural hematoma or abscess** may include localized back pain, radicular pain, back tenderness, leg weakness or numbness, bladder/bowel dysfunction, fever, and elevated white blood count. The presence of neurologic deficits from a hematoma and/or the presence of an epidural abscess is a surgical emergency. Decompression within 6 hours of onset of neurologic dysfunction is usually associated with at least partial return of function.

4. Cauda equina syndrome refers to the small nerve fibers of the terminal spinal cord being affected by chemical irritation from drugs, trauma, infection, or scarring, with resultant autonomic dysfunction of the bladder/bowel and sensory changes in the sacral dermatomes.

5. Use in patients with **elevated intra-abdominal pressure** may unexpectedly increase the level of analgesia achieved (e.g., pregnancy, ascites, obesity). This can usually be prevented with gentle titration of the dose to the desired effect.

F. Technique of Epidural Catheter Placement

1. The patient may be seated, be prone, or be in the decubitus position. The patient must be able to flex the back to make the spinous processes prominent and to open the interspinous spaces through which the needle passes.

2. The proper level for needle insertion is the midpoint of the dermatomes that one wants to block, because the analgesic mixture will spread both cephalad and caudad. Approximately 1.5 mL per segment is needed in the lumber epidural space in the adult. The skin is prepared and draped. A skin wheal is placed and the ligaments infiltrated in the conscious patient. A 17- to 19-gauge needle is used, with a variety of needle tips available.

3. The **loss of resistance technique** usually is used to identify the epidural space, though a hanging drop technique is possible in thoracic or cervical placements.

4. A **test dose** of 3 mL is given. The injectate contains 1:200,000 epinephrine (5 µg/mL) to identify intravascular placement of the drug (>20 percent increase in heart rate) *and* LA drug of sufficient concentration to result in spinal anesthesia if subarachnoid placement is present. Usually, the LA used for catheter placement is more potent than that required for analgesia (e.g., bupivacaine 0.25% for testing versus 0.125% or less for analgesia).

5. The **dose of epidural drug** is given incrementally (e.g., 5 mL every 1 to 2 min) while vital signs are observed and questions indicating intravascular injection or the onset of spinal anesthesia asked. The dose through the needle distends the epidural space, minimizing the risk of trauma to the epidural veins. Further, the dose is chosen according to the desired therapeutic effect. When the catheter is to be used solely for analgesia, a smaller dose (e.g., 6 mL) of LA is used to confirm position in the epidural space. This dose should provide a band of decreased sensory perception (e.g., pinch, pin prick, ice) several dermatomes wide. As the patient's responses guide the injection of drug, it is important to have a responsive patient, if at all possible.

6. A **catheter is inserted** 2 to 3 cm into the epidural space and the needle is withdrawn. An additional test dose is usually injected through the catheter to rule out a subarachnoid or IV catheter position. Special attention should be given to securing the epidural catheter, since it will be needed for therapy for a number of days. Notation of the markings on the catheter that appear at the skin level should be made, so that its position can be confirmed on a regular basis.

G. Drugs

1. **Local anesthetics** such as lidocaine or bupivacaine are commonly used in dilute concentrations and as an infusion. **Bupivacaine** in concentrations of 0.0625% to 0.125% is frequently used, and produces a mild sympathectomy and some sensory changes without impairing motor function. The addition of epinephrine *may* increase the duration of drug effect, though using an infusion obviates the need for this. It is common to add bicarbonate to LA solutions to modify the pH and enhance the onset time, but this is generally not an issue in the management of established epidural

Table 13-4 Perispinal drug effects

Local anesthetics		Narcotics
+ +	Sympathetic block	− −
+ +	Sensory block	− −
+ +	Weakness	− −
+ +	Urinary retention	+ +
− −	Pruritus	+ +
− −	Nausea, vomiting	+ +
− −	Respiratory depression	+ +

analgesia in the postoperative or posttrauma period. (See Chapter 10.) Table 13-4 compares the effects of LAs with those of narcotics placed in the perispinal area.

2. **Opioid drugs** can be bolused (Table 13-5), but are more commonly added to the bupivacaine infusion to block pain at the spinal cord level and to minimize the concentration of LA drug needed. Frequently used drugs include **fentanyl** (Sublimaze), **hydromorphone** (Dilaudid), and **preservative-free morphine** (Duramorph). Intermittent boluses of morphine are sometimes used (e.g., 2 to 5 mg every 6 to 24 h, depending on the age and size of the patient, as well as the location of the catheter tip).

3. **Combined infusions** of LA and opioid allow the use of lower concentrations of each class of medication, which minimizes side effects and risks while maximizing pain control. Further, epidural PCA has been used in many institutions with excellent success. In either case, adjunctive analgesics (nonsteroidal anti-inflammatory drugs [NSAIDs], opioids, and/or narcotic agonist–antagonists) are generally made available to the patient for "breakthrough pain" or pain generated from sites not covered by the epidural (e.g., nasogastric tubes, spit fistulas, etc). Common combined infusions and rates are listed in Table 13-6. Epidural PCA doses are listed in Table 13-7.

Table 13-5 Bolus injections of epidural narcotics

	Dose	Interval, h
Morphine	2–5 mg	6–24
Hydromorphone	200–300 μg	6–10
Meperidine	25–100 mg	6–8
Fentanyl	50–100 μg	4–6
Sufentanil	10–60 μg	2–6

Subarachnoid dose is approximately 1/10 of the epidural dose.

Table 13-6 Suggested drugs and doses for epidural infusions

	Concentration*	Rate, mL/h†	
		Thoracic	Lumbar
Bupivacaine	0.0625–0.25%	4–8	6–15
Fentanyl	1–10 µg/mL	6–10	8–15
Morphine	20–60 µg/mL	6–10	8–15
Hydromorphone	3–12 µg/mL	6–10	8–15
Meperidine	1 mg/mL	6–10	8–15

*When used as the sole agent, concentrations will often need to be at the higher end of the range, but when used in combination (e.g. bupivacaine plus morphine), the lower concentration of each is often adequate.

†Subarachnoid rates are approximately 1/10 of the above rates.

H. Epidural Versus Spinal Analgesia

1. **The advantages of epidural analgesia,** as compared with subarachnoid techniques, include:

   a. The presence of the catheter that allows for continuous infusion *and* titration of drug dose and concentration to the desired effect. Once stabilized, this is less labor intensive than intermittent injections.

   b. The combination of opioids with LA drugs such that lower doses of two drugs are used and the side effects of both classes of drugs minimized.

   c. A lower incidence of side effects and complications.

2. **The disadvantages of epidural analgesia,** when compared with subarachnoid techniques, include:

   a. The presence of the catheter with an injection site and relevant problems with disconnections and accidental injection of inappropriate medications (e.g., antibiotics intended for an IV injection port).

   b. A risk of catheter migration into the subarachnoid space and a subsequent increase in the density and level of blockade.

Table 13-7 Epidural PCA doses and settings

	SAD, mL	LOP, min	Basal rate, mL/h
Bupivacaine 0.0625% plus fentanyl 5 µg/mL	2–5	10–15	2–10
Bupivacaine 0.125% plus fentanyl 5 µg/mL	2–4	12–15	4–6
Fentanyl 10 µg/mL	2–3	10	2–3
Sufentanil 2 µg/mL	2–4	10	1–4
Morphine 20–40 µg/mL	0.1–0.4	10	1–3

Subarachnoid dose is approximately 1/10 of the epidural dose.

c. The risk of catheter tip avulsion if an improper technique is used when the catheter is removed, and the possible need for surgical retrieval.

   d. The potential for LA toxicity from an infusion of analgesic drugs, especially if the catheter migrates into an epidural vein, although with low concentrations of LA, seizures are unlikely.

IV. SUBARACHNOID (SPINAL) ANALGESIA

A. Description

Spinal analgesia is achieved by the instillation of LA drug of sufficient concentration into the CSF to produce sympathectomy, sensory change, and, frequently, motor paralysis. Intrathecal opiates can also be used to avoid these effects. There will be few circumstances in which spinal analgesia will be chosen as a primary technique. Most commonly, patients who have received spinal anesthesia and also some intraspinal opioid for an operative procedure will be returned to the ICU or postsurgery ward.

B. Anatomy

The needle passes through the same structures as listed above for epidural analgesia, with the exception that the spinal needle is intentionally advanced through the epidural space and then through the dural and arachnoid membranes into the subarachnoid space. The free return of CSF confirms the placement.

C. Indications and Contraindications

The **indications** and **contraindications** for spinal analgesia are similar to those listed for epidural analgesia.

D. Complications

The **complications specific to spinal analgesia** include the following.
   1. **Bleeding** can result from trauma to the epidural or dural vessels.
   2. **Neural injury** can be caused by **needle trauma** to the nerve roots. This could include persistent paresthesia or chronic neuralgic pain. Due to this risk, it is recommended that spinal injections be performed below the L1 level (i.e., below the conus medullaris). Concern has been expressed about the possibility that some of the **drugs** used can cause neural injury, either as a direct effect or as a result of the vehicle or preservatives. For instance, anterior spinal artery syndrome is characterized by necrosis of the central gray matter and degeneration of the spinal cord. Some believe this results from

intense vasoconstriction of the anterior spinal artery when epinephrine is added to spinal anesthetic drugs to extend the duration of the anesthesia.

3. Catheters are not usually used in spinal anesthesia, although continuous techniques have been described. Of recent interest has been the use of 25- to 27-gauge **microcatheters.** There has been the concern that spinal drugs do not mix well with the CSF when administered through these catheters. The persistence of a high concentration of LA has been considered a possible causative factor in cases of cauda equina syndrome reported in patients receiving continuous spinal anesthesia with such equipment. Due to their minute size, these catheters are also fraught with technical problems, including kinking and high back pressure, causing infusion pumps to fail and alarm frequently.

4. The incidence of **post–dural-puncture headache (PDPH)** is higher in younger patients, females, patients who required multiple passes of the needle, cases in which large-gauge needles are used, and cases in which the bevel of the needle is not parallel to the longitudinal axis of the dural fibers. Common **symptoms** include occipital and frontal headaches that are worse with sitting or standing, but abate when lying down; photophobia; nausea and vomiting; and tinnitus. **Treatment** may include oral hydration with caffeine-containing liquids, IV caffeine (500 mg caffeine sodium benzoate in a liter of IV fluid given over an hour), bed rest, minor analgesics, the application of an abdominal binder, epidural saline infusion, or epidural blood patch.

E. Technique

1. The patient can be in the seated, decubitus, or prone (jackknife) position. It is crucial to the success of the procedure that the patient's spine be flexed to open the interspinous spaces. A midline approach is usually taken, although a paramedian entry may be helpful if the patient's ligaments are calcified or the proper position is difficult to obtain.

2. An 18- to 32-gauge needle is passed through properly prepared skin and a skin wheal. For needles smaller than 23 gauge, an introducer needle is anchored in the ligaments before the spinal needle is used. The bevel of the needle should be oriented parallel to the longitudinal axis of the dural fibers so that the fibers are separated rather than cut. Attention to this small detail lowers the risk of PDPH.

3. The free flow of CSF indicates proper location of the needle. Sporadic return of CSF, even with aspiration, may indicate location in a root sleeve. A catheter is passed or the chosen drugs given. The catheter should be securely taped, as it can be used for days.

F. Drugs

1. The **drugs commonly used** include lidocaine 0.5 in 1 percent, and bupivacaine 0.0625 to 0.125 percent.

2. Epinephrine 200 µg or phenylephrine 5 mg may be added with the intent of increasing the duration of the anesthetic drug by 50 to 100 percent.

3. Opioids such as fentanyl 5 to 10 µg or morphine 200 to 500 µg may be used with or without an LA drug.

4. As a rule, doses required for spinal anesthesia or analgesia are about one-tenth of the dose required for epidural analgesia (Tables 13-5 through 13-7).

G. Pros and Cons of Spinal Analgesia

1. **The advantages of spinal analgesia** include the small amount of drug used, the absence of a catheter, and the easy identification of the subarachnoid space.

2. **The disadvantages of spinal analgesia** include the single-shot nature of most of the use and the higher incidence of opioid side effects (pruritus, nausea, vomiting, urinary retention, and respiratory depression) than when epidural opioids are used.

V. SYMPATHETIC NERVE BLOCKS

A. Cervicothoracic (Stellate Ganglion) Block

A stellate block will usually provide a sympathectomy to the ipsilateral upper quadrant of the body (above T8), including the upper extremity. The stellate ganglion (SG) is formed by the fusion of the lower cervical and first thoracic sympathetic ganglia. It is located in a fascial plane at approximately the C7 level in the neck and lateral to the vertebral spine.

1. An **anterior paratracheal approach** is usually taken with the patient in the supine position, the head extended over a small pillow, and the mouth open in a relaxed posture to decrease the tension in the neck musculature.

2. **The anterior tubercle of the C6** vertebrae is palpated and the overlying skin prepped. A 25-gauge, 1½-inch needle is passed through the skin to rest on the tubercle. The needle must be pulled back 1 mm to get the tip out of the longus colli muscle and prevertebral fascia.

3. After aspiration for CSF and blood, a 1 mL **test dose** of 1% lidocaine or 0.25% bupivacaine is given. If no adverse response results in 60 s, a total of 10 mL of the drug with or without 1:200,000 epinephrine is injected incrementally with aspiration performed after each 2 mL.

4. An **SG block is indicated for** improving blood flow to the upper extremity and diagnosing and treating sympathetic mediated pain (SMP), including that related to malignancy or limb ischemia, herpes zoster, angina, and phantom limb pain.

5. The **advantages** of stellate block as compared with other upper extremity blocks include the absence of sensory and motor block and improved blood flow.

6. **Disadvantages** include possible spillover of LA to affect the recurrent laryngeal nerve and limited duration of action. If prolonged sympathetic blockade is needed (e.g., limb reimplantation or distal emboli), consideration should be given to a brachial plexus catheter and LA infusion (see plexus blocks below). Temporary miosis may interfere with the neurologic evaluation of a patient with an elevated intracranial pressure.

7. The **potential complications** include spinal or epidural block, toxic reaction to the LA drug due to vertebral artery injection, bradycardia (with right-sided blocks), pneumothorax, and recurrent laryngeal nerve block that causes temporary hoarseness.

B. Lumbar Sympathetic Block

1. A lumbar sympathetic block (LSB) interrupts the sympathetic outflow to the ipsilateral lower extremity. The sympathetic chain at the L2–4 level is located anterolateral to the vertebral column and adjacent to the aorta and vena cava.

2. A **posterior or posterolateral approach** is taken with the patient in a prone or decubitus position. The needle is inserted 7 to 12 cm from the midline at the L2, L3, or L4 level at a 30- to 45-degree angle off the perpendicular to the skin and aimed toward the lateral aspect of the L2–4 vertebral body. Once contacted, the tip is 'walked" into a position that is anterolateral to the spine. The needle has passed through the skin and the body and anterior fascia of the psoas muscle.

3. Either 6 to 20 mL of 0.5 to 1% **lidocaine or** 0.125% to 0.25% **bupivacaine with 1:200,000 epinephrine** is injected after aspiration of the needle is negative for blood and CSF. Occasionally, a catheter is inserted to maintain the effects of the block, or a **neurolytic drug** (e.g., alcohol or phenol) is injected in the hope of achieving a long-lasting block. (*Note:* The patient *must* be fully capable of understanding the risks and benefits of neurolytic block before this is considered.)

4. The indications for **LSB** are to improve blood flow to the lower extremity, to manage phantom pain, and to diagnose and treat SMP syndromes. When an extended sympathectomy is indicated, continuous sympathetic blockade can be readily achieved with an epidural infusion of LA.

5. The complications of **LSB** include spinal or epidural anesthesia, injection into a root sleeve, lumbar plexus block, intravascular injection precipitating a toxic reaction, and L2, L3, or L4 neuralgic pain.

C. Celiac Plexus Block

1. The celiac plexus is a grouping of sympathetic ganglia located approximately at the L1 level of the body, anterior to the aorta, anterolateral to the celiac artery, and posterior to the pancreas. Blockade of the celiac plexus provides **intra-abdominal visceral analgesia.**

2. The patient is placed in a **prone position** with a pillow under the lower abdomen to reduce the lumbar lordosis. A needle is inserted 7 to 10 cm from the midline at the L2 landmark, as for LSB. In addition to the 30- to 45-degree angle off the perpendicular to the skin, for celiac plexus block (CPB), the needle must also be directed 45 degrees cephalad. The tip is 'walked' off the lateral aspect of the L1 vertebral body to an additional depth of 2.5 to 3 cm.

3. When aspiration of the needle is negative for blood, CSF, and urine, 15 to 25 mL of 0.5% **lidocaine or** 0.125% to 0.25% **bupivacaine** can be injected incrementally. When **neurolytic blocks** are done, **50% alcohol** is used. (See neurolytic blocks in Chapter 32.)

4. **Indications for CPB** include the management of pain associated with chronic pancreatitis and as a diagnostic tool to rule out a visceral cause for abdominal pain. It could be used to manage postoperative pain selectively after abdominal surgery. Neurolytic CPB is usually reserved to treat visceral pain of abdominal malignancy. **Contraindications** are the same as those listed in the Introduction.

5. **The complications of CPB** include spinal or epidural anesthesia, intravascular injection, neuralgic pain in the upper lumbar roots, postural hypotension, urinary difficulties or renal trauma, pneumothorax, and hemorrhage.

D. Intravenous Regional (Bier) Block

1. This is a technique for producing anesthesia of an extremity using ischemic isolation with a tourniquet and refilling the vascular system with LA. With **LAs,** the duration of action is only minutes longer than the tourniquet time. When **sympathetically active drugs** (e.g., bretylium) are added, peripheral sympathectomy that lasts for 1 to 2 weeks can be obtained, even without the use of LAs.

2. An IV is placed in a peripheral vein of the extremity that is to be blocked. The extremity is elevated and an Esmarch elastic wrap applied to achieve the necessary exsanguination. Elevation of the extremity for 5 to 15 min can be substituted for exsanguination when the latter is impractical due to pain. The upper cuff of a double tourniquet placed above the elbow or knee is inflated to exceed the systolic blood pressure by 100 torr.

3. For surgical anesthesia, 0.5 mL/kg of 0.5% lidocaine is injected through the previously placed IV. When sympathectomy is the goal, 1 to 3 mg/kg bretylium or 10 to 20 mg guanethidine is injected along with the LA. Other possible additives include steroids, ketorolac, and opioids.

4. Bier block is **indicated for** anesthesia of the distal extremity for orthopedic or soft tissue surgery and for providing peripheral sympathectomy in patients with SMP syndromes. It is **contraindicated in** patients who do not have an intact venous system, those with infection in the extremity, and those for whom a tourniquet is a poor choice.

5. The **complications** of Bier blocks involve LA toxicity if the tourniquet fails or if the tourniquet is deflated before 30 min have elapsed since the primary injection. Tourniquet leak is manifest in tinnitus, circumoral numbness, and dizziness, but the dose of LA (e.g., 0.5% lidocaine, 200 mg in the average adult) is not usually high enough to cause seizures. If patients have received a sympathetic blocking drug, orthostatic hypotension is possible following systemic distribution. If such a drug can also cross the blood–brain barrier, headache is possible.

VI. PLEXUS BLOCKS

A. Brachial Plexus

Brachial plexus block techniques will provide sensory, motor, and/or sympathetic blockade of the ipsilateral upper extremity, depending on the concentration of LA drug used.

1. **The brachial plexus is made up of nerves from C5–8 and T1.** Occasionally, there are contributions from C4 and T2. The nerves are **enclosed in fascia** from their origin at the cervical vertebrae to their peripheral ramification in the axilla. All techniques for blocking the brachial plexus are predicated on inserting a needle into this fascial tube and letting the volume of LA injected determine the extent of the block. Some note that there are septa that divide the fascial tube and isolate the nerves in compartments as the plexus goes more distally. The exact significance of this possibility is not known.

2. The details for **interscalene, supraclavicular, subclavian perivascular, infraclavicular,** and **axillary approaches** to brachial block are described in routine textbooks. Varying the concentration of the LA will determine the physiologic consequences of the block. Obesity may interfere with the identification of the landmarks for certain approaches, so it is reasonable to be familiar with more than one technique.

3. Patients may receive brachial plexus blocks with 1% to 1.5% **lidocaine or mepivacaine with 1:200,000 epinephrine or** 0.25% to 0.5% **bupivacaine** in the operating room for surgery. Some critically ill patients may benefit from the placement of a **catheter for the continuous infusion** of LA (e.g., 0.0625% to 0.125% bupivacaine) to provide **sympathetic block** for the purposes of maximizing blood flow or 0.125% to 0.25% bupivacaine to provide more **profound analgesia** that enhances patient comfort without the need for other analgesic drugs (and their side effects) and permits physical therapy.

4. Brachial plexus blocks are **contraindicated** for patients with active infection in the extremity or area of needle/catheter insertion. Other general contraindications for regional analgesia are listed at the beginning of the chapter.

5. It is noteworthy to mention that **with the interscalene and supracla-**

vicular techniques, there is a high likelihood of getting **ipsilateral phrenic nerve block.** This will be of little consequence in patients who are being mechanically ventilated. There is also a risk of pneumothorax with these two approaches to the brachial plexus. There is a risk of LA toxicity with the axillary technique, especially when a transarterial approach is used, as a result of intravascular injection of LA.

B. Cervical Plexus

Cervical plexus block (superficial and deep) provides sensory and/or motor block of the distal C1–4 nerves. The technique is normally used for surgery in the neck and supraclavicular area. Since muscle relaxation is usually not an issue, 1% lidocaine or mepivacaine or 0.25% bupivacaine is used. For **superficial block,** 10 mL of LA is placed at the midpoint of the posterior border of the sternocleidomastoid muscle with the patient's head turned to the opposite side. For **deep plexus block** (and motor block), the C4 transverse process is palpated in the lateral neck and 10 to 20 mL of LA given. It is important to note that at least a partial phrenic nerve block can accompany deep cervical plexus block.

C. Lumbar Plexus

Lumbar plexus block can provide sensory and/or motor block of the anterior thigh and quadriceps muscle (L1–L4). A concentration of lidocaine, mepivacaine, or bupivacaine consistent with the clinical need is chosen. From 15 to 30 mL of the drug is injected into the area posterior to the psoas muscle and anterior to the L5 vertebrae. Given the proximity to the central neural canal and major vessels, spinal, epidural, and intravascular injections are possible.

VII. PERIPHERAL NERVE BLOCKS FOR ANALGESIA

A. Infiltration of Wound Margins or Incision Irrigation

Infiltration of the wound margins or irrigation of the wound with long-acting LAs such as bupivacaine will decrease incisional/wound pain. The extent to which this limits the amount of other analgesic medications needed and enhances the patient's comfort will vary among patients and the sizes and locations of the wounds or incisions. It should be noted that LAs injected into an infected area will be less effective due to altered ionization caused by the acidic milieu, which limits the amount of LA able to pass through the neuronal membrane. However, more proximal blockade of the same nerve will provide adequate analgesia.

B. Paravertebral Blocks

Paravertebral blocks provide sensory analgesia of selected spinal nerves by the placement of LA distal to the intervertebral foramen. A needle is inserted through the skin one to two finger breadths lateral to the midline and one segment above the nerve level to be blocked. The needle is angled 45 degrees off the perpendicular to the skin *and* 45 degrees caudad, and advanced until contact with the transverse process of the targeted vertebrae is made. Then 5 to 7 mL of LA is placed.

C. Intercostal Nerve Blocks

Intercostal nerve blocks (INBs) provide analgesia in a dermatomal distribution of the chest wall and the parietal pleura. This block can be of tremendous benefit in patients with postoperative thoracic or abdominal pain, rib fractures, or indwelling chest or gastrostomy tubes. The LA must be placed near the nerve before it divides into its cutaneous branches. The usual location for an INB is at the lateral border of the paraspinal muscles or the posterior axillary line. The nerves are blocked as they course along the underside of the ribs. Some 3 to 5 mL of 1% to 1.5% lidocaine or mepivacaine or 0.25% to 0.5% bupivacaine with 1:200,000 epinephrine is injected at each rib. As there are many blood vessels in the vicinity of these nerves, and because multiple nerves are frequently blocked at one time, there is a high risk of LA toxic reaction, particularly within the first 30 min after injection. The risk of pneumothorax is also prominent. Disadvantages include the limited duration of action of a single dose of LA (6 to 8 h) and the subsequent need for repeated injections, which are painful for the patient and labor intensive for the physician.

D. Intrapleural Administration of LA

Intrapleural analgesia is based on the concept that LA drugs infused into the intrapleural space can simulate the effect of multiple intercostal blocks and reduce the labor intensiveness of repeating INBs every 6 to 8 h. This technique is applicable to many patients who would qualify to receive INBs. A catheter is placed through an epidural needle inserted *over* the T7 or T8 rib at the posterior axillary line and directed posteriorly toward the spine. Then 20 to 30 mL of 0.25% to 0.5% bupivacaine with 1:200,000 epinephrine is injected every 8 to 12 h. The effectiveness of the technique is enhanced if, when the catheter is injected, the patient can be temporarily placed with the injected side uppermost and rolled slightly toward the back, and chest tube suction is interrupted for approximately 20 min. There is a small risk of pneumothorax with catheter placement, and because the pleura is a vascular absorptive surface, all patients must be monitored for signs of LA toxicity.

E. Ilioinguinal Nerve Block

Ilioinguinal nerve block with 1% to 1.5% lidocaine or mepivacaine or 0.25% bupivacaine would provide sensory analgesia of the ipsilateral groin area. Use of 2% lidocaine or 0.5% bupivacaine will result in motor block, and can relieve muscle spasm due to pain in the lower abdominal wall.

F. Femoral Nerve Block

Femoral nerve block can relieve the pain of femur fracture and reflex muscle spasm in the quadriceps. The nerve is blocked with 10 to 20 mL of LA placed lateral to the femoral artery and just below the inguinal ligament.

G. Suprascapular and Intrabursal Blocks

Suprascapular nerve block will relieve shoulder pain and spasm of the supra- and infraspinatus muscles of the scapula. This may be helpful to patients who have suffered musculoskeletal trauma, been confined to bed for a period of time, or have recovered enough to begin participating in rehabilitative physical therapy. The nerve is blocked with 6 to 8 mL of 0% to 25% bupivicaine injected superior to and at the midpoint of the scapular spine. **Intrabursal block** with LA and depot steroid may be a useful adjunct to treat subacromial/deltoid bursitis in selected patients as they resume ambulatory activities.

H. Occipital Nerve Block

Occipital nerve block is a technique that provides analgesia in the distribution of the posterior division of the C2 spinal nerve. Patients who have suffered musculoskeletal trauma or have endured prolonged bed rest may complain of occipital headaches. This block uses 5 mL of 1.5% lidocaine or 0.5% bupivacaine with or without 1:200,000 epinephrine and, in some cases, depot steroids injected at the point of insertion of the paraspinal muscles at the nuchal line.

VIII. TRIGGER POINT INJECTIONS

The etiology and pathology of trigger points are discussed in Chapter 32. It is worth repeating here the recommendation that when trigger points are identified, simple infiltration with LA drugs (e.g., bupivacaine 0.5%, 3 to 6 mL) can be of marked benefit in the management of the patient's pain. Occasionally, trigger points also require the injection of depot steroid compounds to prolong the favorable response to such therapy.

SUGGESTED READINGS

Bonica JJ: *The Management of Pain,* 2nd ed. Philadelphia, Lea & Febiger, 1990.
Brown DL: *Atlas of Regional Anesthesia.* Philadelphia, Saunders, 1992.
Carron HC, Korbon GA, Rowlingson JC: *Regional Anesthesia: Techniques and Clinical Applications.* Orlando, Florida, Grune & Stratton, 1984.
Cousins M, Bridenbaugh PO: *Neural Blockade in Clinical Anesthesia and Management of Pain,* 2nd ed. Philadelphia, Lippincott, 1988.
Raj PP: *Handbook of Regional Anesthesia.* New York, Churchill Livingstone, 1985.
Sinatra RS: *Acute Pain Management: Mechanisms and Management.* St Louis, Mosby, 1992.
U.S. Department of Health and Human Services: *Acute Pain Management: Operative or Medical Procedures and Trauma.* Autor, February 1992.

CHAPTER 14

ADJUNCTIVE THERAPY FOR PAIN

John C. Rowlingson
Rodger S. Kessler
Joseph R. Dane
Robin J. Hamill

STIMULATION-INDUCED ANALGESIA
Transcutaneous Electrical Nerve Stimulation
  I. Introduction
  II. Indications for TENS
  III. Contraindications
  IV. Complications
     A. Most Common Complications
     B. Other Concerns
  V. Application of TENS
     A. Understanding the Unit
     B. Modes of Stimulation
Acupuncture
  I. Introduction
  II. Indications for Use
  III. Contraindications
  IV. Potential Complications
     A. Needle-Related Complications
     B. Technique-Related Complications
  V. Applications
SELF-REGULATION TECHNIQUES
  I. Introduction
     A. Goals of Psychological Intervention
     B. Patient Training
     C. Choice of Technique
  II. Characteristics of Specific Self-Regulation Techniques
     A. Overlap Between Techniques
     B. Differences
     C. Levels and Types of Psychological Intervention
     D. Manipulation of the Patient's Focus of Attention

E. Meditation
   F. Imagery
   G. Relaxation Training
   H. Biofeedback
   I. Stress Inoculation Training
   J. Brief Psychotherapy
   K. Hypnosis
III. Limitations and Caveats with Self-Regulation Techniques
   A. Minimal Risk of Negative Outcomes
   B. Structural Issues
   C. Clinical Issues
IV. Case Examples
Suggested Readings

The use of additional therapeutic modalities to supplement those traditionally or commonly applied to control the acute pain of illness, trauma, or the postoperative period is desirable. The contemporary concept that "pain" is caused by and experienced as the combination of many, perhaps diverse, factors makes it reasonable that attacking the pain with a multitude of treatments will result in a more satisfactory degree of pain control. The coordinated use of medication *and* nonmedication techniques gives the healthcare professional an enviable amount of latitude for dealing with a patient's changing needs for pain regulation. If one modality affords an ineffective response, there will be little delay in providing pain relief because other options are readily available. Techniques that give the patient a real or perceived sense of control over their use can mitigate the anticipatory anxiety that immediate steps won't be taken to relieve incident or breakthrough pain. Finally, some patients will have a greater capacity to apply self-regulation strategies or simply to cope with the pain than others, so not all patients need the same prescriptions. This chapter discusses some common options for adjunctive, nonpharmacologic therapy. They can be grouped under the major categories of stimulation-induced analgesia and self-regulation techniques.

STIMULATION-INDUCED ANALGESIA

TRANSCUTANEOUS ELECTRICAL NERVE STIMULATION

I. INTRODUCTION

   A. Transcutaneous electrical nerve stimulation (TENS) is the technique of applying controlled, low-voltage electrical impulses to the nervous system through electrodes attached to the skin.

B. TENS is best used as a component of a therapeutic program, although some patients will achieve complete relief with TENS alone. It has been shown to be effective for symptomatic relief and the management of selected acute and chronic pain problems.

C. TENS is used to help control the pain, and not to eliminate it.

D. The **mechanism of effect** is postulated to be either of the following:

1. The gate control theory states that the balance between the input from large (myelinated) and small (unmyelinated) fibers to the dorsal horn of the spinal cord will determine the intensity of the stimulation that passes on to the higher levels of the central nervous system (CNS). When TENS stimulates the large, myelinated fibers, this input overrides that transmitted by the A-delta and C fibers that carry many of the "pain" impulses. The "gate" is proposed to be at the level of the substantia gelatinosa of the dorsal horn where an inhibition of responses occurs through a complex network of relay neurons and neurochemicals.

2. At more intense levels of neural stimulation, **endorphin release** is triggered. This results in the activation of descending pathways that exert an inhibitory effect on ascending nerve impulses, in part by increasing the threshold for stimulation of the dorsal horn cells, though this process may also occur at many levels in the CNS.

II. INDICATIONS FOR TENS

A. The advantages of TENS use include:
1. It is a noninvasive therapy.
2. It is patient controlled after the patient is oriented to it.
3. It has no systemic side effects.
4. It does not interfere with other ongoing therapy.
5. It is nonaddictive, safe, and reasonably convenient.
6. It can decrease the need for analgesic medications, thereby limiting the risk of undesirable side effects (e.g., nausea, constipation, sedation, confusion, respiratory depression).

B. TENS is indicated for use in the following situations:

1. An important use is as an **adjunctive treatment** of posttraumatic and postoperative acute pain. Research has shown that up to 25 percent of postoperative patients will need little else for pain control when TENS is used, and that 50 percent of patients exhibit a decreased need for potent opioids with concurrent TENS therapy. Reducing the amount of narcotic in the postoperative period should lessen the incidence of drug-related side effects as noted above.

2. Another use is for the **symptomatic relief of chronic pain.** Patients with active chronic pain problems need some or all of their usual therapy continued while management of the acute pain situation is ongoing.

C. Data reveal that when TENS is used as a component of a comprehensive chronic pain management program, 65 to 70 percent of patients find benefit with it early in treatment, while only 50 percent continue to benefit after a year. When TENS is used in a more isolated fashion, 50 percent of patients claim initial success, and this drops to 30 to 35 percent after a year.

III. CONTRAINDICATIONS

A. The efficacy of TENS is markedly enhanced when the prospective patient can be given a detailed explanation of the unit's operation and function. This discussion helps the patient to form realistic expectations about TENS and reinforces its use as an adjunctive therapy. Unfortunately, patients who are critically ill may not be able to process information adequately about TENS use, whereas postoperative patients can be given an orientation to the unit preoperatively, and even the chance to experiment with its operation.

B. **TENS is not recommended** in:
1. Patients with demand pacemakers in place.
2. Patients with an undiagnosed pain source or those deemed psychologically nonpredisposed to want control of the pain therapy.
3. Patients with skin anesthesia or numbness at the site of electrode placement.
4. Patients who would need stimulation over the carotid sinus, laryngeal/pharyngeal muscles, or eyes.

IV. COMPLICATIONS

A. Most Common Complications

The most **common complications** of TENS include the following.
1. **Skin irritation** may occur at the site of electrode placement due to:
   a. Allergic reaction to the contact gel or the metal snap connector.
   b. Chemical reaction to the gel.
   c. Mechanical stress on the skin caused by sheer forces between the tape on the electrode and the skin.
2. **Burns of the skin** may be caused by excessive stimulation or poor electrode placement (i.e., the patch is in only partial contact with the skin, causing areas of higher density current).
3. There may be **electrical interference** with monitors (e.g., electrocardiograms).

B. Other Concerns

1. The patient must be able both physically *and* emotionally to interact with the TENS unit, as well as to process the explanation offered concerning its use. Active participation and compliance are factors in the treatment's success. The patient's capacity for this may be particularly impaired in the setting of the intensive care unit (ICU) for many reasons, including the concomitant use of sedating medications, sleep deprivation, metabolic disturbances (e.g., hepatic encephalopathy, severe uremia), or intracranial pathology (e.g., trauma, infection, bleeding).
2. The patient may accommodate to the stimulating effects of repetitious TENS at constant settings.
3. The use of sedatives may hamper the benefit of TENS by modifying its physiologic effects in the CNS.
4. TENS may be less effective in patients with a history of alcohol or drug dependncy.

V. APPLICATION OF TENS

A. Understanding the Unit

1. The **parameters** that can be set include:
   a. The **rate** = the number of pulses per second.
   b. The **amplitude** = the strength of the stimulation.
   c. The **pulse width** = the duration of the pulses.
2. The amplitude and duration of the stimulation must meet or exceed the threshold for excitability of the tissue stimulated.
3. The placement of the electrodes depends on the pathologic process being treated. They may be used along dermatomes, over muscles that are in spasm, or over vascular channels to augment blood flow.
4. To decrease the incidence of accommodation to the stimulation, a pattern of stimulation should be chosen that rhythmically varies the parameters (e.g., modulation mode) or the unit should be used intermittently (e.g., 1 h on, 1 h off).

B. Modes of Stimulation

The **modes of treatment** are varied to improve both the therapeutic effect and the patient's compliance, as well as with respect to the nature and location of the pain and the patient's condition.

1. **Conventional TENS**
   a. Conventional TENS is often used for acute, soft tissue, localized pain (e.g., incisional pain, rib fractures).

  b. Electrodes can be placed bracketing the painful area or over the paraspinous region of the involved dermatome(s).
  c. Settings are listed in Table 14-1.
  d. TENS provides quick relief during the treatment time and has a short carryover analgesic effect. Thus it is used on an as-needed basis.
  e. Accommodation is common, so variation in the settings is important to maintain the therapeutic effect.
 2. Acupuncture-like TENS
  a. Acupuncture-like TENS is often used for deep, aching, chronic pain.
  b. Electrodes are placed along acupuncture meridians. (See "Acupuncture," I-C.)
  c. Settings are listed in Table 14-1.
  d. Intensity is adjusted to the level required for muscle activation. This mode is uncomfortable and is not well tolerated by some patients. Further, because this mode **releases endorphins,** the onset of effect is not as rapid as with conventional TENS, but the carryover analgesia is greater.
 3. Brief, intense TENS (burst mode)
  a. Brief TENS is used for more intense analgesia for wound debridement, joint manipulation, and other brief treatments.
  b. Electrodes are placed along the course of the dermatomes or peripheral nerves to the involved area or proximal and distal to the wound.
  c. Settings are listed in Table 14-1.
  d. The intensity of stimulus is adjusted as tolerated by the patient, to just below the muscle twitch threshold. This modality is also perceived by some as uncomfortable.
 4. Modulation mode
  a. The modulation mode is used for patients with a variety of pain problems who need more undulation in the nervous system stimulation, who have not responded to conventional TENS, and for whom a change in stimulus intensity is more comfortable or tolerable.
  b. Electrodes are placed to surround the area of pain, along dermatomes with the pads proximal and distal to the region of pain, or over muscles that are in spasm.
  c. The settings are listed in Table 14-1.
  d. The amplitude, pulse width, and/or rate are rhythmically increased and decreased by 25 to 50 percent to provide the patient with a sensation that is not unlike a massage. Wider pulses stimulate more fibers and enhance the therapeutic effect without the need for increasing the amplitude, while giving the patient the sense that stimulation is occurring over a larger area. The soothing and relaxing nature of these sensations enhances patient compliance.

Table 14-1 Transcutaneous electrical stimulation modes and parameters

Mode	Pulse width, ms	Pulse rate, pulse/s	Amplitude	Diagram
Conventional	60–100	80–125	Low, perceptible sense of vibration	
Acupuncture	200–300	7–10	High, to patient tolerance	
Brief intense	200–250	2–7 beat bursts	High, to patient tolerance	
Modulation	Varies: 30–250	Varies: 5–125	Varies from 75% to 100% of setting, maximal intensity to patient tolerance	

and enhance the therapeutic effect without the need for increasing the amplitude, while giving the patient the sense that stimulation is occurring over a larger area. The soothing and relaxing nature of these sensations enhances patient compliance.

ACUPUNCTURE

I. INTRODUCTION

   A. **Acupuncture** is the technique of stimulating specific points on or near the skin by the insertion of needles. Other methods of stimulation that have been or are being used include suction, heat, cold, burning, low-voltage current, pressure, ultrasound, and lasers.

   B. Acupuncture was founded in ancient Chinese philosophy. The concept of disease was based upon there being a **balance of yin** (female, passive, accepting) **and yang** (male, aggressive, forceful) forces in the body, represented as **Chi**. The flow of Chi is blocked by stresses such as injury and illness. This results in an imbalance of yin and yang, and, subsequently, pain and disease.

   C. The acupuncture points are distributed along **meridians** on the surface of the body. Meridians are hypothetical lines through which the life force Chi flows. There are 12 paired and two unpaired meridians. (See Fig. 14.1.)

   D. The **mechanism of action** of traditional acupuncture is the insertion of needles into the acupuncture points to release the blockade of Chi flow and restore harmony to and health in the body. In spite of the contemporary understanding of neural stimulation, debate over the true mechanism of action of acupuncture continues. There are clearly biochemical (although not necessarily just endorphin) and neurophysiologic (increased heart rate and blood pressure, altered gastrointestinal function and blood chemistry) effects of acupuncture. Given the invasive nature of acupuncture and its capability to stimulate medium-sized afferent nerve fibers in muscles, the concept of large-fiber stimulation blocking small-fiber input (the gate control theory) is certainly plausible. Other mechanisms commonly mentioned include a placebo effect, distraction, counterirritation and psychological bias.

II. INDICATIONS FOR USE

   A. This technique is useful as an adjunctive form of therapy in selected patients with many different acute and chronic pain syndromes.

CHAPTER 14   ADJUNCTIVE THERAPY FOR PAIN

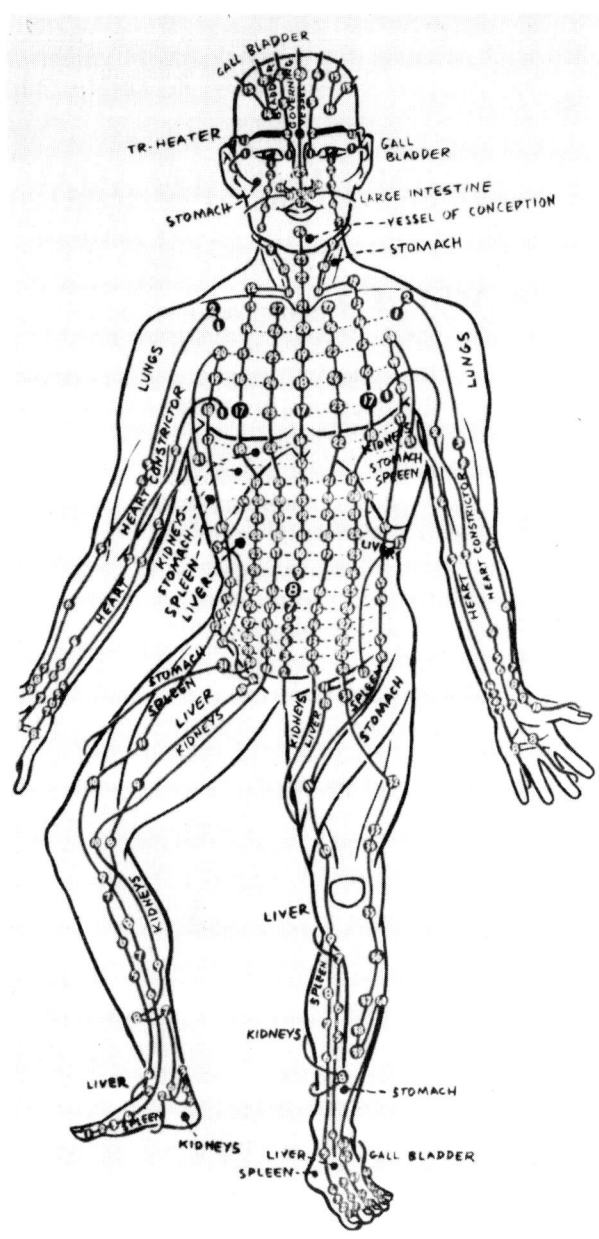

Figure 14-1

B. Data reveal that 50 to 80 percent of patients may exhibit a short-term benefit.

C. Studies find no statistically significant difference between acupuncture and other methods of stimulation, except when it is used as a component of a comprehensive treatment program.

III. CONTRAINDICATIONS

A. Acupuncture is an invasive therapy. It is not recommended in patients who are anticoagulated, have infection at the site of needle insertion, or have active, blood-borne infection.

B. Consideration needs to be given to the complications listed below. Acupuncture would not be advised in patients for whom a complication could have drastic consequences, for example, a patient with severe chronic obstructive pulmonary disease in whom a pneumothorax might be life-threatening.

C. Patients with a high degree of nonphysical pain are poor candidates for acupuncture.

IV. POTENTIAL COMPLICATIONS

A. The **needle-related complications** include:
1. Breaking a needle.
2. Causing bleeding.
3. Creating local infection.
4. Transmitting disease, such as hepatitis B, AIDS, or cytomegalovirus.
5. Invading nontargeted tissue, as by causing pneumothorax, paresthesias, or nerve damage.

B. The **technique-related problems** include:
1. Vasovagal reactions and fainting.
2. Contact dermatitis.
3. Lack of therapeutic effect.
4. Delay in providing more conventional therapy.

V. APPLICATIONS

A. The number of acupuncture points used and the number of treatments provided depend on the patient's preference, type of pain, chronicity, and seriousness of the problem.

B. To implement the technique, 26- to 30-gauge needles are inserted a few millimeters into the skin to create a feeling of warmth, heaviness, soreness, or local numbness. They can be untouched, twirled, or have low-voltage current applied. Some forms of the therapy intentionally penetrate deep enough to stimulate muscles.

C. Though the length of each treatment can vary, periods of 20 to 30 min are common.

SELF-REGULATION TECHNIQUES

I. INTRODUCTION

A. Goals of Psychological Intervention

The **goals of psychological intervention** in acute pain are to establish an effective patient/caregiver alliance rapidly and to enhance patient comfort, compliance, and active participation in the recovery process. These goals are best facilitated through a variety of "self-regulation" techniques that train patients to regulate spontaneously the various cognitive, affective, and physiologic components of pain perception and response to pain. The context for utilizing these techniques and training patients in their use is all important. The reader is referred to Chapter 5 for ways to establish and maintain an appropriate context.

B. Patient Training

Effective **training in the use of self-regulation techniques** involves five basic phases (see "Coping Skills Training" in Chapter 5). Such training typically elicits:

1. Heightened internal awareness of physiologic events and the ability to influence these independently.

2. Reduction of cognitive and affective distractions and distortions ("worry and preoccupation"), which could interfere with this awareness.

3. Practice in using this awareness and acquired skill of self-regulation to maintain or reestablish the desired outcomes when needed.

C. Choice of Technique

The choice of a particular self-regulation technique depends on the unique characteristics of the patient and the clinical setting, combined with the desired outcome goals. When outcome goals are limited (e.g., compliance with a specific procedure), guidance in the use of cognitive strategies which are initiated and sustained by the caregiver is often sufficient. When emotionality is an issue, more global strategies, such as imagery and dissociative phenomena, are more useful. In most instances, it is desirable to include strategies which evoke deep physiologic relaxation. This provides decreased autonomic reactivity, lowered heart rate, and increased oxygenation, along with increased ease and a decreased rate of respiration. When repeatedly evoked or maintained by the patient over time, these changes typically result in increased compliance and comfort with injury-related immobility, while maximizing healing processes and eventual readiness for increases in activity.

II. CHARACTERISTICS OF SPECIFIC SELF-REGULATION TECHNIQUES

A. Overlap Between Techniques

Self-regulation techniques overlap to some extent and vary in how much they depend on:

   1. The use of specific **cognitive strategies** (e.g., positive or encouraging self-statements, or refocusing of attention through distraction, imagery, music, or humor).

   2. Patient practice of specific **physiologic activities** (e.g., deep breathing and muscle relaxation).

   3. Active manipulation of **dissociative phenomena** (e.g., hypnosis).

   4. An integration of items 1 through 3.

   5. The use of **external paraphernalia,** either for generation of external feedback about internal physiologic states such as muscle tension or skin temperature (e.g., biofeedback equipment), or as an aid to practice of the technique (e.g., audiotapes and tape recorder/playback units for self-hypnosis or relaxation training).

   6. The presence of **ongoing interaction** with a caretaker or instructor.

B. Differences

Self-regulation techniques also vary in:

   1. Ease of **training** for independent use by the patient, including the amount of patient/caregiver time and energy required for instruction, learning, and practice of the techniques in which the patient is being trained.

   2. Degree of **impact** provided on specific affective, cognitive, and physiologic changes.

   3. Degree of **"portability"** across clinical settings.

C. Levels and Types of Psychological Intervention

The reader is directed to Table 5-4 of Chapter 5 for a summary of the various **levels and types of psychological intervention** available. This table organizes interventions and teachable coping skills into categories of "brief/rudimentary" and "extended/complex," based roughly on the time required for delivery of the intervention and the amount of specialized training necessary for the staff to utilize the intervention.

D. Manipulation of the Patient's Focus of Attention

All psychological techniques for managing pain **manipulate the patient's focus of attention,** and to this extent, are characterized by some form of "distraction" from the pain. However, techniques vary in their degree of sophistication and complexity in eliciting and utilizing the various effects possible through manipulation of attention. In general, hypnosis is the most broadly effective and efficient of all available techniques. A continuum of techniques, however, is delineated below.

E. Meditation

Meditation is probably the oldest and broadest tradition, and the one from which contemporary techniques draw most heavily. The goal of meditation is to shape the capacity for dispassionate observation and avoidance of "attachment" (e.g., attachment to awareness of painful sensation). Many meditative techniques consist of focusing attention on some aspect of one's experience, such as the in-and-out flow of one's breath. The focus may be active, such as focusing on a particular word or phrase, or passive, such as merely observing the passage of one's thoughts or the flow of one's experience throughout the day's activities. **Yoga** (which refers to "yoking" of the mind and the body) is also a form of meditation whose focus of attention is on disciplined physical exertion involving stretching and balance. Rudimentary aspects of meditation can be readily taught and require no external equipment. Effective practice generally necessitates a quiet setting free of distractions. Physiologic relaxation generally occurs spontaneously, but is not usually targeted as specifically as with other techniques.

F. Imagery

Imagery may also be part of meditative practice, but is treated separately here since "guided imagery" is frequently referred to as an independent technique in contemporary pain literature. Individuals vary widely in the vividness or intensity of their imagery, and few are capable of a "Polaroid picture" or "360-degree-surround" type of imagery. However, since the capacity to become absorbed in internal fantasy is one of the few demonstrable correlates of measured hypnotic capacity, it may be that individuals who respond well to imagery alone are also capable of generating a wide range of medically useful hypnotic phenomena if the caretaker is trained to recognize and take advantage of them (see below).

G. Relaxation Training

Relaxation training combines the focused attention of meditation with the conscious intent to alter physiology through the addition of instructions about specific physiologic procedures. These procedures may utilize soothing images, but focus primarily on alterations in breathing, alterations in muscular contractions (e.g., **progressive muscle relaxation**), or alterations in proprioception and sensation (e.g., **autogenics training**). Physiologic relaxation is specifically targeted by these techniques, with the assumption that affective relaxation is likely to follow automatically. However, without sufficient rapport and preparation, the blatant focus in these techniques on relaxation per se may initially seem ludicrous or impossible to patients in significant acute pain.

H. Biofeedback

Biofeedback uses equipment to monitor and translate the physiologic experience of relaxation (e.g., changes in muscle tension) into external cues (e.g., tones or lights) which are more readily discriminable than internal estimates of that experience. Its great advantage is the specificity of feedback provided in terms of parameters which can be monitored (e.g., muscle tension, heart rate, blood pressure, skin temperature, galvanic skin response), as well as in the degree of change in each parameter. Its great disadvantages for acute situations are the reliance on specialized and expensive equipment which requires application and removal of sensors for each utilization, and the lack of opportunity to train the patient before application is needed. Although portable units are available, the need for specially trained technicians usually precludes the use of biofeedback in medical inpatient settings.

I. Stress Inoculation Training

Stress inoculation training was developed by Meichenbaum as a way to alter attitudes and affect the patient's sense of "self-efficacy," or the perceived ability to carry out specific coping strategies. It is a three-step process involving (1) patient education about the cognitive and affective principles governing pain perception, (2) collaboration with the patient in developing effective coping strategies from an array of available techniques, and (3) practice with these techniques until a sense of mastery is achieved. This program is grounded in solid research, and shows promise of good results with some patients. It is particularly appropriate when preparation time is available in advance of the patient's undergoing the painful procedure.

J. Brief Psychotherapy

Brief psychotherapy refers to extended discussions with patients about the thoughts, feelings, and behavior patterns affecting their pain or illness, all of which can affect their ability and motivation to utilize self-regulation techniques. **Cognitive-behavioral** approaches focus on altering current thoughts and behaviors, such as by training in the use of positive self-statements and by analyzing the behavioral components of particular emotional responses. **Psychodynamic** approaches address internal conflicts and drives which may be out of the patient's conscious awareness, but which are amenable to alteration with appropriate treatment. These approaches can be particularly helpful in addressing arrested grief reactions, which so frequently go unrecognized in acute medical settings, but which can interfere significantly with adequate pain management (see "The Grieving Process" in Chapter 5).

K. Hypnosis

Hypnosis is often confused with the simplistic use of one or more of the above techniques, particularly distraction, relaxation, and imagery. It is true that in its application, hypnosis resembles many aspects of these other techniques. Likewise, similar types of physiologic outcomes are often equally well accomplished with either hypnosis or one of the other techniques. However, the unique contribution of hypnosis is its recognition and use of a phenomenon known as **dissociation,** and its appreciation for individual differences in the capacity to experience this phenomenon.

    1. **Dissociation** is a function of highly focused attention, but is quite distinct from mere distraction, in the same way that a daydream differs from a full-blown hallucination. Dissociation refers to a profound reorganization of perceptual and informational processing, which allows undeniably personal experience (e.g., the pain of surgery) to occur for the individual as if it were happening separately from the individual's experience—that is, as if it were happening to "someone else" or not happening at all. In its extreme forms, dissociation helps to explain so-called multiple personality disorders, where a child's innate capacity for dissociation becomes reinforced over time as a primary defense system to protect the child from conscious awareness and memory of repeated, prolonged abuse. The individual's various "personalities" are simply congruent attitudes, beliefs, emotions, and behaviors which the individual has developed over time and which he or she experiences as appropriate to certain circumstances or stimuli, but which remain totally separate ("dissociated"), one from the other, within the person's internal experience. We mention this rather exotic form of dissociation here merely to emphasize the point made earlier in Chapter 5 (see "Hyp-

notic Capacity"). Namely, "hypnosis" is a naturally occurring phenomenon which has profound implications for human experience that can be helpful or disruptive, depending on whether they are recognized and utilized appropriately.

2. The great clinical advantage of **training in hypnotic strategies** is that one learns to elicit, shape, and maximize whatever level of hypnotic capacity an individual patient may possess. This capacity may range from simple relaxation and mild pleasant imagery to profound surgical anesthesia. A capacity for amnesia can help reduce anticipatory anxiety related to repeated painful procedures, such as burn debridement. The capacity to respond to posthypnotic suggestions can permit the recurrence of pain to become a cue for the patient that automatically triggers the use of an effective coping strategy. Moreover, the hypnotically trained clinician is able to "start with patients where they are." For example, with patients in acute discomfort, purely rational instructions for progressive muscle relaxation can be quite frustrating, and even counterproductive. Hypnotic strategies, on the other hand, can use the patient's attentional focus on pain as the beginning focal point in the hypnotic induction process, gradually shaping the patient's attention by suggesting and eliciting a variety of hypnotic experiences that move toward relaxation and analgesia as the hypnotic state progresses. One can then use positive suggestion and reframing of the patient's experience, evoking the patient's awareness of existing coping skills which have become lost in the terror of the moment, or even eliciting a capacity for sensory alteration which the patient had never realized could be accomplished.

3. Another important advantage of hypnosis is its **impact on interpersonal rapport.** Research has confirmed the "pull for regression" that often accompanies hypnotic interactions. This simply means that the hypnotized person is likely to attribute parentlike qualities to the hypnotic facilitator. Properly utilized, these attributions can contribute enormously to patient comfort and compliance and to positive clinical outcome. Further, because it makes use of suggestion, hypnosis is simultaneously an active mode of psychotherapeutic intervention and a vehicle for training in specific coping skills.

4. In summary, hypnosis is a broadly effective and efficient technique that has the following characteristics.

    a. It permits a **rapid focus** on the problem at hand, whether behavioral, attitudinal, or a question of altering physiologic response.

    b. It **facilitates and enhances rapport.**

    c. It allows both **active treatment** and **patient education.**

    d. It has **maximum "portability"** across clinical settings, while providing multiple intervention strategies. In many individuals, hypnosis can promote alterations in physiology, sensation, memory, affect, and time perception, all of which constitute the subjective matrix within which pain is perceived. As discussed in Chapter 5, altering this matrix can significantly alter an individual's experience of pain.

5. It should be acknowledged that the experimental literature demonstrating the **validity of hypnoanalgesia** and its relationship to hypnotic capacity is quite strong. However, controlled clinical studies of hypnosis are infrequent and often poorly designed, so that most reviewers unfamiliar with its use tend to dismiss it as "unproven." As medical science continues to grow in its awareness of the impact of psychological factors on comfort and healing, it is expected that the use of these techniques will become more commonplace. In the meantime, the clinical impact of effectively delivered hypnotic suggestion with hypnotically responsive patients remains quite remarkable.

III. LIMITATIONS AND CAVEATS WITH SELF-REGULATION TECHNIQUES

A. Minimal Risk of Negative Outcomes

The use of these techniques generally involves a **minimal risk of negative outcomes,** but there are certain issues and activities which must be addressed to ensure optimal results and the lowest risk of negative outcome.

B. Structural Issues

1. **Time and setting**

   a. Training patients in self-regulation techniques requires an **investment of staff time** beyond that required by traditional medical care. However, this time is usually more than offset by the reduction in both frustration and total care time ultimately required by such patients, given their increased sense of well-being and their motivation to participate as a partner in their own care.

   b. Again, hypnosis is a most efficient tool in this regard, since it is both a form of direct intervention and a methodology for training patients. However, it is **crucial that the overall setting be supportive of and conducive to patients' having time** to practice their self-regulation techniques, and that the predictable need for fine-tuning and reinforcement of this practice not be interpreted as proof that the techniques "just aren't working."

2. **Training of staff**

   a. Appropriate use of self-regulation training **requires specialized training** for providers. Optimally, a trained mental health professional who specializes in pain treatment can serve as a consultant to help identify training needs and resources.

   b. Issues of **training in hypnosis** deserve special attention. Almost anyone can readily be taught to do hypnotic inductions effectively. The question is knowing what to do (and what not to do, see "Caveats—Adverse Reactions" below) once the hypnotic state is established. Hypnosis is a powerful modality of treatment, but not a treatment in itself. It should only be used clinically by personnel with a level of training appropriate to the problem being treated. The most senior licensed professional credentialing possible is that of Diplomate in either Medical, Psychological, or Dental Hypnosis, as conferred by the American Board of Clinical Hypnosis, Incorporated. Certification of basic and advanced hypnosis training for licensed professionals is available through the American Society of Clinical Hypnosis.

C. Clinical Issues

1. Selection of technique

a. General considerations in selecting psychological strategies for pain management are discussed in Chapter 5 under "Selection of Intervention Strategy." The following remarks are limited to specific categories of self-regulation techniques.

b. Laboratory research has demonstrated that relaxation techniques have a greater **impact on the affective or distress component of pain** (i.e., "How much does the pain bother you?") **than** they do **on the sensory component** (i.e., "How intense is the pain?"). Physiologic relaxation clearly interrupts the well-recognized pain/tension cycle, decreases muscle spasm, decreases pressure and strain on pain-sensitive structures, and increases the patient's sense of available energy. Relaxation can also facilitate sleep onset and enhance the general quality of sleep. Relaxation techniques are, therefore, especially helpful with pain that is enduring but relatively low in intensity, such as that following surgery. In addition, relaxation techniques are best introduced either before the pain has become terribly intense, or after severe pain has been brought under control with medication sufficient to allow mental concentration. However, it is also clear that **brief discussions** and simply providing written instructions on how to relax, as opposed to interpersonally mediated demonstration, instruction, and reinforcement, are **not sufficient** to elicit the desired benefits.

c. For the more intense pain associated with procedures ranging from intravenous catheter insertion to bone marrow aspiration, relaxation alone does not reduce pain perception. Nevertheless, it does provide excellent preparation and can help reduce the anxiety associated with these procedures. During such procedures, however, it is important to add the use of cognitive strategies which **promote disattention** to the pain (e.g., counting; naming objects in the room), which help counter the tendency to "catastrophize" (e.g., repeating positive coping statements such as, "This won't last forever; I've made it through this before, and I can make it through this now"), or which redefine the pain via ideas or imagery (e.g., tolerating the pain as one would tolerate an injury and keep on playing in order for one's team to win).

   d. Research has also clearly shown that for both relaxation techniques and techniques involving cognitive attentional shifts, there is a clear interaction with the patient's **locus of control** (LOC) (see Chapter 5). Patients with an external LOC respond better to more directive techniques, while those with an internal LOC prefer and benefit more from interventions in which they feel in control.

   e. Laboratory research has also clearly demonstrated that **hypnotic responsiveness** involves something other than mere relaxation and cognitive shifts in attention. For example, high hypnotic responders do not get as much pain relief with stress inoculation training as with hypnoanalgesia, even when they are told that it is the same thing as hypnosis. That is, the only way to optimize pain control in hypnotically responsive individuals is through the use of specific hypnotic techniques which are adapted to the individual's personal style and preferences.

2. Caveats

   a. While the risks associated with self-regulation techniques are minimal, practitioners should be aware of **three potential adverse reactions.**

   b. The first potential adverse reaction is known as **relaxation-induced anxiety.** This involves a reaction of dysphoric psychophysiologic arousal (e.g., increased heart rate, palmar sweating, palpitations) that is sometimes accompanied by generalized anxiety and negativistic preoccupations, all of which occur, paradoxically, in certain patients when they attempt to relax. This reaction is usually conceptualized psychophysiologically as a type of parasympathetic "rebound," which can usually be overcome by simply slowing down and proceeding very gradually with the relaxation process. If this is not effective, then a psychodynamic formulation of the problem (e.g., that muscular relaxation has in some parallel fashion relaxed the patient's usual defenses against previously repressed dysphoric material) may be more accurate and may indicate the need for psychological treatment.

   c. The second potential adverse reaction is relatively rare, but is important to recognize when it occurs. This involves the **spontaneous abreaction** (i.e., revivification or reliving) **of emotional trauma** which had previously been repressed from memory. When present, this is most commonly seen in patients with a history of physical or sexual abuse, where the pain generated by the current injury or medical procedure is in some way reminiscent of the earlier abuse, either by virtue of its location (e.g., groin or abdomen), or by virtue of the circumstances in which it occurs (e.g., perceived caregivers inflicting pain). It appears that with such individuals, attentional focus and relaxation techniques can provoke a state of dissociation similar to that used as a defense by the patient at the time of the trauma, thereby "uncapping" or reactivating memories of the trauma. While simple reassurance and reorienting to the present time can be helpful with these patients, such reactions often require consultation with mental health professionals.

d. A third potential adverse reaction involves patients who have **trouble distinguishing between internal fantasy and external reality.** Actively psychotic patients are obviously poor candidates for techniques which would heighten such difficulties, unless the caregiver is already experienced in working with such populations, and is well trained in the use of self-regulation techniques. At the same time, a history of psychosis should not automatically preclude the use of self-regulation training, but it does signal the need for closer monitoring of the patient's experience as he or she proceeds through the training process.

e. It should be emphasized that all of the adverse circumstances described above are relatively rare, and all can be effectively managed by the appropriately trained clinician who is aware of their existence.

IV. CASE EXAMPLES

Two extended **case examples** of adjunctive self-regulation training in acute care settings are provided at the end of Chapter 5.

SUGGESTED READINGS

TENS and Acupuncture

Carman D, Roach JW: Transcutaneous electrical nerve stimulation for the relief of post-operative pain in children. *Spine* 13:109–110, 1988.

Evans D: Acupuncture, in Raj PP (ed): *Practical Management of Pain,* 2nd ed. St. Louis, Mosby, 1992, pp 934–944.

Gersh MR, Wolf SL: Applications of transcutaneous electrical nerve stimulation in the management of patients with pain: state-of-the-art update. *Phys Ther* 65:314–322, 1985.

Mannheimer JS, Lampe GN: *Clinical Transcutaneous Electrical Nerve Stimulation.* Philadelphia, Davis, 1984.

McLean B, Fives HE: Stimulation-induced analgesia, in Warfield CA (ed): *Principles and Practice of Pain Management.* New York, McGraw-Hill, 1993, pp 413–425.

National Council Against Health Fraud: Acupuncture: the position paper of the National Council Against Health Fraud. *Clin J Pain* 7:162–166, 1991.

Richardson PH, Vincent CA: Acupuncture for the treatment of pain: a review of the evaluative research. *Pain* 24:15–40, 1986.

Tulgar M, McGlone F, Bowsher D, Miles JB: Comparative effectiveness of different stimulation modes in relieving pain. Part I. A pilot study. *Pain* 47:151–155, 1991.

Ulett GA: Acupuncture treatments for pain relief. *JAMA* 245:768–769, 1981.

Vincent CA, Richardson PH: The evaluation of therapeutic acupuncture: concepts and methods. *Pain* 24:1–13, 1986.

Self-Regulation Techniques

Alman B, Lambrou P: *Self-Hypnosis: A Complete Manual for Health and Self Change,* San Diego, International Health Publications, 1983.

Ewin DM: Hypnosis in surgery and anesthesia, in Western WC, Smith AH (eds): *Clinical Hypnosis: A Multidisciplinary Approach.* Philadelphia, Lippincott, 1981, pp. 210–235.

McCafree M, Beebe A: *Pain: Clinical Manual for Nursing Practice,* St. Louis, Mosby, 1989.

Meichenbaum DH: *Cognitive Behavior Modification: An Integrative Approach,* New York, Plenum Press, 1977.

Pratt GJ, Wood DP, Alman BM: *A Clinical Hypnosis Primer.* La Jolla, California, Psychology and Consulting Associates Press, 1987.

Sacerdote P: Techniques of hypnotic intervention with pain patients, in Barber J, Adrian C (eds): *Psychological Approaches to the Management of Pain.* New York, Brunner/Mazel, 1982.

CHAPTER
15

PHYSICAL AND OCCUPATIONAL THERAPY IN THE PREVENTION AND MANAGEMENT OF PAIN IN THE INTENSIVE CARE UNIT

Kathleen Henahan
Leslie D. Baruch

Case
  I. Consequences of Pain
     A. Effect of Pain
     B. Effects of Pain on the Musculoskeletal System
     C. Pain as a Result of Immobilization
 II. Normal Musculoskeletal Function
     A. Musculoskeletal System
     B. Normal Muscle Function
     C. Factors Influencing Range of Motion
III. Physical and Occupational Therapy Management of Pain
     A. What Does a Physical Therapist Do?
     B. What Does an Occupational Therapist Do?
     C. Role of Physical and Occupational Therapy
 IV. Therapeutic Intervention
     A. Respiratory Function
     B. Cognitive Assessment
     C. Positioning and Splinting
     D. Range-of-Motion Activities
     E. Strategies to Decrease Pain and Perception of Pain
     F. Prefunctional Activities
     G. Retraining in Activities of Daily Living
     H. Functional Mobility

V. Modalities
   A. Heat
   B. Cryotherapy
   C. Electrotherapy
Conclusion
Suggested Readings

CASE

J.C. is a 70-year-old right-hand-dominant white male who was involved in a motor vehicle accident. He was an unrestrained driver in a vehicle that was hit broadside on the driver's side by a truck, and he was ejected from the car. His injuries included facial lacerations, right-upper-extremity brachial plexus stretch injury, right rib fractures with a pneumothorax, right displaced femur fracture, loss of consciousness, and road burn of the right axilla and flank. J.C.'s course was complicated by pneumonia and renal failure. His past medical history is significant for obstructive airway disease and arthritis. Following stabilization of his medical condition, physical and occupational therapy consultation is indicated.

I. CONSEQUENCES OF PAIN

A. Effect of Pain

The experience of acute or chronic pain affects a person's functional independence, as well as psychological state. Pain can make a patient reluctant to move and/or encourages the patient to assume the least painful position. Initially, pain may be perceived as a protective response to prevent further injury. Eventually, however, the pain may develop into a self-propagating process of noxious stimuli. The experience of acute or chronic pain slows the healing process, as illustrated in Fig. 15-1. It is necessary to decrease a patient's pain before increasing function. Consequently, premedication for pain may facilitate physical and occupational therapy intervention, which in itself results in increased mobility and decreased pain.

B. Effects of Pain on the Musculoskeletal System

1. In the presence of acute or chronic pain, the musculoskeletal system often responds with protective **muscle spasms and splinting of movement**. For example, J.C. may demonstrate muscle spasm in the anterior and medial muscles of the thigh at rest or with active muscle contraction following surgical repair of the fracture. When attempting to move the affected

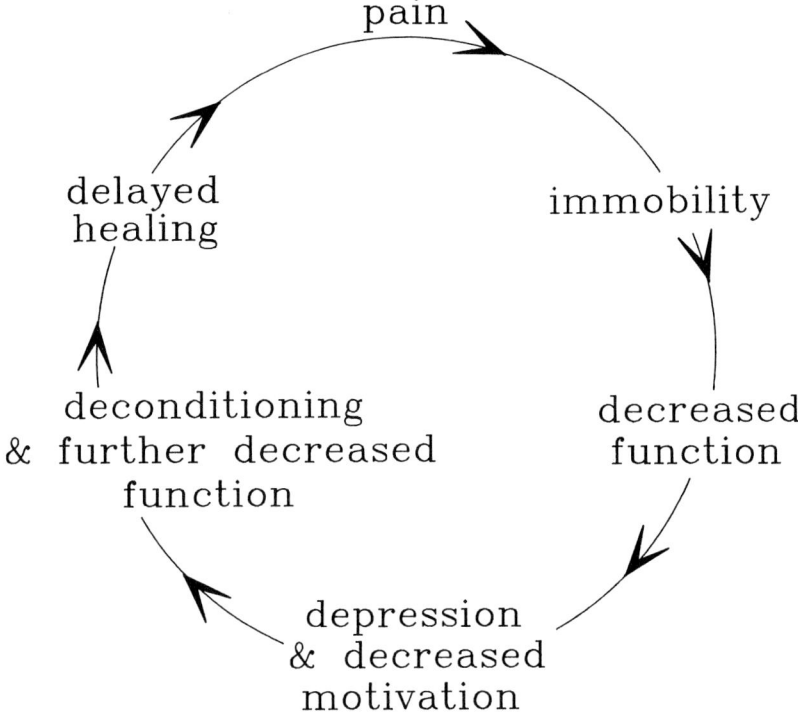

Figure 15-1 Pain and immobilization cycle

extremity, J.C. may demonstrate increased muscle tension, resistance to range of motion (ROM), and splinting of movement.

2. **Abnormal postures or movement patterns** are exhibited secondary to muscle fibers working in either an abnormally shortened or lengthened range. This will affect the speed, coordination, and strength of movement, as well as the antagonist muscle function. Joint capsule and skin tightness, contractures, and, in severe cases, deformities may also develop.

C. Pain as a Result of Immobilization

1. Multiple medical problems often require a patient, such as J.C., to be immobilized for long periods. Strict bed rest for 2 weeks, even without associated injury or illness, results in the loss of up to 25 percent of strength and 50 percent of endurance in a muscle. J.C. will be limited by his impaired respiratory and kidney function and femur fracture. This could induce

many **secondary complications,** including respiratory failure, skin ulceration, muscle atrophy, and deep vein thrombosis, all of which will lengthen the patient's hospital stay.

2. The physiologic **effects of prolonged immobility** include decreased bone density, orthostatic hypotension, decreased endurance, muscle shortening and atrophy, and joint capsule tightness.

II. NORMAL MUSCULOSKELETAL FUNCTION

A. Musculoskeletal System

The musculoskeletal system provides support to the body and facilitates movement. To have coordinated movements, the body must first have postural support and control of the proximal muscles and joints.

B. Normal Muscle Function

Muscle function involves full passive physiologic length, strength in the tonic muscles for control, strength in the **phasic muscles** for movement, and the endurance to maintain all postures and movements. **Tonic muscles,** which are usually classified as extensor muscles, are located proximally and are composed primarily of small, slow-twitch motor units that are resistant to fatigue. Phasic muscles are generally considered flexors, and are composed of large, fast-twitch motor units that fatigue easily.

C. Factors Influencing Range of Motion

Among the factors that influence ROM are the contours of the articulating surfaces of the joints, the direction of ligamentous fibers, and normal neuronal input. The age of the patient, as well as any preexisting condition, may also affect ROM.

III. PHYSICAL AND OCCUPATIONAL THERAPY MANAGEMENT OF PAIN

A. What Does a Physical Therapist Do?

1. A physical therapist evaluates a patient's musculoskeletal, neurologic, and cardiopulmonary systems. This may include an assessment of ROM, strength, sensation, endurance, tone, bed mobility, and ambulation as appropriate. The therapist then develops a therapeutic regimen designed to maximize functional independence, in accordance with the patient's ability to participate in and tolerate treatment.

B. What Does an Occupational Therapist Do?

1. An occupational therapist evaluates a patient's ability to perform functional tasks, which may include feeding, bathing, dressing and transfers; cognition and perception; upper-extremity ROM; and strength, coordination, and sensation. The therapist then develops a treatment plan that translates those abilities, no matter how limited, into activities that are purposeful and meaningful to the patient. Independence with age-appropriate functional activities is the ultimate goal.

C. Role of Physical and Occupational Therapy

1. Evaluation and treatment After establishing the patient's baseline level of function, the physical and occupational therapist will take steps to decrease or eliminate pain in order to prevent the loss of and to increase function. In the case of J.C., the initial evaluation results in instructions to the nursing staff to implement a regimen of passive interventions related to respiratory function, positioning, splinting, and ROM. Treatment interventions progress commensurate with J.C.'s ability to participate. Next steps may involve manual therapies, adaptive equipment, sensory stimulation or desensitization activities, training in activities of daily living, and therapeutic exercise to enhance functional mobility. This last stage of treatment might involve the use of electrical modalities. The interaction between the patient and the therapist provides additional psychosocial support and positive reinforcement of progress.

2. Consultation and referrals The therapists also assist the multidisciplinary team in making appropriate referrals to other specialties. Early intervention may dramatically affect the patient's short- and long-term prognosis. Mobilizing the critically ill patient can have a positive impact on all body systems, and can decrease the length of hospitalization by preventing many of the secondary complications of prolonged immobilization. Table 15-1 lists the negative effects of immobility.

VII. THERAPEUTIC INTERVENTION

A. Respiratory Function

1. Pulmonary hygiene Aggressive pulmonary toilet is crucial to the critically ill patient, for whom the negative physiologic effects of immobility are intensified. The physical therapist's primary objectives are to decrease the effects of immobility on the patient's recovery and to decrease the length of stay in an intensive care unit (ICU). Aggressive pulmonary toileting can be used prophylactically as well as therapeutically. Percussion, vibration,

Table 15-1 Negative effects of immobility and prolonged bed rest (6 to 10 days)

Function	Negative effects
Cardiovascular	Orthostatic hypotension: secondary to loss of general muscle tone and decreased efficiency of orthostatic neurovascular reflex control Increased work load: secondary to increase in cardiac output in supine position and deconditioning Thrombus formation: secondary to venous stasis with lack of muscle contraction in legs, and secondary to increased viscosity of blood with bed rest Hypovolemia: secondary to the fluid shifts that take place in the body as horizontal posture is assumed
Respiratory	Slowed respiratory rate: to compensate for reduced demand of gaseous exchange Oxygen/carbon dioxide imbalance: resulting in hypoxemia Decreased respiratory movement: secondary to prolonged counterresistance of a bed or chair on the rib cage Stasis of secretions: threatening patient airways, resulting in bronchitis, pneumonia, medium for bacterial growth
Motor	Contractures: secondary to lack of active movement, ROM Muscle atrophy: secondary to lack of active muscle contraction Decubitus ulcers: secondary to lack of weight shifting off bony prominences; most likely to appear in malnourished persons with negative nitrogen balance Osteoporosis: secondary to lack of stress on bone with muscle contraction and weight bearing
Metabolic	Decreased metabolic rate: secondary to decreased energy requirements Accelerated catabolic activity: leading to protein deficiency and negative nitrogen balance and excretion of electrolytes Change in body temperatures: increasing perspiration with loss of fluids and electrolytes Decreased production of adrenocortical hormones: changing metabolism of carbohydrates, protein, and fat, and changing electrolyte balance of sodium, potassium, and chloride
Gastrointestinal	Ingestion: within 6 to 10 days of bed rest, nitrogen balance reverses to a negative state, accelerating catabolic activity, which results in protein deficiency and eventually anorexia Elimination: immobility interferes with visceral reflex; diminished expulsion power results in constipation, fecal impaction

From Greenleaf JE: *Bed rest studies: fluid and electrolyte responses.* Laboratory of Human Environmental Physiology, Biomedical Research Division/NASA AMES Research Division (unpublished internal report), 1983; and Olsen E: The hazards of immobility. *Am J Nursing* 67(4):780–797, 1967.

and autogenic drainage are adjunctive techniques that mechanically mobilize secretions and subsequently facilitate clearance through the use of endotracheal sunctioning or coughing. Postural drainage can be discontinued once a patient is up regularly, sitting or ambulating, and is able to breathe deeply and cough.

Pulmonary hygiene becomes a more complex task for the ventilated patient. The weaning of a critically ill patient from prolonged mechanical ventilation is generally a slow process due to catabolic wasting, weakness, and fatigue of the respiratory muscles. **Weakness** refers to the "failure to generate an expected force or a chronic reduction in the contractile force" of respiratory muscles (Shekleton, 1987). **Muscle fatigue** refers to the inability to maintain the force needed repeatedly to sustain a contraction.

a. Signs of fatigue that affect a physical therapy treatment may include tachypnea, dyspnea, increased minute ventilation, and a discoordinated respiratory pattern. The treatment of fatigue focuses on resting respiratory muscles and restoring their contractility. Finally, the strength and endurance of the respiratory muscles are increased with gradual, graded conditioning plans.

b. Strengthening and endurance conditioning of the inspiratory muscles involves high-pressure, low-volume work for strengthening and low-load, high-repetition work for endurance. This process may be accomplished by brief periods of fatiguing exercise alternated with periods of rest. Facilitation of the intercostal muscles to improve inspiration can be used in breathing retraining. Also, accessory muscles help maintain respiration in the critically ill patient, and it is important to address them during retraining. Accessory muscles include the sternocleidomastoid, anterior and middle scalene, serratus anterior, pectoralis major and minor, and trapezius. Strengthening these muscles in their primary muscle function positively affects their accessory function in the respiratory system and can aid in the weaning process.

c. Gravity has a significant impact on weak muscles. Strengthening should begin in a gravity-eliminated or -assisted position. Proper positioning of a patient with weak muscles or neurologic impairment, such as with a high-level spinal cord injury, will help prevent deformity of the chest wall and maintain good respiratory muscle position. When a patient is chronically placed in a supine position, gravity becomes the main force acting on the chest wall. Due to the absence of resistive muscular forces, a flattening or flaring of the anterior rib cage may occur. The use of an abdominal binder will support the abdominal viscera and help to maintain the diaphragm in an elevated position to assist effective respiration.

d. The goals of breathing retraining/exercise are to improve ventilation, improve cough, correct abnormal breathing patterns, mobilize and maintain chest wall mobility, and improve the strength and endurance of the respiratory muscles.

2. Diaphragmatic breathing This is a normal breathing pattern. The patient should be instructed initially in the supine position, with progression through gait and elevation activities. Segmental breathing patterns and manual techniques can be used for more specific problems, including atelectasis, and with muscle splinting from pain.

3. Relaxation Relaxation, a state of lessened tension or strain, is a prerequisite to breathing retraining. Signs and symptoms of tension or strain include irritability, pain, insomnia, decreased flexibility, and an irregular breathing pattern. Patient education is an essential part of the treatment in tension reduction. Relaxation may involve guided imagery, rhythmic movement, or a series of isometric contractions followed by relaxation. By incorporating relaxation into a treatment session, one can alter respiratory patterns, as well as minimize muscle tension, which improves ROM.

B. Cognitive Assessment

The ICU is a highly technical, stressful environment that contributes to sleep disturbances, sensory deprivation, and isolation, and in which daily living routines are disrupted. These may lead a patient to a state of generalized disorientation, thought disorganization, and even delirium.

The occupational therapist uses a variety of tools to assess and improve a patient's cognitive status. Orientation, memory, thought processing, and organizational skills are a few of the areas assessed. Treatment is based on the deficits found in any of these areas, with the goal of returning the patient to his or her baseline cognitive and visual/perceptual status and promoting safety awareness.

C. Positioning and Splinting

Intensive care is usually associated with limited mobility. Patients are critically ill, attached to lifesaving equipment, and often in some degree of pain. They are reluctant to move, even if they can, for fear of increasing their pain, dislodging their many lines and catheter, or making their condition worse by participating in activities.

1. Indications Mobilizing a patient and encouraging participation in self-care and functional tasks is not always possible because of the patient's medical status. Proper positioning is crucial to prevent soft tissue and joint contractures, maximize respiratory function, prevent the formation of decubitus ulcers, and reduce edema.

a. Contractures can develop when a body part is not frequently moved through its full ROM. After a tissue injury, such as a burn or amputation, the patient may assume a position of comfort with the involved body part. The neurologically impaired or chemically paralyzed patient is also susceptible to contractures due to the loss of voluntary motor control and the resulting muscular imbalance. Positioning is crucial to help prevent fixed deformities, minimize subsequent loss of function, and preserve skin integrity. In J.C.'s case, it would be important to position his right upper extremity with his wrist extended and with the metacarpal phalangeal joints (MCPs) and proximal interphalangeal joints (IPs) partially flexed. Refer to Table 15-2 for the most common positions.

  b. Respiratory function can be enhanced by positioning, and this also will prevent deformity of the chest wall, which can impair the effectiveness of the respiratory musculature.

  c. Decubitus ulcers are costly iatrogenic sequelae of immobilization, and are **preventable**. Patients with impaired sensation or mobility should not be left in one position or weight bearing on any bony prominences for extended periods in either a bed or a chair. These potential areas include the sacrum, the greater trochanters, the ischial tuberosities, and the calcaneous. **Pressure relief** is essential in the prevention of decubitus ulcers. If the patient is able, he or she is taught how to perform pressure relief. If the patient is unable to assist or perform pressure relief, the nursing staff is primarily responsible for changing the patient's position. When seating a patient at risk for breakdown, the patient should be evaluated for and provided with an appropriate cushion to decrease static pressure on the bony prominences. Pressure relief should be provided while the patient is sitting, even when a cushion is present—30 s for every 15 min of sitting. When in bed, patients need to be positioned in alternating side-lying positions, and be helped to sit up when possible several times during the day. Some patients may require aggressive positioning programs which cannot be achieved through normal, manual positioning techniques. Kinetic beds, such as the Rotorest or the Biodyne II, can be passively rotated at regular intervals for pressure relief and pulmonary hygiene. Fluid air (sand) beds are also used for pressure relief for those patients who are at high risk of or have skin breakdown.

  d. Edema management is crucial to the healing process. If left unchecked, edema (anasarca) can lead to musculoligamentous fibrosis, ongoing pain, and loss of ROM and function. To decrease edema, the involved body part is elevated above the heart level. Retrograde massage, compression garments, and intermittent compression pumps can also be used when positioning alone is not sufficient.

D. Range-of-Motion Activities

  1. Joint structure and integrity and the elasticity of soft tissue affect the amount of motion available between any two bones. When moving an extremity, all structures in the region are affected: muscles, articulating surfaces, nerves, fascia, joint capsules, ligaments, tendons, and blood vessels.

Table 15-2   Proper positioning for the patient with decreased mobility*

Area involved	Position of contracture and associated complications	Proper position	Method of positioning
Anterior neck/ upper chest	Flexed, with impaired respiratory status	Extended	No pillow Roll at scapulas Neck splint
Axilla	Adducted Internal rotation Brachial plexus impingement	Abducted to 90° External rotation	Bedside table Abduction tray Airplane splint
Elbow	Flexed Cubital tunnel syndrome	Extended	Pillow Abduction tray Elbow splint
Wrist	Flexed Carpal tunnel syndrome	Extended	Hand resting on pillow Wrist splint
Hand	MCPs extended IPs flexed Thumb adducted or clenched fist	MCPs and IPs flexed 30° or MCPs flexed and IPs extended for dorsal hand burn Thumb abducted	Hand open on pillow Roll-in palm Hand splint
Hips	Flexed External rotation "Frog legged" Peroneal nerve palsy	Extended Neutral rotation Slight abduction	Pillow at lateral thigh Side-lying or prone if medically able
Knees	Flexed	Extended	No pillow under knees Out of bed with legs extended and elevated Knee or leg splint
Ankles	Plantar flexed Foot drop	Dorsiflexed No pressure on heels	Pillows under calves Heels off the bed Foot board Short leg splint

*Common positions of contracture along with associated impairments are listed. The proper joint positions are noted, as well as suggestions for implementing these positions.

To prevent the loss of normal ROM, segments must be moved through their available ranges. Many factors can lead to decreased ROM. These include, but are not limited to, systemic, joint, neurologic, or muscular diseases; traumatic or surgical insult; immobilization; or inactivity.

2. Types of range of motion

   a. **Passive ROM** is the movement of a segment by an external force (the therapist or a mechanical device such as a continuous passive motion machine, CPM). No voluntary muscle contraction occurs.

   b. **Active-assistive ROM** is the movement of a segment by both an internal and an external force. In this instance, the muscle, the internal force, is too weak to complete the motion independently and requires assistance, an external force.

   c. **Active ROM** is the movement of a segment by internal forces; a voluntary contraction of the muscles that cross the joint.

   d. **Active-resistive ROM** is the use of resistance, manual or weights, to strength a muscle with a muscle grade of fair or higher. Table 15-3 shows the indications for and types of ROM.

3. **The goals of ROM exercise** are to maintain joint and soft tissue mobility, to prevent the formation of contractures, to prevent the loss of mechanical elasticity of muscle, and to assist in promoting good circulation. Active ROM will not increase the strength of muscles that have greater than

Table 15-3 Types of range of motion

Type	Definition	Indications
Passive ROM	No voluntary muscle contraction present	Patient unable to or restricted from actively moving segment
Active-assisted ROM	Weak active muscle contraction External force needed to complete ROM	Patient demonstrates poor to fair-minus muscle grades Used to achieve full ROM
Active ROM	Isometric: static muscle contraction in which muscular tension is developed	Muscle recruitment without movement across the joint
	Isotonic: dynamic concentric or eccentric muscle contraction	Movement is present through full range
Resisted ROM	Active muscle contraction in which resistance is added	Used to strengthen a muscle with a fair muscle grade or higher

Adapted from Kisner C and Colby LA: *Therapeutic Exercise: Foundations and Techniques.* Philadelphia, F.A. Davis Co., 1985.

a fair muscle grade. If stronger than a fair muscle grade, an active-resistive ROM is needed. Table 15-4 shows the muscle-strength grading system.

E. Strategies to Decrease Pain and Perception of Pain

1. Manual therapies Manual therapies are used to reduce pain through the restoration of normal joint and tissue mobility. They include massage, myofascial release, deep massage, and joint mobilization. Modalities are discussed later since they are less likely to be used during the acute phase of the patient's critical illness.

    a. Massage is the manipulation of soft tissue. It can produce beneficial effects on the nervous and muscular systems and improve the circulation of blood and lymphatic fluid.

    b. Myofascial release and deep massage are techniques used to restore normal tissue and fluid exchange, improve soft tissue pliability and extensibility, and reduce scarring. The improved blood flow to the involved area aids in the removal of metabolic waste products and reduces painful ischemia.

    c. Deep massage is especially useful over **"trigger points,"** which can result from muscle trauma, disease, or emotional stress. Muscles can go into spasm when the trigger points are active. The spasm tightens the muscle and more pain occurs. Pain messages are transmitted through nociceptive pathways to the thalamus and cortex, which have efferent inhibitory pathways to the spinal cord. The thalamus and cortex send back impulses that cause muscles to contract further. This is called **splinting** and produces a vicious cycle of pain. Deep pressure and vibration applied over trigger points can help break up the pain cycle by altering neuronal input and reflex responses.

    d. Joint mobilization involves mobilizing a joint in a manner that decreases adhesions surrounding the joint capsule and permits improved motion and less pain with movement.

Table 15-4 Muscle-strength grading system (scale of 0 to 5)

Normal (5) Good (4)	Complete ROM against gravity	With full resistance at end range With some resistance at end range
Fair (3) Poor (2)	Complete ROM	Against gravity with no resistance With gravity eliminated
Trace (1) Zero (0)	No ROM	Slight contraction No contraction

Adapted from Daniels L and Worthingham C: *Muscle Testing Techniques of Manual Examination,* Philadelphia, Saunders, 1986.

2. **Stress management and relaxation techniques** are incorporated into the therapy program to decrease pain and its perception. They may include, but are not limited to, deep breathing, visual imagery, and isometric contractions.

F. Prefunctional Activities

Prior to or in conjunction with participation in the activities of daily living, **prefunctional activities** are often used by the occupational therapist. These activities may include pencil-and-paper tasks for cognition, fine motor tasks or simple crafts designed to improve dexterity, and grippers and exercise putty to improve strength. All of these activities are carefully monitored and are graded as ability improves or declines.

G. Retraining in Activities of Daily Living

   1. After a patient's **level of function is assessed** by the occupational therapist, the patient is encouraged to participate in a program of graded self-care activities designed to break the pain cycle and dependence. Initially patients may be instructed only to wash their faces, brush their teeth, or comb their hair. Activities progress to promote independence and self-esteem further as the patient's medical status allows.
   2. **Adaptive devices,** such as long-handled sponges, reachers, button hooks, sock donners, built-up utensils, and raised toilet seats, can be used to allow patients to perform activities they might otherwise be unable to carry out.
   3. **Specialized splints** for the upper extremity can be fabricated to assist function mechanically. For example, to encourage functional independence, J.C. would benefit from a dorsal wrist support with a built-in pocket to hold a utensil in view of his wrist and hand weakness.
   4. It is important to allow patients to participate in as many of the activities of self-care as possible. Those who are unable to participate should be allowed to make decisions regarding their care so that the routine may resemble that which is most familiar to them.

H. Functional Mobility

   1. The **transition** from being supine to standing and ambulating usually requires the initiation of a sitting program in which the patient must tolerate having the lower extremities in a dependent position. Sitting is limited when a vascular access catheter is placed in a femoral vessel, which impedes the patient's ability to flex the hip. Standing and ambulation are limited when intravenous lines are placed in the feet.

2. If sitting is not possible or patient weakness indicates the need, a standing program can be preceded by the use of a tilt table. In J.C.'s case, he might be unable to work on sitting activities if a femoral vein Sorenson catheter were used for dialysis. A **tilt table** is a passive standing apparatus used to promote the positive effects of standing and lower-extremity weight bearing. Use of the tilt table is a prudent step to reintroduce vertical posture, if the patient has been supine for a long time. Precautions should be taken to prevent orthostatic hypotension through the use of antiembolism support stockings or Ace wraps and an abdominal binder. Standing maintains muscle length improves the position of the internal organs (i.e., aids in bowel and bladder function), decreases the chance of decubitus ulcers by relieving pressure on the sacrum, assists in circulation, and may diminish osteoporosis.

3. **Ambulation** of the critically ill patient, if not contraindicated, can benefit the patient both physiologically and psychologically. The patient should be involved in an active sitting and standing program and exercise regime. Ambulation requires a minimum of at least fair strength in major muscle groups (see Table 15-4). It is important not to overstress the cardiopulmonary system when initiating a gait program.

V. MODALITIES

As a patient's condition improves, the use of modalities may augment the patient's ability to participate in the therapy program. These interventions may not be introduced in the ICU, as they are more frequently used as part of a rehabilitation or an outpatient treatment program.

A. Heat

Heat as a modality involves the use of physical agents to increase tissue temperature. Two types of heat generally are considered: superficial heat and deep heat. Effectiveness depends on the type of agent and the duration of use.

1. **Localized physiologic effects of heat** include increased metabolic activity, which is temperature dependent; increased blood flow secondary to the reflex effect on the arterioles; decreased viscosity of fluids; and increased extensibility of collagenous tissue, which can lead to improved ROM and an analgesic effect due to the change in neuronal activity (decreased firing of alpha-motor neurons).

2. **Effects on the musculoskeletal system**   Heat's effects on this system include decreased spasm, relief of local ischemia, release of endorphins, and

acceleration of the healing process secondary to vasodilation, which increases phagocytosis.

3. **Superficial heat** warms the dermal layers of the skin to the depth of approximately 1 cm. The skin controls the body temperature. Heat applied to the skin has a limited effect on the deeper tissues because cutaneous vasodilation will dissipate the heat. An erythmic response will be visible as a result of using superficial heat.

   a. Superficial heat can be classified as either **moist heat** or **dry heat**. Paraffin and hot packs provide moist heat via conduction. Infrared lamps provide radiant dry heat. Fluidotherapy is a dry heat through forced convection.

   b. **Clinical indications** for the use of heat may include, but are not limited to, reduction of pain and stiffness, decreased muscle spasm (therefore, increased ROM), and improved healing due to an increase in blood flow.

   c. **Precautions** must be taken in the application of heat in cases of impaired sensation, arterial insufficiency, hemophilia, or long-term steroid use. It is important to carefully monitor the effect of heat therapy on the patient's skin, especially if there is a known sensory impairment. With arterial insufficiency, heat accumulation is associated with increased metabolic demands and increased potential for a tissue burn. Capillary fragility is a side effect of steroid use, and this also increases a patient's risk of injury.

4. **Deep heat** penetrates to the depth of approximately 3 to 6 cm. Examples of deep heat are ultrasound and diathermy.

   a. Although effective as a heat modality, **diathermy** has limited clinical application in the ICU setting because of the precautions it involves. Diathermy is contraindicated for patients with acute inflammatory conditions, hemorrhage, known sensory impairment, or other conditions in which there is fluid buildup, drainage material, or metallic implants, including pacemakers. Patients must not be in contact with metallic objects during the treatment (bed, bed frame).

   b. **Ultrasound** is the mechanical oscillation of sound waves with a depth of penetration of 4 to 6 cm. Absorption varies in relation to the density of the tissue. For example, a fatty area has decreased absorption of ultrasonic energy and an associated decreased heating of the area.

   c. The **physiologic effects** of ultrasound are divided into four groups: (1) **chemical**—ultrasonic vibrations stimulate surrounding tissues and increase chemical reactions; (2) **biologic**—the permeability of the membrane is changed to allow the transfer of nutrients; (3) **mechanical**—the high frequency of oscillation/vibration of ultrasound deforms the molecular structure of loosely bonded substances which can be associated with a reduction in muscle spasms, the breakup of calcium deposits, and the mobilization of scar tissue; (4) **thermal** effect—the rapid oscillation of the molecules allows for the buildup of heat (Kahn, 1991).

d. Clinical indications for the use of ultrasound may include muscle spasm associated with musculoskeletal or neuromuscular conditions, scar tissue, and athletic injuries. Another application of ultrasound is **phonophoresis,** or the introduction of medication through the skin using ultrasonic energy. Drugs commonly used are the antiinflammatories hydrocortisone and salicylate and local analgesics such as lidocaine. Precautions must be taken when using phonophoresis in case of allergies or sensitivities to the substance being used on the skin.

e. Precautions should be taken in the use of ultrasound when applying it directly over growing epiphyses, bony prominences, and pacemakers, and during pregnancy. Ultrasound is to be used with caution over any appliance implanted in the body; it is believed that the vibration of the ultrasonic waves may disrupt the chemical bonding of the cement and loosen it.

B. Cryotherapy

Cryotherapy involves the use of physical agents to reduce tissue temperature. These may include cold/ice packs, ice cubes for ice massage, ice-soaked towels, cold baths, cold units with thermal controls, and vapocoolant sprays. Its effectiveness depends on the length of time applied and the temperature of the agent. The estimated depth of penetration is 4 cm.

1. Physiologic effects of cryotherapy include vasoconstriction, decreased metabolism, decreased inflammation, and an analgesic effect due to an elevation of the pain threshold.

2. Pattern of vasoconstriction and vasodilation Following the application of cold, there is an initial decrease in vascular flow with reduced nerve conduction velocity. This results in muscle relaxation and ischemia, which cause a reflex vasodilation to preserve tissue viability. This is followed by vasoconstriction to maintain core temperature.

3. Clinical indications Indications **for cryotherapy** may include acute musculoskeletal pain, myofascial pain, spasticity, and inflammatory processes.

4. Precautions must be taken **in the use of cryotherapy** for patients with cold sensitivity syndromes (i.e., Raynaud's phenomenon), areas of compromised circulation (i.e., peripheral vascular disease), or significant hypertension.

C. Electrotherapy

Electrotherapy involves the use of electricity to obtain a desired physiologic response for treatment purposes.

1. Physiologic effects of electrotherapy can be divided into four categories: (1) **cellular,** in which there are excitation of the peripheral nerves, changes in membrane permeability, and tissue remodeling (2) **tissue,** in which smooth muscles relax and changes in blood flow occur; (3) **segmental,**

in which muscle group contraction affects joint mobility and synergist muscle activity; (4) **systemic,** in which analgesic effects are seen.

   2. Clinical indications   Electrical stimulation can be effective for joint swelling, in tissue healing, in muscle reeducation, for circulatory impairments, and in the relaxation of muscle spasms.

   3. Precautions   Cases requiring precautions include new fractures, active hemorrhaging, the presence of pacemakers, pregnancy, and metal implants.

   4. Neuromuscular electrical stimulation   involves the activation of muscle tissue through stimulation of the peripheral nervous system. **Clinical indications** for neuromuscular electrical stimulation include strengthening muscles below a fair grade (see Table 15-5), facilitating voluntary motor control, and providing temporary relief of spasticity.

   5. Transcutaneous electrical nerve stimulation (TENS)   is a technique that may be an effective adjunct to pain management in the critical care setting, but needs to be used with caution with the hemodynamically unstable patient as the electrical activity may interfere with the quality of electrocardiograms. It is discussed in detail in Chapter 14. **Clinical indications for TENS** include pre- and postsurgical or trauma pain, nonunited fracture pain and bone healing, labor pain, and temporomandibular joint pain.

Table 15-5   Indications for physical therapy modalities

Modality	Indications/uses
Superficial heat	Reduction of pain and stiffness Decreased muscle spasms Increased ROM Increased localized blood flow Increased extensibility of collagenous tissue
Deep heat	Increased blood flow Increased temperature of deeper tissues Reduction of muscle spasms
Cryotherapy	Vasoconstriction Decreased inflammation Reduction in acute musculoskeletal pain, inflammatory processes
Electrotherapy	Decreased muscle spasm Increased blood flow Muscle reeducation Tissue healing Pain management

   Adapted from Nelson R, Currier D: *Clinical Electrotherapy.* Norwalk, Connecticut, Appleton & Lange, 1987; Kahn J: *Principles and Practice of Electrotherapy,* 2d ed. New York, Churchill Livingstone, 1991.

VI. CONCLUSION

The physical therapist and the occupational therapist are an integral part of the multidisciplinary team treating the critically ill patient. The goal of physical and occupational therapy is to help treat existing pain, as well as to prevent painful syndromes from arising and to facilitate the patient's participation in purposeful activities that promote physical and mental well-being and functional independence.

Therapeutic pain-control measures are essential early in the patient's hospital course. Pain is reduced and healing promoted before acute pain can progress to a chronic pain syndrome.

SUGGESTED READINGS

Afflect A: Providing occupational therapy in an intensive care unit. *Am J Occup Ther* 40:5, 1986.

Alon G: Principles of electric stimulation, in Nelson R, Currier D (eds): *Clinical Electrotherapy.* Norwalk, Connecticut, Appleton & Lange, 1987, chap 3, pp 54–55.

Bengston R, Warfield C: Physical therapy for pain relief. *Hosp Pract,* Aug 1984.

Boughton A, Ciesla N: Physical therapy management of the head-injured patient in the intensive care unit. *Top Acute Care Trauma Rehab* 1:1, 1986.

Dean E: Bedrest and deconditioning. Neurology Report, *Am J Physical Therapy* 17:1, 1993.

Frownfelter: *Chest Physical Therapy and Pulmonary Rehabilitation: An Interdisciplinary Approach,* 2d ed. Yearbook Publishers, 1987, chap 9, pp 218–230.

Imle C, Boughton A: The physical therapist's role in the management of acute spinal cord injury. *Top Acute Care Trauma Rehab* 1:3, 1987.

Innocenti D: Physiotherapy in intensive care. *Radiography* 52:605, 1986.

Kahn J: *Principles and Practice of Electrotherapy,* 2d ed., 1991, chap 3, pp 51–70.

McCormack GL: Pain management by occupational therapists. *Am J Occup Ther* 42:5, 1988.

Malick M, Carr J: *Manual on Management of the Burn Patient* Harmarville Rehabilitation Center, 1982.

PART FIVE

CLINICAL PROBLEMS

CHAPTER
16

NEUROLOGIC INJURY AND DISEASE

Karen J. Schwenzer
Robin J. Hamill

Case
Chapter Focus
  I. Differential Diagnosis of Headache
     A. Migraine
     B. Tension or Muscle-Contraction Headache
     C. Sinus Headache
     D. Posttraumatic Headache
     E. Post–Dural-Puncture Headache
     F. Temporal Arteritis
     G. Headache Secondary to Infection of the Central Nervous System
     H. Headache of Subarachnoid Hemorrhage
     I. Headache of Increased Intracranial Pressure
     J. Headache of Acute Epidural Hematoma
     K. Headache of Acute Subdural Hematoma
     L. Headache of Chronic Subdural Hematoma
     M. Headaches Related to Medical Disorders
 II. Head Injury and Increased Intracranial Pressure
     A. Neurophysiology
     B. Management of Patients
III. Alcohol Withdrawal Syndrome
 IV. Pain Associated with Spinal Cord Compression
     A. Neoplastic Spinal Cord Compression
     B. Spinal Epidural Abscess
     C. Spinal Epidural Hematoma
     D. Traumatic Spinal Cord Compression
     E. Autonomic Hyperreflexia

V. Pain Associated with Upper Motor Neuron Lesions
  A. Thalamic Pain Syndrome or Poststroke Central Pain
  B. Multiple Sclerosis
  C. Amyotrophic Lateral Sclerosis
VI. Pain Associated with Peripheral Nerve Lesions and Lower Motor Neuron Lesions
  A. Peripheral Neuropathies
  B. Pathogenesis of Generalized Neuropathies
  C. Guillain-Barré Syndrome or Acute Inflammatory Polyradiculoneuropathy
  D. Diabetic Neuropathy
  E. Toxic Neuropathies
  F. Vasculitic Neuropathy
  G. Acute Anterior Poliomyelitis (Infantile Paralysis)
  H. Postherpetic Neuralgia
  I. Reflex Sympathetic Dystrophy
VII. Neuromuscular Junction Disorders Associated with Pain
  A. Myasthenia Gravis
  B. Botulism
  C. Tetanus
  D. Hypocalcemic Tetany
  E. Duchenne Type and Other Muscular Dystrophies
  F. Inflammatory Myopathies
VIII. Pain Management in the Presence of Neurologic Disease
  A. Disease Components That Alter Analgesic Options
  B. Analgesic Medications (Drugs)
  C. Analgesic Modalities
Case Discussion
Suggested Readings

CASE

A 54-year-old alcoholic male was hit by a pickup truck while walking in the road four nights earlier. He suffered: a closed-head injury and a subdural hematoma, which was surgically drained; multiple facial fractures and lacerations; and a five-rib flail chest with an associated pulmonary contusion. Confounding problems include preexisting end-stage liver disease from alcoholic cirrhosis manifested as ascites, hypoproteinemia, and a mild coagulopathy; mild to moderate organic brain syndrome, which also was felt to be alcohol related; and a 120-pack-a-year history of cigarette abuse. Currently the patient is awake but confused, though his intracranial pressures have been normal for 48 h. The patient's pulmonary contusion has resolved, but he shows significant pain-related behavior with any motion, suctioning, or coughing. The plan is to attempt weaning him from the ventilator. You are consulted for pain management.

CHAPTER FOCUS

The diagnosis and treatment of painful conditions associated with neurologic injury and disease are an important part of critical care medicine. This chapter presents an overview of certain painful conditions and their treatment.

I. DIFFERENTIAL DIAGNOSIS OF HEADACHE

A. Migraine

1. **Neurologic, or classic, migraine** is characterized by an aura accompanied by a disturbance of neurologic function (hemianopsia or central blindness, hemiparesthesia, slight speech abnormality or aphasia, or hemiparesis), followed by the sudden onset of unilateral, throbbing headache, nausea, and vomiting, all of which last for hours or for as long as a day or two.

2. The other syndrome, **common migraine,** is characterized by an unheralded onset of unilateral or generalized headache with or without nausea and vomiting, but following the same temporal pattern as neurologic migraine.

3. **Treatment** Both syndromes respond to ergot preparations, if administered early in the attack. The dose of **ergotamine** (Cafergot, Wigraine) is 2 mg orally or sublingually given as soon as the headache starts. Doses of 2 mg may be administered at intervals of 30 min thereafter if necessary, until a total of 6 mg has been taken. No more than 10 mg should be ingested per week.

Ergotamine may also be administered by oral inhalation. A single inhalation (0.36 mg) is given and repeated at intervals of 5 min, to a total of 6 doses in 24 h. The maximal dosage in 1 week is 5.4 mg (about 15 inhalations).

Rectal ergotamine suppositories, 2 mg, are another option.

Ergotamine can be administered by intramuscular (IM) injection (1 mg, repeated at 1 h intervals to a total of 3 mg) or, in some circumstances, intravenously (IV), 2 mg maximum. No more than 6 mg should be given parenterally in 1 week.

Propranolol (Inderal) is the preferred drug for the prophylaxis of migraine. Fewer and less intense attacks occur when 80 to 240 mg of propranolol are taken daily in divided doses. Atenolol (Tenormin, 50 mg daily), nadolol (Corgard, 40 mg daily), and timolol (Blocadren, 10 mg bid) are also effective.

B. Tension or Muscle-Contraction Headache

1. A tension headache is characterized by bilateral, nonthrobbing, constant head pain that begins in the occipital area and spreads to the frontal area. It is not worsened with a Valsalva maneuver. The sensation may be described as pain, but fullness, tightness, or pressure on which waves of aching pain are superimposed are better descriptors. The onset is more gradual

than for migraine. Headache may occur acutely under conditions of emotional excitement or intense worry, and lasts for hours or a day or two, though some persist unremittingly for weeks or months. The pain is quite severe, but patients rarely complain of nausea, vomiting, or malaise. Modest dizziness, blurring of vision, and tinnitus sometimes occur.

2. Treatment

    a. Tension headaches are very difficult to treat. Traditional analgesics have benefit only if the pain is intense and of the aching type. An individual headache may be treated with **aspirin** or nonsteroidal anti-inflammatory drugs **(NSAIDs)**. Ergotamine is of no benefit.

    b. Many patients with tension headaches, particularly chronic ones, are depressed and respond to antidepressants, such as **amitriptyline** (Elavil), 50 to 150 mg daily.

    c. Some patients are tense and anxious and respond to antianxiety drugs such as **diazepam** (Valium), 5 mg tid for 2 to 3 weeks. These drugs help break the cycle of anxiety–muscle tension–anxiety, so that a short course may give prolonged relief.

C. Sinus Headache

1. Sinusitis is characterized by frontal, nonthrobbing head pain with tenderness to percussion over the sinuses. The pain is dull and aching, made worse by changing head position, and seldom associated with nausea and vomiting. The most common predisposing factor of acute purulent sinusitis is viral infection of the upper respiratory tract, which may lead to obstruction of drainage of the paranasal sinuses and the development of localized pain, tenderness, and low-grade fever. Typically, sinus headache begins in the morning and subsides in the early evening.

2. The presence of gastric and endotracheal tubes in the nasopharynx of critically ill patients will also obstruct the normal drainage of paranasal sinuses and lead to sinusitis. Left untreated, sinusitis may lead to osteomyelitis, bacterial meningitis, the formation of brain abscesses, and the septic syndrome.

3. The diagnosis is made when constitutional manifestations are present, such as fever, pain and tenderness of the involved sinuses, and recurrent headaches. Persistent purulent discharges should be cultured and appropriate antimicrobial drugs employed. Radiographic views of opacified sinuses aid in the diagnosis in acutely injured patients.

4. Treatment

    a. Sinusitis is best treated with a combination of **decongestants** (oxymetazoline, Afrin nasal spray, 0.025 to 0.05%) and **antibiotics** (penicillin G, 10 to 20 million units daily). Needle aspiration or, when severe, surgical drainage may be indicated.

    b. Nasal tubes should be removed to help normalize drainage.

c. Headache persisting after surgical drainage of a diseased sinus is evidence of extradural and possible subdural infection.

D. Posttraumatic Headache

1. Posttraumatic headache may be indistinguishable from chronic, recurring tension headache. It may persist up to 6 to 12 months after head trauma. It may be associated with dizzy spells and be part of a postconcussion syndrome, which is also characterized by fear, anxiety, fatigue, irritability, and inability to concentrate.

2. **Treatment**

a. Mild analgesics, NSAIDs, acetaminophen, and aspirin provide some relief.

b. **Diazepam** (Valium, 5 mg orally tid) can decrease anxiety and restlessness, but dependence may develop with chronic use.

c. **Propranolol** (Inderal, 80 to 140 mg daily, in divided doses) and **amitriptyline** (Elavil, 10 to 25 mg daily, increased by 10 mg every 5 to 7 days to a maximum of 150 mg), have also been used for chronic headache, along with psychological support and reassurance.

E. Post–Dural-Puncture Headache

1. "Spinal headache" is characterized by severe, aching pain in the occiput, radiating downwards and toward the shoulders following a lumbar puncture (LP) or dural puncture for other reasons. The headache more or less disappears when the patient lies recumbent. It increases dramatically when the patient is in an upright position, can be incapacitating, and may be associated with deep venous thrombosis (because of bed rest), hearing loss, tinnitus, visual disturbances, cerebral vein thrombosis, and compression of the brainstem at the foramen magnum. Post–dural-puncture headache is more often seen in younger patients and women.

2. It is caused by low cerebral spinal fluid (CSF) pressure resulting from leakage through the puncture hole in the dura. Smaller needles reduce the incidence of this problem.

3. **Treatment**

a. A conservative approach includes bed rest and generous hydration, via the IV route, if necessary.

b. Analgesics are usually ineffective.

c. Caffeinated beverages and parenteral **caffeine** (500 mg in a liter of fluid given over 1 h) increase CSF production and can speed the resolution of symptoms.

d. In very severe cases, blood injected into the epidural space (blood patch) at the puncture site has shown great success.

F. Temporal Arteritis

1. Temporal arteritis is characterized by severe, continuous, unilateral head pain. Patients are commonly older than 55 years of age. It affects women more often than it does men. It is associated with an increased erythrocyte sedimentation rate (ESR). Tender, swollen nonpulsatile temporal arteries are often present. Ischemic injuries can lead to blindness and focal deficits. A diagnosis can be obtained by biopsy 2 to 3 days after presentation.

2. Treatment

   a. Temporal arteritis represents an emergency as ischemic injuries will occur if left untreated.

   b. A large bolus of steroids, **prednisone** 60 to 80 mg orally, should be administered, and continued until the ESR returns to normal.

G. Headache Secondary to Infection of the Central Nervous System (Brain Abscess, Encephalitis, or Meningitis)

1. Any headache associated with fever and an altered mental status should be considered as attributable to infection of the central nervous system (CNS) until proved otherwise. It is characterized by a subacute or acute onset of constant, increasingly severe pain, which is usually generalized and increases with physical activity. It is associated with nuchal rigidity, nausea and vomiting, irritability, restlessness, altered level of consciousness, photophobia, strabismus, ptosis, and pupillary inequality.

2. Meningitis is caused by a wide variety of bacterial, viral, fungal, and parasitic agents, as well as by noninfectious irritants. Brain abscesses are caused by a wide variety or organisms as well, and arise from contiguous spread (e.g., sinusitis) or hematogenous spread (e.g., endocarditis). The prognosis depends on a rapid diagnosis and initiation of appropriate therapy.

3. The diagnosis is established by LP and analysis of CSF. If the physician suspects that the patient is suffering from acute bacterial meningitis, LP must be done immediately. In patients suspected of harboring an intracranial mass lesion with increased intracranial pressure, such as with a brain abscess, a computed tomography (CT) scan of the brain should be performed first and LP deferred due to the risks of herniation. In such situations, the CSF sample will not grow the causative organism of the brain abscess, unless the abscess has ruptured into a ventricle or into the subarachnoid space.

4. Treatment

   a. Treatment is geared toward correct identification of the infectious agent and the prompt use of appropriate antimicrobials.

   b. When a brain abscess is identified on CT scan, a combination of antibiotics and surgical drainage is indicated.

c. Efficacy of treatment is determined by resolution of neurologic symptoms and/or repeated LPs.

H. Headache of Subarachnoid Hemorrhage

1. When rupture of an intracerebral aneurysm occurs, blood enters the subarachnoid space under high pressure, and several clinical patterns may emerge.

　　a. The patient may lose consciousness immediately, develop decerebrate rigidity and signs of brainstem ischemia (respiratory and circulatory collapse), and die.

　　b. The patient may complain of sudden, severe excruciating headache with no previous history of headache. Headache is either occipital or generalized, associated with nuchal rigidity, dizziness, nausea and vomiting, irritability, restlessness, convulsions, and drowsiness, A depressed level of consciousness is common.

2. About one-fourth of patients will have had a less severe "warning" bleed within the previous several months.

3. A CT scan of the brain demonstrates subarachnoid blood in many cases. Cerebral angiography of all major intracranial vessels detects the location of the aneurysm(s).

4. Treatment

　　a. Conservative medical therapy is aimed at regulation of systemic blood pressure, sedation, and provision of a quiet, nonstimulating environment.

　　b. Mild analgesics are of some benefit, especially the prostaglandin inhibitors, such as **ketorolac** (Toradol, 30 mg IM or 15 mg IV every 6 h).

　　c. As one of the most devastating events is rebleeding, early clipping of the aneurysm has gained favor over the more conservative approach of waiting and clipping later.

I. Headache of Increased Intracranial Pressure

A headache resulting from increased intracranial pressure (ICP) is initially mild and intermittent, then increases in severity to steady, bilateral, nonthrobbing pain. It is worsened with a Valsalva maneuver, and, when severe, is associated with vomiting. It is paramount that the cause of the increased ICP be found and treated. See below for general management of patients with increased ICP.

J. Headache of Acute Epidural Hematoma

1. Acute epidural hematoma is characterized by head pain that develops a few hours or days after a head injury. The patient may have a normal neurologic exam initially, but then develops a headache of increasing severity,

as well as vomiting, drowsiness, confusion, seizures, and hemiparesis. The level of consciousness continues to decrease and bilateral Babinski's signs appear, as may spasticity or decerebrate rigidity. Death will occur if the clot is not evacuated.

    2. Diagnosis is made by a CT scan of the brain.

    3. Treatment is surgical drainage, identification of the bleeding vessel, and ligation.

K. Headache of Acute Subdural Hematoma

    1. Acute subdural hematoma may present immediately after an injury or be delayed in presentation for days to weeks. It is characterized by headaches, drowsiness, agitation, slowness in thinking, and confusion that get progressively worse. Focal or lateralizing signs are late and tend to be less prominent than the disturbance of consciousness.

    2. Diagnosis is made by a CT scan of the brain.

    3. Treatment is surgical evacuation of the clot.

L. Headache of Chronic Subdural Hematoma

    1. Chronic subdural hematoma is characterized by headache and dizziness of fluctuating severity, followed by drowsiness, stupor, coma, and hemiparesis. The head injury may have been minor and forgotten by the patient and family. The headaches are deep-seated, steady, unilateral or generalized, and of increasing frequency and severity over several weeks or months.

    2. Diagnosis is made by a CT scan of the brain.

    3. Treatment

        a. The headache responds to traditional analgesics, such as aspirin, acetaminophen, NSAIDs, and narcotics.

        b. Surgical evacuation may be indicated.

M. Headaches Related to Medical Disorders

Headaches can arise from many medical disorders, including, but not limited to, fevers of any cause, carbon monoxide exposure, chronic lung disease and hypercapnia, hypothyroidism, Cushing's disease, withdrawal of corticosteroids, chronic nitrate exposure, acute anemia, and acute rises in blood pressure (pheochromocytoma).

II. HEAD INJURY AND INCREASED INTRACRANIAL PRESSURE

A. Neurophysiology

    1. Intracranial pressure is a reflection of the intracranial and intraspinal volume of fluid and tissue and the restriction on it by the rigid skull and the partially distensible spinal subarachnoid space. The intracranial volume is made up of the brain, CSF, interstitial fluid, and intravascular blood. As intracranial volume increases, ICP increases. The relationship between ICP and intracranial contents is called cerebral compliance (C = $\Delta V/\Delta P$) and is an exponential relationship. Cerebral perfusion pressure (CPP) is the difference between mean systemic blood pressure (MAP) and ICP.

   2. Control of cerebral blood flow

   a. Autoregulation refers to the intrinsic capacity of the cerebral circulation to alter its resistance to maintain cerebral blood flow (CBF) constant over a range of MAP changes (50 to 150 mmHg). Autoregulation is modified by cerebral disease states. High sympathetic tone, such as that encountered during hemorrhage or shock, results in lower than normal CBF at a given MAP, rendering the brain more susceptible to the ischemic effects of hypotension. When autoregulation is lost, there is also a passive increase in CBF and cerebral blood volume when MAP goes up, as in an agitated, head-injured patient.

   b. There is strict **coupling in the normal brain of metabolism and blood flow.** For instance, seizure and fever greatly increase CBF whereas pharmacologic coma and hypothermia decrease CBF.

   c. The major extracerebral physiologic factors contributing to overall cerebral perfusion are arterial blood gas tensions. The CBF varies directly with $Paco_2$ and inversely with Pao_2. The response is attenuated below a $Paco_2$ of 25 mmHg and above a $Paco_2$ of 100 mmHg. Below a Pao_2 of 50 mmHg, CBF increases toward its maximum value. Systemic hypoxia also causes tissue lactic acidosis and a decrease in cerebral vascular resistance.

   3. As ICP increases (expanding intracerebral hematoma, brain tumor, cerebral edema, etc.), MAP will increase to maintain CPP. When elevations in ICP continue unabated, CPP will eventually decrease. If CPP decreases to less than 40 to 60 mmHg, CBF is dangerously compromised and brain ischemia occurs. The major goal of ICP therapy is to maintain an adequate difference between ICP and MAP.

B. Management of Patients

In patients who have suffered severe craniofacial trauma or intracranial hemorrhage, sedation and analgesia may be essential to prevent ICP elevation or occurrence of **plateau waves** (periodic elevations in ICP associated with decreased cerebral compliance). When used, careful monitoring of the physiologic impact on the respiratory status and a neurologic exam are essential. If doubt as to the integrity of either of these systems exists, an endotracheal tube should be placed for airway protection and the ventilation assisted.

1. **Effects of analgesics and sedatives**
    a. **Barbiturates** cause a dose-dependent reduction in CBF and ICP. The mechanism of action includes lowered cerebral metabolic rate with resultant decreased CBF, blockage of the generation of oxygen-free radicals, and a direct vasoconstricting effect on the cerebral vasculature. When given at a dose to produce an isoelectric electroencephalogram (EEG), barbiturates reduce CBF and cerebral metabolic rate (CMR) by 50 percent, and further increases in dose have no additional effect. **Thiopental** (0.5 to 5 mg/kg as an IV bolus) rapidly lowers ICP and is helpful in situations of acute increases, such as with intubation, suctioning, radiography, and other short procedures. **Pentobarbital** can be given in a bolus of 5 to 10 mg/kg and followed by a continuous infusion of 1 to 5 mg/kg/h. Profound hypotension is not unusual due to myocardial depressant effects with both of these barbiturates. Intravascular volume resuscitation and inotropic support are commonly required to maintain CPP.
    b. **Etomidate** (Amidate, 1 to 2 mg/kg as an IV bolus), a carboxylated imidazole derivative, decreases ICP. It has minimal cardiovascular depressant effects as compared with thiopental and allows better support of CPP. The high incidence of myoclonic activity may be mistaken for seizures and lead to inappropriate treatment. Etomidate inhibits adrenal steroidogenesis, limiting the patient's adrenocortical response to stress. Long-term use as a sedative has been correlated with increased mortality in critically ill patients.
    c. **Narcotics** are very useful in managing agitation and pain in head-injured patients. Though these drugs interfere with the pupillary response, they can be reversed with small doses of naloxone (0.04 mg IV, doubled incrementally). Naloxone is also useful if there is concern that the patient's depressed sensorium is due to narcotics.

    Morphine sulfate (0.05 to 0.2 mg/kg IV) has little effect on ICP, though large doses may produce histamine release and result in decreased MAP and CPP. In normovolemic patients, morphine can be used as intermittent boluses or as a continuous infusion.

    Fentanyl (Sublimaze, 1 to 5 μg/kg IV) has little effect on ICP and may be the ideal narcotic to give patients with increased ICP or abnormal cerebral compliance due to its rapid onset and relatively short half-life. Fentanyl infusions may be beneficial for long-term use in multitrauma patients.

    The use of sufentanil (Sufenta) has been associated with an increase in ICP. The effects of alfentanil (Alfenta) are intermediate between those of sufentanil and fentanyl, producing a small increase in ICP.
    d. **Benzodiazepines** are used to relieve anxiety and agitation, and to treat the alcohol withdrawal syndrome (see below). They have no analgesic properties. They produce minimal cardiovascular depression and mild respiratory depression, especially when used in conjunction with narcotics. **Diazepam** (Valium, 2 to 10 mg IV) has been shown to decrease CBF and

cerebral blood volume without changing ICP. **Midazolam** (Versed, 1 to 2 mg IV), like diazepam, has been shown to decrease CBF and may possibly decrease ICP in patients with increased ICP.

    e. Lidocaine, an amide local anesthetic, causes a decrease in cerebral metabolism and CBF. Intravenous lidocaine (1 to 1.5 mg/kg) is used to blunt the sympathetic nervous system response to laryngoscopy, tracheal intubation, and suctioning. It is also an effective cough suppressant. The peak effect occurs 60 s after IV administration. Intratracheal lidocaine (1 to 1.5 mg/kg) can provide topical anesthesia to the tracheobronchial tree to facilitate suctioning of the intubated patient; however, the instillation of lidocaine down an artificial airway may actually precipitate bucking and coughing, actions that acutely increase ICP. Intravenous lidocaine would avoid this, and lead to blood levels of lidocaine that block ICP elevations during suctioning.

    f. Propofol (Diprivan) produces a dose-dependent decrease in CBF, cerebral metabolism, and ICP in head-injured patients. However, propofol-induced hypotension may be poorly tolerated, as with thiopental, especially if hypovolemia has not been completely corrected.

    g. Ketamine, an arylcyclohexylamine, is a potent cerebrovasodilator that causes an increase in CBF that is not dependent on an increase in systemic blood pressure. *Ketamine increases ICP and should not be used in patients with intracranial hypertension.*

  2. Airway management and other procedures

    a. Often when neurologic injury is severe and airway reflexes are blunted or absent, it becomes necessary to intubate patients with increased ICP.

    b. Laryngoscopy and intubation in unsedated patients increase MAP and lead to large increases in ICP, which can be catastrophic in patients with decreased intracranial compliance. Coughing and straining also increase ICP, and all attempts should be made to gain control of the airway without increasing ICP.

    c. Moderate to large doses of thiopental, etomidate, or propofol will help blunt the responses to intubation, but may be contraindicated if rapid intubation cannot be accomplished. Lidocaine, narcotics, and benzodiazepines are suitable alternatives, especially in the face of hypovolemia.

    d. It is not unusual to use **muscle relaxants** such as atracurium (Tracrium, 0.5 mg/kg) or vecuronium (Norcuron, 0.2 mg/kg) to accomplish smooth laryngoscopy and intubation. Succinylcholine has been shown to increase ICP and should be used with extreme caution in patients with decreased cerebral compliance. This risk must be weighed against the benefit of succinylcholine's rapid onset, which may aid in the placement of an endotracheal tube and correction of hypoxia and hypercarbia, both powerful stimuli that increase ICP.

3. **Blood pressure control**

a. Head-injured patients have marked systemic hypertension. It is essential that CBF and CPP be maintained, but severe hypertension needs to be treated as long as CPP remains above 60 mmHg. Ideally, the goal of treatment is to lower ICP first, and then decrease blood pressure.

b. Ensuring **adequate analgesia** with narcotics in head-injured patients will help control blood pressure. Using IV lidocaine or moderate doses of thiopental before suctioning or positioning the patient will also help.

c. **Labetalol** (Trandate, 5 to 20 mg IV, repeated as needed) is a useful agent in the acute management of severe hypertension associated with head trauma. If greater than first-degree heart block or bradycardia exist, **hydralazine** (Apresoline, 10 to 20 mg IV) is a useful alternative.

d. Vasodilating drugs, such as sodium nitroprusside, can be dangerous because of the effects of increasing cerebral blood volume and decreasing CPP.

III. ALCOHOL WITHDRAWAL SYNDROME

A variety of neurologic symptoms may occur in the chronic drinker after a period of relative or absolute abstinence from ethanol.

A. The most common symptom is **tremulousness,** associated with general irritability, mild autonomic hyperactivity, anorexia, nausea, and vomiting. These symptoms begin early and may last for several days.

B. The second major symptom is **disordered perception** and **hallucinosis,** which may occur in 10% to 25% of tremulous patients. This can begin on day 1 and can last up to a week.

C. The third main symptom is **withdrawal seizures,** which occur within 8 to 48 h following the cessation of drinking, with a peak incidence between 12 and 24 h. Generalized motor seizures occur with loss of consciousness.

D. The fourth manifestation of the withdrawal syndrome is **delirium tremens (DTs),** which are a rare, serious state of profound confusion, vivid hallucination, tremors, sleeplessness, and signs of increased autonomic nervous system activity with fever, tachycardia, dilated pupils, and profuse sweating. Mortality remains high at 5% to 10%.

E. Treatment

1. Management includes ruling out other causes of neurologic symptoms, such as CNS infection or subdural hematoma, by using CT, LP, EEG, etc.

2. Fluid and electrolyte replacement, thiamine, multivitamins, and other nutritional supports are indicated.

3. Benzodiazepines and other sedatives are administered in order

to calm the patient without putting him or her to sleep. A cumulative dose effect can be seen with delayed metabolism of such drugs, so caution is urged. No sedative drug should be given to a sleeping patient.

    4. A variety of sedatives may be given. **Chlordiazepoxide** (Librium, 25 to 50 mg IV every 2 to 4 h) and **diazepam** (Valium, 10 mg PO or IV every 2 to 4 h) are commonly given. Alternatives include **lorazepam** (Ativan), **prochlorperazine** (Compazine), **chlorpromazine** (Thorazine), **promethazine** (Phenergan), **hydroxyzine** (Vistaril), and **paraldehyde.**

IV. PAIN ASSOCIATED WITH SPINAL CORD COMPRESSION

Acute spinal cord compression is a neurologic emergency requiring prompt diagnosis and treatment. Most frequently, cord compression is caused by trauma or tumors, and less frequently by abscesses, hematomas, or herniating disks. Regardless of the etiology of cord compression, the lesion must be treated promptly to prevent complete and permanent paralysis.

A. Neoplastic Spinal Cord Compression

    1. Metastases are the most common cause of neoplastic cord compression, though primary intraspinal neoplasms can be seen. The patient presents with **pain** as the initial symptom, followed by weakness, sensory loss, and autonomic dysfunction. The pain is usually a constant, deep ache. It may be associated with radicular pain which radiates into the arms or legs (common with tumors in the cervical and lumbosacral regions) or as a dermatomal band or girdle from back to front around the chest or abdomen. A very characteristic feature of the pain of cord compression is that it may be worse in the recumbent position.

    2. The second most common symptom of acute cord compression is **weakness.**

    3. Patients also complain of **numbness** and **paresthesias.**

    4. Diagnosis is made by magnetic resonance imaging (MRI), CT scan of the spine, and/or myelography.

    5. Treatment

        a. **Mannitol** and **steroids** decrease cord edema. Dexamethasone (Decadron, 40 to 100 mg IV) is effective in rapidly ameliorating pain.

        b. Adjuncts include **NSAIDs** (especially ketorolac, Torodol, 15 to 30 mg IV or IM every 6 to 8 h), **amitriptyline** (Elavil, 50 to 150 mg daily), and **narcotics,** though tolerance may develop with chronic use.

        c. **Surgical decompression** and **radiation therapy** are the definitive treatments.

B. Spinal Epidural Abscess

1. Epidural abscess is a frequently overlooked cause of acute spinal cord compression. It is characterized by intractable aching back pain that progresses to radicular pain within a day or several days and is usually accompanied by fever, headache, and nuchal rigidity. Rapidly progressive paresthesias and paraplegia develop.

2. Diagnosis is made by MRI, CT scan of the spine, and/or myelography.

3. Treatment is surgical drainage and a prolonged course of appropriate antimicrobials.

C. Spinal Epidural Hematoma

1. Epidural hematoma is a rare cause of spinal cord compression resulting from spontaneous or traumatic rupture of epidural veins. Typically, a previously healthy adult develops sudden back or neck pain. Symptoms may include radicular pain and weakness that evolve over several hours.

2. Diagnosis is made by MRI, CT scan of the spine, and/or myelography.

3. Treatment is surgical evacuation of the clot.

D. Traumatic Spinal Cord Compression

The incidence of acute spinal cord injury (SCI) in the United States is approximately 30 new cases per annum per one million population. About half are caused by motor vehicle accidents and a quarter by falls. In the multitrauma patient, SCI is associated with many other injuries and 15 to 50 percent of patients have concomitant head injury. An SCI patient may not appreciate abdominal pain, making the diagnosis of abdominal trauma more difficult.

1. If pain is present, it is often radicular in nature due to the involvement of sensory spinal nerves at the level of the lesion. Pain seldom involves the trunk or extremities below the level of the injury.

2. There can also be severe, incapacitating muscle spasms.

3. The patient may experience increased sensitivity above the level of the lesion; therefore, painful procedures, such as phlebotomy, should be done below the level of the lesion whenever possible.

4. Treatment

    a. Antispasticity agents such as **baclofen** (Lioresal, 5 mg bid initially, which may be increased up to 60 mg daily) and **dantrolene** (Dantrium, 25 mg daily initially, increasing every 3 or 4 days by 25 mg) are useful. The dosage may be increased until the therapeutic goal is reached. Liver function tests should be checked for evidence of hepatic toxicity. **Benzodiazepines** such as diazepam (Valium, 5 to 10 mg IV) may be necessary for severe muscle spasms.

      b. Amitriptyline (Elavil, 25 to 75 mg at night) can be given to facilitate sleep and to improve neuralgic or phantom pain through its serotonergic effects. Major depression and emotional lability will require higher doses (up to 150 mg daily).

E. Autonomic Hyperreflexia

      1. Transverse lesions of the cord above T7 functionally separate the sympathetic outflow of the spinal cord segment below the lesion from the modulating, vasodilating effect of the brainstem and hypothalamus. Activity below the lesion subsequently becomes reflexive in nature and is characterized by autonomic hyperreflexia, a syndrome of unbridled sympathetic discharge in response to pain, bladder and rectal distension, or surgical stimulation.

      2. A mass reflex characterized by rigidity and spasticity of muscles, pilomotor erection, nausea, agitation, sweating, flushing of the face and neck, severe headache, congestion of mucous membranes, bradycardia, heart block, ventricular arrhythmias, and hypertension can occur. If uncontrolled, the hypertension can lead to loss of consciousness, convulsions, and death from cerebral hemorrhage.

      3. Autonomic hyperreflexia usually reaches a peak 4 weeks after spinal cord injury and then subsides. It can recur at any time, and is usually initiated either by noxious stimuli applied below the level of the lesion, or by bladder or bowel distension.

      4. Treatment

         a. Control is achieved by a cessation of the stimulus. Bladder distension can be readily corrected with catheterization. Autonomic hyperreflexia from fecal impaction should not be treated with emergency disimpaction, as disimpaction may worsen the hyperreflexia. Alternatively, blood pressure should be managed pharmacologically and disimpaction accomplished under more controlled circumstances.

         b. Reflex muscle spasm and autonomic hyperreflexia are effectively prevented by spinal and epidural anesthesia, which block afferent visceral pathways.

         c. Sodium nitroprusside and alpha-adrenergic blocking agents are generally effective in treating the severe hypertension of autonomic hyperreflexia if a clear response is not noted very soon after removing the initiating stimulus.

V. PAIN ASSOCIATED WITH UPPER MOTOR NEURON LESIONS

A. Thalamic Pain Syndrome or Poststroke Central Pain

1. Supratentorial occlusive stroke is the most common cause of thalamic pain syndrome, occurring in one of 15,000 strokes. It is characterized by spontaneous, intermittent, lancinating pain that develops weeks to months following the stroke and involves some portion of the affected side of the body. Pain is described as burning, shooting, stabbing, or gnawing, and is associated with hyperpathia and allodynia. Pain is usually constant, subject to exacerbations for no apparent reason, or evoked by light touch, heat, cold, movement, auditory or visual stimuli, anxiety, and by visceral activity such as micturation.

2. Atrophic changes of skin, muscle, or bone are present.

3. Anxiety and depression occur with the syndrome.

4. Treatment

  a. Treatment is frustrating because the pain does not yield to conventional analgesics, though narcotics may be effective in selected patients.

  b. Phenytoin (Dilantin, 100 mg tid), **baclofen** (Lioresal, 5 mg bid initially, which may be increased up to 60 mg daily), **dantrolene** (Dantrium, 25 mg daily initially, increasing every 3 to 4 days by 25 mg), and **diazepam** (Valium, 5 to 10 mg tid) may relieve the jabbing or lancinating pain.

  c. Tricyclic antidepressants may help the burning dysesthetic pain and allodynia.

  d. A wide range of **neurosurgical procedures,** including ablative techniques and the use of electrical stimulation of the thalamus, internal capsule, and periaqueductal gray do not produce sustained pain relief. Peripheral **transcutaneous electrical stimulation** (TENS) has not proved effective either.

  e. To avoid the atrophic changes of skin, muscle, and bone, intensive **physical therapy** and **desensitization techniques** (heat or cold, vibration, or merely increased usage of the affected parts) are indicated. Psychotherapy, biofeedback, and self-hypnosis may be useful in helping the patient gain some control of the pain.

B. Multiple Sclerosis

1. Multiple sclerosis (MS) is an intermittent, progressive disorder of ambulation, vision, coordination, and bladder control that affects young adults. Pathophysiologically, it is characterized by recurrent attacks of demyelination in widely distributed areas of the CNS, which result in a variety of clinical symptoms.

a. Visual problems include nystagmus, monocular visual loss, and diplopia.

b. Motor signs include paresis, spasticity, and excessive fatigue.

c. Cerebellar dysfunction includes ataxia, incoordination, and dysarthria.

d. Urinary urgency and frequency are common.

e. Sensory problems include paresthesia, hyperesthesia, hypoesthesia, dysesthesia, and hyperpathia.

2. Pain is not a common symptom. L'Hermitte's sign (tingling or electric shocklike paresthesias on neck flexion) can be viewed as a nonspecific manifestation of MS within the cervical spinal cord.

3. **Treatment**

a. Antispasticity agents such as **baclofen** (Lioresal, 5 mg bid initially, which may be increased up to 60 mg daily) and **dantrolene** (Dantrium, 25 mg daily initially, increasing every 3 to 4 days by 25 mg) are very useful. Check liver function tests for hepatic toxicity.

b. **Amantadine** HCl (Symmetrel, 100 mg once or twice a day) improves fatigue.

c. **Steroids** can be used short-term to decrease the duration of flareups.

d. **Amitriptyline** (Elavil, 25 to 75 mg at night) can be given to facilitate sleep. Major depression and emotional lability will require higher doses, up to 150 mg daily.

C. Amyotrophic Lateral Sclerosis

1. Amyotrophic lateral sclerosis (ALS) is a fatal, degenerative disease of the CNS characterized by progressive paralysis of the voluntary muscles involving the limbs, trunk, and respiratory and pharyngeal muscles. Clinical symptoms include weakness, wasting, fasciculations, cramps, stiffness, and slowness of movement and speech.

2. No sensory or intellect abnormalities occur.

3. **Treatment**

a. No treatment is effective in stopping or slowing ALS. The clinician should remember that the patient has an intact sensory nervous system, including pain sensation.

b. Antispasticity agents such as **baclofen** (Lioresal, 5 mg bid initially, which may be increased up to 60 mg daily) and **dantrolene** (Dantrium, 25 mg daily initially, increasing every 3 to 4 days by 25 mg) are very useful. Check liver function tests for hepatic toxicity.

c. **Amitriptyline** (Elavil, 25 to 75 mg at night) can be given to facilitate sleep. Major depression and emotional lability will require higher doses, up to 150 mg daily.

VI. PAIN ASSOCIATED WITH PERIPHERAL NERVE LESIONS AND LOWER MOTOR NEURON LESIONS

A. Peripheral Neuropathies

The peripheral nervous system (PNS) encompasses those parts of the nervous system that lie outside the confines of the brain, brainstem, and spinal cord. It consists of the primary sensory neurons, lower motor neurons, and autonomic neurons that are outside the CNS. All parts of the PNS are associated with Schwann cells or the comparative ganglionic cells, the satellite cells.

   1. If nerves to muscles are disrupted, weakness may be present and atrophy of muscle fibers occurs, as does attenuation of the reflexes. Cramping and fatigue are common.

   2. If sensory nerves are injured, alterations in sensation are common. Complete anesthesia is rare, and more typically hypoesthesia, hyperesthesia, paresthesia, and dysesthesias occur. Pain is one of the major features of generalized neuropathies, though not all neuropathies are associated with pain. For those patients with pain, suffering can be extreme and very difficult to manage.

   3. Autonomic dysfunction may be present.

B. Pathogenesis of Generalized Neuropathies

Pathogenesis of damage to nerve fibers in generalized neuropathies includes metabolic abnormalities, amyloid deposition, ischemic injury of the vasa vasorum, and inflammatory demyelination. Regardless of the etiology of the neuropathy, the nature of the pain is quite similar. Intermittent, burning, lancinating dysesthetic pain may dominate the clinical presentation, though aching, boring, deep, continuous pain can also be a component of the patient's suffering.

C. Guillain-Barré Syndrome or Acute Inflammatory Polyradiculoneuropathy

   1. The Guillain-Barré syndrome (GBS) is one of the most common peripheral nerve diseases and frequently requires intensive care unit admission. It is an acute or subacute syndrome characterized by weakness more than by sensory symptoms. The cranial nerves and radicular nerves are commonly affected. Occasionally, the autonomic nervous system is affected. The usual history is one of previous good health interrupted by a mild respiratory or gastrointestinal febrile illness. Patients develop symmetrical leg weakness, followed by arm weakness and respiratory failure.

   2. Associated with the weakness is an ascending numbness that begins in the distal extremities and progresses proximally. Although such dyses-

thesias are considered to be painful (burning, aching, raw), severe neuropathic pain is unusual. Sensory loss is variable, but usually mild. Pain sensation is least affected by the disease.

    3. Over half of patients experience aching discomfort in their proximal muscles and back during the early stages of the illness.

    4. Treatment

        a. The patient has intact pain sensation, but is unable to move or respond to a painful stimulus. Every attempt should be made to communicate with the patient regarding analgesic needs.

        b. Frequent orientation to time and place and adequate sleep will improve motor function.

        c. Peripheral-nerve-pressure palsies should be avoided by frequent repositioning and attention to potential nerve exposure points.

        d. The illness is self-limited, and intensive and respiratory care have helped decrease mortality. **Plasmapheresis** to remove complement-dependent myelinotoxic antibodies and circulating immune complexes has shown some benefit in shortening the duration and severity of symptoms.

D. Diabetic Neuropathy

    1. Diabetic neuropathy is a metabolic neuropathy characterized by symmetrical, primarily sensory, polyneuropathy. The usual presentation is painless foot trauma, though it can present with burning, hyperesthesias, or paresthesias of the distal extremities.

    2. Treatment

        a. Strict blood glucose control is the key in diabetic neuropathy.

        b. **Amitripytline** (Elavil, 25 to 150 mg daily) or a combination of **fluphenazine** (Prolixin, 2 to 4 mg daily) and amitriptyline is suggested.

        c. The anticonvulsants **phenytoin** (Dilantin, 100 mg tid), **carbamazepine** (Tegretol, 200 mg qid), and **valproic acid** (Depakene, 250 to 750 mg daily) may be helpful.

        d. The underlying etiology is hypoxia due to an altered peripheral nerve–blood barrier. The use of hyperbaric oxygen has shown temporary improvement in diabetic neuropathies.

        e. Narcotics and other analgesics are not indicated.

E. Toxic Neuropathies

    1. **Mercury poisoning**

        a. **Acute ingestion** causes severe inflammatory pain of the oropharynx, abdominal cramps, nausea, and vomiting, leading to dehydration, and progressive damage to renal tubules causing anuria. Death may occur due to dehydration and uremia.

        b. **Chronic poisoning** is manifested by a variety of neurological symptoms such as tremors of the extremities, dysarthria, ataxia, apprehensions, and depression.

c. **Treatment**

   i. **Penicillamine** 250 mg qid orally) is an excellent chelating agent of heavy metals, which promotes their excretion in the urine, and has the additional advantage of being well absorbed from the gastrointestinal tract, while the alternative medications, BAL and EDTA, require systemic injection. Penicillamine has much less toxicity than BAL, but has the disadvantage of acute sensitivity reactions.

   ii. **BAL** (British antilewisite, 2,3-dimercaptopropanol, dimercaprol) also combines with heavy metals. BAL is most effective if given early after exposure, 5 mg/kg body weight IM (a single dose should not exceed 300 mg), repeated every 4 h on the first day and every 6 h on the second day. Thereafter, it should be given three times daily for several days. Doses should be tapered and discontinued about 10 days after acute poisoning. Overdosage results in nervousness, hyporeactivity, muscle twitching, and hyperreflexia. BAL is renally excreted and should be administered with caution in anuric or oliguric patients.

   iii. **EDTA** (ethylenediaminetetraacetate) is another chelating agent that is useful for heavy metal poisoning. Use 1 g in 250 mL 5% dextrose IV every 12 h for 5 days.

2. **Arsenic poisoning**

   a. Arsenic poisoning is characterized by a sensory neuropathy with severe pain, numbness, tingling, and burning of the feet and hands; followed by muscular weakness. Red feet and hands with hyperhydrosis are a characteristic sign.

   b. Diagnose with a 24 h urine analysis, hair analysis, and blood arsenic level.

   c. Treat with **penicillamine, BAL,** or **EDTA.**

3. **Lead poisoning**

   a. Lead poisoning is characterized by colic, encephalopathy, peripheral neuritis, anemia, and painful joints. Lead colic, or "painter's cramps," is characterized by agonizing, wandering, poorly localized abdominal pain, which is often accompanied by spasm and rigidity of the musculature of the abdominal wall.

   b. **Treatment** Narcotics have little effect on lead colic. The IV injection of **calcium** affords transient relief. The definitive treatment is with **BAL** and **EDTA,** followed by **penicillamine.**

4. **Thallium poisoning**

   a. Thallium poisoning is characterized by vomiting, diarrhea, and leg pains, followed by a severe, and sometimes fatal, sensorimotor polyneuropathy.

   b. Treatment is symptomatic.

F. Vasculitic Neuropathy

1. Vasculitic neuropathy is a generalized neuropathy associated with connective tissue diseases that result in ischemic injury to the vascular sup-

ply of peripheral nerves. Included in this category are polyarteritis nodosa, rheumatoid arthritis, lupus erythematosus, systemic sclerosis, cranial arteritis, and Wegener's granulomatosis. It is characterized by shooting pains, as well as dysesthesias, in the distribution of the affected nerve(s).

   2. Treatment

   a. Treating the underlying process is key to the management of a systemic vasculitis of the vasa vasorum.

   b. Amitripytline (Elavil, 25 to 150 mg daily) or a combination of **fluphenazine** (Prolixin, 2 to 4 mg daily) and amitriptyline is suggested.

   c. The anticonvulsants **phenytoin** (Dilantin, 100 mg tid), **carbamazepine** (Tegretol, 200 mg qid), and **valproic acid** (Depakene, 250 to 750 mg daily) may be helpful.

   d. Narcotics and other analgesics are not indicated.

G. Acute Anterior Poliomyelitis (Infantile Paralysis)

   1. Poliomyelitis is an acute illness caused by poliovirus, which selectively destroys the motor neurons of the spinal cord and brainstem and results in flaccid, asymmetric weakness.

   2. The incubation period from exposure to the neurologic phase lasts between 4 and 10 days. The major illness begins with fever and malaise, and is followed by headache, vomiting, nuchal rigidity, drowsiness, irritability, and apprehension. If paralysis develops, it usually begins on the second to fifth day after headache.

   3. Discomfort may occur early in the course, and is likened to the muscular pain experienced after heavy or unaccustomed exertion.

   4. Treatment is purely supportive, with specific attention directed to preventing contractures and respiratory complications.

   5. Postpolio syndrome presents many years after the acute disease with progression of weakness in muscles previously thought not to be affected. Treatment is supportive.

H. Postherpetic Neuralgia

   1. Herpes zoster is a disease of individuals who have previously had varicella infection (chicken pox). It is caused by reactivation of the varicella zoster virus that has remained dormant in spinal ganglia since the initial episode of varicella. Perhaps due to age- or neoplasm-related depression of cell-mediated immunity, the virus reerupts in the sensory ganglion to cause an inflammatory reaction and reinfection of the skin and mucous membranes. The virus affects the thoracic (55 percent of cases), cervical (20 percent), lumbar, and sacral nerves (15 percent), and the ophthalmic division of the trigeminal nerve. Herpes zoster is characterized by fever and rash and pain that are localized to the dermatomes of the affected nerves. Pain can be severe, but usually subsides as the rash heals, within 2 to 3 weeks.

2. If pain persists beyond 1 month or recurs after the rash heals, it is referred to as **postherpetic neuralgia** (PHN), and may last for several months or years. The pain is described as burning, nagging, gnawing, and lancinating. Hyperesthesia, dysesthesia, and allodynia have also been described.

3. Treatment

  a. Pain relief for patients with acute herpes zoster and preemptive therapy for the prevention of PHN in patients with herpes zoster have been reasonably successful with **prednisone** (60 mg daily, taper after 2 weeks) and **amantadine** HCl (100 mg bid for a month). Vidarabine, interferon, and the combination of levodopa and benserazide, as well as sympathetic block with local anesthetics, have resulted in variable results in the relief of symptoms and prevention of PHN.

  b. For established PHN, a reduction in pain from severe to mild can be achieved with **amitriptyline** (Elavil, 10 to 25 mg daily, increased by 10 mg every 5 to 7 days to a maximum of 150 mg), **fluphenazine** (Prolixin, 2 to 4 mg daily), and **topical capsaicin** (Zostrix, the substance of hot chili peppers). Combining these modalities with **anticonvulsants** (carbamazepine, phenytoin, and valproic acid), TENS, or topical anesthetics has been suggested.

I. Reflex Sympathetic Dystrophy

1. Reflex sympathetic dystrophy (RSD) can follow any soft tissue injury. Pain may begin within minutes or hours of the injury, is usually burning in quality, is often disproportionately intense with respect to the nature or extent of the injury, and persists even after presumed healing of the injury. RSD is characterized as having no associated major nerve damage. When its symptoms are associated with nerve damage and neurologic deficits (e.g., brachial plexus injury after a gunshot wound), the syndrome is classified as **causalgia** (see Chapter 32).

2. The **acute stage** lasts several weeks, starts within hours or days of the injury, and is characterized by aching and burning pain, hyperpathia, erythema, edema, increased diaphoresis, and altered hair and nail growth. These changes are usually restricted to a nondermatomal, vascular, or peripheral nerve area.

3. The **dystrophic stage** begins about 3 months later. The skin over the affected area becomes smooth and glossy, and cutaneous vasoconstriction and subcutaneous atrophy may be present. The affected extremity is often cooler than the normal extremity. The pain occupies a greater area, the hyperpathia and swelling are more pronounced than in the acute stage, and there are muscle wasting, osteoporosis, and functional loss of the extremity due to pain and pericapsular fibrosis of joints.

4. The **atrophic stage** is the end stage of RSD and usually occurs 6 months or longer after the injury. This stage is characterized by an atrophic,

contracted extremity. The pain is frequently less intense or has "burned out."

   5. Treatment

   a. Blocking efferent sympathetic fibers supplying the involved body area is the mainstay of therapy for RSD pain. Temporary **local anesthetic blockade of sympathetic ganglia,** such as the stellate ganglion or cervicothoracic ganglion block (for head, trunk, and upper extremity), celiac plexus (for abdominal pain), or the lumbar sympathetic ganglia (for lower extremity), can be accomplished with lidocaine or bupivacaine. Alternatively, single-dose epidural injections and bretylium Bier blocks can be used for the extremities (see Chapters 13 and 32). Success is better the sooner the block is performed after the onset of symptoms. Pain relief usually occurs within minutes of the block and may persist for days or weeks. Continuous blockade can be accomplished by infusing bupivacaine (0.125 to 0.25%) near sympathetic and somatic nerves supplying the affected body area.

   b. Systemic **sympatholytic drugs** can be tried as alternatives to sympathetic block. Propanolol (Inderal), guanethidine (Ismelin), prazosin (Minipress), and phenoxybenzamine have all been used to manage RSD pain.

   c. The calcium channel blocker **nifedipine** (Procardia) will increase peripheral blood flow and antagonize the effects of norepinephrine on arterial smooth muscle, and can provide some relief.

   d. Corticosteroid therapy may be helpful, especially when joint involvement is marked.

   e. NSAIDs may provide some relief. The use of narcotics in the management of chronic sympathetic pain is usually not indicated.

   f. Tricyclic antidepressants (amitriptyline [Elavil] 10 to 25 mg daily, increased by 10 mg every 5 to 7 days to a maximum of 150 mg) and **anticonvulsants** (phenytoin [Dilantin] 100 mg tid, or carbamazepine [Tegretol] 200 mg qid) may help in the management of neuropathic RSD pain.

   g. Over vascular areas, **TENS** is particularly effective in early RSD and in the treatment of pediatric patients. **Physical therapy** is a vital component of the treatment plan. Other adjunctive therapies include myofascial trigger point injections, biofeedback, and self-hypnosis (see Chapter 32).

VII. NEUROMUSCULAR JUNCTION DISORDERS ASSOCIATED WITH PAIN

A. Myasthenia Gravis

   1. Myasthenia gravis is a failure of synaptic neuromuscular transmission due to autoimmune-mediated abnormalities of the postsynaptic membrane. It occurs in all age groups. Symptoms are muscle fatigue in ocular, bulbar, limb, and trunk musculature with partial or complete recovery after rest. The disorder can be acute and fulminating, but more commonly it is characterized by a slow progression of symptoms with frequent remissions and relapses. Sensory nerves are not affected.

   2. Myasthenic crisis is the sudden exacerbation of weakness precipitated by infection, surgical procedures, pregnancy, or emotional upset. The weakness may be profound and lead to respiratory failure.

   3. Treatment

   a. **Anticholinesterase drugs** are the mainstay of therapy. **Cholinergic crisis** results from toxic levels of anticholinesterase drugs causing overdepolarization of the postsynaptic membrane. Muscarinic effects are then prominent and include abdominal cramps, diarrhea, and excessive pulmonary secretions. Nicotinic drug effects cause fasciculations, weakness of voluntary muscles, and bronchospasm. Cholinergic crisis can mimic an acute abdomen and lead to unnecessary surgical exploration.

   b. Thymectomy, steroids, and plasmapheresis are beneficial in selected cases.

   c. The advent of modern intensive and respiratory care has decreased the morbidity and mortality of this disease.

B. Botulism

   1. Botulism is an acute neuromuscular disease caused by a group of protein toxins produced by *Clostridium botulinum,* an anaerobic, gram-positive soil organism. Botulinum toxins are the most potent neurotoxins known. Ingestion of food containing preformed toxin is the most common route of infection.

   2. The disease is characterized by subacute paralysis of extraocular muscles with involvement of pharyngeal muscles that usually appears within 2 days of toxin ingestion. The presenting complaints often reflect cranial nerve dysfunction: diplopia or blurred vision, ptosis, dysphagia or dry mouth, and dysphonia. The neurologic manifestations of the disease are bilateral and follow a descending pattern, with peripheral muscle weakness following cranial nerve dysfunction.

   3. Botulism may be diagnosed by isolating the toxin from the patient's blood, feces, or food. An electromyogram aids in the diagnosis.

   4. Treatment The treatment includes use of
   a. a botulinum antitoxin,
   b. respiratory support,
   c. symptomatic analgesia and sedation.

C. Tetanus

   1. Tetanus is caused by *Clostridium tetani,* an anaerobic gram-positive bacillus. The organism forms spores which are commonly found in the soil. If introduced into a wound, the spores produce a potent neurotoxin.

2. Diagnosis is made by clinical criteria. The disease is characterized by severe, painful, incapacitating muscle spasms. The patient has a fixed smile with the teeth clenched (trismus) and the rest of the muscles in constant contraction. Severe spasms can cause vertebral fracture and airway obstruction. Symptoms can appear 1 to 54 days after injury. Autonomic disturbances may occur, resulting in cardiac dysrhythmias, lability of blood pressure and heart rate, and profuse diaphoresis. Pulmonary complications and cardiac dysrhythmias are the major causes of mortality.

3. Treatment

a. **Airway protection** is critical and the patient should be intubated at the first sign of dysphagia or laryngospasm. **Ventilatory support** is almost always necessary in conjunction with sedatives and certainly so with nondepolarizing neuromuscular blocking agents.

b. **Diazepam** (Valium, 2 to 20 mg every 2 to 8 h), **chlorpromazine** (Thorazine, 50 to 150 mg every 4 to 8 h), or **meprobamate** (Deprol, 400 mg every 3 to 4 h) may be titrated to reduce muscle spasms. However, continuous infusions of nondepolarizing neuromuscular blocking agents (**metacurine** [Metubine] 0.3 mg/kg loading dose followed by 5 to 10 mg/h or **tubocurare,** 0.3 mg/kg loading dose followed by 3 to 10 mg/h) are required to prevent spasms in all but the mildest cases. Prolonged use of the steroid-like nondepolarizing neuromuscular blocking agents (pancuronium, vecuronium) is not recommended because of reports of prolonged muscle weakness and atrophy following long-term use.

c. **Analgesics,** including narcotics, are warranted.

d. **Human tetanus immunoglobulin** (TIG-H, 3,000 to 10,000 units) should be administered IM at several sites, including the area of presumed injury. The TIG will bind free toxin, although it will not affect toxin already incorporated into nerve fibers.

e. **Penicillin G** (1 to 10 million units a day) should be given for 10 to 14 days. Tetracycline, erythromycin, and chloramphenicol may be used in penicillin-allergic patients.

D. Hypocalcemic Tetany

1. Hypocalcemia is another cause of painful, intractable muscle spasms, but is characterized by a milder tetany than is tetanus. The presence of Chvostek's and Trousseau's signs aids in the diagnosis.

2. Treatment is the intravenous administration of 20 to 30 mL 10% calcium gluconate.

E. Duchenne Type and Other Muscular Dystrophies

1. Muscular dystrophies are inherited myopathies of unknown etiology associated with progressive muscle weakness, destruction of muscle fibers, and eventual replacement of fibers with fibrous and fatty connective tissue. Duchenne's muscular dystrophy is characterized by weakness of the lower

extremities, tight heel cords, lumbar lordosis, mild mental retardation, and an enlarged tongue. By 9 to 12 years of age, the patient suffers frequent falls and increasing proximal weakness. Once in a wheelchair, painful contractures develop in all joints, the feet invert, and progressive kyphoscoliosis develops.
   2. **Treatment**
      a. There is no specific treatment for any of the muscular dystrophies.
      b. Rehabilitation is paramount in easing discomfort in these patients.

F. Inflammatory Myopathies

   1. Inflammatory myopathies make up a heterogenous group of disorders characterized by diffuse weakness, though focal symptoms can be present. Some are caused by bacterial, parasitic, or viral infections. Others are more clearly autoimmune in etiology.
   2. Polymyositis and dermatomyositis are characterized by subacute onset of proximal weakness and muscle pain. Diagnosis is made by increased creatine phosphokinase (CPK) and ESR.
   3. **Treatment**
      a. **Prednisone,** 100 mg every other day, is effective in relieving pain.

VIII. PAIN MANAGEMENT IN THE PRESENCE OF NEUROLOGIC DISEASE

A. Disease Components That Alter Analgesic Options

There are several consequences of neurologic disease that significantly alter one's choice of analgesic modalities for nonneurologic pain. These include elevated ICP, altered mental status, perispinal malignancy or infection, syringomyelia, and some neuromuscular diseases such as multiple sclerosis.

B. Analgesic Medications (Drugs)

   1. **Opioid agonist and agonist–antagonist medications** cause some element of respiratory depression, although the latter drugs offer a ceiling effect as opposed to the dose-dependent effect of the pure agonists (see Chapter 8). In the spontaneously breathing patient with diminished intracranial compliance, these drugs can cause an increase in carbon dioxide which results in a critical rise in ICP. In the face of controlled ventilation, narcotics will decrease cerebral metabolic rate ($CMRo_2$) and, when delivered by infusion, can be titrated to a level where relative comfort can coexist with an interpretable neurologic exam. In addition, in the event of a decline in mental

status, these medications can be *gently* reversed with naloxone to rule out excessive narcotization as a cause. It should be noted that the agonist–antagonist drugs do not reverse as easily as the pure agonists due to avid binding to the opioid receptors.

  2. Benzodiazepines decrease CMR_{O_2}, but can also cause respiratory depression. The confusion and/or sedation caused by benzodiazepines may make interpretation of the neurologic exam difficult. With the availability of flumazenil, this is less of a concern.

  3. Ketamine is a direct cerebral vasodilator and increases ICP in patients with decreased intracranial compliance. Because it is a potent analgesic, ketamine can be used in patients with other neurologic problems who are undergoing brief painful procedures, but should be avoided in those patients in whom sympathetic stimulation is undesirable.

  4. Local anesthetics, in excessive doses, can cause neuroexcitation. This can be manifest as confusion and seizures. Low doses of local anesthetic are actually antiepileptogenic and can be given safely.

C. Analgesic Modalities

  1. The **PO** and **PCA** administration of analgesic medications is limited to patients who are neurologically able to manage them. **Intravenous bolus dosing** (prn or scheduled) can cause swings in mental status from alert, agitated, and in pain to sedated and less responsive. In the face of intracranial pathology, these effects can be confusing at best. Once equilibrated, **IV infusions** offer a "steady state" of analgesia and sedation, allowing easier interpretation of the neurologic exam. Concerns related to this mode of delivery include gradual accumulation of drug, as well as the development of tolerance.

  2. Epidural analgesia should not be used in the face of elevated ICP or CNS infections. Further, it should be used with extreme caution in patients with syringomyelia and perispinal malignant disease. Concerns include increases in CNS pressure by the addition of volume to the epidural space that further elevates ICP and the possible seeding of malignant cells into the CSF.

  a. Local anesthetics are discussed above. **Peridural local anesthetics** should not be used in patients with demyelinating diseases such as multiple sclerosis or Guillain-Barré. Demyelinated nerves are very sensitive to even low concentrations of local anesthetic, and the clinical effect is likely to be more profound (e.g., motor blockade) and of significantly longer duration than expected.

  b. Outside of the general risks mentioned above, the primary risk of **peridural narcotics** is that of delayed respiratory depression which is related to the levels of narcotic in the CSF causing depression of the brainstem respiratory centers.

3. Pleural catheters can be used in patients with neurologic disease with little risk, except as noted above regarding toxic levels of local anesthetics. The technique is described in Chapter 13.

4. Plexus blocks and **peripheral nerve blocks** can be safely administered in neurologic disease, though there are some theoretical concerns about the toxicity plexus blocks shown in patients with peripheral demyelinating processes. Plexus blocks can be administered via intermittent injections or by infusion after placement of a catheter in the appropriate location (e.g., a supraclavicular catheter for the brachial plexus). The precautions associated with local anesthetic administration are well delineated above.

5. TENS is a safe adjunctive pain therapy which has no contraindications in this patient population. It should be noted that the TENS impulses will interfere with EEG monitoring, however.

6. Self-regulation techniques are limited to patients who are alert and cooperative. These techniques can be very useful in patients with spinal cord injuries and progressive neuromuscular diseases. They not only offer a pain management strategy for the discomfort associated with the specific disease, but one that is also beneficial for the repeated painful procedures associated with routine hospital care (e.g., IVs, venipunctures, lumbar punctures, dressing changes).

CASE DISCUSSION

Good pulmonary toilet is critical to the successful weaning of this patient, and this, to a large extent, depends on adequate analgesia. This patient's premorbid organic disease, as well as the residual confusion from his head injury, influences the choice of options available to manage his pain.

Narcotics would be of benefit for his baseline pain, but would be less helpful for incident pain (e.g., coughing). PCA administration is not a likely option because of his altered mental status, but an IV infusion of narcotic could be used. As most narcotics are primarily metabolized in the liver, one must watch for a gradual accumulation of drug and the associated sedation and respiratory depression. Intermittent boluses of opioids are possible, but tend to be inadequate due to our inability to assess pain effectively and because they carry the risks of wide swings in levels of pain relief and sedation. Fentanyl is felt by many to be preferable to morphine for patients with hepatic failure. The NSAIDs, such as ketorolac, although very effective in treating pleuritic pain, should not be used in this patient given the underlying coagulopathy.

A regional analgesic technique would be desirable to avoid or minimize requirements for medications that alter mental status, such as narcotics. Epidural analgesia (local anesthetic with or without narcotic) would be very effective, but is contraindicated in the face of a coagulopathy and pathology where intracranial compliance may be altered. Intrapleural administration of local anesthetic would provide significant pain relief with minimal risk, can be used in the face of mild to moderate coagulation disturbances, and would cause little or no alteration in mental status. Bupivacaine 0.25% can be administered through an epidural or pigtail catheter placed in the pleural space aseptically (see Chapters 13 and 24 for details). Small doses of IV narcotics can be used as a supplement.

SUGGESTED READINGS

Adams RD, Victor M: Headache and craniofacial pain, in *Principles of Neurology.* New York, McGraw-Hill, 1989, pp 134–154.

Adams RD, Victor M: Diseases of peripheral nerve and muscle, in *Principles of Neurology.* New York, McGraw-Hill, 1989, pp 1009–1168.

Alderson JD, Frost EAM: *Spinal Cord Injuries: Anaesthetic and Associated Care.* London, Butterworths, 1990.

Ducker TB, Saul TG: The polytrauma in spinal cord injury, in Tator CH (ed): *Early Management of Acute Spinal Cord Injury.* New York, Raven Press, 1982, pp. 53–58.

Fields HL: *Pain Syndromes in Neurology.* London, Butterworths, 1990.

CHAPTER 17

PAIN AND CARDIOVASCULAR DISEASE

Kenneth R. Greer
John W. Hoyt

Case
I. Introduction
II. Clinical Manifestation of Pain in Cardiovascular Disease
    A. Hypothesis of the Transmission of Cardiac Pain
    B. Cardiac Ischemia and Chest Pain or Angina Pectoris
    C. Theories of Cardiac Muscle Pain
    D. Modulation of Cardiac Pain
    E. Effect of Systemic Disease on Myocardial Pain
III. Painful Cardiovascular Syndromes
    A. Myocardial Ischemia
    B. Myocardial Infarction
    C. Pericarditis
    D. Other Thoracic Processes Causing Chest Pain
    E. Pain After Thoracic Surgery
    F. Vascular Pain
IV. Impact of Preexisting Cardiac Disease on Pain Management in the Critically Ill Patient
    A. Physiology of Cardiac Disease
    B. Effects of Analgesic and Sedative Medications on Patients with Cardiovascular Disease
    C. Routes of Administration of Analgesic and Sedative Medications in Critical Care
Case Discussion
Suggested Readings

CASE

An upper gastrointestinal bleed related to the administration of nonsteroidal anti-inflammatory drugs (NSAIDs) for osteoarthritis precipitated an admission to the intensive care unit (ICU) for a 68-year-old male with a history of coronary artery disease and previous inferior-wall myocardial infarction. Mr. M. required the transfusion of eight units of blood before going to the operating room for a gastrectomy in order to control bleeding. The postoperative course was marked by a short period of mechanical ventilation, followed by extubation and severe incisional and abdominal pain. On the third postoperative day, the patient was noted to complain of chest pressure and pain radiating down the left arm and into the neck. Vital signs revealed a heart rate of 120 and a blood pressure of 160/96. An electrocardiogram (ECG) showed ST depression and T-wave inversion across the precordium. Auscultation of the chest suggested early pulmonary edema.

I. INTRODUCTION

One of the primary missions of the cardiovascular system is the uptake and distribution of oxygen to meet the metabolic needs of the cells in the various tissues and organs of the body. This mission can be compromised by three etiologies of low cardiac output: (1) **pump failure** from poorly functioning cardiac muscle, as seen in myocardial ischemia and infarction; (2) **preload failure** from inadequate left ventricular end diastolic volume secondary to hypovolemia from hemorrhage or intravascular volume depletion; and (3) **afterload failure** from excessive resistance to left ventricular ejection, which might be valvular (aortic stenosis) or vasoconstrictive (elevated systemic vascular resistance) in nature. Pain, cardiac in nature, can result from a disturbance of the delicate balance of myocardial-muscle oxygen demand and supply. The management of this pain resulting from cardiac ischemia and infarction is one of the major themes of this chapter. Patients with preexisting cardiac disease who experience pain after trauma or surgery as seen in the case presentation can develop cardiac pain because of inadequate cardiac reserves. The effect of pain on patients with cardiac disease is the second major theme of this chapter.

II. CLINICAL MANIFESTATION OF PAIN IN CARDIOVASCULAR DISEASE

A. Hypothesis of the Transmission of Cardiac Pain

1. The heart is innervated by both the sympathetic and parasympathetic nervous systems.

2. The **sympathetic nervous system** arises from the first four or five thoracic segments. Preganglionic fibers synapse in the three cervical sympa-

thetic ganglia and the upper four or five thoracic sympathetic ganglia. Postganglionic fibers travel to the cardiac plexus and innervate the heart. Sympathetic stimulation increases heart rate and contractility. Visceral afferent fibers are carried in these sympathetic nerves.

   3. The **parasympathetic system** starts in the dorsal motor nucleus of the vagus nerves in the brainstem. Preganglionic fibers travel to the cardiac plexus and then to the heart and synapse with postganglionic cell bodies and fibers. Parasympathetic stimulation through the vagus nerve slows heart rate.

   4. The **sensation of pain** from the heart seems to be mostly detected and transmitted by sympathetic afferents that enter the left side of the spinal cord at the first thoracic level. Thus pain from the heart is referred to a first thoracic dermatome distribution, which includes the anterior chest and the inside of the upper left arm.

B. Cardiac Ischemia and Chest Pain or Angina Pectoris

   1. **Myocardial oxygen supply** that is inadequate to meet the metabolic oxygen demand of cardiac muscle usually causes substernal chest pain or pressure. This pain may radiate into the left arm, the neck, or the jaw. The heart normally extracts 70 to 75 percent of available oxygen from blood passing through the coronary arteries. Additional oxygen demand by cardiac muscle cannot be met by increased extraction. Only increased cardiac-muscle oxygen transport can meet the needs of increased myocardial oxygen consumption. If there is a restriction in cardiac-muscle oxygen transport, chest pain or angina pectoris occurs.

   2. **Angina pectoris** is a clinical syndrome characterized by exertional substernal chest pain, pressure, squeezing, tightness, heaviness, or choking. Chest pain comes on with exertion or emotion and is relieved by rest. Patients will commonly develop pain at exactly the same point in their daily activity. Clinicians have known for years that angina pectoris leads to decreased cardiac output, ventricular irritability with ventricular ectopy, and myocardial infarction.

   3. **Angina decubitus** is chest pain at rest or in the recumbent position. Angina at rest commonly follows an increase in the frequency of exertional angina, and is commonly viewed by clinicians as a worsening of the imbalance between myocardial oxygen demand and supply. Patients complain of waking up with chest pain that is identical to the pain experienced during exertion.

   4. **Direct stimulation** of the heart does not cause pain. Cardiac pain is limited to certain portions of the heart under very specific conditions—usually ischemia. A patient can have left ventricular dilatation during congestive heart failure and experience no pain. Bacterial endocarditis can destroy heart valves, and yet the patient will perceive no painful sensation.

5. Cardiac pain is caused by an imbalance of myocardial oxygen supply and demand. **Myocardial oxygen supply is dependent on coronary vessel pressure and diastolic time,** since most coronary blood flow occurs during diastole. Increased cardiac muscle pressure during systole prevents blood flow in most myocardial muscle, particularly the endocardial area. In addition, **hemoglobin** and **oxygen saturation** of hemoglobin will determine myocardial oxygen supply.

6. Myocardial oxygen demand is determined by heart rate, systolic blood pressure, and tension of contractility of cardiac muscle. Increased heart rate or tachycardia increases myocardial oxygen demand and decreases myocardial oxygen supply, since diastole shortens with tachycardia while systole stays the same. At a heart rate of 90, the time in systole and diastole is approximately equal. At heart rates above 90, there is progressively less time in diastole than in systole. By a heart rate of 120, two-thirds of the time is spent in systole and one-third is spent in diastole.

7. In the presence of coronary artery disease with narrowing of the vessel lumen, there is a restriction of flow. During exertion, heart rate and blood pressure increase. Partial occlusion of a coronary vessel limits increases in cardiac-muscle oxygen transport. When myocardial muscle oxygen demand from exertion is greater than myocardial muscle oxygen transport, ischemia occurs and chest pain is perceived.

C. Theories of Cardiac Muscle Pain

1. Specificity theory suggests a specific nociceptor. Ischemia causes the release of local and hormonal mediators. The subsequent release of catecholamines, epinephrine and norepinephrine, further increases heart rate and blood pressure.

2. At the tissue level, there are local muscle metabolic changes. This causes alterations in the concentration of adenosine, bradykinin, calcium, carbon dioxide, oxygen, and vasodilator metabolites. With tissue hypoxia there is a decline in cellular adenosine triphosphate (ATP) and an increase in adenosine monophosphate (AMP), adenosine, inosine, hypoxanthine, and xanthine. Lactate is formed and increases in tissue concentration.

3. Bradykinin may be the mediator of ischemia pain activating sympathetic afferent fibers which transmit through the spinal cord in the high thoracic area. This path causes the referred pain of angina pectoris to the anterior chest wall and the inside of the left arm.

4. Thus a specific mediator gives rise to specific pain through the sympathetic nervous system. Research has shown that thoracic sympathectomy will block pain-related behavior in the animal model when ischemia is created.

5. The intensity theory is an alternative hypothesis for cardiac pain. This theory proposes excessive stimulation of a general receptor apparatus rather than a specific nociceptor.

6. The **modified intensity theory of Malliani** is a combination of specificity theory and intensity theory. This proposal suggests that cardiac pain results from the intense stimulation of a spatially restricted group of afferent nerve fibers.

7. Mechanical forces such as traction on coronary vessel ligatures have been shown to cause chest pain.

8. The vagus nerve seems to transmit some aspects of pain associated with cardiac ischemia. When thoracic sympathectomy relieves substernal and left arm pain with cardiac muscle ischemia, pain in the neck and jaw, thought to be vagal in origin, becomes more prominent.

D. Modulation of Cardiac Pain

1. Vagal afferents seem to be able to modulate both the threshold and the characteristics of pain due to cardiac muscle ischemia.

2. The **spinal cord** is the center for the convergence of fibers that are capable of increasing or decreasing nociception.

3. Transcutaneous electrical nerve stimulation (TENS) or dorsal column stimulation can decrease nociception via the spinal cord.

4. There can be a **cognitive modulation** of chest pain depending on the level of anxiety, agitation, and the patient's understanding of the problem and the environment. The treatment of cognitive co-factors can significantly lower the patient's perception of cardiac pain.

E. Effect of Systemic Disease on Myocardial Pain

1. Diabetes causes a dysfunction of the sympathetic nervous system. Myocardial infarction can occur in 30 to 42 percent of diabetic patients without chest pain.

2. Silent ischemia is a common problem in diabetic patients. There are histologic alterations in the autonomic nerve fibers of cardiac muscle in patients with diabetes.

III. PAINFUL CARDIOVASCULAR SYNDROMES

A. Myocardial Ischemia

1. Patients with arteriosclerotic cardiovascular disease may experience several episodes of **exertional angina** per day. These are relieved by rest or sublingual nitroglycerin, and appear to be of no long-term physiologic significance.

2. Chest pain unrelieved by rest or nitroglycerin represents a medical emergency which requires immediate evaluation in a hospital Emergency Medicine Department. The pain as described above, crushing or squeezing substernal pain, usually radiates to the inside of the left arm and occasionally to the neck or jaw.

3. **Persistent ischemia** manifested by unrelieved chest pain leads to poor contraction of the affected muscle with **wall motion abnormalities** seen on echocardiography. Cardiac output falls, cardiac muscle becomes irritable as shown by the onset of **ventricular ectopy,** cardiac muscle **compliance decreases** with an increase in left ventricular end diastolic pressure and pulmonary capillary wedge pressure, **pulmonary edema** begins with shortness of breath and diaphoresis, and the ECG shows ST depression and T-wave inversion.

4. In response to the chest pain and decline in cardiac output, there is a generalized **release of catecholamines,** with an elevation of blood pressure and heart rate. The hypertension and tachycardia aggravate the imbalance of myocardial oxygen supply and demand and further accelerate the angina and ischemia process. With worsening pulmonary edema, the patient develops respiratory failure and hypoxia, which worsens the myocardial ischemia, since there is less oxygen uptake and myocardial oxygen transport declines.

5. If unreversed, the physiologic disturbance of cardiac ischemia will lead to a stunned myocardium. Cardiac cellular energy stores are depleted and the cell membrane is less able to maintain electrolyte gradients, such as for calcium and sodium. If the process is reversed at this point, several days of cardiac muscle support with afterload reduction and inotropic therapy will be necessary to return to a previous level of cardiac muscle function. If the process is not reversed at this point, ischemia will progress to infarction or to a fatal arrhythmia and death.

6. The patient with **refractory angina** commonly presents with substantial chest discomfort, shortness of breath, and a correct sense of impending doom. The clinical picture must be differentiated from that of other causes of chest pain, such as dissecting thoracic aortic aneurysm, esophageal pain, pleural pain as from a pulmonary embolus, or musculoskeletal pain. Examination of the whole patient with a history of medical problems and laboratory tests such as an ECG will usually allow a swift diagnosis of ischemia and initiation of urgent treatment.

7. The immediate **life-threatening aspects of refractory angina** are pulmonary edema with hypoxia and low cardiac output syndrome with poor peripheral perfusion. The patient commonly will be focused on the pain and shortness of breath, but the medical emergency is to restore oxygen transport to the cells of various body tissues and organs.

8. The immediate treatment on admission to the Emergency Medicine Department is **oxygen,** either by face mask or endotracheal tube. Subsequent management includes intravenous (IV) morphine, 5 to 10 mg, depending on the size and age of the patient, the degree of hypotension, and the level of consciousness. **Morphine** will relieve pain and sedate the patient,

reducing circulating catecholamines that are causing hypertension and tachycardia and aggravating the ischemia. Morphine is also a vascular preload and afterload reducer that improves cardiac output and peripheral perfusion.

9. A continuous infusion of **nitroglycerin** IV should be started at 0.5 μg/kg/min, which will reduce preload and afterload, and provide some coronary artery dilatation. Pain relief is often immediate with IV nitroglycerin, though the mechanism is not clear other than the improvement of the balance of myocardial oxygen supply and demand. **Furosemide** (Lasix) is commonly given by the IV route, 20 to 40 mg, to improve pulmonary edema. This loop diuretic will lower intravascular volume by increasing urine output in the fluid-overloaded patient. Most important, furosemide will decrease pulmonary capillary wedge pressure almost immediately, since it is a pulmonary capillary vasodilator. This improves the pulmonary edema pathology and helps to correct the oxygenation problem.

B. Myocardial Infarction

1. A prolonged ischemic event as described above will commonly lead to a small increase in cardiac enzymes, creatine phosphokinase (CPK-MB; the MB isoenzyme of CPK is most specific for myocardial necrosis) and lactate dehydrogenase (LDH-1) isoenzyme. This is a **non–Q-wave myocardial infarction,** and is to be distinguished from a transmural infarction.

2. Occlusion by thrombosis at the site of an atheromatous plaque of either the right or left coronary artery or a branch of the left main vessel will lead to a **transmural infarction** in the distribution of the occluded vessel. Right coronary artery occlusions commonly lead to an inferior or right-sided infarct and left coronary artery occlusions lead to an anteroseptal and/or lateral wall infarction.

3. The **pain of infarction** is not to be differentiated from the pain of refractory angina. The ECG will demonstrate ST elevation with the evolution of a Q wave at the site of the infarction. The clinical picture will be quite similar to, or identical in all respects to, persistent unrelieved ischemia.

4. The **management of infarction** is initially similar to that for ischemia, including oxygen, nitrates, and morphine for pain management. When the ECG fails to show correction of ST elevation abnormalities with nitrates, there are four principles to be remembered for correcting the physiologic abnormalities of myocardial infarction and treating cardiac pain.

5. The first principle is to **treat the underlying cause** of the chest pain. It is clearly understood now that rupture of an atheromatous plaque into the lumen of a coronary vessel initiates a coagulation cascade that results in a clot at the site of the plaque and an occlusion of the vessel. The vessel must be opened within 4 to 6 h of the occlusion by the use of a thrombolytic agent if significant cardiac muscle is to be saved from the infarction process.

Agents such as **tissue plasminogen activator (TPA)** given as a bolus and then as a continuous infusion will start the thrombolysis process and remove the clot, restoring perfusion and relieving chest pain. One of the cardinal signs of reperfusion is the relief of pain. **Heparin** as a bolus and continuous infusion must be started immediately with the TPA in order to prevent reocclusion of the vessel and recurrence of chest pain.

   6. The second principle in managing the chest pain of myocardial infarction is to **employ the physiologic principles of myocardial oxygen supply and demand.** Tachycardia and hypertension, a common part of myocardial infarction because of the pain and systemic release of catecholamines, worsen the pain because of an increase in myocardial-muscle oxygen demand and a decrease in cardiac-muscle oxygen supply. **Beta-blockers** have been shown to substantially decrease the acute and long-term morbidity and mortality of transmural myocardial infarction. **Metoprolol** (Lopressor), given IV at the time of diagnosis of a myocardial infarction, slows heart rate, which increases diastolic time and improves myocardial oxygen supply. Beta-blockers also decrease blood pressure, which reduces myocardial oxygen demand. An improved balance of cardiac oxygen supply and demand relieves chest pain.

   7. The third principle in treating cardiac pain is to **take advantage of some of the physiologic effects of analgesic medications. Morphine,** for example, as mentioned above, has both a direct analgesic effect for relieving chest pain and an indirect analgesic effect by improving cardiac function. By reducing preload and afterload, there are an improvement in oxygen transport and a balancing of myocardial oxygen supply and demand.

   8. The fourth and last principle in treating cardiac pain is to **optimize ventricular function.** The use of **nitrates** and **inotropic agents,** such as **dobutamine** (Dobutrex) and **amrinone** (Inocor), increases contractility and reduces preload and afterload. In both refractory angina and transmural infarction, the insertion of the **intra-aortic counterpulsation balloon** (IACB) commonly will bring immediate relief of chest pain. The IACB empties during systole, creating a mechanical afterload reduction, and inflates during diastole to push oxygenated blood back up the aorta and to facilitate diastolic coronary blood flow. The major physiologic cardiac improvement appears to be afterload reduction, which reduces the stress on the heart, lowers cardiac oxygen consumption, and relieves chest pain.

C. Pericarditis

   1. Anatomy of the pericardium
      a. The heart and the beginning of the great vessels are surrounded by a fibroserous sac known as the pericardium.
      b. The outer layer is very thick and strong and provides a protective covering over the heart. The phrenic nerves run on the surface of this fibrous layer.

c. The inner layer of the pericardium is thin and serous and wraps around to cover the epicardium of the heart. The serous membrane on the inside of the fibrous sac is the visceral layer. The thin layer on the surface of the heart is the parietal portion of the pericardium.

d. The space between the visceral and the parietal layers of the pericardium is the pericardial cavity. The two serous membranes create a fluid to lubricate the movement of these two layers on each other. When the heart contracts, the visceral and parietal layers of pericardium slide on each other without friction or additional work to the heart.

e. The pericardium is attached to the diaphragm and sheath of the inferior vena cava inferiorly; to the esophagus, aorta, and four pulmonary veins posteriorly; to the great vessels superiorly; to the pleura of the right and left lung laterally; and to the sternum anteriorly.

f. It receives sensory **innervation from the phrenic and intercostal nerves** and autonomic innervation to its blood vessels from the esophageal plexus. There may also be innervation from the vagus nerve, cardiac plexus, and stellate ganglia.

2. **Etiologies for the pain of pericarditis**

a. The visceral and parietal pericardia, particularly on the upper part of the heart, are insensitive to pain. The lower parietal pericardium may originate painful stimuli with severe inflammation.

b. **Noninfectious pericarditis,** as associated with uremia, usually is not painful. **Infectious pericarditis,** as from a viral infection, causes marked inflammation and a pleuritic type of pain. Afferent fibers for this pain run through the phrenic nerve, and enter the spinal cord at the levels of the third to fifth cervical nerves. As a result, pain from inflammation of the lower parietal pericardium is referred to the tip of the shoulder, trapezius ridge, and neck.

c. Infectious pericarditis often spreads laterally and involves the attached pleural surfaces. This area is innervated by the sixth to the ninth thoracic intercostal nerves. The pain of pericarditis from this area is referred to the anterior chest and upper abdomen, and from time to time to the back in the same thoracic dermatome region.

d. The **most common pain** of pericarditis is **pleuritic** in nature or related to respiratory movements and markedly aggravated by cough or deep inspiration. This pain can be provoked by swallowing, since the esophagus is behind the heart. A change in bodily position will also worsen the pain. This pain is sharp and referred to the neck or flank. It is not relieved by nitroglycerin and lasts much longer than the pain of angina pectoris. This type of pain is classic for the combined pleural and pericardial inflammation of an infectious etiology.

e. A **second form of pericarditis pain is steady and severe,** often described as **crushing** and is very difficult to distinguish from the pain of myocardial infarction. Inflammation of afferent nerves on the surface of the heart in the parietal pericardium may be responsible for this pain.

f. The **last type of pericardial pain** is the least common, and is **associated with each beat of the heart.** It is usually perceived at the left border of the heart and the left shoulder.

g. A **diagnosis of pericarditis** is made by a combination of a careful history; auscultation of the chest, listening for a friction rub; and echo analysis of the heart, looking for pericardial fluid.

h. The **treatment** of pericarditis and efforts to improve the pain should be directed at the underlying etiology. **Aspirin, indomethacin** (Indocin, 25 to 75 mg four times a day), intramuscular (IM) or IV **ketorolac** (Toradol, 30 to 60 or 10 to 30 mg per dose, respectively, up to four times per day), or **prednisone** may be helpful for pain relief while the underlying etiology is being addressed.

i. For the ICU patient, the use of the new NSAID ketorolac given IV may be quite helpful for pain management. If the patient has renal insufficiency, the dosing interval should be lengthened to minimize accumulation of the drug and to decrease the risk of gastric ulceration.

D. Other Thoracic Processes Causing Chest Pain

1. Pulmonary embolus is known to cause chest pain. A massive pulmonary embolus can cause substernal chest pain similar to that of myocardial infarction. A less substantial embolus can cause a pleuritic type of chest pain that is more lateral in location. **Systemic narcotic** administration may be helpful with pain management, but attention must be directed to the primary disease, considering thrombolysis to dissolve the clot in the pulmonary artery and heparin to limit the formation of further clots in the venous circulation. Ketorolac may also be an effective adjunct acutely, but probably is not desirable after systemic anticoagulation has been established.

2. Endocarditis of a bacterial nature can be quite destructive to the heart without being painful. Some peripheral embolization to the extremities may cause pain of a vascular nature, but the heart is largely spared any pain process.

3. Tietze's syndrome is characterized by pain in the anterior chest wall due to **costochondritis.** The chest wall is usually painful upon palpation, and there are several areas in the costochondral or chondrosternal articulations that are very tender. This pain is frequently sharp and neuritic or darting in nature, lasting only a few seconds. There can also be a chronic aching type of chest pain, as well as a sense of chest tightness if there is associated muscle spasm. For the acute form, oral analgesics will usually be helpful. There is a chronic form associated with arthritis of the spine that can be more difficult to manage. A combination of antiinflammatory therapy and analgesic therapy will usually control the pain.

4. Postcardiac-injury syndrome causes chest pain and occurs after some form of injury to the myocardium. This syndrome is seen after traumatic myocardial injury of a penetrating or blunt nature; after cardiac surgery, when it is known as **postpericardiotomy** or **postcommissurotomy syndrome;** and after a myocardial infarction, when it is known as **Dressler's syndrome.** Symptoms commonly begin 2 weeks after injury, and are associated with pericarditis, pleuritis, and fever. This is a form of fibrinous pericarditis that responds to steroids and analgesics. The clinical dilemma is to distinguish this clinical entity from refractory angina or myocardial infarction.

   5. Acute blunt trauma to the chest can cause muscle injury and low cardiac output syndrome from myocardial contusion. In the absence of inflammation or pericarditis, there is no cardiac pain associated with this injury. Chest pain from myocardial contusion is associated with injury of the anterior chest wall. Analgesic agents, intercostal nerve blocks, or a thoracic epidural with a narcotic with or without a low-dose local anesthetic (e.g., bupivacaine, 0.0625 to 0.125%) administration will control pain. See Chapter 24 for a detailed discussion.

E. Pain After Thoracic Surgery

   1. Pain after **thoracotomy** for lung surgery can be intense and is known to markedly limit pulmonary function. Intercostal nerve blocks performed inside the chest may be initially helpful. Epidural narcotics with or without low-dose local anesthetics through a thoracic epidural catheter can provide a very high quality of pain relief and allow for much more normal postoperative lung function. Other alternatives include patient-controlled analgesic (PCA) (Chapter 13) or a pleural catheter with local anesthetic installation (e.g., 0.25% bupivacaine, 20 mL every 4 to 6 h). NSAIDs may supplement narcotic-mediated analgesia and decrease the total dose of narcotic required (thus with fewer side effects). TENS can be applied paraspinously or paraincisionally as an additional adjunct (see Chapter 25).

   2. Sternotomy for cardiac surgery is associated with much less pain. Patients commonly complain more of pain from pleural chest tubes and mediastinal drainage tubes than from the actual incision. Narcotics by IV bolus or continuous infusion provide excellent pain relief that normally permits extubation within 24 to 36 h after cardiac surgery. Ketorolac (10 to 30 mg IV every 6 to 8 h) may be very beneficial in the management of chest tube–induced pleuritic pain.

F. Vascular Pain

   1. Acute vascular occlusion, common in the lower extremities, can cause ischemic pain. This is best managed by correcting the underlying problem. An arteriogram is helpful diagnostically. This can be followed by thrombectomy, intra-arterial thrombolytic therapy and heparin, or vascular surgery. Reperfusion usually relieves the extremity pain, but IV narcotics are helpful in controlling pain. Pharmacologic sympathectomy, by the use of epidural local anesthetics or lumbar sympathectomy, can control pain and lead to some therapeutic vasodilatation.

2. Chronic extremity hypoperfusion or ischemia leads to chronic pain. Narcotics in this setting may not be very helpful, particularly for long-term treatment. As in the case of acute vascular occlusion pain, surgical or pharmacologic sympathectomy may reduce pain and improve blood flow.

3. Reimplantation of an extremity or part of an extremity can lead to vascular or ischemic pain. In the case of an upper extremity, an axillary or supraclavicular block may be helpful. The use of local anesthetics in this setting will provide sensory blockade for pain relief, as well as sympathectomy and vasodilatation for improved blood flow. A continuous brachial plexus block with a catheter could be considered if there is a good response to the injection of local anesthetics. In the case of the lower extremities, a continuous epidural or the spinal administration of local anesthetics and narcotics could be very helpful. Vasospasm is a common part of the clinical picture of reimplantation surgery, and the use of local anesthetics may be quite helpful in reducing vasospasm and improving blood flow.

IV. IMPACT OF PREEXISTING CARDIAC DISEASE ON PAIN MANAGEMENT IN THE CRITICALLY ILL PATIENT

A. Physiology of Cardiac Disease

1. Ischemic heart disease with myocardial infarction leads to poorly functioning cardiac muscle. As noted, one of the main tasks of the cardiovascular system is to deliver oxygenated blood to the cells that make up the tissues and organs of the body. This permits aerobic metabolism and the efficient production of high-energy phosphates. In the absence of adequate oxygen delivery, many cells switch to anaerobic metabolism, producing lactate and metabolic acidosis. The loss of cardiac muscle from ischemia and infarction reduces cardiac output and ejection fraction. There may be a compensatory vasoconstriction to maintain blood pressure and little ability to increase cardiac output in the face of vasodilatation.

2. Valvular heart disease, most commonly of an aortic or mitral nature, will create limitations of cardiac output, peripheral perfusion, and oxygen transport. **Aortic stenosis** chronically leads to hypertrophied muscle that is very demanding of an oxygen supply via the coronary arteries. Because of the obstruction at the aortic valve, there is a limitation on cardiac output. Agents that cause a reduction in systemic vascular resistance, as seen with some narcotics, can provoke uncompensated hypotension, since cardiac output is unable to increase to maintain blood pressure. On the other hand, narcotics and afterload reducing agents may be helpful in the presence of

aortic insufficiency, while untreated pain and sympathetic stimulation will increase afterload and subsequently, regurgitant flow. Mitral valve disease with **mitral stenosis** or **mitral regurgitation** can create an unstable picture in which patients are sensitive to analgesic agents. A patient with mitral stenosis will have a limited ability to move blood from the left atrium across a restricted mitral valve into the left ventricle.

B. Effects of Analgesic and Sedative Medications on Patients with Cardiovascular Disease

   1. Narcotics may have a quite variable effect on the patient with cardiac disease, depending on the degree of cardiac or vascular stimulation or depression of the drug. Notably, narcotics may release histamine and cause vasodilatation and hypotension, particularly if the patient has a limited cardiac output as a result of ischemic or valvular disease.

   a. Morphine has no direct effect on cardiac muscle, and has a long history of safe use in critically ill patients. Morphine does cause histamine release and hypotension, particularly in the hypovolemic patient, the patient with limited cardiac reserves, or the upright patient. This is most prominent when the drug is given as an IV bolus. Fluid administration to compensate for the vasodilatation and the continuous infusion of narcotics to maintain a stable blood level are well tolerated by critically ill patients.

   b. Meperidine (Demerol) has seen little use in the modern ICU, particularly in patients with cardiac disease. This agent causes direct myocardial depression and tachycardia. The increase in heart rate decreases diastolic time and reduces coronary blood flow, which may be poorly tolerated by patients with coronary artery disease. Meperidine has no advantage for critically ill patients, particularly those with ischemic or valvular heart disease.

   c. Fentanyl (Sublimaze) is a short-acting synthetic narcotic with essentially no histamine release and, as a result, little or no hypotension, particularly in the supine patient with an adequate vascular volume. It tends to decrease heart rate and has no myocardial depression. In critical care, fentanyl is best given by continuous infusion at rates of 50 to 250 μg/h and titrated to analgesic effect to maintain a steady blood level. The short duration of action limits the value of bolus IV fentanyl administration in critical care.

   d. Alfentanil (Alfenta) and **sufentanil** (Sufenta), also synthetic narcotics with which there has been vast experience in the operating room, have had little or no use in critical care. Fentanyl is an inexpensive and very effective narcotic that has not been replaced by these newer agents.

   e. Narcotic antagonists such as **naloxone** (Narcan) have some value in critical care when there has been excessive administration of a narcotic agent. Naloxone often leads to sympathetic stimulation with hypertension and tachycardia which may be quite detrimental to the patient with cardiac disease. The use of narcotic antagonists in critical care should be quite limited, with a constant concern for the complications of sympathetic stimulation. The severity of sympathetic response can be limited by titrating small, frequent doses of naloxone (e.g., 40 μg IV every 2 min) until the desired effect has been achieved. Many critically ill patients receive significant narcotic doses. Tolerance and physical dependence can develop within days. The administration of narcotic antagonists (or agonist–antagonists) can precipitate **withdrawal.**

2. **Sedatives** can be quite valuable in critical care for patients with cardiac disease who are experiencing pain. The central nervous system, as noted above, has a modulating effect on the perception of pain. Admission to the ICU can cause anxiety and increase the perception of pain. Benzodiazepines are the most commonly used sedatives in critical care. They have few detrimental effects on the cardiovascular system, and can be given IV without hypotension or a decrease in cardiac output.

   a. **Diazepam** (Valium) has the longest history of use in critical care. It cannot be diluted and given as a continuous infusion. It is painful to inject and should be given as a bolus through a central venous catheter. There are active metabolites of diazepam and a prolonged action when drug elimination is compromised, particularly in elderly patients. Despite the fact that it is inexpensive, the use of diazepam in the ICU is declining.

   b. **Midazolam** (Versed) has become much more popular than diazepam. It is safely used in patients with cardiac disease. Because of its short duration of action, it is best administered in the ICU as a continuous infusion, usually at a rate of 1 to 5 mg/h. Midazolam can be diluted for IV administration and is not painful to inject. Midazolam does not have problems with prolonged duration of action or elimination. Midazolam and fentanyl, both given as continuous infusions, are common in critical care for patients with pain and anxiety.

   c. **Lorazepam** (Ativan) is somewhat more potent than midazolam, with 1 mg equivalent to 3 to 6 mg of midazolam. It can be diluted in IV fluid and likewise given as a continuous infusion. The absence of active metabolites and a small volume of distribution make this a short-acting sedative when used as a continuous IV infusion in the ICU. It has little cardiovascular effect, particularly as a continuous infusion. The drug is well tolerated by patients with preexisting cardiac disease.

   d. Other sedatives, such as **barbiturates** and **phenothiazines,** are seldom used in the ICU. The **butyrophenones, haloperidol** (Haldol) and **droperidol** (Inapsine), are of some value in critical care. Haloperidol is a valuable sedative for patients with a psychotic level of agitation. This agent has some alpha-blocking properties, as do the **phenothiazines,** and can lead to hypotension, particularly in patients with depletion of the intravascular volume.

3. The **IV general anesthetics** as yet have seen little use in the ICU. **Ketamine** (Ketalar), the oldest, causes hypertension and tachycardia, which could be quite harmful for patients with cardiac disease. Hypovolemic and hypotensive trauma patients may benefit from ketamine, but patients with ischemic heart disease are likely to develop acute myocardial ischemia from the hypertension and tachycardia the agent produces. The analgesic properties of ketamine are quite good when used for patients with traumatic injuries.

Propofol (Diprivan) is a new short-acting IV general anesthetic that sometimes is used in critical care for deep sedation. This agent is a potent vasodilator with some myocardial depression, and would not be recommended for patients with moderate to severe ischemic or valvular heart disease. The agent works well for patients in sympathetic storm (delirium tremens) who have substantial cardiac reserves. (See Chapter 9 for a detailed discussion.)

4. **Neuromuscular blocking agents** are receiving more use in the ICU because of new forms of ventilation, such as pressure control and inverse ratio ventilation. Intensivists are concerned about the trauma of large tidal volumes to the lung of the respiratory failure patient. Agents such as **curare** that cause histamine release would be detrimental to the patient with cardiac disease because of hypotension. **Pancuronium** (Pavulon) does the opposite, leading to hypertension and tachycardia, which may cause ischemia in patients with coronary artery disease. **Vecuronium** (Norcuron) is neutral in the cardiovascular system, and has become the most common muscle relaxant used in critical care. Repeated doses or an infusion of vecuronium can lead to prolonged neuromuscular blockade.

5. **Local anesthetics** are used in two forms in the ICU. First, they are used IV to control cardiac rhythm disturbances. Second, they are used for analgesia, as in peripheral nerve blocks, spinal and epidural blocks, or IV for analgesia of the airway before suctioning. They provide good pain relief when used for conduction anesthesia, but the sympathectomy resulting from spinal or epidural local anesthetics can lead to wide fluctuations in blood pressure. For that reason, epidural narcotics are much more popular for pain relief in the ICU. The clinician must be constantly aware of the dose of local anesthetic being given to avoid toxicity, which will lead to seizures, a most detrimental complication for the patient with cardiac disease. Local anesthetics should usually be given without epinephrine to ICU patients with cardiac disease to avoid hypertension and tachycardia.

C. Routes of Administration of Analgesic and Sedative Medications in Critical Care

1. The **enteral administration** of analgesic and sedative agents is very rare in critical care. The oral route is particularly rare. The enteral route via

a nasogastric tube or nasoduodenal tube would be somewhat more common. There is a growing emphasis in critical care on the use of early nasoduodenal feedings and a decline in the use of total parenteral nutrition. In ICU patients with a functioning gastrointestinal tract on enteral nutrition, the nasoduodenal tube is an excellent route of administration for sedative agents such as diazepam, which is formulated as an elixir. There has been little experience with administering analgesic agents by this route.

2. The **IM route** is another uncommon route of administration of analgesics and sedatives in critical care. Both narcotics such as morphine and meperidine and sedatives such as midazolam are frequently administered by the IM route in the general hospital setting, but not in the ICU. Cardiac patients with alterations in cardiac output and peripheral perfusion have a very unpredictable absorption of and response to IM medications.

3. **Parenteral delivery** of analgesic and sedative drugs is the preferred route in critical care because of the more reliable uptake and distribution and subsequent response to the dose.

    a. **Bolus administration** of IV agents provides a rapid onset, but in the case of sedatives and analgesics, may lead to substantial fluctuations in blood pressure. This route may also lead to a variable quality of analgesia. Post–bolus-injection high blood levels provide excellent analgesia, but trough levels prior to the next dose may lead to substantial pain.

    b. **Continuous IV administration** of analgesics and sedatives is much preferred to obtain a stable blood level. This blunts some of the hypotensive effects of bolus administration and provides a much more stable level of analgesia and sedation. Morphine infusions at 1 to 5 mg/h and fentanyl infusions at 50 to 250 μg/h titrated to analgesic effect by the bedside nurse promote a stable cardiovascular profile and excellent analgesia in ICU patients with pain and a history of cardiac disease. Sedation should be considered to reduce anxiety, using a continuous IV infusion of midazolam at 1 to 5 mg/h or lorazepam at 1 to 3 mg/h.

    c. The use of a **PCA** pump in more alert ICU patients is most effective for the delivery of IV narcotics to achieve high-quality pain relief. This is another form of bolus administration, but with the patient in control of dosing. Small doses are given at short intervals to maintain a steady blood level and simulate some of the effects of a continuous infusion. There is the elimination of painful intervals when low blood levels of analgesic lead to severe pain, as has been reported with nurse-administered bolus analgesic medication.

    d. **Peridural administration** of narcotics has been shown to provide excellent pain relief and to reduce the ICU length of stay, complications, and cost after major surgery in high-risk patients. **Morphine** (5 mg every 8 to 12 h) or **fentanyl** (2 to 5 μg/mL at 6 to 16 mL/h) delivered through an epidural catheter is an excellent analgesic prescription for patients with preexisting cardiac disease. This technique provides excellent cardiac stability, a low dose of analgesic, and superb pain relief. **Local anesthetics** can also be dosed through an epidural catheter in the ICU. The administration of local anesthetics in the high lumbar and lower thoracic areas leads to a sympathectomy, with the possibility of a widely fluctuating blood pressure. This effect is less marked when low doses and/or concentrations of local anesthetic are used. If there is an advantage of sympathectomy in improving lower extremity blood flow, this technique may be valuable in the ICU. Under usual circumstances, the peridural administration of narcotics is preferred to local anesthetics.

e. Other analgesic techniques in critical care may include the use of **pleural catheters** for delivery of local anesthetics or **sympathetic block,** such as stellate ganglia, celiac plexus, or lumbar block. These approaches are rare in critical care, but may have some advantages for patients with cardiovascular disease who have special pain problems, such as pancreatic pain or upper/lower extremity ischemic pain (see Chapter 13).

CASE DISCUSSION

Mr. M. is in congestive heart failure and pulmonary edema, most likely resulting from the catecholamine release and hypertension/tachycardia of inadequate postoperative analgesia and exacerbated by perioperative fluid shifts. His blood pressure of 160/96 and heart rate of 120 are elevating myocardial oxygen demand. In this patient with a history of coronary artery disease and previous inferior-wall myocardial infarction, there is a limit on coronary artery oxygen transport. When demand exceeds supply, ischemia occurs. The left ventricle becomes stiff when ischemic, and leads to an elevated left ventricular end diastolic pressure, pulmonary capillary wedge pressure, and pulmonary edema. On day 3 postoperatively, it is likely that Mr. M. was mobilizing fluid, leading to intravascular fluid overload and further increasing myocardial oxygen consumption.

Postoperative pain management with the epidural administration of narcotics with or without a low-dose local anesthetic would have improved his pain control and decreased the sympathetic response, perhaps preventing the development of myocardial ischemia. At the present time, the patient needs oxygen first, and then IV morphine and nitrates to correct the pulmonary edema. A single dose of IV furosemide may help to reduce pulmonary capillary pressure and to improve pulmonary edema. An agent with beta-blocking properties, such as labetalol, could be used to control the blood pressure and heart rate, if the first-line agents fail to control the situation, but may worsen pulmonary edema through myocardial depression. If the pulmonary edema and chest pain are not readily improved with the above therapies, endotracheal intubation and controlled ventilation would increase oxygenation, decrease myocardial work, and allow more generous administration of morphine. At this point, morphine by continuous infusion would be most appropriate to maximize sedation and minimize metabolic rate with the least hemodynamic fluctuation.

SUGGESTED READINGS

Cote P, Gueret P, Brersassa M: Effects of diazepam in patients with normal and diseased coronary arteries. *Circulation* 50:1210–1216, 1974.
Crafts RC: *A Textbook of Human Anatomy.* New York, Ronold Press Cy, 1966, pp 143–158.

Dajezam E, Gorden A, et al: Long term post thoracotomy pain. *Chest* 99:270–274, 1991.

Droste C, Roskamn H: Pain mechanisms in symptomatic and silent ischemia. *Israeli J Med Sci* 25:287–492, 1989.

Faerman I, Faccio F, et al: Autonomic neuropathy and painless myocardial infarction in diabetic patients. Histologic evidence of their relationship. *Diabetes* 26:1947–1958, 1977.

Guzman F, Braun C, Lim RKS: Visceral pain and the pseudoafferent response: intraarterial injection of bradykinin and other analgesic agents. *Arch Int Pharm* 136:353, 1962.

Lewis T, Kellgrer JH: Observations related to referred pain in viscero-motor reflexes and other phenomena. *Clin Sci* 44:47–71, 1939.

Malliani A: The elusive link between transient myocardial ischemia and pain. *Circulation* 73:201–204, 1986.

Michalelis L, Hickes P, Clark T, et al: Ventricular irritability associated with the use of naloxone hydrochloride. *Ann Thorac Surg* 186:608–614, 1974.

Tuman KJ, McCarthy RJ, March RJ, et al: Effects of epidural anesthesia and analgesia on coagulation and outcome after major vascular surgery. *Anesth Analg* 73:696–704, 1991.

Wilson JD, Braunwald E, Isselbacher KJ, et atl: *Harrison's Principles of Internal Medicine.* New York, McGraw-Hill, 1991, pp 93–105, 938–970, 980–987.

Yeager MP, Glass D, Neff RK, et al: Epidural anesthesia and analgesia in high-risk surgical patients. *Anesthesiology* 729–736, 1987.

CHAPTER
18

RESPIRATORY DISEASE

Richard B. Becker

Case
  I. Pathophysiology of Respiratory Failure
    A. Etiology
    B. Gas Exchange
    C. Pulmonary Mechanics
  II. Pathophysiology of the Adult Respiratory Distress Syndrome
    A. Etiology
    B. Physiologic Effects
  III. Pain and Respiratory Failure
    A. Pathophysiology of Pain in Respiratory Failure
    B. Painful Pulmonary Disorders
    C. Effects of Pain on Lung Function
  IV. Pain from Therapy of Respiratory Failure
    A. Types of Pain
  V. Analgesia in the Management of Respiratory Failure
    A. Analgesic Therapy
    B. Nonanalgesic Therapy
  VI. Routes of Anesthesia and Analgesia in Respiratory Failure
    A. Intravenous Route
    B. Epidural/Intrathecal Opioid Analgesia
Case Discussion
Suggested Readings

CASE

    A 60-year-old male with a history of chronic obstructive pulmonary disease (COPD) develops the adult respiratory distress syndrome (ARDS) after sustaining multiple rib fractures, a pulmonary contusion, and an unstable pelvic fracture due to a motor vehicle accident. He is in the intensive care unit (ICU) following a splenectomy and massive blood loss. He is intubated, is on a ventilator, and requires sedation and pain control.

I. PATHOPHYSIOLOGY OF RESPIRATORY FAILURE

A. Etiology

The state of respiratory failure occurs when there is insufficient oxygenation or ventilation to maintain cellular homeostasis. Pathologic processes affect either pulmonary mechanics (compliance) or gas exchange, and result in arterial blood gas values that meet established criteria for acute respiratory failure.

1. The addition of such **clinical findings** as a respiratory rate of less than 6/min or greater than 30/min, cyanosis, and discoordinate movements of the thorax and abdomen (so-called paradoxical respiration) is useful when the presence of respiratory failure is suspected, but the diagnosis rests on arterial blood gas analysis.

2. A **Pa_{O_2}** less than the normal age-predicted value for a given patient or a **Pa_{CO_2}** greater than 50 mmHg constitutes respiratory failure in the acute setting. These numbers do not hold true for the patient with preexisting, but physiologically compensated, pulmonary disease; the presence of an acute respiratory acidosis as demonstrated by a **pH** of less than 7.35 will alert the physician to the presence of an acute or chronic state of respiratory failure. Table 18-1 lists pathophysiologic causes of respiratory failure.

Table 18-1 Etiology of respiratory failure

Primary pulmonary disorders	Extrapulmonary disorders

Pneumonia
  Infectious
  Aspiration
Atelectasis/secretions
	Central nervous system
	  Respiratory center depression
	
	Peripheral nervous system
	  Quadriplegia, Guillain-Barré

ARDS	Respiratory muscle weakness Atrophy, myasthenia gravis
Asthma/bronchospasm	Chest wall restriction Incisional pain, obesity, kyphoscoliosis

Pulmonary edema
  Cardiogenic
  Noncardiogenic
	Pleuritic disease

Pulmonary embolism
  Blood
  Fat
  Amniotic fluid
	Upper airway obstruction
	  Epiglottitis, tracheal obstruction/foreign bodies

B. Gas Exchange

Respiratory failure on the basis of abnormalities of the lung parenchyma that cause problems in gas exchange results in hypoxia, hypercarbia, or both. An ideal match of alveolar ventilation and pulmonary capillary perfusion results in the most efficient lung function. Any mismatch of ventilation and perfusion (V/Q) may result in hypoxia, hypercarbia, and, if severe, respiratory failure. Usually, however, such mismatching is readily corrected with supplemental oxygen therapy. Pulmonary edema and COPD are common causes of V/Q mismatch. There are two extremes of V/Q mismatch.

   1. Shunt occurs when mixed venous blood enters the systemic circulation after bypassing exposure to alveolar gas. Atelectasis, pneumothorax, and lobar pneumonia are all examples of shunt, and, unlike V/Q mismatch, are usually refractory to supplemental oxygen therapy.

   2. Dead space consists of those portions of the lung unit that are ventilated but not perfused. It has two main components.

   a. **Anatomic dead space** is composed of the volume of the gas-conducting passages that do not participate in gas exchange, and, while fairly constant, can be influenced by many factors, including the age, size, and posture of the subject; the position of the neck and jaw; lung volume; endotracheal intubation or tracheostomy; hypoventilation; drugs; and temperature (Table 18-2).

   b. The **alveolar dead space** represents that part of the inspired gas at the alveolar level which does not participate in gas exchange. Upright position, air or pulmonary embolism, COPD with destruction of alveolar septa and contained vessels, hyperinflation of the lung, hypovolemia, and other sources of pulmonary arterial obstruction all result in an increased alveolar dead space.

   c. The total of anatomic and alveolar dead space results in **physiologic dead space,** which, in simple terms, is that part of the tidal volume that does not participate in gas exchange.

   d. The ratio of **dead space to tidal volume (V_D/V_T)** remains relatively constant at various tidal volumes and simplifies calculations of alveolar ven-

Table 18-2 Factors influencing anatomic dead space

Increased dead space	Decreased dead space
Old age	Youth
Obesity	Thin body habitus
Sitting position	Supine position
Neck extension, jaw protrusion	Neck flexion, chin depressed
High lung volumes at end inspiration	Endotracheal intubation, tracheostomy
Atropine, trimethaphan	Pneumonectomy
Hypothermia	Hypoventilation (small tidal volumes)

tilation from minute volume. A normal physiologic dead space is approximately 2 mL/kg body weight, which results in a V_D/V_T of about 0.3. Values exceeding this may result in hypercarbia and respiratory failure. A V_D/V_T greater than 0.6 is usually inconsistent with the ability to maintain spontaneous ventilation, or with weaning of the ventilated patient.

3. **Diffusion abnormalities** result from a thickened alveolar-capillary membrane, but due to the relatively rapid diffusion of oxygen and carbon dioxide, decreased diffusion is rarely a cause of hypoxemia or hypercarbia.

4. The **minute ventilation** of the lung is that volume of gas entering the lung each minute and depends grossly on respiratory rate and tidal volume. The volume that is available for gas exchange is the **alveolar ventilation,** or the total ventilation less the physiologic dead space. When the alveolar ventilation is abnormally low, the P_{AO_2} falls and the $PaCO_2$ rises to produce the state of hypoventilation. The relationship between the fall in P_{AO_2} and the rise in $PaCO_2$ is predicted by the **alveolar gas equation:**

$$P_{AO_2} = (P_B - P_{H_2O})F_{IO_2} - Pa_{CO_2}/RQ + f$$

where P_{AO_2} = alveolar oxygen tension
P_B = barometric pressure
P_{H_2O} = water vapor pressure = (3 to 6)
F_{IO_2} = the inspired fraction of oxygen
Pa_{CO_2} = the arterial concentration of carbon dioxide
R = the respiratory quotient or the carbon dioxide production/oxygen consumption
f = a small correction factor

C. Pulmonary Mechanics

Disorders of pulmonary mechanics, the forces that move the lung and chest wall and the resistances they overcome, are important factors in the pathophysiology of respiratory failure.

1. The slope of the pressure–volume curve of the lung, the so-called **compliance curve,** changes with various disease states, and reflects the increase or decrease in the work of breathing. The normal lung is extremely compliant, requiring only minimal pressures (-2 to -10 cmH$_2$O) for adequate expansion during ventilation. Atelectasis, fibrosis, and edema all create a stiffer lung that requires more force to expand to a given volume and, therefore, has decreased compliance. Processes such as aging and emphysema, which represent a loss of elastic lung tissue, decrease the force required for lung inflation, and thus increase the compliance of the lung.

2. Aside from the compliance of the lung parenchyma itself, **chest wall compliance** plays an important role in determining the net compliance of the lung. At a volume that is approximately 75 percent of the vital capacity, the chest wall rests in equilibrium with atmospheric pressure—a reminder of the chest wall's natural tendency to expand in opposition to the lung

parenchyma. Disease processes such as rib fractures, tight bandages, obesity, and splinting from chest and upper abdominal incisions all limit the ability of the chest wall to expand, decrease the total compliance of the lung, and ultimately increase the work of breathing. This sets the stage for respiratory failure.

   3. The **surface tension of the lung,** or the force at the alveolar air–fluid interface, is another factor that, when altered, affects pulmonary compliance. Cells lining the alveoli secrete **surfactant,** a complex phospholipid that acts to decrease surface tension at the alveolar level and thereby increases overall lung compliance. The absence of surfactant results in the respiratory distress syndrome, which is discussed in more detail later in this chapter.

   4. The balance between **airway resistance** and pulmonary compliance is what ultimately determines the overall **work of breathing.** Airway resistance peaks at the level of the medium-sized segmental bronchi (fourth generation) and drops off to a nadir in the terminal bronchioles (16th generation). This paradoxical pattern of resistance, low in the smaller airways and high in the larger airways, is best explained by cross-sectional areas, which remain largest at the level of the terminal bronchioles. Resistance in all conducting airways is subject to several factors: dynamic compression of airways by intrathoracic pressure, high or low lung volumes, bronchial smooth muscle contraction, and the density and viscosity of the inspired gas (least important clinically)—all of which increase airway resistance. Pneumothorax, bronchospasm, COPD, and mucous plugging of airways all increase airway resistance, as well as the work of breathing, and thus predispose to respiratory failure.

   5. The work of breathing is accomplished by the **muscles of respiration.**

      a. Of these, the **diaphragm** is the most important, moving about 1 cm with normal tidal breathing and up to 10 cm with forced breathing efforts. Paradoxical or discoordinate movement of the diaphragm indicates paralysis or exhaustion of this muscle and impending respiratory failure.

      b. The **intercostal muscles** assist in inspiration (external intercostal muscles) and active expiration (internal intercostal muscles), and paralysis does not greatly affect breathing unless the diaphragm is failing.

      c. The **accessory muscles** of inspiration include the scalene muscles and sternocleidomastoid muscles, which raise the first two ribs and the sternum. Normally inactive during quiet breathing, these muscles become important and clinically noticeable during exercise or in situations of increased work of breathing.

      d. **Expiration** during quiet breathing is passive, with the elastic lung parenchyma returning to its functional residual capacity without further energy expenditure. Exercise, or forced expiration, as in obstructive lung disease, requires muscle activity and the abdominal wall musculature to act in concert with the diaphragm to produce a forced expiration. Failure of these muscles presents as paradoxical or discoordinate movements of the abdominal wall during respiration.

   6. The body's ability to compensate for the detrimental effects of diseases that cause respiratory dysfunction ultimately depends on the central and peripheral **control of respiratory drive.**

      a. Centrally, three main groups of neurons act to establish an appropriate respiratory pattern. The **medullary, apneustic, and pneumotaxic centers** in the medulla and lower and upper pons, respectively, receive multiple inputs to produce involuntary respirations. The **cortex** can override this to some extent. The most important stimulus to the central control of breathing, however, is the **cerebrospinal fluid (CSF) pH,** which is inversely proportional to the $Paco_2$. A fall in the CSF pH results in an increased minute ventilation. The ventilatory response to carbon dioxide is reduced, however, if the work of breathing is increased.

      b. Peripheral chemoreceptors are the most sensitive mechanisms to increase ventilation in response to hypoxemia. The **carotid bodies** located at the bifurcation of the carotid arteries and the less important **aortic bodies** in the aortic arch begin their response to hypoxia at a Pao_2 of less than 100 mmHg and fire rapidly in response to a Pao_2 of less than 60 mmHg. These peripheral receptors are much less sensitive to changes in pH and $Paco_2$ than are the central receptors.

      c. The combined central and peripheral controllers or respiratory drive in concert with pulmonary mechanics produce respiratory patterns common to various pathophysiologic states.

II. PATHOPHYSIOLOGY OF THE ADULT RESPIRATORY DISTRESS SYNDROME

Our understanding of ARDS has evolved over the past 25 years, since it was first recognized as a clinical and pathophysiologic entity. The contemporary definition is based on four criteria: evidence of pulmonary edema on CXR, exclusion of heart failure as a cause of pulmonary edema, hypoxemia requiring high levels of inspired oxygen and/or positive end-expiratory pressure (PEEP) to maintain adequate Pao_2, and reduced lung compliance.

A. Etiology

As a syndrome, there are multiple inciting factors in ARDS, but the resultant lung damage is clinically, and even histologically, the same. Damage to the alveolar-capillary unit with subsequent deposition of water, solutes, and collagen results in heavy, noncompliant lungs and hypoxemia from increased venous admixture. Acute neutrophilic inflammation and the release of inflammatory cytokines are thought to be contributing factors, but the appearance of ARDS in neutropenic patients argues for the existence of neutrophil-independent pathways as the mechanism of injury. There are, most likely, several different pathways of lung injury that result in ARDS, starting with those that attack the lung endothelium (sepsis, trauma, pancreatitis) and including those that damage the alveolar epithelium (aspiration pneumonia, inhalation injury) or directly injure the pulmonary microvasculature (toxic oxygen). Table 18-3 lists risk factors associated with the development of ARDS.

B. Physiologic Effects

Pulmonary edema, hypoxemia, and multisystem organ failure (MSOF) or systemic inflammatory response syndrome (SIRS) are the three most significant clinical manifestations of ARDS.

1. Increased lung microvascular permeability, combined with a major **disruption in alveolar epithelium** or small airway permeability, while difficult to document, is the most likely cause of the lung edema in this disease process. Persistent areas of elevated **shunt** and **physiologic dead space,** combined with an **increasingly noncompliant lung,** perpetuate respiratory failure in ARDS.

2. Hypoxemia in ARDS results not just from the flooding of alveoli with edema fluid, but also from the continued perfusion of these liquid-filled alveoli, resulting in ventilation and perfusion mismatch. Inhibition of the normal defense mechanism of hypoxic pulmonary vasoconstriction by endogenous mediators such as prostacyclin and abnormalities in airway reactivity often result in severe hypoxemia in ARDS, the extent of which depends on the magnitude and duration of the initial lung insult.

3. The majority of patients who die of ARDS succumb to **MSOF** and not to ARDS alone. In ARDS, MSOF is characterized by extrapulmonary

Table 18-3 Risk factors for ARDS

Shock	*Trauma*
Hemorrhagic	Long bone fractures
Septic	Pulmonary contusion
Cardiogenic	Burns
Anaphylactic	Near drowning
	Cardiopulmonary bypass
	Multiple transfusions
Infection	*Obstetric complications*
Bacterial, viral, fungal pneumonia	Eclampsia/severe preeclampsia
Gram-negative sepsis	Air or amniotic fluid embolism
	Endometritis
Inhalation injury	*Intravenous drug abuse*
Gastric aspiration	
Smoke or toxic gas inhalation	*Pancreatitis*
Oxygen toxicity	

organ dysfunction that includes a decline in mental status, renal insufficiency and failure, gastrointestinal (GI) hemorrhage, and liver failure, to name a few. Once MSOF is established, the mortality rate is high. It is likely that many of the mediators released during the initial pulmonary insult act at other tissue sites in addition to lung. This would explain the generalized permeability defect often seen in MSOF. Development of suprainfection in ARDS is not unusual, and, it is, in fact, these subgroups that develop sepsis and, ultimately, fatal ARDS with MSOF.

III. PAIN AND RESPIRATORY FAILURE

A. Pathophysiology of Pain in Respiratory Failure

The structures of the lung are richly innervated such that diseases of the tracheobronchial tree, the pulmonary circulation, the lung parenchyma, or the parietal pleura may be manifest as painful syndromes of the thorax. The absence of pain, however, does not necessarily indicate a disease-free respiratory system, as such diseases as ARDS and asthma result in pain more from therapeutic medical interventions than from the diseases themselves.

1. The **innervation of the pulmonary system** is complex and, while a detailed description is beyond the scope of this text, an overview of the primary sympathetic and parasympathetic innervations at various levels of the lung is given in Table 18-4.

2. The **nerve supply to vessels** within the lung varies in richness as follows: the small bronchial arteries $>$ pulmonary arteries $>>$ pulmonary veins. Pulmonary nerves and plexi contain both myelinated and unmyelin-

Table 18-4 Innervation of the tracheobronchial tree

	Structure			
System	Trachea	Main bronchi	Smaller bronchi—respiratory bronchioles	Alveolar ducts and sacs
Sympathetic	Stellate and T1- ganglia	Subepithelial and deep pulmonary plexi	Combined pulmonary plexus	Afferent from combined plexus
Parasympathetic	Superior laryngeal nerve, upper thoracic vagal rami	Subepithelial and deep pulmonary plexi	Combined pulmonary plexus	Afferent from combined plexus

ated fibers, which, in the pulmonary circulation, are involved in reflex vasoconstriction and vasodilation.

   3. **Nociceptive function** in the lung depends on two types of receptors: **type J receptors** of afferent nerves and **lung-irritant receptors** of A-delta afferents, all running in the **vagus nerves**. The J receptors are located within the pulmonary interstitium near the capillaries, whereas the lung-irritant receptors appear in the epithelial lining of the lung and its airways. Pain caused by mechanical distortion or mechanical and chemical damage to the lung is probably mediated by these A-delta fibers. **Sympathetic afferents** may contribute to the transmission of painful stimuli, but are mostly involved in the reflex control of the pulmonary circulation and the tracheobronchial tree. Nociceptive transmission from the tracheobronchial tree, however, occurs through afferent fibers of the ipsilateral vagus nerve.

   4. The **parietal pleura** is richly supplied by sensory fibers that relay nociceptive information via the specific nerves related to the region of the pleura involved (mediastinal and diaphragmatic pleura via the phrenic nerves, apical pleura via brachial plexus, chest wall pleura via intercostal nerves). The visceral pleura and the pulmonary parenchyma, while richly innervated, contain no nociceptive fibers. Disease processes affecting these structures become painful only when J or lung-irritant receptors are stimulated.

B. Painful Pulmonary Disorders

The disorders of the pulmonary system that result in pain via the above mechanisms are best divided into processes involving the tracheobronchial tree, the lung itself, the pulmonary circulation, or the parietal pleura.

   1. **Tracheobronchitis,** whether infectious or irritative in etiology, results in a mild to moderate soreness and irritability of the airway. Inhalation of steam from a vaporizer and the administration of nonsteroidal anti-inflammatory drugs (NSAIDs) are useful in pain management.

   2. **Bronchiectasis** is not often associated with pain. Those patients who develop pain with bronchiectasis often have associated osteoarthritis (so-called rheumatic bronchiectasis) and present with chest and upper limb pain, as well as cutaneous and deep hyperalgesia of these areas. This pain is usually managed with NSAIDs in moderate to high doses, with the addition of trigger point injections with local anesthetic should myofascial pain persist.

   3. **Pneumonia,** with its symptoms of cough, fever, chest pain, dyspnea, and sputum production, causes pain through several different pathways. Chest wall pain and hyperalgesia result from pneumonia that involves the peripheral lung tissues (i.e., lobar pneumonia), with **pleuritic pain** from inflammation of the pleura occurring early in the process. The exact location of chest pain secondary to an inflamed pleura depends on the area of the involved pleura. A diaphragmatic pleura, for example, may refer pain to

C3–C5 or T9–T11 dermatomes, whereas upper lobe pneumonia results in T2–T6 dermatomal involvement. Pain management involves NSAIDs as an initial therapy, with the addition of narcotics such as codeine or other potent narcotics as needed. Patient-controlled analgesia (PCA) is a highly effective means of delivering narcotics in doses that assure maximum patient comfort to allow necessary pulmonary toilet maneuvers to be carried out efficiently while minimizing the risk of excessive sedation and hypoventilation. Patients with severe pain that is not adequately relieved by systemic analgesics are candidates for intercostal block of the segments involved with pain using a long-acting local anesthetic, or, alternatively, for the placement of a catheter for continuous thoracic epidural analgesia (see Chapter 13).

4. **Lung abscesses,** usually the result of aspiration of infected material, result in chest pain from pleuritic involvement. Most patients have a moderate to severe dull, aching pain referred to the dermatome of the inflamed pleura that is involved. As in pneumonia, cutaneous and deep hyperalgesias are common, and the management of pain is as described for pneumonia.

5. **Uncomplicated ARDS** is not associated with pain, but suprainfection of the lung, MSOF, and iatrogenic supportive maneuvers during the course of ARDS are all associated with various types of pain, discussed elsewhere in this text.

6. **Pulmonary hypertension,** either acute or chronic, is a common cause of severe chest pain similar to that of acute myocardial infarction, but without radiation to the arms, jaw, or back. The **acute syndrome** is associated with severe, crushing chest pain and a sense of impending death, whereas those patients with **exacerbations of chronic pulmonary hypertension** have symptoms similar to those of exertional angina. Elimination of the causative factor, if possible, is the best treatment, but inhalation of high concentrations of oxygen, a potent vasodilator, is effective in treating the high pressure, and consequently the pain. Patients with pain from chronic pulmonary hypertension are managed quite easily using NSAIDs with or without codeine.

7. **Pulmonary embolism** usually arises from thrombi forming in the deep veins of the leg or pelvis, and commonly presents with the acute onset of chest pain, dyspnea, and tachypnea. The chest pain is usually pleuritic in nature and results from pulmonary infarction, which produces inflammation of the pleural surfaces. Pleuritic pain, however, is usually a late finding because of the time required for pulmonary infarction to occur. Patients with large pulmonary emboli experience severe retrosternal crushing pain that does not radiate. This results from a sudden distension of the pulmonary artery and right ventricle, and may reflect some component of right ventricular ischemia. While pain management is secondary to therapy of the acute event with oxygen, heparin, and circulatory support, if necessary, morphine or other potent narcotics should be titrated parenterally to the relief of pain. If repeated doses are required, PCA is a viable option for coop-

erating patients. Those patients unable to gain relief from reasonable doses of narcotics may require ipsilateral stellate ganglion block with bupivacaine; this will provide relief for up to 6 to 10 hs. Pleuritic pain is usually treated with NSAIDs and a potent narcotic administered orally or parenterally, but intercostal nerve blocks with bupivacaine may also be useful in patients with persistent pain.

   8. **Pleuritis** can occur with many different underlying pulmonary diseases, as discussed above. Pleural pain in the absence of physical or radiologic (CXR) findings or a known underlying disease suggests early malignancy, bacterial infection (empyema) or viral infection of the pleura (epidemic pleurodynia), or a connective tissue disorder. Pain management is as described above, progressing from NSAIDs and oral/parenteral narcotics to intercostal nerve blocks, and, if necessary, thoracic epidural analgesia.

   9. **Pneumothorax,** either complete or partial, presents with an acute onset of pleuritic chest pain, dyspnea, and tachypnea, although the severity of the symptoms is not necessarily indicative of the size of the pneumothorax. Management ranges from conservative observation with serial CXR to more aggressive tube thoracostomy. The conservative approach, from a pain management point of view, usually requires only oral analgesics, but a more aggressive approach that includes a chest tube may require parenteral narcotics or intercostal nerve blocks. The use of NSAIDs is very effective in managing the irritation and pain associated with chest tubes.

C. Effects of Pain on Lung Function

Both somatic and visceral pain often result in altered lung function and significant pulmonary morbidity. Much of this pathophysiology has been learned from studying postoperative patients who, with thoracic or upper abdominal incisions, typically display a **restricted pattern of breathing**, with rapid, shallow breaths.

   1. **Splinting** results from incisional pain and reflex diaphragmatic dysfunction, and is characterized by a shift from the usual abdominal to compensatory rib cage breathing with the loss of the diaphragmatic contribution to tidal volume. Shallow breathing, the absence of spontaneous sighs, and mechanical disruption of the coordination of the thorax and abdomen for breathing all promote these postoperative changes in lung function that are not related to the reduction in lung volumes that occurs during anesthesia.

   2. **A progression from decreased compliance to decreased vital capacity (VC), and ultimately to decreased functional residual capacity (FRC),** results in a maximal reduction in FRC of 70 to 80 percent of the preoperative volume. If severe enough, clinically significant atelectasis, lobar collapse, pneumonia, and air trapping due to an increase in the ratio of closing capacity (CC) to FRC may result in hypoxic or hypercapnic respiratory failure.

3. **Restoration of lung function** normally begins 2 to 3 days postoperatively, with full function returning at 1 week or more after surgery.

4. Extrapolation of these postsurgical data to other disease processes in which pain produces splinting, shallow breathing, and an overall restrictive pattern of respiration yields similar pathophysiologic changes, in addition to changes specifically due to the underlying disease process.

IV. PAIN FROM THERAPY OF RESPIRATORY FAILURE

A. Types of Pain

Pain in the setting of respiratory failure in the ICU consists of several components: pain caused by the underlying pathology, pain that results from physical procedures such as endotracheal intubation or suctioning, and "pain" that is associated with a stress syndrome induced by a host of factors, including fear, anxiety, sleep deprivation, light, nearly constant noise, temperature variation, unpleasant physical surroundings, and the absence of day and night cycles.

1. Anesthesia or sedation for **intubation** is beyond the scope of this text, and the reader is referred to a multitude of anesthesia tests on this subject.

2. Pain from an **indwelling endotracheal tube** is more likely to be associated with anxiety or with ventilator management that is inadequate for a patient's needs than with actual painful stimulation from the tube itself. Oropharyngeal, laryngeal, and tracheal irritation and inflammation, when present, are easily treated with small doses of topically applied local anesthetic.

3. Endotracheal tube **suctioning** is the source of moderate discomfort, much of which is abated with a small (2 to 3 mL) volume of local anesthetic instilled through the tube 30 to 60 s prior to suctioning. Intravenous (IV) lidocaine (1 mg/kg) also causes significant short-term analgesia, which peaks 60 to 90 s after injection. Small doses of short-acting narcotics (fentanyl, 25 to 50 μg) are effective too, but one must be cautious about producing oversedation and blunting of the cough reflex, because expectoration is a major part of clearing secretions via endotracheal tube suctioning and requires that the patient have intact reflexes.

4. Much of the anxiety associated with respiratory failure disappears when adequate ventilatory support is provided. Some patients may remain agitated even after an appropriate respiratory rate and rhythm are established on the ventilator. This may result from the **anxiety** factor just discussed, or, perhaps, from **stimulation of the stretch (J) receptor** by positive pressure ventilation of the lung or by increased interstitial fluid in the lungs

of those patients with pulmonary edema. **PEEP** contributes to this agitation via the same mechanism, and these patients benefit from parenteral sedation, as discussed below.

V. ANALGESIA IN THE MANAGEMENT OF RESPIRATORY FAILURE: RISKS, BENEFITS, AND CHOICE OF AGENT

A. Analgesic Therapy

In the critically ill population, any drugs used to produce relief must be directed specifically at those symptoms causing stress. There are different sets of drugs to treat pain, anxiety, insomnia, and psychosis, and therapy should be tailored toward individual needs. The commonly used analgesic drugs include narcotics, nonnarcotic analgesics, and local anesthetics.

   1. **Narcotics** are easy to administer, relatively inexpensive, and result in euphoria as well as analgesia. Hence they remain the gold standard in pain relief.

   a. The most frequent route of administration in hospitalized patients is intramuscular (IM), and a multitude of studies have shown that irregular absorption from IM depots usually results in inadequate serum levels of narcotic and an uncomfortable patient. Many doctors and nurses interpret pain relief to mean the minimal dose of analgesic that produces a tolerable level of pain, based on a fear of overdose as well as of addiction; consequently, a large proportion of patients receive too little narcotic to produce true relief of pain. In the critically ill patient, prediction of the effect of analgesics and the need for them is complicated by variable physiologic and psychological factors, as well as pharmacokinetics, altered by age and impaired hepatic and/or renal function.

   b. Table 18-5 compares the various narcotics commonly used in the critical care setting. Morphine is probably the most commonly used narcotic analgesic in the ICU because of its reliability, low cost, high therapeutic index, and familiarity. The relatively recent reduction of the cost of fentanyl (Sublimaze) has resulted in an increase in its usage. Its marked advantages of rapid onset and short duration make it an ideal agent for the critically ill patient who may require analgesia that is more rapidly titratable. Still, there are no conclusive studies that show a statistically significant advantage of one drug over another.

   c. The **undesirable side effects** of respiratory depression, drowsiness, cough suppression, nausea, vomiting, decreased GI motility with increased GI secretions, increased biliary sphincter tone, and the potentiation of the cardiovascular and respiratory effects of other analgesics or sedatives are

Table 18-5 Narcotics in the ICU

Drug	Equipotent dose, mg	Peak onset, min	Duration, h	Dosage scheme Load: µg/kg Infusion rate: µg/kg/min	Relative cost, $/dose equivalent
Meperidine	100	10–15	3–4	500–1000 2.5–5.0	0.41
Methadone	15	10–15	18–20	150–450 0.75–2.5	2.39
Morphine	10	15–20	4–5	100–300 0.5–1.5	0.49
Hydromorphone	1.25	10–15	5	125–375 0.6–1.9	0.59
Alfentanil	0.3	1	0.1–0.2	10–25 0.25–1.0	1.49
Fentanyl	0.1	5	0.5–1.0	1–3 0.005–0.03	0.47
Sufentanil	0.01	5	0.5–1.0	0.1–0.3 0.0005–0.003	1.80

similar among the drugs in this group. The presence of active metabolites of morphine and meperidine (Demerol) that rely on renal excretion makes the pharmacokinetics of these narcotics less predictable in the patient with renal insufficiency, whether acute or chronic. The presence of significant hepatic disease prolongs the duration of all the narcotics listed above.

2. The **agonist–antagonist opioid analgesics**—pentazocine (Talwin), propoxyphene (Darvon), butorphanol (Stadol), nalbuphine (Nubain), buprenorphine (Buprenex), and dezocine (Dalgan)—have limited usefulness for pain relief in the ICU because of their analgesic ceiling. All produce only a limited degree of respiratory depression, which is a useful feature in a patient with mild to moderate pain who is not relying on mechanical ventilation. Most of these drugs can antagonize the analgesia produced by any opioid agonist, as well as prolong and potentiate the desired *and* undesired effects, including respiratory depression, of nonnarcotic hypnotics such as diazepam. Nalbuphine, however, is not a sigma receptor agonist and, therefore, lacks the dysphoria associated with the other agonist–antagonist opioids. In the critical care setting, it is desirable to provide analgesia during weaning from ventilatory support, as it has a minimum of undersirable clinical side effects.

3. **Local anesthetics** in therapeutic doses, given either subcutaneously, for regional nerve block, or for conduction anesthesia, are a tremendous adjuvant therapy for pain relief in the ICU. Characteristics of some commonly used local anesthetics are shown in Table 18-6.

The **toxic effects** of all of the local anesthetics listed progressively

Table 18-6 Characteristics of some local anesthetics

Drug	Onset	Potency	Penetration	Duration	Toxicity
Chloroprocaine	Short	Low	Poor	Very short	Low
Procaine	Short	Low	Poor	Short	Low
Lidocaine	Intermediate	Intermediate	Good	Intermediate	Intermediate
Bupivacaine	Long	High	Good	Long	High
Etidocaine	Long	High	Good	Long	High

include dizziness, tinnitus, circumoral numbness, restlessness, muscle twitching, convulsions, cardiorespiratory depression, cardiac arrest, and coma.

B. Nonanalgesic Therapy

Patients in an intensive care setting often require pharmacologic sedation for reasons other than pain management. Anxiety and sleeplessness, leading to fear and psychosis, may result from being in a frightening environment, the use of restraints, unusual and disturbing sounds, and, in the case of the intubated patient, an inability to communicate.

    1. Drugs used for the purpose of **alleviating anxiety and sleeplessness** include sedative/hypnotics and amnesics. **These drugs do not provide analgesia, and, in fact, when used alone, may cause hyperalgesia, a paradoxical excitement, delirium, or agitation.** Therefore, a combination of an analgesic agent and a nonanalgesic sedative is recommended for the optimal management of pain and agitation in the critical care setting. Such combinations, however, may result in dangerous cardiovascular and pulmonary depression which are not present when these agents are used alone. The most commonly used of the sedative/hypnotics are the benzodiazepines, which produce sedation, drowsiness, amnesia, and unconsciousness, depending on the dose. Table 18-7 lists the common characteristics and recommended doses of the more commonly used benzodiazepines.

Table 18-7 Commonly used benzodiazepines

Drug	Dose Load: $\mu g/kg$ Infusion: $\mu g/kg/min$	Onset, min	Duration, h	Clearance, mL/min/kg	Cost, $/dose equiv
Midazolam	0.0025–0.1 0.25–1	6–30	1–4	4.4–11.1	6.40
Lorazepam	0.01–0.08	20–40	12–24	1.1	6.03
Diazepam	0.1–0.4	30–40	24–57	0.24–0.53	1.41

2. **Antipsychotic and neuroleptic drugs** exert a pronounced anxiolytic effect, thereby reducing agitation and restlessness.

a. Chlorpromazine (Thorazine) is the most often used of the **phenothiazines;** it produces sedation without hypnosis and is useful in the ICU patient who has lost the ability to perceive ICU therapeutics as beneficial or necessary. In addition to its antipsychotic and sedative properties, chlorpromazine exhibits degrees of alpha-adrenergic blocking, muscarinic blocking, and adrenergic agonist activity, all of which may interfere with other hemodynamically active drugs administered in the ICU. Respiratory complications at therapeutic doses of this drug are unusual and infrequent. The therapeutic index of chlorpromazine is low, with many undesirable effects present at therapeutic doses. Dosing usually begins with 2 mg IV at 2-min intervals until the desired effect is reached. These drugs carry the risk of triggering the neuroleptic malignant syndrome in approximately 0.5 to 1.0 percent of patients to whom these drugs are administered.

b. The **butyrophenones** suppress spontaneous neural movements and complex motor behavior patterns, such as ataxia, incoordination, or dysarthria, with minimal central nervous system depressant effects. Haloperidol (Haldol), the more frequently used butyrophenone, produces little sedation and has very little effect on heart rate, blood pressure, or respiration, while at the same time it possesses a strong antipsychotic mechanism. Starting dose for mild agitation is 1 to 3 mg IV.

c. Extrapyramidal reactions occur frequently with haloperidol and consist of parkinsonianlike symptoms that are dose related. Therapy includes diphenhydramine (Benadryl) 50 mg, followed by benztropine (Cogentin) 1 to 2 mg qd for 48 h to prevent recurrence of symptoms. Up to 975 mg of haloperidol per day has been reported as safe for treatment of agitation and was not associated with side effects.

VI. ROUTES OF ANESTHESIA AND ANALGESIA IN RESPIRATORY FAILURE

A. Intravenous Route

Adequate pain control to allow comfortable respiration and pulmonary toilet is an important part of avoiding pulmonary complications. The patient requiring mechanical ventilation is best managed, from both physiologic and nursing points of view, with a level of sedation and analgesia that permits the patient to rest free of the unpleasant sensation of an endotracheal tube and positive pressure ventilation. The IM route of administration of narcotics or sedatives for this purpose is uncomfortable, unpredictable, and inefficient. The most titratable and effective means of administering sedatives or narcotics to the patient requiring mechanical ventilation is via continuous IV infusion. Drugs with short elimination half-lives and few active metabolites prove the most predictable for use in a continuous infusion.

   1. Many critically ill patients, however, have some degree of **end organ failure** that may result in prolongation of the half-life and exaggerated clinical effects of almost any sedative or narcotic drug, even those with short half-lives (see Chapter 6).

   2. In addition, short-acting narcotics and the infusion mode of delivery are both associated with the more rapid development of **tolerance** than with long-acting narcotics or the utilization of intermittent dosing. In no way is this meant to suggest that fentanyl infusions are inappropriate. On the contrary, they are a very effective therapeutic tool. The caregiver must keep in mind, however, that the dose may need to be increased almost daily to maintain the same level of analgesic effect.

   3. Acute administration of narcotics has been associated with **chest wall rigidity** when used for the induction of anesthesia, but this problem is seldom seen with constant IV infusions for the mechanically ventilated patient in the intensive care setting.

   4. The appropriate dose of IV narcotic is difficult to determine in the intensive care setting, as there are no good objective monitors of analgesic effect, and **clinical assessment** can be complicated. The concept of PCA, whereby patients maintain their own analgesic level on demand, within preset limits, is fast becoming popular because of the more accurate and appropriate titration of sedative or narcotic drug that it allows. Most PCA devices allow for the administration of a background continuous infusion, which, when combined with patient-administered bolus medication, readily produces adequate analgesia. The PCA device may be useful even in the patient requiring heavy sedation, as bolus medication may be administered by the bedside nurse via the PCA pump, reducing nurse response time and obviating the need for repeated signouts of medication prior to delivery to the patient.

B. Epidural/Intrathecal Opioid Analgesia

The epidural and intrathecal routes of administration of opioids produce profound levels of analgesia with relatively small doses of narcotic and little sedative effect. Epidurally administered opioids reach, via diffusion across the dura mater, opioid receptors in the substantia gelatinosa of the spinal cord, where they exert antinociceptive effects. The extent and duration of analgesia are determined by a combination of the lipophilicity of the drug versus its relative affinity for opioid receptors. Table 18-8 lists some of the more commonly used epidural opioids, with their recommended doses and expected duration of action.

   1. Improved analgesia is attained with combinations of epidural opioids and dilute concentrations of **local anesthetics,** such as 0.06% to 0.125%

Table 18-8 Commonly used epidural narcotics

Drug	Dose, mg	Onset, min	Duration, h
Meperidine	30–100	5–10	4–20
Methadone	5	15–20	6–8
Morphine	3–5	30–60	12–18
Hydromorphone	1	10–15	7–15
Fentanyl	0.05–0.10	5–20	3–5
Sufentanil	0.005–0.01	3–5	2–4

bupivacaine, when compared with analgesia from epidural opioids alone. Side effects such as hypotension, muscle weakness, and numbness can occur, but almost all routine postoperative patients are neurologically intact at this dosage range, and usually are able to ambulate without difficulty while the infusion is running. On the other hand, even dilute solutions of epidurally administered local anesthetics may result in hypotension from a **pharmacologic sympathectomy** in the patient who is hypovolemic or unable to maintain adequate systemic arterial resistance, as in sepsis syndrome. Judicious patient selection is, therefore, essential when employing local anesthetics for postoperative epidural analgesia in the ICU.

2. The critically ill patient with pulmonary or thoracic disease may find great benefit from epidural analgesia. In multiple studies, epidural opioid analgesia has been demonstrated to be superior or equal to other parenteral opioid techniques with respect to the degree of sedation, improvement in postoperative pulmonary function, early ambulation, and postoperative pulmonary morbidity. When compared with conventional analgesic techniques, specific advantages seen in the ICU are decreased intubation and ventilator-dependency time, a decreased incidence of nosocomial pneumonia, a lower incidence of tracheostomy, and reduced ICU and hospital stays.

3. **Side effects** include a **dose-dependent, delayed respiratory depression** that is most common with morphine. There is a well-documented biphasic peak occurrence of epidural morphine-induced respiratory depression: 1 to 2 h after the initial administration of the drug secondary to epidural venous uptake, and then 8 to 10 h after administration of the drug, associated with a cephalad rise in the level of analgesia and high CSF concentrations of the drug. Other side effects include **urinary retention, itching, nausea, and vomiting,** all of which are antagonized by IV naloxone, which can be added to the maintenance IV fluid (0.8 mg naloxone per liter at 75 to 150 mL/h). Nalbuphine in 5 mg IV doses also can be used, but care must be taken when drugs with narcotic antagonist properties are given to patients who have been receiving opioids routinely for any length of time because of the risk of initiating withdrawal.

CASE DISCUSSION

This 60-year-old man has a number of issues related to pain and anxiety. Pain from his rib fractures will impede weaning in a patient with preexisting respiratory dysfunction. The pelvic fracture will cause pain as well as interfere with the patient's mobility, further impeding pulmonary toilet. As the ARDS develops, elevated anxiety and discomfort associated with mechanical ventilation require the employment of sedative and antianxiety medications.

The patient's course can be divided into three phases, each with its own clinical dilemmas. During the acute phase, attention is focused on achieving hemodynamic stability and adequate oxygenation. Due to the severity of the patient's injuries and significant blood loss, immediate analgesia is most appropriately achieved through use of parenteral opioids. Small doses of a sedative medication such as midazolam will help control agitation. Once the patient is stabilized and any coagulopathy corrected, the patient's pain could be managed with PCA opioids or a thoracic epidural catheter infused with a dilute solution of local anesthetic and opioid (e.g., $\frac{1}{16}$% bupivacaine with 2 to 5 μg/mL of fentanyl or 6 to 9 μg/mL hydromorphone). An epidural infusion would be most beneficial if the patient were doing well clinically and appeared ready to begin weaning, as the analgesia provided by an epidurally administered combination of local anesthetic and opioid improves pulmonary function and toilet while offering little risk of respiratory depression.

If the patient enters the subacute phase and develops ARDS with the associated increases in airway pressures, hypoxemia, and respiratory distress, he will likely require higher doses of narcotic and sedative medications to facilitate the tolerance of mechanical ventilation. These can be administered as intermittent boluses or as an infusion. Occasionally, patients with mild ARDS can control their anxiety and discomfort with a PCA, but often, especially when there is severe respiratory dysfunction, they require doses that cause marked sedation to obtundation, making PCA impractical.

The severity of his ARDS and the duration of ventilatory support will influence the patient's analgesic requirements during the convalescent phase, primarily depending on the extent to which fractures have healed and the degree of pain generated with activity. If his rib fractures still cause severe pain and subsequent compromise of pulmonary function and toilet, an epidural infusion is the best choice. The pelvic fracture, while uncomfortable, will have less influence on his respiratory function. If pain is mild to moderate, a combination of oral (or parenteral) opioids and an NSAID (PO or IV) can very effective. Further pain relief can be achieved with TENS placed bracketing the rib fractures or paravertebrally on the affected side. Further augmentation might include a low-dose TCA at bedtime to improve sleep and increase the level of serotonin, an inhibitory neurotransmitter active in the modulation of pain. If weaning from the ventilator is associated with significant anxiety, self-regulation techniques such as self-hypnosis or relaxation exercises can be very helpful.

SUGGESTED READINGS

Crews JC: Epidural opioid analgesia, in *Crit Care Clin N Am* 6(2):315–342, 1990.
Dantzker DR: *Cardiopulmonary Critical Care,* 2d ed. Philadelphia, Saunders, 1991.
Dehring DJ, Arens JF: Pulmonary thromboembolism: disease recognition and patient management. *Anesthesiology* 73:146–164, 1990.
Stanley TH, Allen S, Bryan-Brown CW: Management of pain and pain-related problems in the critically ill patient, in Shoemake WC (ed.): *Critical Care: State of the Art,* Vol. 6, Society of Critical Care Medicine, 1985.
Zapol WM, Lemaire F: *Adult Respiratory Distress Syndrome.* New York, Marcel Dekker, 1991.

CHAPTER
19
RENAL DISEASES

Timothy B. Gilbert
John F. Williams

Case
  I. Pathophysiology of Renal Failure
     A. Acute Renal Failure
     B. Chronic Renal Failure
     C. Treatment
 II. Renal Failure and Pain
     A. General
     B. Bone and Joint Pain
     C. Neuropathy
     D. Pruritus
     E. Drug-Associated Pain
III. Dialytic Management
     A. Physiology of Dialysis
     B. Sources of Pain
 IV. Other Renal Syndromes
     A. Renal Colic
     B. Loin Pain Hematuria Syndrome
  V. Pain Management Strategies for the Critically Ill Patient
     with Renal Insufficiency
     A. Determination of Extent of Renal Insufficiency
     B. Effect of Renal Failure on the Choices of Drugs to Treat Pain
     C. Impact of Hemodialysis

D. Choice of Drugs
E. Choice of Techniques
Case Discussion
Suggested Readings

CASE

A 64-year-old female on chronic hemodialysis for 12 years is admitted to the intensive care unit (ICU) following respiratory arrest during dialysis treatment. The patient had complained of severe abdominal, muscle, and joint pain, particularly in her right arm (which contained the arteriovenous fistula). She had received repeated doses of intramuscular (IM) morphine sulfate with minimal relief over the preceding 2 h. Her respiratory rate had progressively declined throughout dialysis. Although currently intubated and on mechanical ventilation, she is awake and alert, but appears uncomfortable and restless.

I. PATHOPHYSIOLOGY OF RENAL FAILURE

A. Acute Renal Failure

1. Any abrupt loss of renal function is labeled as acute renal failure (ARF). Up to 5 percent of hospitalized patients will exhibit an episode of ARF. Potential etiologies are divided into **prerenal** (inadequate perfusion to the kidneys because of decreased intravascular volume and/or cardiac output), **intrarenal** (intrinsic damage to the renal glomerular and/or tubular structure from disease or toxins), and **postrenal** (distal obstruction to urine flow). If intravascular volume and cardiac output are maintained, the most common cause of renal failure in the critical care environment is **acute tubular necrosis (ATN)**, often iatrogenically induced with the administration of nephrotoxins such as antibiotics (aminoglycosides) and iodine-containing contrast materials. Comorbidities that appear to place patients at particular risk for ATN are preexisting renal insufficiency, hypertension, vascular disease, diabetes mellitus, and dehydration. Regional renal hypoperfusion, from hypotension and/or intravascular hypovolemia, is most often seen following major surgery or trauma. Sepsis (particularly gram-negative varieties) and rhabdomyolysis may also initiate ATN in the critically ill.

2. The presentation of ARF may be **anuric, oliguric** (<400 mL/day), or **nonoliguric** (>400 mL/day). Initial plasma creatinine and urea levels may be normal, but often rise as renal dysfunction becomes manifest. The hallmarks of established ARF include:

    a. Acute, usually non- or poorly compensated, metabolic acidosis.

    b. Impaired concentrating ability with consequent obligatory sodium, calcium, and glucose losses.

    c. Hypervolemia due to water and sodium retention.

    d. Decreased clearance of renally excreted drugs or toxins.

e. Hyperkalemia, seen only in anuric or severely oliguric patients, due to an inability to excrete the filtered potassium load and/or increased serum potassium from underlying disease (e.g., rhabdomyolysis, hemolytic anemia).

B. Chronic Renal Failure

1. Prolonged damage to the kidneys, regardless of a prerenal, intrarenal, or postrenal etiology, results in a permanent reduction in the glomerular filtration rate (GFR) and a concomitant rise in plasma creatinine and urea. Long-standing diabetes or glomerulonephritis causes most chronic renal failures (CRFs), but hypertension and polycystic and interstitial renal diseases can do so as well. Unresolved ARF in a percentage of critically ill patients will develop into CRF. As the severity of renal insufficiency increases, the clearance of renally excreted substances diminishes, with accumulation of metabolic by-products, primarily urea, uremic toxins (e.g., amines, phenols, indoles, guanidines), and middle-molecular-weight toxins.

2. In addition to those listed above for ARF, features common to CRF include:

   a. Chronic, usually well-compensated, metabolic acidosis from impaired fixed-acid secretion.

   b. Normocytic, normochromic anemia from decreased red cell production, primarily due to decreased production of erythropoietin.

   c. Hyperphosphatemia, hyperuricemia, hypermagnesemia, hypersulfatemia, hypocalcemia, and azotemia from impaired secretion and elevated parathyroid hormone (PTH) levels.

   d. Hyperkalemia is uncommon, except in those patients with severe dysfunction (GFR < 15 mL/min).

   e. Hypertension and edema from volume overload.

   f. Proteinuria and hypoproteinemia from protein wasting.

C. Treatment

The treatment **of renal failure** depends on the severity of azotemia, acidosis, hypervolemia, and patient symptomatology. Prevention of further diminution in renal function is attempted by treating the underlying etiology and any other concurrent disease, such as hypertension, diabetes, or infection, and avoiding nephrotoxic agents. Dietary protein restrictions are imposed to decrease the uremic load. Hyperphosphatemia and hypocalcemia may be controlled with calcium salts and calcitriol (1,25-dihydroxycholecalciferol, vitamin D_3), while allopurinol may improve hyperuricemia. **End-stage renal disease (ESRD)** ultimately requires dialytic management (in the form of hemodialysis or peritoneal dialysis) to manage the uremia, unless renal transplantation becomes practical and available for the given patient.

II. RENAL FAILURE AND PAIN

A. General

Patients with renal dysfunction may develop a myriad of painful symptoms, depending on the severity and duration of their disease, in addition to the types of treatment used (e.g., hemodialysis) to alleviate their uremia. The presence of uremia alone cannot account for all pain symptoms attributed to renal disease, but may be partially responsible for pruritus and gastrointestinal symptoms, such as nausea, vomiting, stomatitis, and abdominal cramps. Electrolyte derangements, primarily those of phosphate and calcium, produce painful bone and joint syndromes. General malaise and weakness are seen in the setting of chronic anemia and iron and vitamin deficiency. Drugs administered to patients with renal failure may have enhanced or abnormal effects, including the production of pain. Psychosocial factors may enhance somatic pain due to the underlying renal disease.

B. Bone and Joint Pain

1. Renal osteodystrophy (ROD) is a generic term which encompasses the complex bone lesions occurring in most ESRD patients that are secondary to abnormal calcium, phosphate, and vitamin D metabolism at osteoid tissue and chronic acidosis. These changes typically require months to several years to become manifest, and are largely prevented by meticulous electrolyte management and vitamin supplementation once renal failure becomes established. Early biochemical changes, such as elevated PTH levels, usually precede symptomatic disease by several years. The development of ROD appears to be determined by the rate of skeletal growth and chronicity of renal dysfunction; therefore, children and those with congenital anomalies are at particular risk. Its primary components are **osteitis fibrosa** and **osteomalacia,** although **osteosclerosis** and **osteoporosis** are infrequently seen. Osteitis fibrosa is distinguished by an increase in osteoclasts and bone resorption with marrow fibrosis, secondary to increased PTH levels (i.e., **secondary hyperparathyroidism**). Osteomalacia refers to decreased mineralization of bone from alterations in vitamin D metabolism. Osteosclerosis is notable for the patchy involvement of bone with increased mineralization and bone density. Osteoporosis is a general term denoting an overall decrease in mineralized bone mass.

2. The clinical manifestations of ROD include bone and joint pain, pruritus, and muscular weakness. Although osteitis fibrosa is almost universal in ESRD patients, only a minority will complain of painful bones. Bone pain is even less frequent in those with osteomalacia. Characterized by vague low back and lower extremity pain (legs, hips, and knees) of varying severity, the typically progressive nature of the pain may eventually impair ambulation and mobility. Severe bone demineralization can ultimately result in frank fracture, a source of acute bone pain in long-term ESRD patients. Joint pain arises from hydroxyapatite deposition, causing swelling and calcific periarthritis. Laboratory confirmation of ROD may include elevation of circulating immunoreactive parathyroid hormone (iPTH) and depression of calcitriol. Hypocalcemia is more common, especially in patients with osteomalacia, although hypercalcemia may occur in severe uremia. Hyperphosphatemia and hypermagnesemia occur as renal dysfunction becomes end-stage. Although moderately elevated uric acid levels are consistently found in CRF, symptomatic gout is infrequent.

3. Treatment is initially aimed at reestablishing normal calcium and phosphate levels. Oral supplementation and (if needed) the addition of calcium to the dialysate bath are used to maintain high-normal plasma levels. To control phosphate, dietary protein and dairy restrictions are enacted, as is the addition of oral phosphate-binding agents (e.g., aluminum hydroxide or carbonate). In order to suppress secondary hyperparathyroidism, in addition to the above calcium-phosphate modifications, calcitriol is added in doses, typically, of 0.5 to 1 g/day. Severe hyperparathyroidism, with bone erosions, persistent hypercalcemia, and pruritus, can require total parathyroidectomy with partial autotransplantation. Symptomatic gout in patients with renal failure may require the use of low-dose allopurinol. Reduced doses of 100 mg/day or 300 mg twice per week usually suffice to reduce serum urate levels.

C. Neuropathy

1. Abnormalities in both the peripheral and central nervous systems are seen in CRF. Manifestations of peripheral neuropathy include limb paresthesias, restless leg syndrome, and sensory deficits. Central symptoms such as agitation, irritability, and depression may accentuate peripheral somatic complaints and lower the pain threshold. Lengthening dialytic periods or using high-surface-area dialysis membranes may afford improvement in symptoms, as does normalization of electrolyte levels. Renal transplantation yields the greatest benefit in reducing symptoms.

D. Pruritus

No single etiologic agent has been documented to cause the frequent and generalized pruritus that accompanies renal failure, particularly CRF. Although no obvious dermatologic lesion is noted, probable offenders include calcium and urea. Secondary hyperparathyroidism causes an increase in the calcium-phosphate product, which in long-standing disease leads to dermal calcium deposition. Urea and uremic by-products have been implicated, since symptoms of pruritus decrease with dietary protein restriction and increased frequency of dialysis. No specific therapy exists, however, some patients benefit from oral histamine type 1 blockers (e.g., diphenhydramine) or topical emolients. Maintenance of proper calcium-phosphate levels, frequent dialysis, and sunlight (or ultraviolet-ray therapy) have been recommended to reduce symptoms. Unresponsive pruritus may be an indication for parathyroidectomy.

E. Drug-Associated Pain

Numerous pharmacologic agents, particular those necessary with long-term therapy, can slowly accumulate and thereby accentuate or produce pain in renal failure patients. Typically musculoskeletal in origin, myalgias, arthralgias, and dermal pains may appear following the administration of many common drugs to patients in renal failure. For example, recurrent myalgias have been associated with cimetidine. Cyclosporine has been suspected of inducing severe arthralgias in conjunction with immunosuppression after renal transplantation. Overdosage of antithymocyte globulin has caused a clinical syndrome of abdominal pain, diarrhea, and fever. Suprofen, a nonsteroidal antiinflammatory drug (NSAID), has been associated with acute flank pain, hematuria, and transient renal dysfunction from an acute uric acid nephropathy, particularly in young males without preexisting renal disease. Discontinuation of the offending agent will almost always reverse symptoms.

Erythropoietin is often administered either intravenously (IV) or subcutaneously to reverse the anemia of ESRD. More effective if given subcutaneously, it causes moderately severe pain in some individuals by that route. The concomitant use of local anesthetics may decrease this source of pain without changing efficacy.

III. DIALYTIC MANAGEMENT

A. Physiology of Dialysis

As renal failure progresses, with increasing impairment of the renal excretory function, accumulating solutes must be removed to prevent the uremic syndrome or death. Most low-molecular-weight solutes, such as electrolytes and urea, can be removed efficiently by dialytic diffusion across a semipermeable membrane separating patient plasma form artificial dialysate. With passive diffusion favoring the various concentration gradients, solutes may move from patient to dialysate (e.g., potassium or urea) or from dialysate to patient (e.g., bicarbonate or acetate). The semipermeable membrane may be a component of an external device attached to the patient's vascular system **(hemodialysis [HD])**, or the patient's peritoneal cavity may be used **(peritoneal dialysis [PD])**. Either form of therapy is inherently limited because of low solute clearances and the failure to provide normal endocrinologic and physiologic functions relative to the native kidney. The use of PD affords greater removal of larger-weight molecules (>500 daltons), preventing the buildup of "middle molecules" responsible for some complications in HD patients. **Continuous arteriovenous hemofiltration (CAVH)** or **continuous venovenous hemofiltration (CVVH)** is occasionally used in critical care areas, in patients unable to tolerate the hemodynamic stress of HD. Using the patient's systemic arteriovenous pressure gradient (CAVH) or an external pump (CVVH) as the hydraulic source, the slow, continuous removal of solute and fluid is achieved across a membrane with increased water and solute permeability.

B. Sources of Pain

Because the ESRD patient must undergo dialytic management to prevent the complications of uremia and death, it is difficult to differentiate symptoms of pain from the progression of CRF versus pain introduced by the dialysis itself. The process of HD may involve painful percutaneous cannulation of the vascular system, impair central and peripheral hemodynamic stability, introduce unwanted substances from the dialysate, and induce musculoskeletal pains. Carpal tunnel syndrome, shoulder pain and stiffness, and other related osteoarticular manifestations are characteristic of the **late dialysis periarticular syndrome,** which typically appears after 6 to 8 years of chronic dialysis. Pain from PD may result from the intraperitoneal catheter or an inflamed peritoneal cavity.

1. Joint pain   Frequent in HD patients, joint pain has been attributed to the accumulation of 2-microglobulin amyloid fibrils in major joints, primarily the shoulders and hips. The use of PD or specialized dialytic techniques such as push/pull hemodiafiltration or polymethyl-methacrylate membranes may decrease its incidence. Joint pain may also arise from ROD (see above) in either dialyzed or nondialyzed patients.

2. Hand pain   Pain, numbness, and cold sensations in the hand have been noted in patients with side-to-side arteriovenous fistulas, due to ischemic steal from major proximal venous collateral vessels. Finger pulse oxymetry has been used to document distal desaturation. Surgical closure of a portion of the venous collaterals improves oxygenation and decreases pain in the hand.

3. Carpal tunnel syndrome   This syndrome can present as a result of amyloid deposits within the synovia and tendons of the wrist. Ischemia distal to the dialysis cannulation is likely to be a facilitating factor, since the syndrome occurs more often on the side of the arteriovenous fistula site. Its incidence increases as the duration of HD increases. Median nerve release by carpal tunnel retinaculectomy results in relief with minimal sequelae, if the intervention is performed as soon as the patient is symptomatic.

4. Cannulation pain The large-bore needles which percutaneously access arteriovenous fistula are a regular source of pain at each dialytic run. Particularly distressing to the pediatric age group, adjuvant topical therapy, such as the eutectic mixture of local anesthetics **(EMLA creme)** or the subcutaneous or iontophoretic administration of lidocaine, notably decreases cannulation pain. The EMLA creme requires prolonged dermal contact (1 h or more) for maximum effectiveness. Minimal systemic absorption or side effects have been noted.

5. Dysequilibrium syndrome This syndrome refers to the occurrence of headache, nausea, vomiting, agitation, and, rarely, seizures or coma during or after HD. The rapid removal of primarily urea and other solutes creates an osmotic gradient capable of increasing brain cell water mass with subsequent cerebral edema. This is especially seen in the initial dialysis in severe ARF with high urea levels. Preventive measures include the use of higher osmolality dialysate, slowing the rate of HD, or infusing hypertonic solutions (e.g., mannitol) into the patient during HD.

6. Dialysis dementia Dialysis dementia or encephalopathy, characterized by personality changes, myoclonic muscle activity, memory and speech disturbances, is a progressive, late, and generally fatal complication of HD. Sporadic, epidemic, and pediatric forms are recognized. High brain aluminum levels have been associated with its development, but treatment with purified water for dialysis, avoidance of aluminum-based antacids, and trials of anticonvulsants or the chelating agent deferoxamine have not been wholly effective.

7. Syndrome associated with first dialyzer use The syndrome of **cramps, nausea and vomiting, headache, pruritus, and chest and back pain is commonly associated with first dialyzer use,** and occurs in up to one-third of dialytic runs. The incidence is increased when a new dialytic membrane is used relative to subsequent repeated uses of the same membrane on different days with the same patient. Although the exact etiology has yet to be elucidated, two points have been noted: (1) new dialyzers contain small quantities of endotoxin, and (2) leukopenia is most severe during the initial use of a dialytic membrane, which can activate the complement cascade and embolize neutrophils. Presumably, this may explain the particularly increased incidence of chest and back pain during the first use of a membrane.

IV. OTHER RENAL SYNDROMES

A. Renal Colic

1. Intense visceral pain may emanate from ureteral and renal pelvis spasm proximal to an obstruction by renal calculi. Variable in intensity and duration, but typically episodic and crescendo in nature, the pain may radi-

ate down the unilateral flank and into the groin. It is often associated with nausea and vomiting, but with only minimal abdominal findings because of the retroperitoneal source. Complete relief occurs when the stone passes distally into the bladder.

2. Potent analgesics, typically opioids, are often required until the stone passes or is removed surgically. Nifedipine decreases the contractility of smooth muscle, and may reduce the spasmodic pain of renal colic. Increased renal prostaglandin synthesis had been described in unilateral ureteral occlusion, and, therefore, nonsteroidal agents (e.g., indomethacin) have been described to reduce ureteral peristalsis; it is not known whether this impedes stone extrusion from the ureter.

B. Loin Pain Hematuria Syndrome

1. Made manifest by recurrent loin pain, episodic hematuria, and angiographically abnormal renal vasculature, this disorder most commonly occurs in young females, especially if they are receiving estrogen therapy. Unilateral or bilateral flank pain in the setting of sterile urine cultures and the absence of any preexisting renal dysfunction often lead to a radiologic workup. These studies reveal abrupt alteration or occlusion of interlobar, arcuate, or interlobular arteries; loss of cortical-medullary definition; and tortuosity of small vessels. Lower poles of the kidneys are more frequently affected. Estrogens are thought to affect platelets, which exhibit decreased life spans, and may sequester in the kidneys.

2. Treatment includes discontinuation of estrogen compounds, use of antiplatelet drugs, and, rarely, renal transplantation in the most severe cases.

V. PAIN MANAGEMENT STRATEGIES FOR THE CRITICALLY ILL PATIENT WITH RENAL INSUFFICIENCY

A. Determination of Extent of Renal Insufficiency

The severity of renal insufficiency cannot be accurately quantified by history and urine output alone. The laboratory evaluation of a patient with suspected renal disease typically is straightforward; the commonly obtained indexes include:

1. Urinalysis
2. Blood urea nitrogen (BUN)
3. Serum creatinine (Crs)

The GFR can then be estimated as follows:

$$\text{GFR}^* \text{ (mL/min)} = [(140-\text{age}) \times \text{weight (kg)}]/72$$

*Multiply by 0.85 for female patients

Creatinine clearance (CrCl) can also be directly measured from timed urine collection of volume (V) and creatinine (Cru), with simultaneous determination of serum values (Crs):

$$\text{CrCl (mL/min)} = \text{Cru (mg/dL)} \times \text{V (mL)}/\text{Crs (mg/dL)}$$

1. Other tests Measurements of serum proteins (i.e., albumin and total protein) are useful in projecting the extent of unbound drugs. In patients with ESRD (CrCl < 5 mL/min or severe oliguria), serum electrolyte measurement may demonstrate hyperkalemia. More detailed testing, such as urine electrolytes, specific gravity, and microbiology, may be indicated for specific clinical scenarios. Radiologic studies may identify obstructive causes for renal dysfunction and detail renal perfusion status.

B. Effect of Renal Failure on the Choices of Drugs to Treat Pain

1. Because the kidneys remain a primary elimination route for many analgesics, it is important to ascertain both the degree of the patient's renal insufficiency and the extent to which the chosen drug depends on renal excretion. Metabolism and redistribution of drugs often terminate the action of lipophilic agents in extrarenal organs, making excretion less important. As glomerular filtration falls and renal clearance is impaired, the elimination half-life of a drug increases, as does the potential for accumulation of either parent compounds or active metabolites. Despite this pharmacokinetic concern for increasing drug dosage intervals, initial doses may actually need to be increased, as the volume of distribution (Vd) can increase significantly in volume-overloaded patients (e.g., prior to HD). If a desired plasma concentration (C) of a given drug is known, a loading dose (Dl) can be calculated:

$$\text{Dl(mg)} = \text{Vd (L/kg)} \times \text{C (g/dL)} \times \text{Wt(kg)} \times 100$$

2. Maintenance doses are typically decreased. Percentage decrease of the maintenance doses (%D) can be estimated if creatinine clearance (CrCl) and the percentage of renal excretion (E) for the drug are known:

$$\%D = E[(\text{CrCl}/125) - 1] + 1$$

3. Alternatively, the dosing interval may be increased to allow greater elimination, instead of using lower maintenance doses. Estimation of the increase in dosing interval (Irf) can be calculated from the normal interval (Inl) and the above information:

$$\text{Irf} = \text{Inl}/\%D$$

4. Additionally, obligate protein wasting from the impaired kidneys leads to hypoalbuminemia and hypoproteinemia, consequently lowering protein binding. Free drug levels, therefore, can be elevated, enhancing bioavailability and drug effect. Most analgesics thus should be titrated to the desired effect with particularly close monitoring in these high-risk patients. Specific agents are discussed below.

C. Impact of Hemodialysis

The use of HD is most effective in removing drugs which are smaller than 500 daltons, not highly protein bound, and have a low Vd. For drugs that fall into these categories (which include most anesthetics, except for muscle relaxants), minimal alteration in dosing may be required, if timing of the next dialytic run is considered. Accumulation will continue to occur between dialysis periods. Minimal drug removal is afforded by PD relative to HD, especially for very-low-molecular-weight substances.

D. Choice of Drugs

Although most analgesics, if appropriately dosed, can be used in patients with renal dysfunction, each class of drug may have theoretical advantages that warrant consideration. In general, drugs with short half-lives and extrarenal metabolism without active by-products will best suffice as the drugs of choice. Table 19-1 lists common drugs, half-lives in normal and ESRD patients, extent of renal excretion, suggested dosage adjustments, and the presence of pharmacologically active metabolites.

1. Pure opioid agonists These remain the standard drugs for producing analgesia.

a. Morphine sulphate undergoes hepatic glucuronidation to morphine-3- and -6-glucuronides, which can produce analgesia, prolonged respiratory depression, and nausea/vomiting in patients with decreased elimination and subsequent accumulation. The parent compound morphine undergoes minimal urinary excretion, with similar levels being noted in patients both with and without renal failure. Its relatively low protein binding is decreased only roughly 10 percent more in CRF. Because of morphine's relatively high Vd in normal patients, renal failure has little impact on its initial dosing. Subsequent maintenance doses should be decreased to prevent the side effects of accumulation.

b. Meperidine (Demerol) exhibits Vd, protein binding, and elimination characteristics similar to those of morphine. However, the hepatic demethylation of meperidine to normeperidine in patients with renal dysfunction has been associated with both prolonged respiratory depression and seizures, limiting its use in these patients.

c. Fentanyl citrate (Sublimaze), a more lipophilic and potent agent, is also hepatically degraded, but appears less likely to accumulate or to produce respiratory depression than morphine or meperidine. More protein

Table 19-1 Drugs commonly used in ICU patients with renal diseases

Drug name	Beta-half-life, normal range (avg), h	Beta-half-life, ESRD, h	Renal excretion of parent compound, %	Decrease dose for ESRD, %	Putative metabolites prolonging effect in ESRD patients due to impaired renal excretion
Fentanyl	2.0–14 (2.0–4.0)	NC	0.3–10	0–25	—
Hydromorphone	2.4–2.6	?	1.3–13.2	→	Dihydromorphine Dihydroisomorphine
Meperidine	2.4–7.0 (3.2–3.7)	NC	2–10	−25–50	Normeperidine Meperidinic acid
Methadone	18–97 (25)	13–55	21–25	−25–50	—
Morphine	2.3–4.7	?	8.5–15	−50	Morphine-3-glucuronide Morphine-6-glucuronide
Sufentanil	2.5–2.7	NC	1–3	→	Desmethylsufentanil
Buprenorphine	1.2–7.2 (3.0)	NC	27–70	0–50	N-Dealkylbuprenorphine
Butorphanol	2.2–4.0	?	0–5	NC	—
Dezocine	2.1–2.8 (2.5)	?	<1	→	—
Nalbuphine	2.1–5.0 (2.1–2.6)	?	7	NC	—
Pentazocine	2.0–6.0 (2.0–3.0)	?	5–12	NC	—
Ketamine	2.5–4.0	?	<4	→	Norketamine
Chlordiazepoxide	5.0–30 (10)	NC	<1	−50	Desmethylchlordiazepoxide Demoxepam
Diazepam	24–55	NC	<1	NC	N-Desmethyldiazepam Temzepam, oxazepam

Drug	t½ normal	t½ ESRD	% excreted unchanged	Dose adjustment	Active metabolite
Lorazepam	8.0–25 (12)	32–70	<1	−50	—
Midazolam	1.2–5.0 (2.5)	↑	<0.03	0–25	1-Hydroxymidazolam, 4-Hydroxymidazolam
Etomidate	1.1–4.6 (2.6)	?	<37	↓	—
Propofol	1.5–6.1 (1.5–1.7)	?	<0.3	NC	—
Thiopental	3.8–10	3.8–18	10–15	−25	—
Chloral Hydrate	7.0–14	?	~0	NR	Trichloroethanol
Chlorpromazine	11–42 (31)	NC	<5	NC	7-Hydroxychlorpromazine
Diphenhydramine	4.0–8.5	?	<4	−25–50	—
Droperidol	2.0–3.0	?	<1	↓	P-Hydroxypiperidine
Haloperidol	10–36 (21)	?	<5	NC	—
Atracurium	0.3–0.4	0.3–0.4	~0	NC	—
d-Tubocurarine	1.4–3.8 (2.0)	2.2–5.0	40–75	NR	—
Metocurine	3.5–6.0	10.7–11.4	46–58	NR	—
Pancuronium	1.7–2.2 (1.8)	4.3–8.2	40	NR	3-Hydroxypancuronium
Pipecuronium	1.8–2.3	3.5–4.4	41	NR	?
Succinylcholine	3.0	?	~0	NC	Succinylmonocholine
Vecuronium	0.9–1.9 (1.1–1.3)	1.4–2.5	10–25	NC	3-Hydroxyvecuronium

NC = Available data suggest no change in maintenance doses required.
NR = Available data suggest drug not recommended for use in ESRD patients.
— = No known clinically significant metabolites.
? = No available data.
↑ = Available data suggest half-life is increased in ESRD patients.
↓ = No recommendations exist in available literature; however, dosage reduction seems necessary, and titration of drug to desired effect is suggested.

bound and exhibiting a greater Vd than morphine, less than 10 percent of fentanyl is excreted unchanged in the urine. By-products of fentanyl are pharmacologically inactive. Its clearance is not significantly changed in renal failure patients. Because of this favorable profile, it may be a preferred narcotic if renal dysfunction is apparent.

  d. Sufentanil citrate (Sufenta), with the greatest potency and lipophilicity of available narcotics, has advantages similar to those of fentanyl. Although it shows minimal urinary excretion of parent compound, one of its o-demethylated metabolites may demonstrate partial activity.

  e. Hydromorphone (Dilaudid), a hydrogenated ketone of morphine and roughly 8 to 10 times more potent, is metabolized primarily by the liver. Excreted mainly as the glucuronidated conjugate, small amounts of both the parent compound and 6-hydroxylated reduction metabolites are also found in urine. Compared with morphine, hydromorphone may produce greater sedation and less euphoria, possibly decreasing the incidence of physical dependence. Its high potency in a small volume affords easy subcutaneous or IM injection, which is useful if the patient has poor venous access.

 2. Opioid agonist–antagonists These were developed as high-potency analgesics, while attempting to decrease unwanted side effects, such as respiratory depression, physical dependence, and abuse potential. Because of chronic pain, CRF patients often develop tolerance to narcotics, requiring increased doses, with the potential for abuse. Five agents are commercially available: **pentazocine** (Talwin), **butorphanol** (Stadol), **nalbuphine** (Nubain), **buprenorphine** (Buprenex), and **dezocine** (Dalgan). The first three exhibit κ- and σ-agonism while inhibiting μ-receptors. The latter two are partial μ-agonists. Caution must be exercised in patients on previous or chronic narcotic therapy, since agents which have antagonist activity can precipitate withdrawal reactions. Pentazocine undergoes oxidization and glucuronide conjugation, with less than 5 percent renal excretion of the parent compound. Butorphanol is hydroxylated prior to biliary and urinary excretion. Nalbuphine is similarly metabolized by the liver and excreted in the bile. Buprenorphine is mainly excreted unchanged into the bile, while less than one-third is conjugated or metabolized to inactive compounds. Dezocine undergoes glucuronide conjugation, with approximately two-thirds of a dose appearing as the conjugated product and less than 1 percent as parent compound.

 3. Ketamine Ketamine (Ketalar) is a water-soluble derivative of phencyclidine which produces dissociative anesthesia. Because of its minimal protein binding and high lipophilicity, it has extensive extravascular uptake and rapid redistribution. Hepatic clearance occurs by demethylation to less active norketamine, followed by further hydroxylation and glucuronidation prior to urinary excretion. The duration of action of a single loading dose is not changed by renal insufficiency; however, multiple doses may have more prolonged effects due to the accumulation of partially active norketamine.

4. Benzodiazepines The benzodiazepines are highly protein bound and undergo hepatic degradation prior to urinary excretion. Active metabolites are produced from **diazepam** (Valium), flurazepam (Dalmane), and **chlordiazepoxide** (Librium), which may accumulate in patients with renal failure, especially with multiple dosing. Conjugation with glucuronic acid produces by-products of **oxazepam** (Serax) and **lorazepam** (Ativan) with minimal activity. **Midazolam** (Versed) is a unique water-soluble agent which undergoes almost entire hydroxylation to two significantly less potent metabolites which are excreted in the urine. The elimination half-life, Vd, and clearance of midazolam are not altered by renal failure.

5. Other sedatives/hypnotics The **phenothiazines** are highly protein bound, are lipophilic, and have a very large Vd. Metabolism by hepatic degradation is slow, with uremic patients being more susceptible to extrapyramidal symptoms (e.g., myoclonus) or delirium. Because of the availability of less toxic agents, their use in renal failure is limited. **Chlorpromazine** (Thorazine) may potentiate the formation of normeperidine, if concurrently administered with meperidine. The **butyrophenones haloperidol** (Haldol) and **droperidol** (Inapsine), despite minimal urinary excretion of the parent compounds, have potent metabolites which may exhibit prolonged effects in ESRD. The sedative effect of **chloral hydrate** is mainly due to its metabolite trichloroethanol, which requires urinary excretion and should be avoided in ESRD. The induction agents **thiopental, etomidate** (Amidate), and **propofol** (Diprivan) require little change in dosing because of their rapid redistribution and metabolism to inactive compounds. **Diphenhydramine** (Benadryl), with no active metabolites and minimal urinary excretion of the parent compound, similarly requires little dosage change.

6. Nonsteroidal antiinflammatory drugs Typically considered mild analgesics, NSAIDs make up a group of cyclooxygenase inhibitors extensively applied in musculoskeletal, posttraumatic, and inflammatory pain. They have no abuse potential; do not cause dependence, withdrawal, or respiratory depression; and are effective in chronic as well as acute pain. Bleeding time is increased because of qualitative platelet dysfunction, but platelet count and coagulation factors are not affected. They also are beneficial in pain syndromes in which prostaglandins may play a direct role, as in dysmenorrhea, renal colic, biliary duct spasm, and other visceral pains. However, blockade of renal prostaglandins can cause a dose-dependent decrease in renal blood flow and rarely produces overt renal failure. By inhibiting the contraction of smooth muscle, NSAIDs may be more efficacious than narcotics in treating ureteral colic. Until recently, NSAIDs were available only in forms for oral or rectal routes of administration; however, **ketorolac tromethamine** (Toradol) is available for parenteral use. The primary metabolic pathway is conjugation with glucuronic acid, followed by urinary excretion of up to 90 percent of the dose. In patients with Crs levels of 1.5 to 5.0 mg/

dL, the terminal half-life of ketorolac is doubled from control (9.6 versus 4.5 h, respectively) and total clearance is reduced 38 to 50 percent from control. Therefore, in these patients, standard loading doses (30 to 60 mg) may be used, followed by a roughly 50 percent reduction in maintenance doses (typically, 7.5 to 15 mg every 6 h). Use in patients with higher Crs levels or on dialysis has not been extensively studied.

7. **Muscle relaxants** Although devoid of analgesic activity, muscle relaxants are often required in critically ill patients in order to perform procedures, improve ventilation, and prevent undesired motion and injury to the patient. Often administered for prolonged periods, the potential for accumulation is real, especially in the setting of renal dysfunction. Moreover, the pharmacokinetic variability of muscle relaxants in patients with renal failure is greater, possibly related to the multiplicity of associated diseases in these patients. Concurrent disease states (e.g., acidosis, hypothermia, or hypermagnesemia) or drug administration (e.g., aminoglycoside antibiotics) may also accentuate neuromuscular blockade.

a. **Succinylcholine** (Anectine), because of its metabolism by plasma pseudocholinesterase to choline and succinic acid, can be used without modification in single doses. However, because one of its by-products has partial relaxant activity (succinylmonocholine), and may accumulate if sufficient doses of succinylcholine are used, infusions should be avoided in patients with severe renal failure. The depolarizing nature of succinylcholine may additionally exacerbate preexisting hyperkalemia, and must be taken into consideration if the patient is at risk for further elevations of serum potassium.

b. Of the nondepolarizing agents, **atracurium** (Tracrium) is a logical choice for use in patients with severe renal failure. Unique to relaxants, atracurium undergoes **Hoffman elimination** by fission at its aliphatic side chain to **laudanosine,** a central nervous system stimulant devoid of muscle relaxant properties, and other quaternary by-products. Although this reaction is slowed by acidosis, even the moderate acidosis of renal failure is unlikely to prolong the activity of atracurium significantly. Laudanosine, almost totally dependent on hepatic metabolism, has a prolonged elimination half-life and can accumulate if repeatedly dosed. High serum levels are associated with increasing anesthetic requirements and seizures. Those at particular risk would appear to be patients with severe liver disease and those receiving multiple boluses or continuous infusions (e.g., long-term intubated patients).

c. **Vecuronium** (Norcuron), another intermediate-acting agent, is also suitable in renal failure because of its slight dependence on the kidneys for elimination of the parent compound and metabolites. Accumulation can occur with vecuronium upon repeated dosing, but is much less pronounced than with long-acting agents. Beta-elimination half-life and clearance are not changed by renal failure with atracurium, and the half-life is elevated by only 50 percent for vecuronium. An apparent tolerance has been noted in renal failure patients by detecting higher plasma levels of vecuronium at various stages of recovery as compared with control patients. Persistent paralysis has been noted in some critically ill patients after long-term administration of either intermittent boluses or continuous infusions of vecuronium. Patients with renal failure and hypermagnesemia or metabolic acidosis appear to be at increased risk, possibly due to an accumulation of the 3-desacetyl-vecuronium metabolite.

      d. Prolonged effects can be seen with the use of the long-acting agents in renal failure, and, therefore, they should be dosed cautiously. **Gallamine** (Flaxedil) and **pancuronium** (Pavulon) have increased beta-elimination half-lives in ESRD patients, up to six and five times normal respectively. **Metocurine** (Metubine) and **d-tubocurarine** (Curare) have increased half-lives, roughly twice normal, possibly due to prolonged storage in inactive tissue sites and only minor hepatic degradation. Likewise, **pipercuronium** (Arduan) has been shown to have at least a twofold increase in half-life in patients with ESRD.

E. Choice of Techniques

Because of the altered pharmacokinetics in patients with renal dysfunction, the method of administration of drugs can be as important in dictating efficacy and the risk of complications as the specific drug chosen. Interpatient variability with each technique is high, owing to the dynamic state of the patient's renal dysfunction (i.e. chronicity of disease, frequency of dialysis), which can alter acid-base balance, protein binding, and Vd. In addition, patients with renal failure often have concurrent underlying medical diseases or other organ dysfunction, which may further change responsiveness.

      1. Intravenous bolus Historically the most common method, intermittent IV boluses of agents are routinely used in critical care units. Often because the patient is unable to communicate pain (e.g., is intubated or paralyzed), nursing personnel administer drugs on an "as needed" basis. This approach is obviously limited by the inherent difficulty of assessing pain in paralyzed and/or intubated patients. The drugs most often administered by IV bolus include narcotics, sedatives, and muscle relaxants. Rapid onset with high peak levels may accentuate drug response. For narcotics, this may include respiratory depression and hypotension. Duration of effect will depend on the specific clearance and/or metabolism of the drug. Redosing is required when plasma levels of the parent compound and/or active metabolites fall below the therapeutic range.

2. Patient-controlled analgesia When a patient is capable of detecting, comprehending, and responding to pain, the use of patient-controlled analgesia (PCA) can enable the faster administration of narcotics or other analgesics IV or subcutaneously in small incremental doses. The use of these smaller, but more frequent, doses allows efficient titration of the analgesic level by the patient. Lower peak plasma levels are typically and more consistently achieved than with IM or IV bolus dosing. Thus maintenance levels are more frequently near the therapeutic range, balancing pain relief with less frequent or less severe side effects, such as sedation or respiratory depression. Loading doses are commonly used when initiating PCA in order to achieve therapeutic levels quickly. Subsequent maintenance doses usually are 25 to 50 percent lower in renal failure patients, especially if longer-acting agents are used.

3. Epidural analgesia The use of epidural analgesia with local anesthetics and/or narcotics can be a very effective method of controlling pain, if the stimuli emanate from lumbar or lower thoracic spinal cord levels. This technique is relatively contraindicated in certain patients with renal disease, if either coagulopathy (e.g., heparin from dialysis) or platelet defects (e.g., significant uremia) preclude catheter placement. Routine determination of coagulation parameters, including bleeding time, is warranted in severe uremia or if dialysis has been performed recently.

The benefits of the epidural administration of drugs include the fact that smaller doses can be used, with consequently lower systemic absorption and plasma levels (see Chapter 13).

4. Other regional techniques Other techniques may be used for anatomically appropriate pain sources, after the risks of uremia- or heparin-induced coagulopathy are considered. Intercostal, intrapleural, major plexus, or local field and peripheral nerve blocks may effectively attenuate localized sources of pain with minimal risk from systemic absorption. Single injections of standard local anesthetic doses are unlikely to result in toxicity, although the duration of action may be unpredictable in renal failure patients. For example, supraclavicular block duration has been noted to be decreased by roughly 40 percent in renal failure patients, which is thought to be secondary to a high compensatory cardiac output in the face of normal blood volume and reduced hematocrit. Increased tissue blood flow could tend to flush deposits of local anesthetics at a faster rate than in non–renal failure patients. The duration of axillary blocks appears to be less affected by renal failure.

Ester local anesthetics undergo rapid destruction by plasma cholinesterases to para-amino benzoic acid derivatives. Although a decreased synthesis of cholinesterase has been noted in renal failure patients, the change in plasma hydrolysis does not appear to be of clinical significance. Amide local anesthetics are metabolized by hepatic microsomal enzymes to primarily inactive compounds. Clearance, therefore, is mainly dependent on nonrenal mechanisms, although the polar metabolites may accumulate. Lidocaine has a similar clearance and half-life in renal failure patients as compared with controls, with only 20 percent urinary excretion of the parent compound. Its metabolite monoethylglycinexylidide may be elevated twofold or more in renal failure patients, and may be partially responsible for its toxicity.

5. Nonpharmacologic adjuncts Adjuncts such as self-regulation techniques, including hypnosis and relaxation training or transcutaneous electrical nerve stimulation (TENS) units, are particularly suited to the patient with impaired drug elimination. Even if unable to provide complete relief of pain, the addition of these techniques may allow significant reductions in the doses of pharmacologic agents used.

a. Hypnosis is an altered state of consciousness during which a patient is able to exert heightened control over specific sensory modalities through suggestion, imagination, and attention redirection. Appropriately trained practitioners can best induce hypnosis in susceptible patients who have reasonable expectations of its utility as a pain modulator. Useful for both acute and chronic pain syndromes, hypnosis helps the patient to reinterpret pain signals as diminished but tolerable stimuli. Cannulation pain, muscle cramps, joint pains, renal colic pain, or other pains from renal dysfunction may respond to hypnosis.

b. Relaxation techniques lead to a self-induced state of decreased anxiety, muscle tone, and sympathetic activity not related to any depression in consciousness. It can be used to ameliorate pain symptoms temporarily through deep breathing or muscle relaxation—especially if the stimulus is expected (e.g., cannulation pain). Both hypnosis and self-relaxation require an awake patient who can understand and follow instructions, which may not apply to many critically ill patients.

c. TENS may work to down-modulate afferent nociceptive signals, primarily at the spinal cord level. Electrodes can be applied at the site of local injuries producing pain, and regulated by the patient or by nursing personnel, if the patient is not awake or capable. Dual electrodes must be juxtaposed to the injury site, which might be precluded by dressings or other devices. Although TENS rarely achieves complete analgesia, supplementation with pharmacologic agents may be significantly reduced.

CASE DISCUSSION

> The previously described case exhibits several important concepts that must be considered when attempting to treat a patient with painful symptoms in the face of impaired renal function. The major contributor to this patient's somatic complaints most likely is underlying renal osteodystrophy, as typified by osteitis fibrosa and osteomalacia. Most patients with long-standing ESRD develop one or more of the components of ROD, as seen in this patient who was on hemodialysis for more than 10 years. An extensive history of slowly

progressing, vague lower back or joint pain with minimal physical findings is typical. Aggressive attempts at normalizing electrolyte levels—particularly calcium and phosphate—need to include calcium supplementation, phosphate binders, calcitriol or, infrequently, parathyroidectomy. Joint pain may arise from the late dialysis periarticular syndrome, particularly if the hand and shoulder are involved. Hand and wrist pains are more common on the side of an existing fistula, distal to the cannulation. If an ischemic steal secondary to major proximal collateral vessels can be demonstrated, surgical closure of some venous collaterals may decrease pain. Hip and shoulder deposition of 2-microglobulin amyloid fibrils has also been suggested as a source of pain in hemodialyzed patients. Use of PD or specialized HD techniques/membranes may decrease its incidence. Inflamed, swollen, or warm joints with point tenderness are less commonly seen, and may indicate infectious causes which need to be investigated (e.g., by arthrocentesis or radiographic imaging).

Abdominal complaints often arise during HD as urea and other solutes are rapidly removed. The dysequilibrium syndrome typically includes headache, nausea, vomiting, and agitation, which can be lessened by slowing the rate of HD and using higher osmolality dialysates or added parenteral hypertonic solutions. If the HD is performed on a new dialytic membrane, the syndrome associated with first dialyzer use may be responsible for cramps, nausea, vomiting, headache, and pain (usually in the back or chest). The reuse of membranes for subsequent treatments decreases these symptoms. If the patient has an indwelling PD catheter, peritonitis must be considered in the differential diagnosis of abdominal pain, requiring peritoneal culturing, antibiotic administration, and possibly catheter removal.

Respiratory depression in this setting most likely is due to indiscriminate narcotic administration, especially when given by an unpredictable route (IM) from which there may be delayed uptake and the necessity for multiple doses. The use of smaller, IV boluses will achieve therapeutic levels more rapidly and without the delay of IM or subcutaneous deposits, and PCA could then be used to maintain the analgesia. Patient drowsiness would prevent self-overadministration. Morphine sulfate, because of its hepatic glucuronidation to active metabolites, may accumulate in patients with impaired renal function and depress respiratory drive. Although expected to be partially hemodialyzed (low protein binding, low molecular weight, but moderately large Vd), large doses can potentially exceed the rate of HD removal. The use of agents without respiratory depression (e.g., NSAIDs) or without potent metabolites (e.g., fentanyl) may be more appropriate. Even though the patient is currently on mechanical ventilation and respiratory depression is not an issue, ultimately she must be weaned from mechanical support. Pain emanating from areas appropriate for regional or local neural blockade, in the absence of any contraindication (such as coagulopathy), can be controlled effectively with techniques that lessen the risk of respiratory depression.

In light of this patient's chronic underlying disease and symptomatology, and especially with the need for repeated painful procedures, she might have prolonged benefit from adjunct measures such as self-relaxation or hypnosis, in order to reduce her overall need for pharmacologic agents. As long as the patient is able to communicate and interact objectively, intubation and critical illness do not interfere significantly with the use of these techniques.

SUGGESTED READINGS

Alfrey AC, Chan L: Chronic renal failure: manifestations and pathogenesis, in Schrier RW (ed): *Renal and Electrolyte Disorders,* 4th ed. Boston, Little, Brown, 1992, chap 11, pp 539–579.

Aronoff GR, Abel SR: Practical guidelines for drug dosing in patients with renal impairment, in Schrier RW (ed): *Manual of Nephrology,* 3d ed. Boston, Little, Brown, 1990, chap 11, pp 189–201.

Bennett WM: *Drugs and Renal Disease,* 2d ed. New York, Churchill Livingstone, 1986.

Kay J: Renal disorders, in Cheng EY, Kay J (eds): *Manual of Anesthesia and the Medically Compromised Patient.* Philadelphia, JB Lippincott, 1990, chap 4, pp 244–266.

Maher JF: Pharmacokinetic alterations with renal failure and dialysis, in Chernow B (ed): *The Pharmacologic Approach to the Critically Ill Patient,* 2d ed. Baltimore, Williams & Wilkins, 1988, chap 3, pp 47–68.

Steinman TI, Lazarus JM: Organ-system involvement in acute renal failure, in Brenner BM, Lazarus JM (eds): *Acute Renal Failure,* 2d ed. New York, Churchill Livingstone, 1988, chap 21, pp 705–739.

CHAPTER
20

HEPATOBILIARY DISEASE

Catherine K. Lineberger

Case
 I. Pathophysiology of Hepatic Failure
    A. Types of Hepatic Dysfunction
    B. Use of Medications
 II. Pain Syndromes Related to to the Hepatobiliary System
    A. The Liver and Gallbladder
    B. The Pancreas
 III. Effect of Hepatic Failure on Pain Management
    A. Hepatic Clearance
    B. Hepatic Blood Flow
    C. Severe Hepatic Dysfunction
    D. Unpredictability of Drug Effects
Case Discussion
Suggested Readings

CASE

A 52-year-old male alcoholic was admitted to the intensive care unit (ICU) with fever, right-upper-quadrant pain, and jaundice. Broad-spectrum antibiotics were started for a presumed diagnosis of ascending cholangitis, and blood cultures were positive for *Escherichia coli.* The patient's fever defervesced, but he remained jaundiced, and he continued to have midepigastric and right-upper-quadrant pain.

An abdominal computed tomography (CT) scan revealed a pancreatic mass near the ampulla of Vater. Endoscopic retrograde cholangiopancreatography (ERCP) confirmed obstruction of the pancreatic duct at the ampulla, and biopsy was consistent with adenocarcinoma. Surgical resection was deemed inappropriate, as the mass was too extensive. A pain service consultation was requested to assist in managing this patient's pain.

Hepatobiliary disease comprises several major organ systems and includes a whole host of disease conditions. To examine each of these in detail is beyond the scope of this chapter, but some of the major causes of painful conditions related to the hepatobiliary tree that are likely to be encountered in the critical care setting are discussed.

I. PATHOPHYSIOLOGY OF HEPATIC FAILURE

A. Types of Hepatic Dysfunction

Hepatic dysfunction can be classified as follows (see Table 20-1):
   1. **Prehepatic**—The liver is overwhelmed by excessive bilirubin from hemolysis or hematoma resolution, for example.
   2. **Intrahepatic**—Hepatocellular destruction/degeneration results from multiple etiologies, including viral infection, sepsis, cirrhosis, drugs, and hypoxemia.
   3. **Posthepatic**—The liver drainage is obstructed, as with gallstones, sepsis, or pancreatic masses.

B. Use of Medications

Patients who are critically ill and have associated hepatic dysfunction require careful attention when drugs are administered for any reason, since so many of the drugs (pain medications or others) are cleared and metabolized by the liver (see Table 20-2).
   1. **Decreases in hepatic blood flow** will decrease the clearance of many drugs.
   2. **Intrahepatic dysfunction** will result in decreased enzymatic function, which can decrease drug clearance and alter the metabolic transformation of substances normally metabolized by the liver.
   3. If hepatic dysfunction is severe enough to impede the synthesis of albumin and other plasma proteins, **less protein will be available for drug binding,** and, therefore, a greater percentage of free drug will be available at the receptor site.

Table 20-1 Characteristic laboratory findings in hepatic dysfunction

Type of dysfunction	Serum bilirubin	Transaminases	Alkaline phosphatase
Prehepatic	Unconjugated	Normal	Normal
Intrahepatic	Conjugated	Elevated	Normal to slightly elevated
Posthepatic	Conjugated	Normal to slightly elevated	Highly elevated

Table 20-2 Pain management medications with significant hepatic metabolism

Narcotics	Others
Meperidine	Acetaminophen
Morphine	Amide local anesthetics
Methadone	Benzodiazepines
Fentanyl	Droperidol
Alfentanil	Barbiturates
Sufentanil	Diphenhydramine
Hydromorphone	
Nalbuphine	
Butorphanol	
Dezocine	

4. Additionally, the **volume of distribution increases.**

5. Therefore, there is **great potential for exaggerated drug effects and toxicity** from usual drug doses.

II. PAIN SYNDROMES RELATED TO THE HEPATOBILIARY SYSTEM: PATHOGENESIS AND RELATED PAIN MANAGEMENT

A. The Liver and Gallbladder

1. **The anatomy of hepatobiliary pain**

   a. The liver is innervated by branches of the vagus and splanchnic nerves, forming a network of sympathetic and parasympathetic nerve fibers. Afferent sympathetic nerve fibers are felt to be the principal afferent pathway for transmission of hepatic pain to the central nervous system (CNS).

   b. Classically, **hepatic pain** has been attributed to capsular stretch, which can result from enlargement of the hepatic stroma from intrahepatic masses, parenchymal swelling or passive congestion. In some inflammatory processes, somatic pain can be elicited if peritonitis ensues. Hepatic pain is usually localized to the upper abdomen and lower chest. Referred hepatic pain is classically described as radiating to the right shoulder and scapula.

   c. Similarly, **biliary pain** is usually related to distension of the gallbladder itself, or to spasmodic peristalsis of the biliary duct. The pain is usually intense and localized in the right upper quadrant or epigastrium. The gallbladder is richly innervated by both the splanchnic and vagus plexuses, but the predominant afferent pathway is via the sympathetic fibers, much like hepatic pain.

2. Hepatic tumors Tumors may be primary (hepatoma) or secondary (metastases). Although hepatomas may be asymptomatic for years, patients with metastatic hepatic disease frequently present with pain as a predominant symptom. The pain is epigastric, dull and constant, and associated with varying degrees of anorexia, fatigue, epigastric fullness, and weight loss. Jaundice may be an early finding in primary hepatic tumors, but is usually late in onset with metastatic disease, and reflects biliary obstruction from disease in the porta hepatis.

    a. For patients who have **resectable disease,** curative resection should alleviate painful symptoms.

    b. However, the vast majority of patients with hepatic tumors have **widespread disease** at the time of diagnosis, and are not candidates for resection for cure. For these patients, it is imperative to control painful symptoms. Efforts should be made to optimize the patient's overall well-being. For example, consideration should be given to treatment of pruritus with diphenhydramine (Benadryl) or other agents, and uncomfortable abdominal distension from ascites can be alleviated with paracentesis. Prophylaxis against constipation in patients receiving opioids should be achieved with stool softeners and bulk-forming agents. Optimization of nutritional status is of paramount importance. Chemotherapy, either intravenous (IV) or via hepatic artery infusion, may offer some palliative benefit in certain cases.

    c. Initial management for pain associated with hepatic tumors should include nonsteroidal antiinflammatory drugs (NSAIDs) and oral narcotics. Establishing analgesic levels of long-acting oral narcotic (e.g., MS Contin) may require titration over several days, and it is imperative that the patient's acute pain be controlled with rapid-onset oral medication (e.g., MS elixir), or IV narcotics, such as patient-controlled administration of morphine. In patients who are unable to tolerate oral medications, or who require huge doses of opiates, central neuraxial opioid administration via intraspinal or epidural routes can be considered, and may provide excellent pain relief. Implantable pumps and access ports are available for the chronic administration of spinal or epidural opioids and eliminate the need for repeated invasive procedures. Transdermal administration of narcotic (e.g., TTS fentanyl) may also be an option for patients who cannot tolerate oral medications.

    d. Adjuvants such as tricyclic antidepressants may be effective for pain relief, and also to treat the reactive depression often associated with the diagnosis of malignancy.

    e. If all of these measures are unsatisfactory, more **invasive measures** may be considered, such as splanchnicectomy or celiac plexus blockade. (With local anesthetic and/or a neurolytic agent).

3. Hepatitis An acute viral infection of the liver, hepatitis is often associated with dull, achy right-upper-quadrant pain and tenderness of the liver on palpation. This is mediated by hepatic enlargement and stretch of the capsule of the liver. Fever, myalgia, anorexia, and fatigue are the predominant associated symptoms, and jaundice is common.

    a. Therapy for hepatitis is supportive. It is important to avoid hepatotoxins, such as acetaminophen.

    b. The **pain associated with hepatitis** is generally easy to control with IV narcotics if the patient cannot tolerate oral medications. Drug selection for analgesia should be tempered with caution if significant hepatic dysfunction is present (see below).

  4. Biliary colic Cholecystectomy for episodes of painful **biliary colic** accounts for a large percentage of operations performed each year. Most patients with symptomatic gallstones **(cholelithiasis)** present with biliary colic.

    a. This pain is usually nonspecific and midepigastric, and then localizes to the right upper quadrant in most cases. Though the episodes of biliary colic may be sporadic, they are characterized by constant and intense pain. Anorexia, nausea, and vomiting often accompany the episodes. If the obstruction to biliary tract outflow persists, varying degrees of inflammation will occur **(cholecystitis).** This pain is typically located in the right upper quadrant, and palpation of this area intensifies the pain. Fever often accompanies the syndrome.

    b. Cholecystectomy is the treatment of choice for recurrent biliary colic and cholecystitis, and alleviates pain in the vast majority of cases.

      (i) NSAIDs have been shown to decrease smooth muscle tone and greatly improve biliary colic in a significant number of cases, obviating the need for surgery.

      (ii) Many narcotics have been demonstrated to cause spasm of the sphincter of Oddi, and this may exacerbate pain and complicate the interpretation of cholangiograms. However, spasm does not occur in the vast majority of cases, and narcotic-induced spasm can be readily reversed with either naloxone or glucagon. Therefore, it does not seem sensible to withhold narcotic therapy from these patients, if other therapy, such as NSAIDs, is not controlling the pain sufficiently.

      (iii) Other measures for pain relief postoperatively can include intercostal nerve blocks and peridural opiates and/or local anesthetics. The advent of laparoscopic cholecystectomy has decreased the pain and morbidity of cholecystectomy.

      (iv) Patients who continue to have pain following cholecystectomy require a further workup to rule out other disease processes, or complications of cholecystectomy, such as retained common bile duct stones or an incomplete procedure.

B. The Pancreas

1. The anatomy of pancreatic pain

a. The pancreas is a **retroperitoneal organ,** and thus somatic pain does not result from pancreatic disorders unless associated inflammation extends beyond the lesser sac.

b. Like the liver and gallbladder, the **innervation** of the pancreas is both sympathetic and parasympathetic, via the splanchnic nerves and the celiac division of the vagus respectively. Pancreatic pain seems to be mediated via sympathetic afferents, as vagotomy does not produce relief of such pain.

c. The **pain associated with pancreatic disorders** is classically described as severe, boring, or stabbing, and is usually localized to the epigastrium or upper midabdomen. Radiation to the midback or lower thoracic spine is frequent.

2. Acute pancreatitis
In the United States, the two conditions most commonly associated with **acute pancreatitis** are alcoholism and gallstone disease. Less commonly, hypertriglyceridemia and hypercalcemia have been associated with acute pancreatitis. The hallmark of acute pancreatitis, regardless of the causative factor, is extravasation of pancreatic enzymes into the pancreas and surrounding tissues, causing tissue necrosis, edema, and severe inflammation.

a. Upper abdominal **pain,** often with radiation through to the back, and of an unrelenting and severe nature, is the hallmark of acute pancreatitis. The onset of symptoms can be quite rapid. Nausea and vomiting accompany the pain most of the time. Patients are often dehydrated and tachycardic when they present. The severity of the abdominal pain invokes reflex spasm of the abdominal wall musculature, which can be severe enough to compromise ventilation. Hypoxemia is a frequent finding, and some degree of ileus is nearly universal. Acute pancreatitis is a severe, unpredictable disease with a high incidence of complications, morbidity, and mortality. Patients with this disease require aggressive treatment and support.

b. Once the diagnosis of acute pancreatitis has been made, **narcotic analgesics** are the most common pain therapy employed. Oral narcotics are usually avoided as the patients are NPO to minimize pancreatic stimulation. As in gallbladder disease, some concern exists over narcotic-induced spasm of the sphincter of Oddi. Some feel that meperidine (Demerol) is less likely to induce spasm as compared with morphine, but this is controversial. Fentanyl has been shown to cause spasm as well. Epidural or spinal opioids offer the advantage of providing good pain relief at lower doses than needed with systemic narcotics, thereby reducing the risk of spasm of the sphincter of Oddi.

c. Small doses of **narcotic agonist-antagonists** (e.g., nalbuphine

[Nubain], 2.5 to 5 mg IV q4h) can reverse sphincter-of-Oddi spasm caused by narcotic agonists while supplementing their analgesic effects. Agonist–antagonist drugs should be used with extreme caution in patients who have been receiving pure agonists for more than several days as withdrawal can be triggered.

    d. Epidural administration of dilute solutions of **local anesthetics** can provide excellent pain relief, and can improve ventilatory status in patients with abdominal muscle spasm. Additionally, celiac plexus block with local anesthetic has provided temporary relief of the pain associated with acute pancreatitis.

   3. Chronic pancreatitis This is believed to be a distinct entity from acute pancreatitis. In the United States, approximately 90 percent of chronic pancreatitis is caused by alcoholism, with the cause of the remaining 10 percent less clear. Gallstone disease is not felt to be a cause of chronic pancreatitis.

    a. Abdominal pain is the primary characteristic of chronic pancreatitis. Some patients experience constant, unremitting, gnawing epigastric pain, while others have episodic attacks of pain with intervening pain-free intervals. **Anorexia** accompanies the syndrome, as eating often exacerbates the pain. **Weight loss** is a frequent occurrence. Additionally, most patients with chronic pancreatitis have evidence of both endocrine (diabetes mellitus) and exocrine (malabsorption, steatorrhea) pancreatic dysfunction. An association between the amount of pancreatic function and pain has been elucidated. Patients seem to experience persistent and lasting pain relief once pancreatic secretory dysfunction becomes severe. This typically occurs in alcoholic patients after about 5 years.

    b. Therapy for the pain resulting from chronic pancreatitis can be medical or surgical. It should be noted that dietary modification and drugs to decrease pancreatic secretion have not been effective in reducing pain. In most cases, **narcotic analgesia** is required to achieve pain relief, and because of the chronic nature of the disease, this often leads to narcotic dependence.

    c. NSAIDs seem to be of limited value. Transcutaneous electrical nerve stimulation **(TENS)** across the epigastrium or paravertebrally at T5–7 may be of benefit to these patients, providing a nonmedication, patient-controlled modality to reduce pain. **Antidepressant** medication (e.g., amitriptyline [Elavil], 10 to 150 mg qhs) may enhance the analgesia from narcotics, aid in restoring more normal sleep patterns, and modify CNS sensitization to pain processing.

    d. If narcotic therapy is ineffective at controlling pain, various **neurolytic procedures** can be considered. These include celiac plexus blockade and splanchnic blockade, achieved either percutaneously or at the time of laparotomy during surgical therapy. Although pain relief can be quite dramatic initially, the pain frequently recurs weeks to months after neurolytic blockade. This is also true of surgical splanchnicectomy, which can be achieved via laparotomy or thoracoscopy.

     e. Surgical therapy for the pain of pancreatitis involves decompression of the pancreatic duct by performing pancreaticojejeunostomy, or resecting a significant portion of the pancreas to decrease the amount of functioning (and, therefore, pain-producing) pancreatic tissue. After both surgeries, diabetes and malabsorption are common. The success of these procedures in relieving pain (estimated at about 50 percent in some series) must be examined in the context of the natural history of chronic pancreatitis, which tends to "burn out" after several years.

    4. Pancreatic carcinoma   This carcinoma is increasing in incidence, and therapy thus far has not changed the grim statistics that less than 2 percent of patients survive for 5 years.

     a. Pain is the predominant feature of pancreatic carcinoma. The pain is typically characterized as vague and midepigastric, with rapid increases in severity. It is described as gnawing, and frequently radiates to the back. Weight loss and anorexia are often associated with the pain, and jaundice is a frequent finding, though it may develop late in the course of the disease.

     b. Most patients with pancreatic carcinoma cannot undergo curative **resection** of their disease, as it has usually spread beyond the pancreas at the time of diagnosis. **Radiation therapy** is not successful in these patients because of the location of the pancreas and the vulnerability of adjacent organs and the bowel to radiation damage. **Chemotherapy** is merely palliative. Given the extremely poor prognosis associated with pancreatic cancer, the relief of painful symptoms should be the first priority in these patients. Additionally, therapy directed toward **symptomatic relief** of associated problems should be provided, such as stool softeners to prevent constipation from narcotics and biliary decompression to relieve pruritis if biliary tract obstruction occurs. The optimization of the patient's **nutritional** status is important, and steatorrhea can be treated with **pancreatic enzyme replacement therapy.**

     c. Pain management is similar to that described for hepatic neoplasm. **Narcotics** should be the first line of therapy, and most patients can be maintained on oral medication during most of their illness. If oral narcotics become inadequate or high doses induce intolerance or side effects, parenteral or transdermal narcotic therapy can be attempted. Other possibilities include intrathecal or epidural narcotics, either for short-term management or via chronically implanted subcutaneous pumps or reservoirs. If these measures fail to provide adequate pain relief, **neurolytic celiac plexus block** or splanchnicectomy can be considered if skilled personnel are available. The same adjuvant therapies as used in chronic pancreatitis can be employed when managing the pain of pancreatic malignancy.

III. EFFECT OF HEPATIC FAILURE ON PAIN MANAGEMENT

A. Hepatic Clearance

Most of the drugs used in patient care are metabolized and/or cleared by the liver; therefore, it might be expected that severe hepatic dysfunction could affect the eventual disposition of drugs used for pain management. The **hepatic clearance** of a drug depends on hepatic blood flow, hepatocellular uptake and transformation, and the degree of protein binding of the drug (that which is protein bound is unavailable for elimination).

B. Hepatic Blood Flow

If hepatic blood flow is decreased, because of either decreased cardiac output or impaired blood flow due to cirrhosis, for example, drugs with a high hepatic clearance, such as meperidine and local anesthetics, will be cleared less effectively, resulting in higher blood levels of drug. Certain liver diseases can cause impaired hepatocellular enzyme function because of hepatocellular necrosis (e.g., hepatitis), and one could expect reductions in enzymatic function, such as glucuronidation, demethylation, and oxidation.

C. Severe Hepatic Dysfunction

Severe hepatic dysfunction can cause the **decreased synthesis of proteins,** such as albumin and other plasma proteins, thereby decreasing the amount of protein available for drug binding and resulting in higher effective plasma levels for a given drug dose. Impaired hepatic synthesis of **coagulation factors** may affect the advisability of performing regional blocks for pain relief. **Hyperbilirubinemia** associated with hepatic failure may alter the function of the **blood–brain barrier,** resulting in greater and more prolonged activity than usually expected from a single dose of drugs.

D. Unpredictability of Drug Effects

Because of the unpredictability of the effect or toxicity of a given dose of drug in a patient with hepatic failure, a strategy for pain management that employs low doses of safe medication is ideal.

   1. **Spinal and epidural opiates** offer excellent analgesia for a wide variety of postoperative and chronic pain conditions, provided that these routes are not contraindicated by coagulopathy. The addition of dilute amounts of **local anesthetic** to an epidural opiate infusion can reduce the dose of narcotic necessary for adequate analgesia and minimize the side effects of the

narcotic, but the associated sympathetic blockade can complicate the management of a hemodynamically unstable patient.

2. For patients who cannot tolerate oral medication, transdermal fentanyl systems (Duragesic) and hydromorphone (Dilaudid) suppositories can offer **alternative routes of administration.**

3. **Ketorolac tromethamine** (Toradol), a parenterally available NSAID, is useful to provide analgesia without respiratory depression or sedation, unless contraindicated by coagulopathy, peptic ulcer disease, or renal dysfunction, and can be used as an adjunct to minimize the amount of narcotic required for analgesia. The half-life of ketorolac is mildly elevated in liver disease.

4. **Patient-controlled IV analgesia** (PCA) is an attractive option for postoperative pain relief with hepatic disease, although decreased doses of drug or increased lockout interval times may be required to avoid excessive accumulation of the drug and side effects in patients with severe liver failure. Some writers say they avoid morphine sulfate in this patient population because of its long half-life, and recommend fentanyl as the ideal parenteral drug in severe hepatic dysfunction. The use of PCA with subcutaneous hydromorphone may be another effective modality, although each of these drugs is hepatically metabolized and drug accumulation due to decreased metabolism requires careful titration and monitoring of analgesia and sedation levels. The risk of excessive drug response may be limited by eliminating the basal rate.

5. Finally, in patients with severe hepatic dysfunction and coagulopathy, it may be possible to use **peripheral nerve blocks** if appropriate, for the painful condition. Caution must be utilized in choosing the dosage of local anesthetic, as the amide local anesthetics are metabolized by the liver, and elimination may be delayed. Utilization of more dilute solutions than normal and of adjuvants such as ketorolac tromethamine may provide adequate analgesia without significantly increasing the risk of systemic toxicity.

CASE DISCUSSION

The pain management team recommended IV fentanyl delivered by PCA for pain control until the patient was able to take oral medications. This provided the patient with the ability to adjust his dosing to meet his analgesic need. Morphine or hydromorphone could also have been used. Once the patient had established his analgesic requirements and was tolerating oral intake, MS Contin was started. (See Chapter 28 for IV to PO conversion calculations.) Twelve hours after the oral morphine was started, the PCA basal rate was tapered off but the self-administration mode was maintained until the patient had been on MS Contin for at least 24 h. The patient was also given a faster-onset, shorter-duration narcotic medication (e.g., hydromorphone, 2 mg PO q3h prn) for breakthrough pain.

He eventually developed intermittent gastric outlet obstruction and was unable to tolerate pills. The patient refused surgery to relieve his obstruction, and was seen again by the pain team for consideration of celiac plexus block. A diagnostic celiac plexus block with lidocaine provided excellent pain relief, and this was followed by a neurolytic celiac plexus block, which provided pain relief that lasted until the patient's death a few weeks later.

SUGGESTED READINGS

Atron ML, Kalra J: Patient-controlled analgesia for the treatment of oncologic pain, in Ferrante FM, Ostheimer GW, Covino BG (eds): *Patient-Controlled Analgesia.* Cambridge, Massachusetts, Blackwell Scientific Publications, 1990, pp 107–113.

Blendis LM: Abdominal pain, in Wall PD, Melzack R (eds): *Textbook of Pain.* New York, Churchill Livingstone, pp 350–358.

Gardner AM, Solumou G: Relief of the pain of unresectable carcinoma of the pancreas by chemical splanchnicectomy during laparotomy. *Ann R Coll Surg Engl* 66:409, 1984.

Gelman S: Anesthesia and the liver, in Barash PG, Cullen BF, Stoelting PK (eds): *Clinical Anesthesia,* Philadelphia, Lippincott, 1989, pp 1133–1162.

Mulholland MW, Debas HT: Diseases of the liver, biliary system, and pancreas, in Bonica JJ (ed): *The Management of Pain.* Philadelphia, Lea & Febiger, 1992, pp 1214–1231.

Sinatra RS: Pain management in patients suffering from major organ failure, in Sinatra RS, Hord AH, Ginsberg B, Preble LM (eds): *Acute Pain: Mechanisms and Management.* St Louis, Mosby, 1992, pp 399–411.

CHAPTER
21

PAIN MANAGEMENT IN PATIENTS WITH HEMOSTATIC FAILURE

Susan Anderson

Case
 I. Normal Hemostatic Function
    A. Vessels/Tissues
    B. Platelets
    C. Coagulation Factors—Intrinsic and Extrinsic Pathways
    D. Fibrinolysis
    E. Screening Tests
 II. Abnormal Hemostasis
    A. Vessel and Tissue Disorders
    B. Platelet Abnormalities
    C. Coagulation Factor Disorders
    D. Fibrinolytic System
    E. Therapy of Coagulopathies
    F. Thrombotic Disorders
 III. Pain Syndromes Specific to Bleeding Disorders
    A. Bleeding Disorders
    B. Thrombotic Disorders
    C. Vasculitis
 IV. Impact of Coagulopathy on Pain Management
    A. Systemic Narcotics
    B. Invasive Analgesic Techniques
    C. Alternative Analgesic Techniques
Case Discussion
Suggested Readings

CASE

A 19-year-old male is transferred from a small community hospital with a history of severe mononucleosis. Earlier that day, he had been taken to the operating room as an emergency because of a rapidly falling hematocrit and an enlarging abdomen. He had apparently suffered a splenic rupture when he fell on his way to the bathroom. During the laparotomy for exploration, he was noted to be profoundly coagulopathic. Appropriate and massive replacement therapy was administered without improvement, so a splenectomy was performed rather than an attempt made at splenic repair. Laboratory tests confirmed severe disseminated intravascular coagulopathy (DIC). Upon arrival at the tertiary care center, the patient is very pale, still intubated, and somewhat drowsy, but appears to respond appropriately to commands.

I. NORMAL HEMOSTATIC FUNCTION

A. Vessels/Tissues

Subendothelial exposure of collagen in vessel walls following damage promotes the following events:

1. The affected vessels constrict, platelets aggregate and adhere to the injured area, and the coagulation cascade is activated to form thrombin.

2. Thrombin splits plasma fibrinogen into fibrin monomers, which polymerize to form a mesh. This mesh holds the platelet plug in place.

3. Platelet contractile activity draws the fibrin strands together closely.

4. As the vessel is repaired, local production of plasmin hydrolyzes the fibrin mesh into soluble fibrin degradation products (FDPs).

5. Normal vessel endothelium is important for the synthesis of Factor VIII–related von Willebrand's factor (VIII:vWF), which facilitates platelet binding to exposed collagen, and prostacyclin (which vasodilates and prevents excessive platelet plug formation).

B. Platelets

1. The normal platelet count of 150,000 to 350,000/μL is maintained by a balance between platelet utilization and stimulated production by the hormone thrombopoietin. The life span of platelets is about 10 days.

2. Platelets have no nucleus, but contain actin, myosin, and granules. Platelet membranes are able to adsorb circulating plasma coagulation factors, and are a source of arachidonic acid. Once a platelet becomes adherent, arachidonic acid is converted to endoperoxides by cyclooxygenase, which are then converted to thromboxane A_2 by thromboxane synthetase. This causes platelet degranulation, releasing enzymes, proteins, and substrates important for initiating the coagulation cascade and repairing the damaged vessel wall.

C. Coagulation Factors—Intrinsic and Extrinsic Pathways

The final product of both pathways is thrombin (Factor IIa), which is needed to convert circulating fibrinogen into fibrin for the platlet plug. Figure 21-1 gives a simplified outline. The final stage of both pathways is via Factor V, requiring platelets and calcium.

   1. The **intrinsic pathway** is initiated by Factor XII and kininogen, which are adsorbed to the negatively charged subendothelium at damaged areas in the vessel. Factor XI and prekallikrein are also needed.
   2. The **extrinsic pathway** requires a tissue factor produced only when tissue is damaged (tissue thromboplastin). This factor forms a complex with Factor VII.

D. Fibrinolysis

Once bleeding has stopped and vessel repair is under way, the fibrin polymers are lyzed. Plasmin, derived from plasminogen, is the active enzyme which is adsorbed onto the fibrin mesh.

E. Screening Tests

Table 21-1 lists the screening tests used for hemostasis.

II. ABNORMAL HEMOSTASIS

A. Vessel and Tissue Disorders

   1. In **amyloidosis,** amyloid is deposited in the skin and vascular wall, increasing fragility and predisposing to ecchymoses and petechiae. Factor X also adsorbs to the amyloid, and may lead to decreased circulating levels. Despite infiltration of the liver with amyloid, the stigmata of liver disease, including the coagulation defects, are uncommon.
   2. Excessive **corticosteroids** (Cushing's syndrome or exogenous steroids) cause a weakening of the perivascular supporting tissues, which increases the susceptibility to vascular trauma.
   3. **Hereditary disorders of the connective tissue,** such as Ehlers-Danlos syndrome, Marfan's syndrome, or osteogenesis imperfecta, are marked by increased bleeding due to defective connective tissue and perivascular supporting structures. There are also abnormalities of the large vessels. The result is increased vascular fragility and abnormal platelet adhesiveness.
   4. A **drug-induced purpura** can occur in the face of normal platelet number and function. Offending agents include sulfa drugs, penicillins, chlorothiazides, and coumarin derivatives. The purpura resolve with discontinuation of the drug.

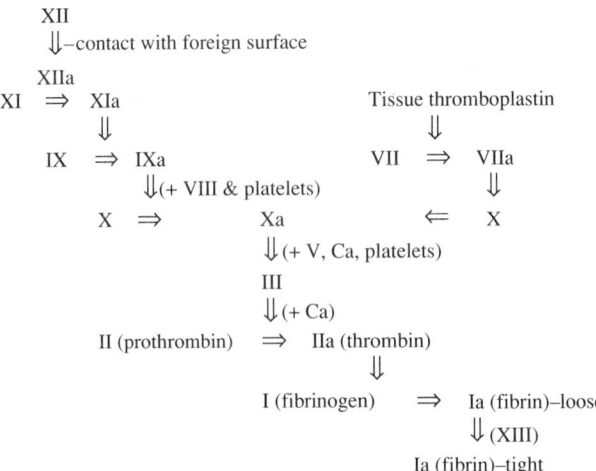

Figure 21-1 The coagulation cascade.

5. **Kaposi's hemorrhagic sarcoma** results from the proliferation of vascular elements. The cutaneous stigmata result from local bleeding and subsequent hemosiderin deposition. This problem is seen in patients with the human immunodeficiency virus (HIV) and in patients who are receiving immunosuppressive therapy.

6. **Schönlein-Henoch purpura** (allergic purpura) occurs primarily in young (2- to 7-year-old) males. The syndrome can include ecchymoses, arthralgias, abdominal pains, and acute glomerulonephritis. Biopsy of skin lesions shows aseptic vasculitis.

Table 21-1 Screening tests for hemostasis

Name	System tested	Abnormality detected
PTT (partial thromboplastin time)	Intrinsic pathway	Low Factors XII, XI, IX, VIII, X, V, II, I; prekallikrein, or kininogen
PT (prothrombin time)	Extrinsic pathway	Low Factors VII, X, V, II, or I; liver disease; vitamin K deficiency; coumadin
TT (thrombin time)	Fibrinogen→fibrin	Fibrin deficiency, inhibition of thrombin by heparin or FDPs
Fibrinogen	Amount of fibrinogen	Hypofibrinogenemia
FDP (fibrin degradation products)	Fibrinolysis	Disseminated intravascular coagulation (DIC)
Bleeding time	Platelet function	Platelet dysfunction, von Willebrand's disease, ASA

B. Platelet Abnormalities

Platelet abnormalities can be separated into low platelet count (from a reduced production or decreased survival time) and platelet dysfunction.

   1. The **reduced production of platelets** by the bone marrow can be caused by infiltration (leukemia, myelofibrosis), marrow hypoplasia (drugs, toxins, radiation), viral infections, or defective maturation of the megakaryocyte (alcoholism, megaloblastic anemia, and thiazide diuretics).
   2. **Decreased survival time** can be due to the destruction, consumption, or sequestration of platelets.

      a. **Destruction** occurs with idiopathic thrombocytopenia purpura (ITP), an autoimmune disorder in which IgG antibodies are produced against platelets. The platelet–Ab complexes are destroyed in the spleen by macrophages. Other causes of platelet destruction include infections and the development of antiplatelet antibodies after transfusion. Increased destruction of platelets may also be secondary to an immunologic disorder (e.g., systemic lupus erythematosus [SLE] or lymphoma) or can be seen with certain drugs (See Table 21-2). Drug-induced immune thrombocytopenia was first described with quinine, but can also occur after therapy with quinidine, heparin, para-aminosalicylic acid (PAS), penicillins, sulfonamides, thiazides, H_2 blockers, methyldopa, and digitoxin. Initial exposure has to be for a minimum of 7 days; subsequent therapy induces an acute fall in platelet count. Platelets can also be destroyed by mechanical interventions such as dialyzers, intra-aortic balloon pumps, and ventricular assist devices. The decreased platelet count can be related to platelet adsorption onto membranes and other surfaces in these devices.

      b. **Consumption of platelets** occurs with DIC and with hemangiomas.

      c. **Hypersplenism** from any cause may result in increased destruction and **sequestration** of platelets in the splenic pool.

      d. **Massive transfusion** (more than 10 units of blood) causes thrombocytopenia by dilution. There may be associated DIC, as well as platelet dysfunction. Platelet count rarely falls below $50,000/\mu L$ in this setting. Tests for DIC should be obtained and appropriate replacement therapy initiated.

Table 21-2 Drugs affecting platelets

Drug	Mechanism
Acetylsalicylic acid (ASA, aspirin)	Irreversibly inhibits cyclooxygenase
Penicillin G, carbenicillin, ticarcillin, ampicillin (not methicillin or cephalosporins)	Adsorbs onto membrane and prevents platelet adherence
NSAIDs (indomethacin, phenylbutazone, ibuprofen)	Inhibits cyclooxygenase
Imidazole antifungal agents	Inhibits thromboxane synthetase

3. **Platelet dysfunction** can be congenital or acquired.

    a. The **congenital disorders** are either defects of platelet secretion or disorders of membrane glycoprotein.

    b. **Acquired dysfunction** is associated with myeloproliferative disorers (e.g., thrombocythemia, polcythemia vera). Clinically, there is a bleeding tendency, prolonged bleeding time, and abnormal platelet adhesiveness and granule content. Thrombotic thrombocytopenic purpura (TTP) is manifested as microangiopathy, affecting the cerebral and intestinal vasculature. Renal, hepatic, and pulmonary involvement are also seen. The etiology and pathophysiology remain obscure; hemolysis and thrombocytopenia may lead to severe hemostatic failure. Renal and liver disease affect platelet function, as do acute and chronic alcohol abuse. The presence of pathologic plasma proteins (e.g., FDPs and macroglobulins) increases bleeding tendencies. Aspirin and the other nonsteroidal anti-inflammatory drugs (NSAIDs) inhibit cyclooxygenase, which impedes the release of dense granules, and subsequently platelet aggregation. Aspirin binds irreversibly to the enzyme, while the other NSAIDs are only competitive inhibitors. As such, aspirin will affect platelet adhesiveness for 7 to 10 days, and NSAIDs for 6 to 24 h, depending on the plasma level. Although these effects are not usually clinically important, in the face of trauma, surgery, or a coagulopathy of another etiology, the platelet effects may be significant.

C. Coagulation Factor Disorders

Coagulation factor disorders can result from either reduced or defective synthesis of coagulation factors, which causes bleeding. The deficit can be either congenital or acquired.

    1. **Congenital disorders** usually involve a single factor deficiency.

    a. **Hemophilia A,** or Factor VIII deficiency, is the most common defect. It is an X-linked recessive disease occurring in one in 10,000 males. Patients may have inadequate or no production of Factor VIII, or may have normal Factor VIII levels that are nonfunctional. Deficient Factor VIII slows thrombin generation via the intrinsic pathway. The clinical severity of the disease usually correlates with the level of Factor VIII, and is classified as severe (less than 1 percent of normal activity), moderate (1 to 5 percent of normal activity), and mild (5 to 25 percent of normal activity). Although bleeding is not usually a clinical problem in patients with a Factor VIII activity level higher than 5 percent of normal, severe trauma or major surgery may necessitate factor replacement. Spontaneous bleeding is rare if activity levels are greater than 1 percent of normal, but bleeding into the joints, muscles (especially after intramuscular [IM] injections), gut, genitourinary tract, and central nervous system (CNS) can occur and requires adequate treatment with cryoprecipitate transfusion. Partial thromboplastin time (PTT) is prolonged; prothrombin time (PT), thrombin time (TT), platelet count, and fibrinogen levels are normal.

     b. Von Willebrand's disease is an autosomal dominant coagulation disorder due to low levels of Factor VIII:vWF. Platelet adherence is affected, resulting in excessive bleeding after trauma, spontaneous bleeding from mucosal membranes, and menorrhagia. Bleeding time is prolonged in spite of a normal platelet count. Available treatment includes cryoprecipitate and DDAVP.

     c. Hemophilia B, or Factor IX deficiency, is an X-linked recessive disease. Clinical features are the same as for hemophilia A, but specific factor assay will distinguish Factor IX abnormalities, and allow correct replacement therapy with fresh frozen plasma (FFP) when required. Epsilon-aminocaproic acid (EACA) can be used with FFP in the face of mucosal bleeding.

     d. Factors XI, X, VII, and V are rare autosomal inherited disorders that can be associated with clinically significant bleeding that may require replacement therapy.

     e. Factor XII, prekallikrein, and high-molecular-weight kininogen deficiencies can occur, but are unusually not clinically significant despite a prolonged PTT.

    2. Acquired disorders

     a. Vitamin K deficiency   Factors II, VII, IX, and X require vitamin K to be converted to a carboxylated form which is able to bind to platelets. These factors are involved in intrinsic and extrinsic pathways. Dietary insufficiency, antibiotic therapy (which kills vitamin K–producing intestinal bacteria), malabsorption (vitamin K is fat soluble), and biliary obstruction may all cause low levels of vitamin K. At levels below 30 percent of normal, PTT and PT become prolonged, and excessive bleeding is a danger. Vitamin K administration corrects the problem within 2 days. Immediate correction can be achieved with plasma or whole blood transfusion.

     b. Anticoagulant-induced bleeding

       i. Coumadin is a water-soluble analog of vitamin K which inhibits carboxylation of Factors II, VII, IX, and X, giving incomplete and ineffective circulating forms of these proteins. The normal therapeutic level is 1.5 to 2 times the PT of normal plasma. Multiple drugs alter the pharmacodynamics of coumadin. Coumadin is displaced from albumin by highly protein-bound drugs such as sulfonamides, sulfonylureas, indomethacin and phenylbutazone, diazoxide, phenytoin, and chloral hydrate. The increased level of free drug can lead to excessive anticoagulation. Barbiturates, chronic ethanol intake, phenytoin, carbamazepine, rifampin, and other enzyme-inducing agents may increase the dose required for adequate therapy. If needed, coumadin can be reversed with FFP or, less rapidly, with vitamin K. Once vitamin K has been administered, further anticoagulation with coumadin will be ineffective for a week.

  ii. Heparin is a naturally occurring negatively charged mucopolysaccharide found in basophils and mast cells. It binds to antithrombin III (AT III), a circulating protease which normally interferes with coagulatin by inhibiting activated Factors X, XI, and II. Heparin increases the action of AT III 2000-fold. The PTT and PT are prolonged. The major unwanted effect is bleeding at sites of surgery, trauma, or damaged organs. **Full anticoagulation** with heparin, as seen in the treatment of pulmonary embolism, is achieved with a loading dose, followed by a continuous intravenous (IV) infusion titrated to keep the PTT twice normal. **Low-dose subcutaneous (SQ) heparin** given as prophylaxis against thromboembolism will not affect the PT or PTT until coagulation factor activity has been reduced by 70 percent. In a limited number of patients, standard SQ dosing will lead to significant elevations in PTT. In most patients, only the TT is prolonged, and AT III is affected enough to afford protection from thrombus formation.

  iii. Protamine, an extract of salmon sperm, is a positively charged substance which binds to heparin and stops the interaction with AT III.

  iv. Heparin-induced thrombocytopenia is an immune reaction which is manifested after 7 to 10 days of therapy. There may be arterial, microvascular, or venous thrombosis, together with platelet aggregation and thrombocytopenia. The incidence of this complication can be reduced by limiting the duration of therapy.

  v. Streptokinase and urokinase activate plasminogen to form plasmin, promoting clot lysis. Streptokinase is used acutely in the therapy of myocardial infarction, in an attempt to induce reperfusion. It is given as an IV infusion over hours. Urokinase can also be used; it acts more quickly, but is more expensive. Therapy is monitored by measuring the TT, which should be two to four times normal.

  vi. Recombinant tissue plasminogen activator (rTPA) has now become available as a more clot-specific agent which has less of an effect on fibrinogenolysis, and carries less risk of allergic reaction than streptokinase. However, FFP, EACA, or aprotinin can reverse treatment if there are complications.

  c. Massive transfusion There are several reasons for hemostatic failure following **massive transfusion.** Coagulation factors and platelets are lost from the circulation or are diluted. Shock affects the ability of the liver and bone marrow to replace the lost moieties, and may cause DIC or fibrinolysis. Stored blood is deficient in factors (especially V and VIII) and platelets. Incompatible transfusion, hypothermia, and citrate toxicity are other factors contributing to abnormal coagulation. As noted above, thrombocytopenia is a common finding, and platelet transfusions are often needed.

   d. Table 21-3 lists **laboratory tests for acquired bleeding disorders.**

D. Fibrinolytic System

   1. **Hepatic disease** is covered in detail in Chapter 20. Pertinent to the hemostatic function, liver disease can be devastating for a number of reasons. Most factors are produced in the liver, including plasminogen, fibrinogen, the vitamin-dependent factors, and the antithrombins. Patients with liver disease can also have an acquired dysfibrinogenemia or increased fibrinolysis due to inadequate synthesis of alpha-2 antiplasmin, or may have a chronic, low-grade DIC. The last can also occur in patients who have received LeVeen peritovenous shunts for ascites. Vitamin K deficiency is not uncommon in alcoholic cirrhosis. Administration of vitamin K and FFP may be needed for correction of the coagulopathy.

   2. Associated with various illnesses, **DIC** is a result of an imbalance of the hemostatic and fibrinolytic systems. The extrinsic pathway is activated by circulating phospholipoprotein membrane fragments released from traumatized tissue, tumor necrosis, destruction of white blood cells in sepsis, ischemic tissue, traumatized or necrotic brain tissue, or obstetric complications. Less commonly, the intrinsic pathway is activated if endothelial damage is severe (dissecting aneurysm). Clotting factors and platelets are consumed, causing microvascular obstruction. Once consumption is established, bleeding becomes a clinical problem. Secondary fibrinolysis follows, making the bleeding worse. Treatment is aimed at correcting the initiating cause and replacing deficient components of hemostasis. FFP contains all coagulation factors, and is the most often used replacement therapy for DIC. Cryoprecipitate (fibrinogen and Factor VIII) and platelet transfusions may also be necessary. Heparin is sometimes used (together with FFP, a source of AT III) to "switch off" the coagulation system; this is usually reserved for the more chronic forms of DIC.

Table 21-3 Laboratory tests in acquired bleeding disorders

	Platelets	PTT	PT	TT	Fibrinogen	FDP
Massive transfusion	Low	High	High	High	Low	High
Vitamin K, coumadin	Normal	High	High	Normal	Normal	Normal
Heparin	Normal/low	High	High	High	Normal	Normal
Liver disease	Normal/low	Normal/high	Normal/high	Normal/high	Normal/low	Normal/high

E. Therapy of Coagulopathies

Therapy is directed toward correcting the primary disorder, when possible, and replacing specific deficiencies.

1. Fresh whole blood (less than 2 days old) contains red cells, functional platelets, and coagulation factors, and is appropriate in hypovolemic patients with coagulopathies.

2. Packed red blood cells (PRBCs) have a hematocrit of 60 to 70 percent, and are used to treat anemia. In the average adult, 1 unit will increase the hematocrit by 2 to 3 percent.

3. Platelets are available as concentrates, and are viable for 3 days after collection. Replacement should be considered when the platelet count falls to $10 \times 10^9/L$ in the absence of active bleeding or $50 \times 10^9/L$ in the face of trauma, spontaneous bleeding, or surgery. There may be clinical situations where platelet transfusion is warranted with significantly higher platelet counts, particularly if the existing platelets are dysfunctional (e.g., aspirin ingestion, von Willebrand's disease). Six units of platelet concentrate raise the count by approximately $30 \times 10^9/L$. These should be administered through an unfiltered infusion set (to prevent trapping).

4. Kept at $-30°C$ in 200-mL bags, **FFP,** once thawed, should be given as soon as possible. All the coagulation factors are present (including fibrinogen and Factors VIII and IX). Compatibility testing is not needed before transfusion.

5. Cryoprecipitate contains Factor VIII, Factor VIII:vWF, fibrinogen, and Factor XIII. It is used for the treatment of hemophilia A, von Willebrand's disease, afibrinogenemia, and Factor XIII deficiency. It has to be stored frozen, and is awkward to make up.

6. Antihemophiliac factor is derived from FFP. It comes as a freeze-dried ampule, and is stable at 4°C for 2 years. It has a more reliable concentration of Factor VIII than does cryoprecipitate. It is used in the treatment of hemophilia, and usually 10 to 15 mL/kg will raise the Factor VIII level to over 30 percent.

F. Thrombotic Disorders

Thrombotic disorders also occur in congenital and acquired forms.

1. Inherited deficiencies of the anticoagulants **protein C, protein S, major antithrombin** (AT III), and **minor antithrombin** (heparin cofactor II) should be considered in young patients or those with unusual thrombotic events (e.g., dural sinus thrombosis). Most patients with thrombotic events have acquired, predisposing factors, such as obesity, pregnancy, prolonged bed rest, myeloproliferative disorders, malignancy, or lupus anticoagulant. Of those where no predisposing factor can be identified, 1 to 2 percent will have AT III deficiency, 5 percent will be deficient in protein C, and 5 percent will be deficient in protein S.

2. **Treatment** of acute thrombotic events in patients with protein C or protein S deficiency includes anticoagulation with heparin, and subsequently an oral warfarin compound. Anticoagulation is not indicated in the heterozygote who does not have a history of thrombosis.

III. PAIN SYNDROMES SPECIFIC TO BLEEDING DISORDERS

A. Bleeding Disorders

The **pain associated with bleeding diatheses** is usually related to abnormal bleeding. The treatment of these pain syndromes is generally aimed at correcting the bleeding disorder. Supplemental analgesic therapy is also often warranted while the clinical situation improves. A few of the potential pain problems are discussed in the following as samples of the approach to pain management in patients with inadequate coagulation.

1. **Schönlein-Henoch purpura** can often have associated arthralgias, abdominal pain, gastrointestinal bleeding, and glomerulonephritis. Acetaminophen can be used to supplement narcotics as the primary mode of analgesia. Peridural techniques are contraindicated due to the risk of epidural bleeding. NSAIDs are also inappropriate in the face of significant bleeding. A transcutaneous electrical nerve stimulation (TENS) unit might be applied if pain complaints are localized (e.g., to a single extremity).

2. Patients with **bone marrow infiltration** and pathologic fractures from leukemia, myelofibrosis, or multiple myeloma may have bony pain that responds well to NSAID therapy, but the decision to administer these drugs must take into account the presence of defective coagulation. Again, TENS may be very useful in localized disease, as with a compression fracture. Narcotics and acetaminophen are generally safe to administer. Pathologic fractures may require surgical stabilization.

3. **Acute splenic and/or hepatic enlargement** causes pain from capsular stretch. The pain is visceral in quality, and would respond best to peridural analgesic techniques. However, placement of a catheter in the epidural space should only be considered in those whose coagulopathy has been treated and who are hemostatically stable, because of the risk of damaging an epidural vein and causing an epidural hematoma. If the patient's coagulopathy has been corrected temporarily but carries a reasonable likelihood of recurring, a catheter should not be placed because removal of epidural catheters in the face of a coagulopathy also carries the risk of bleeding. Other analgesic options are as noted above.

4. **Hemarthroses,** seen commonly in hemophiliacs, are usually treated with narcotics and acetaminophen. Peripheral nerve blocks (e.g., femoral, sciatic) with a long-acting local anesthetic (e.g., bupivacaine) might be considered after factor replacement. These offer a significantly lower risk of

bleeding complications than does the placement of an epidural catheter. Surgical drainage is occasionally indicated.

5. **Spontaneous CNS bleeding** can occur in the face of a significant coagulopathy or with excessive anticoagulation. Headache is a common complaint, but the clinical condition can deteriorate very rapidly and become a surgical emergency. Correction of coagulation is paramount. Treatment of increased intracranial pressure is discussed in detail in Chapter 16.

B. Thrombotic Disorders

The **pain with thrombotic disorders** relates to thromboembolic phenomena. These include peripheral thrombi which create painful ischemic tissue, visceral thromboses, or embolic events such as pulmonary embolism. The pain is specific to the site affected, so that treatment must be directed by the specific site and symptoms.

1. Pain from thrombotic events or infarction (e.g., splenic infarcts seen in sickle cell disease, ITP, TTP) requires treatment of the coagulation problem and mild to moderate analgesics.

2. Hypercoagulable states are not usually considered to be contraindications to **peridural analgesia,** but, if anticoagulation is to be initiated, these are not recommended. However, if the patient had, for example, a heterozygote protein C deficiency and was scheduled for elective surgery, peridural analgesia may be beneficial. Epidural analgesia has been shown to decrease thromboembolic complications in patients undergoing major vascular surgery, despite the fact that this patient population is premorbidly relatively hypercoagulable. By dilating blood vessels, epidural local anesthetics have been shown to improve the arterial inflow and the rate of venous emptying.

C. Vasculitis

Syndromes causing **vasculitis** may require steroid therapy in addition to analgesics.

IV. IMPACT OF COAGULOPATHY ON PAIN MANAGEMENT

A. Systemic Narcotics

1. **Injections by the IM route** are contraindicated in patients with a significant coagulation disturbance due to the risk of hematoma formation, and should be avoided in preference to other routes of administration (IV, PR, PO) whether or not there is a coagulopathy.

2. **Narcotics given IV** are excellent analgesics in patients with bleeding disorders. For patients who are alert and cooperative enough, patient-con-

trolled analgesia **(PCA)** is an effective method which allows the patient to titrate the medication to meet his or her needs. Any type of narcotic may be used (see Chapters 8 and 13). Because many of these patients have chronic problems that require frequent hospital visits and invasive interventions, they are at risk of developing the personality style of a chronically ill patient. Every effort should be made to provide adequate analgesia for acute episodes and with a minimum of inconvenience. The PCA technique offers the patient a sense of control in an otherwise threatening and incapacitating situation.

B. Invasive Analgesic Techniques

1. Coagulopathies and systemic anticoagulation are generally contraindications to **peridural techniques.** The risk of spinal cord compression from intraspinal hematoma leading to paraplegia is very real. Patients with significant coagulation deficiency should be offered systemic analgesia as a safer alternative to regional analgesia. Patients with chronic pain syndromes who are on anticoagulants have received **caudal** morphine through a small-gauge needle with no neurologic sequelae. A single-shot spinal injection using a small-gauge needle and only opiates may be atraumatic, and allow the onset of cord compression to be noticed quickly; administration of local anesthetic may mask the early symptoms of peridural bleeding. Severe back pain, meningismus, or local tenderness in such patients merits magnetic resonance imaging (MRI) or a computed tomography (CT) scan. If a hematoma is found, but the coagulopathy has been corrected and there are no neurologic symptoms, only close observation is indicated. However, if the coagulopathy is not under control, or if there are any signs suggestive of neurologic compromise, immediate decompressive laminectomy is indicated.

2. Patients receiving **partial anticoagulation with SQ heparin or daily oral aspirin** are at a mildly increased risk of hematoma formation, but this is only a relative contraindication to epidural or spinal techniques. A midline approach and injection of saline or local anesthetic through the epidural needle to dilate the epidural space prior to insertion of the catheter (no more than 3 to 4 cm into the epidural space) will minimize the likelihood of trauma to the epidural veins. Short-acting local anesthetics will allow frequent evaluation of neurologic status as the block wears off. Opiates would be the drugs of choice for injection, for the reasons discussed above. If there is an abnormal PTT or ACT in patients on SQ heparin, regional analgesia should be avoided or the effects of the drug allowed to subside before catheter placement is attempted. The bleeding time has been advocated by some as a measure of platelet dysfunction. However, coagulation studies in preeclamptic obstetric patients have been found to be inconsistent and not helpful in predicting bleeding potential. The best predictor of bleeding risk appears to be the presence of current bleeding (e.g., epistaxis, hematuria, oozing around vascular catheters). Unless there is a distinct clinical advan-

tage to the patient (e.g., thoracic epidural for patients with flail chest), peridural anesthetic techniques should probably be avoided when there is any question.

3. **Pleural catheters** dosed with local anesthetic (either by bolus or infusion) may be a reasonable alternative to peridural analgesia in the coagulopathic patient. These will be most effective if the pain is unilateral and involves the thorax or upper abdomen. Local anesthetic is rapidly absorbed from the pleural space and the bilateral administration of local anesthetic carries the risk of local anesthetic toxicity due to the achievement of high blood levels (see Chapter 13).

4. **Peripheral nerve blocks** may be useful for focal pain. Use of a small-caliber needle and an application of direct pressure over the site minimize the risk of hematoma formation.

C. Alternative Analgesic Techniques

1. **Adjunctive medications** can be used to limit narcotic requirements and improve the patient's sense of well-being. **NSAIDs** such as ketorolac have been administered IV, but the effect on platelet adhesiveness needs to be considered. Tricyclic antidepressants **(TCAs)** will facilitate sleep while elevating CNS/neural serotonin levels and enhancing analgesia. **Sedatives and/or amnestics** such as midazolam may also be helpful supplements for patients whose pain is exacerbated by anxiety or for patients undergoing painful procedures. **Ketamine** is a potent analgesic of short duration that can be very useful for painful invasive procedures such as bone marrow biopsies.

2. The use of **self-regulation techniques** such as hypnosis should be evaluated for any patient with a chronic, painful illness, and particularly for those requiring repeated hospitalizations or invasive procedures. Patients hospitalized with acute problems requiring frequent painful procedures, such as dressing changes, venous access procedures, or physical therapy, should also be considered for these modalities (see Chapters 5 and 14).

3. As mentioned above, **TENS** units offer an adjunct for the management of localized pain, and carry very little risk regardless of the severity of the coagulopathy.

CASE DISCUSSION

In light of the severity of the patient's coagulopathy and the massive fluid shifts necessitated by its treatment, the decision was made to retain the artificial airway and mechanical ventilation. As such, parenteral narcotics were chosen, as they offer both sedation and analgesia. After several IV boluses of fentanyl (50 μg) precipitated hypotension, it was elected to begin a fentanyl infusion. Supplemental doses of midazolam were ordered for sedation.

Over the next 36 h, the patient received 110 units of PRBCs, 52 units of FFP, 60 units of platelets, and 23 units of cryoprecipitate, with almost complete resolution of his coagulopathy (PT 14.7, PTT 46). Although his coagulopathy was improving and he was awake, he had significant tissue edema and had evidence of n ld adult respiratory distress syndrome, so that immediate extubation was not possible. He complained bitterly of abdominal pain and made frequent demands for supplementa IV pain medication.

Ketorolac was felt to be inappropriate in light of a mild residual coagulopathy. The idea of an epidural was rejected for similar reasons. A unilateral pleural catheter was felt to offer inadequate coverage for a midline incision, although this technique was not contraindicated by his hemostatic status. The nurse felt that the patient had significant anxiety about control of his analgesia, so PCA morphine was ordered, with a basal rate of 2 mg/h and intermittent doses of 3 mg with a lockout of 6 min. These doses were somewhat higher than those used for the usual narcotic-naïve postoperative patient, and reflected an expectation that some tolerance to narcotics had developed while the patient was receiving the fentanyl infusion. A bedtime sedative was also administered. After education about the use of the pump, the patient dosed himself frequently over the next several hours (four to six doses per hour with 15 to 20 attempts per hour, which made the nurses a bit nervous), but then he settled down to one to three self-administered doses per hour. He also learned to facilitate his care by dosing himself before suctioning, physical therapy, and other pain-provoking activities.

Over the next several days, the ventilatory support was weaned and the patient extubated. He gradually tapered himself to rare PCA doses by the tenth postoperative day. Since he was allowed to start clear liquids, oxycodone with acetaminophen (Percocet) was ordered. The basal rate was discontinued, but the self-administered doses were retained until it was clear that the patient was able adequately to absorb his oral analgesics. At that time, the PCA was discontinued.

SUGGESTED READINGS

L Kaufman (ed): Haemostasis in anaesthesia and intensive care, in *Anaesthesia Review.* 6 Ed. New York, Churchill Livingstone, 1989.
Macdonald R: Aspirin and extradural blocks. *Br J Anaesth* 66:1, 1991.
Mosher DF. Disorders of blood coagulation, in Wyngaarden (ed): *Cecil Textbook of Medicine.* Philadelphia, Saunders, 1988, p 1060.
Oh TE (ed): Hemostatic failure, in *Intensive Care Manual,* 3rd ed. London, Butterworths, 1990.
Owens EL, Kasten GW, Hessel EA: Spinal subarachnoid hematoma after lumbar puncture and heparinization: a case report, review of the literature, and discussion of anesthetic implications. *Anesth Analg* 65:1201, 1986.

CHAPTER
22

SEPSIS AND MULTIPLE SYSTEM ORGAN FAILURE

Mark O. Daugherty

Case
  I. Introduction
 II. Pathophysiology of MSOF
     A. Systemic Inflammatory Response Syndrome
     B. The Cascade of MSOF
     C. Typical Scenario
III. Pain Syndromes Associated with MSOF
     A. Incidence of Pain in the ICU
     B. Difficulty of Pain Assessment and Monitoring
     C. Problems Associated with Prolonged Bed Rest
     D. Recurrent Sepsis
     E. Surgical and Nonsurgical Procedures
     F. Organ System Dysfunction
 IV. Effect of MSOF on Pain Management
     A. General Principles
     B. Medications
     C. Specific Modalities
Case Discussion
Suggested Readings

CASE

A 58-year-old obese, diabetic female presents to the emergency room with abdominal pain, hypotension, tachycardia, tachypnea, and cyanosis. Abdominal films reveal free air. She is taken to the operating room for an emergency exploratory laparotomy, which reveals a perforated diverticulum with gross fecal spillage. Intraoperatively, the patient has wheezing and high airway pressures and is difficult to oxygenate. Her urine output is less than 10cc/h despite aggressive fluid replacement and a central venous pressure of 14 cm H_2O. The patient is taken to the surgical intensive care unit (ICU) postoperatively. Over the ensuing 2 days, she develops severe adult respiratory distress syndrome, anuric renal failure, and hepatic insufficiency with an associated coagulopathy. Her hemodynamic function is supported by dobutamine and norepinephrine. She requires daily irrigations of her peritoneal cavity in the ICU as she is too ill to be transported to the operating room.

I. INTRODUCTION

A. Dealing with the management of pain in a patient with multisystem organ failure (MSOF) requires an astute mind. With the progressive development of the syndrome, the need for adequate analgesia and sedation increases as the choice of drugs and of routes of administration diminishes.

B. The natural history of MSOF results in this group of patients' being the sickest and most labor- and time-intensive patients in the ICU. With so many factors to consider, pain management is often given a low priority. Particularly in the early stages, this may be detrimental to the patient's overall outcome. In addition to reducing the degree of pain and discomfort, blunting the stress response with effective analgesic techniques may affect the course of the developing syndrome.

II. PATHOPHYSIOLOGY OF MSOF

A. Systemic Inflammatory Response Syndrome

MSOF is the end result of a host of predisposing causes. Sepsis is generally considered to be the most common, but whether it is the initiating factor or merely a catalyst is not clear. Many other factors have been implicated, and in 1992 at the Society of Critical Care Medicine Consensus Conference, the terminology **systemic inflammatory response syndrome (SIRS)** was proposed to replace sepsis syndrome. SIRS encompasses the inflammatory response to both infectious and noninfectious causes. Examples of noninfectious causes include pancreatitis, ischemia, multitrauma, burns, hemorrhagic shock, and immune-mediated organ injury.

B. The Cascade of MSOF

The **cascade of events in MSOF** appears to proceed along two pathways—one in series and the other in parallel.

  1. **In parallel,** it is postulated that some mediator of multisystem dysfunction exists which circulates freely. The various cytokines and the endogenously derived mediators of inflammation have been implicated in this role.

  2. **In series,** clinical experience suggests that failure or dysfunction in one organ system facilitates the development of dysfunction in others.

C. Typical Scenario

  1. The typical scenario starts with a 48- to 72-h period of relative hemodynamic stability following the **resuscitative phase** of the initial insult. The patients who may then go on to develop MSOF enter part of a **systemic injury response pattern** known as the **hypermetabolic state.** This is usually associated with some form of lung injury, which ranges from mild capillary leak to fulminant **adult respiratory distress syndrome (ARDS).** Primary lung pathology, such as pneumonia or lung contusion, may further contribute to the development of ARDS. The patients generally require ventilation at this time, and further deterioration is manifest clinically as decreasing lung compliance, mismatching of ventilation and perfusion, along with arterial hypoxemia. (See Chapter 18.)

  2. With increasing tissue injury, the **peripheral demand for oxygen rises,** resulting in an increase in cardiac output and a decrease in systemic vascular resistance. Failure of the heart to respond, due either to inadequate preload, preexisting cardiac disease, or acquired cardiac dysfunction, significantly increases the overall mortality. **Inadequate preload** may result from inadequate volume resuscitation or underestimated volume loss due to endothelial injury with interstitial sequestration of the vascular volume. **Acquired cardiac dysfunction** is common in MSOF and is thought to be due to **myocardial depressant factors** (MDFs), cytokines that seem to have a selective cardiac effect. This stage requires adequate fluid volume therapy to maintain filling pressures, along with inotropes and vasopressors to improve oxygen delivery to the tissues.

  3. The **gastrointestinal (GI) tract** has been implicated as both a target organ and a potential effector of MSOF. Ischemia leads to stress-induced gastritis, GI bleeding, ileus, and diarrhea. As a consequence of this underperfused state, and altered bowel flora due to the intensive use of antibiotics, the GI tract becomes increasingly permeable to toxins, which are then released into the systemic circulation.

  4. **Renal blood flow** is maintained early in the course of MSOF, but as

the process continues, there is a progressive fall in glomerular filtration rate and acute renal failure ensues. The renal insult may also be the result of hypotension, hypoxemia, or the aggressive use of diuretics and other toxins, such as the aminoglycoside group of antibiotics.

   5. **Biliary dilatation and bile stasis** are common and frequently occur, even in the absence of extrahepatic obstruction. Clinical **hepatic failure** develops with rising levels of bilirubin and hepatic enzymes, reduced hepatic protein synthesis, and disordered amino acid metabolism.

   6. **Coagulopathy, impaired platelet function, and disseminated intravascular coagulation** become manifest as the hypermetabolic state progresses.

   7. **Neurologic dysfunction** may be a direct result of the sepsis syndrome, a consequence of the metabolic disarray seen with hepatic and/or renal dysfunction, due to hypoperfusion, related to sedative medications, or caused by specific intracranial pathology such as meningitis. Depending on the etiology of the encephalopathy, a peripheral motor and/or sensory neuropathy may also be part of the clinical picture. The alteration in mental status limits the patient's ability to communicate information regarding the extent, location, and severity of pain. It may also alter the patient's memory of the painful experience. However, it is likely that the segmental and suprasegmental responses to the pain (see Chapter 4) remain operational, and even in an obtunded patient, some level of integrative functioning (i.e., perception, interpretation, subconscious and possibly conscious memory) is likely to occur.

III. PAIN SYNDROMES ASSOCIATED WITH MSOF

A. Incidence of Pain in the ICU

A 1987 survey of hospitalized medical and surgical patients found that 58 percent reported excruciating pain at some stage during their stay. The **incidence of pain** must be far greater in the ICU, especially in patients with MSOF. They may experience pain related to their primary injury or pathology, such as major trauma, burns or GI tract perforations, as well as that related to the invasive procedures required in their frequent assessment and management. Arterial and central venous cannulae, dialysis catheters, and endotracheal and tracheostomy tubes are commonly cited as pain generators in such patients.

B. Difficulty of Pain Assessment and Monitoring

It not only is **difficult to assess and monitor pain** in the very ill, but it also is easy to focus on other aspects of their management, particularly those perceived as imminently life-threatening. Inadequately treated pain may lead to **profound behavioral and physiologic disturbances.** These can cause anxiety, interference with sleep, severe confusion, agitation, and feelings of hopelessness and depression, resulting in a decreased tolerance for pain. Many of these responses may also diminish the patient's ability to cooperate with his or her care, and may themselves be life-threatening. For example, the confused patient is at significant risk of self-extubation, the removal of vascular access catheters, or even attempts to climb out of bed. Furthermore, anxiety and agitation increase metabolic demands in an already stressed and hypermetabolic patient. Those with preexisting organ dysfunction, such as ischemic cardiac disease, may be unable to compensate adequately for this additional increase in metabolic demand.

C. Problems Associated with Prolonged Bed Rest

Immobility requires frequent nursing attention and changing of positions to prevent decubiti. Prolonged bed rest causes pain from prolonged direct pressure on bony prominences, joint stiffness, and low back discomfort, even in young patients. Every movement is potentially painful.

D. Recurrent Sepsis

Even when sepsis is not the initiating event, it is normally a problem as the illness progresses. Recurrent episodes of sepsis from abscess formation, urinary tract infections, vascular access infections, and especially pneumonias characterize the process and are all associated with pain.

E. Surgical and Nonsurgical Procedures

Surgical procedures are often necessary, such as the drainage and removal of infected tissues, exploratory laparotomy, thoracostomy tube placement, and tracheostomy formation. **Nonsurgical procedures,** such as bronchoscopy, magnetic resonance imaging, echocardiography, and ultrasound studies, may also cause discomfort. Even the movement associated with routine chest radiographs is unpleasant and causes a substantial increase in metabolic rate in the average ICU patient.

F. Organ System Dysfunction

Dysfunction in each organ system may contribute to the pain experience. This is addressed in detail in the relevant chapters.

IV. EFFECT OF MSOF ON PAIN MANAGEMENT

A. General Principles

1. Optimal pain control is vital to allow **adequate spontaneous ventilation.** The use of regional analgesia with continuous infusions of narcotics or local anesthetics has dramatically improved the problem of pain-induced hypoventilation following chest trauma and thoracic and upper abdominal surgery.

   a. **Progressive deterioration in pulmonary function** with acute lung injury in the form of ARDS frequently heralds the onset of MSOF. This usually necessitates intubation and mechanical ventilation to maintain oxygenation, clear secretions, and prevent alveolar collapse.

   b. **Ventilation difficulties** usually require sedation, analgesia, and possibly the use of neuromuscular blocking agents to provide optimal oxygenation. Sedation and paralysis may contribute to the signs of neurologic failure, complicating the subjective assessment of pain.

2. As mentioned earlier, **myocardial depression** frequently occurs with severe sepsis and is usually associated with peripheral vasodilation and a low systemic vascular resistance, all contributing to **hypotension.** Furthermore, **high levels of positive end-expiratory pressure (PEEP),** sometimes needed to oxygenate patients with ARDS, impede venous return and can cause overdistension of the right ventricle, creating the picture of **right heart failure.** These phenomena may make the patient particularly susceptible to the myocardial depressant effects of various sedative and analgesic medications.

3. **Hepatic and renal dysfunction** commonly follow the onset of ARDS. Most analgesic agents require both hepatic clearance and biotransformation, followed by renal excretion in order to be eliminated. As such, pharmacokinetics will be altered by impaired organ function, making a drug's effect and duration less predictable.

4. MSOF is frequently associated with **sepsis and/or coagulopathy.** Both are relative contraindications to the use of invasive modalities such as epidural catheters. However, in this situation, the use of a 25- or 26-gauge spinal needle for intrathecal opioid placement may be considered. In the presence of new-onset sepsis, indwelling epidural catheters are usually treated like other invasive catheters (e.g., central lines) and removed or changed. Because of the availability of alternative analgesic regimens that do not carry such significant, if infrequent, risks (epidural abscess and subsequent surgical drainage), epidural catheters are usually simply removed.

B. Medications

1. **Opioids** The **opioids** are used predominantly for their sedative effects, especially in patients on mechanical ventilators, and for analgesia. In

addition, opioids suppress the cough reflex, which increases the tolerance of endotracheal tubes and suctioning. Intravenous (IV) infusions are the most common mode of delivery. Epidural catheters permit the use of a much lower total dose of opioid, and they also provide superior analgesia, but little or no sedation, as compared with the parenteral administration of an equianalgesic dose. Bioavailability and metabolism differ among the different subclasses and, depending on the degree of organ failure present, will influence the choice of drug, mode of delivery, and dose.

    a. An IV dose of **morphine** is rapidly cleared from plasma. Most of the drug undergoes hepatic glucuronidation to morphine-glucuronides, which are eliminated through the kidneys. Approximately 10 percent is eliminated unchanged. Morphine-glucuronide has weak opioid activity. Cerebrospinal fluid (CSF) levels of morphine may be substantially higher in patients with an altered blood–brain barrier, resulting in significant depression of the central nervous system (CNS). For these reasons, hepatic, renal, and neurologic dysfunction necessitate an adjustment of dose. When administered peridurally, morphine, a relatively hydrophilic drug, enters the CSF to a significant degree. The cephalad circulation of the CSF places the patient at risk of delayed respiratory depression 12 to 24 h after the initial injection. On the other hand, a single epidural dose of 3 to 5 mg of preservative-free morphine (Duramorph) (or 0.3 to 0.5 mg subarachnoid) can provide up to 24 h of analgesia. Morphine causes a variable degree of histamine release, which may result in hypotension, bronchospasm, and pruritus (usually localized to the IV site, but in the case of peridural administration, the entire body may be involved). It thus should be avoided in cases of preexisting chronic obstructive pulmonary disease (COPD) or asthma. Other side effects include dose-dependent spasm of the sphincter of Oddi, nausea, constipation, and urinary retention.

    b. Hydromorphone (Dilaudid) and **oxymorphone** (Numorphan) are more lipophilic, have a more rapid onset of action, and are 6 to 10 times more potent than morphine. Profound analgesia with minimal side effects can be produced with far lower doses of drug when administered via the epidural route. Hydromorphone has no active metabolites, and the duration of action is minimally affected by hepatic or renal dysfunction.

    c. Fentanyl (Sublimaze) is a good choice for patients with hepatic and renal dysfunction. It has high analgesic potency, its major metabolites are inactive, and it can be eliminated in the bile and urine. It does not cause histamine release, and it does not depress the myocardium. However, its high lipid solubility results in rapid penetration into the CNS, causing depression of the level of consciousness and respiration. This can be late in onset if the drug has accumulated within adipose tissue. Other side effects include vagomimetic effects, such as bradycardia and nausea. It can be given by IV infusion that is titrated to individual patient need, by patient-controlled analgesia (PCA), by the epidural route, or by using a transdermal patch (Duragesic) which provides a low dose of 25, 50, or 100 μg/h. Limitations of the transdermal patch include slow onset (12 to 24 h), slow offset (12 to 18 h), and unreliable cutaneous blood flow in the critically ill patient, with subsequent variable uptake from the application site. This modality is much more useful during the convalescent phase.

   d. **Alfentanil** (Alfenta) has a smaller volume of distribution and a shorter elimination half-life, making it useful for MSOF patients. It can be given as an infusion or as a single bolus to cover short procedures. Alfentanil is much more expensive than the older narcotics. But although infusions of alfentanil may represent an unnecessary expense, its shorter duration of action may be desirable for brief, painful procedures.

   e. **Meperidine** (Demerol) is generally not indicated in MSOF because of its active metabolite, **normeperidine.** Normeperidine has a prolonged half-life and significant CNS stimulant effects, which include progressive hyperreflexia, myoclonus, and seizures. Irritability of the CNS is most likely to occur with prolonged administration and/or in patients with renal dysfunction.

   f. **Dezocine** (Dalgan), a narcotic agonist–antagonist, is as potent as morphine and has a more rapid onset, but a shorter duration of action. Like the other agonist–antagonists (see Chapter 8), it has a ceiling effect for the depression of respiration, and so it may be useful in patients for whom respiratory compromise is a concern. It has been noted that moderate doses may cause excessive sedation. Dezocine should be used with extreme caution (if at all) in patients with opioid tolerance, as its administration can precipitate withdrawal.

2. **Local anesthetics (LAs)**

   a. Amide-type local anesthetics are more commonly used for regional nerve block techniques and in epidural infusions than are ester LAs. They are all metabolized by the liver. Renal excretion of free drug is minimal. Systemic toxicity is related to the dose, extent of plasma binding, redistribution kinetics, and the rate of hepatic clearance.

   b. **Bupivacaine** (Marcaine) has the slowest rate of hepatic metabolism. The bupivacaine dose should be carefully calculated and adjusted in patients with cardiac and liver dysfunction, because toxic levels carry a significant risk of myocardial depression and arrhythmias which can be resistant to treatment.

   c. **Lidocaine** (Xylocaine) is more readily metabolized in the liver than is bupivacaine. In renal failure, however, the total lidocaine dose should be restricted, since active metabolites accumulate and pose the risk of systemic toxicity. Cardiac toxicity occurs at higher blood levels than neurotoxicity, and so seizures precede cardiovascular collapse with lidocaine, whereas with bupivacaine, their occurrence will nearly coincide.

   d. **Mepivacaine** (Carbocaine) has a more rapid hepatic metabolism.

Like lidocaine and prilocaine, it is a relatively safe alternative in hepatic-failure patients, especially when dilute concentrations are used. A 0.5% solution works effectively in continuous intrapleural, femoral, and axillary blocks.

     e. Prilocaine (Citanest) is the most readily metabolized amide LA and may produce **met-hemoglobinemia,** especially when doses greater than 500 mg are used. This is caused by the accumulation of a metabolite o-toluidine.

     f. Chapter 10 reviews LAs in greater detail.

    3. Nonsteroidal anti-inflammatory drugs (NSAIDs) Ketorolac (Toradol), a potent NSAID, has a high analgesic ceiling as compared with morphine, as well as additional, moderate anti-inflammatory activity. Ketorolac has an advantage over other NSAIDs in that it is available in a parenteral formulation. NSAIDs as a class offer antiprostaglandin-mediated analgesia and modulation of inflammation. They are particularly useful for musculoskeletal pain, burns, and pain secondary to smooth muscle spasm (e.g., biliary, uterine, ureteral). Further, they have little to no sedative effect and do not cause respiratory depression. The adverse effects associated with the NSAIDs are usually dose and duration related. NSAIDs are contraindicated in patients with a history of peptic ulceration and those with a coagulopathy or the risk of acute bleeding (e.g., splenic or hepatic lacerations, pelvic fractures). Hepatic dysfunction has a minimal effect on elimination. In renal impairment and in the elderly, plasma clearance is reduced and elimination half-life prolonged. Dosing intervals should be increased in proportion to the degree of renal dysfunction. In general, NSAIDs should be used with caution or avoided in patients with renal impairment where recovery of renal function is possible.

    4. Benzodiazepines These sedatives are frequently used in the critically ill population. The ICU is an active, well-lit, and noisy environment. Sedation is an important part of the care, as agitation, anxiety, sleep deprivation, and confusion can exacerbate pain syndromes. All of the benzodiazepines, in sedative doses, have minimal respiratory and cardiovascular depressant effects. When used with narcotics, however, depression of both the cardiovascular system and the respiratory system is augmented. Paradoxical excitement (disinhibition) and confusion can occur with benzodiazepines, particularly in the elderly.

     a. The benzodiazepine most commonly used in ICUs is **midazolam** (Versed). This can be given as a bolus for short procedures or as an infusion. It is a water-soluble, highly protein-bound drug with a large volume of distribution (Vd). Hepatic clearance is the main route of metabolism, with elimination in the bile and urine. The dose, therefore, should be restricted in patients with hepatic dysfunction. Renal failure does not affect the metabolism and clearance of midazolam.

b. **Diazepam** (Valium) is lipid soluble, is metabolized in the liver to active metabolites (e.g., oxazepam), and has a prolonged elimination half-life. Most of the drug is bound to albumin, and so, in hypoalbuminemic states, diazepam-related side effects are common. The dose should be restricted in hepatic disease, COPD, and CNS dysfunction.

c. **Lorazepam** (Ativan) offers a longer duration of action than midazolam, but without the risk of accumulation of active metabolites seen with diazepam. As such, it is the drug of choice for longer-acting, intermittently dosed sedation.

5. **Intravenous anesthetic agents**

a. **Propofol** (Diprivan) is being used more and more frequently for sedation in the ICU, for both short- and long-term patients. Compared with midazolam, propofol has been shown to decrease significantly the mean recovery time to extubation, thereby shortening the stay in the ICU. Concerns related to the use of propofol in the critically ill include myocardial depression and vasodilation, which may cause profound hypotension when the drug is administered as a bolus to patients with limited myocardial reserve or hypovolemia. Administration as an infusion causes minimal cardiovascular changes. The high lipid content of propofol (i.e., intralipid vehicle) may cause hypertriglyceridemia in patients receiving large doses, particularly if they also are receiving a substantial proportion of their nutritional requirements as parenteral fat calories (IV lipid). Consideration should be given to the number of fat calories being provided by the propofol infusion. Furthermore, normal triglyceride values usually return upon discontinuation of the propofol infusion. Another disadvantage has been the high cost of propofol. While more expensive than intermittent IV boluses such as lorazepam, propofol infusion costs significantly less than a midazolam infusion.

b. **Ketamine** (Ketalar) is a dissociative anesthetic agent which has potent analgesic effects with minimal respiratory depression. In addition, ketamine has sympathomimetic cardiovascular effects, whereas all other IV anesthetic agents cause myocardial depression and/or vasodilation. Thus ketamine can be a very useful and well-tolerated drug in septic or hypovolemic patients. The dose required to produce this analgesic effect is much less than the dose required for the induction of anesthesia (0.25 to 0.5 mg/kg versus 1 to 5 mg/kg every 5 to 15 min). Emergence delirium and hallucinatory phenomena are a problem. The use of ketamine should be limited to providing analgesia for short procedures.

c. **Etomidate** (Amidate) causes adrenal suppression. Higher mortality rates have been shown to result in ICU patients, so it is no longer used for continuous sedation.

d. **Barbiturates** (thiopental, pentobarbital) can be useful in single bolus doses for brief procedures (e.g., intubation), but hypotension is likely to occur in hypovolemic or septic patients due to myocardial depression and, sometimes, histamine release. Less often, they are used as continuous infusions in select cases of status epilepticus or refractory intracranial hypertension (e.g., closed-head injury). Problems associated with their long-term use include myocardial depression, loss of thermoregulatory control (poikilothermia), and decreased leukocyte function. Although patients may have better control of seizures or intracranial pressure when on barbiturate infusions, they often die of infection.

    6. Neuromuscular blocking agents In severe pulmonary failure with marked hypoxia present, or in severe head trauma, paralysis may be necessary to prevent the patient from coughing or breathing against the ventilator. In all cases, appropriate sedation and analgesia *must be* used concurrently. The degree of neuromuscular block should be monitored to avoid accumulation. (See Chapter 12.)

C. Specific Modalities

    1. Peridural analgesia

        a. Epidural or intrathecal administration of opioids offers an excellent form of analgesia with reduced systemic effects as compared with parenterally administered narcotics, including less sedation, an attenuation of the stress response, improved pulmonary function, and reduced duration of ventilator dependence. The doses required are generally 5 to 20 percent of parenterally administered opioids, the lower end of the range representing the intrathecal route.

        b. Intrathecal administration of a small dose of morphine (0.25 to 0.5 mg) can provide up to 24 h of analgesia, depending on the age and perfusion status of the patient. For example, elderly vasculopathic patients may exhibit more than 24 h of relief with a single dose, whereas young, well-hydrated patients may receive only 8 to 10 h of analgesia.

        c. Placement of an **epidural catheter** would enable prolonged analgesia with either intermittent bolus doses or a continuous infusion. The opioids of choice are the less lipophilic drugs, such as morphine and hydromorphone. Doses should be adjusted in MSOF to approximately half normal; for example, **morphine** (3 to 6 mg bolus dose or 0.4 to 0.6 mg/h as an infusion) or **hydromorphone** (1 to 1.5 mg bolus and 0.1 to 0.2 mg/h as an infusion). The lipophilic agents fentanyl and sufentanil may be less desirable in this patient population in continuous infusions because the dose requirements are high, and deposition in epidural fat stores can result in accumulation and the potential for unpredictable drug levels, depending on tissue perfusion and patient activity.

        d. There are **potential complications and side effects,** and one must evaluate the risks and benefits.

            (1) In the earliest stage of MSOF, severe **sepsis** is considered a relative contraindication to the placement of an epidural catheter or breach of the dura. There is a risk that an **epidural abscess** or **septic meningitis** will develop. However, the evidence is not conclusive, and if appropriate antibiotics are being given at the time, the risk is probably theoretical. As the disease process progresses from a systemic inflammatory response to lung involvement and ARDS with renal failure, the epidural and intrathecal routes can be used so long as there are no signs of active infection or of a coagulopathy.

(2) In the **presence of CNS pathology** that can be associated with an **increased CSF or intraspinal pressure** (e.g., head trauma, intracranial malignancy, hepatic encephalopathy, syringomyelia), peridural techniques should be avoided due to the risk of further increasing the CNS pressure through drug (volume) administration or the hazard of herniation of the brainstem after inadvertent dural puncture, both of which result in further neurologic injury.

(3) Placement of an epidural catheter in the presence of a **coagulopathy** carries the risk of causing an epidural hematoma, a complication that may require surgical decompression. In the patient with clinical signs of coagulopathy (hematuria, epistaxis, bleeding around IV cannulas), the peridural route is absolutely contraindicated. If hepatic dysfunction is evident, the risk of developing an associated clotting disorder further precludes the epidural route. Subarachnoid injections carry a somewhat smaller risk of significant bleeding due to the smaller needle caliber (17 to 19 gauge versus 24 to 25 gauge). The degree of coagulopathy and the risk/benefit ratio must be assessed before proceeding.

2. Nerve blocks Either used alone or in combination with IV opioids and ketorolac, **nerve blocks** can be performed for painful procedures in the ICU or in critical care patients requiring surgery. The techniques available are generally the same as for healthy patients, but in this group, positioning may be a problem. It may be more beneficial to use continuous techniques with an infusion via a pleural catheter or a catheter placed near the femoral nerve or the brachial plexus. (See Chapter 13.) Single-shot peripheral nerve blocks and intercostal nerve blocks can be performed, but their usefulness is limited by the duration of LA activity. The choice of LA used and the concentration will need to be adjusted according to the degree of organ dysfunction. (See Chapter 10.)

3. Patient-controlled analgesia At various stages of the disease process, PCA techniques may be useful. During the acute phase of MSOF, most patients are too ill or neurologically depressed to use PCA effectively, but in those recovering from MSOF who are sufficiently alert, the technique offers many benefits. It gives patients a sense of control over some aspect of their care in a situation in which they often suffer from a frightening loss of control. Further, with appropriate patient training, PCA allows the patient to titrate the analgesic dose effectively to match his or her needs.

a. Useful situations for PCA use include weaning from the ventilator or providing effective analgesia for chest physiotherapy, invasive interventions in the ICU setting, or postoperative pain control.

   b. The **choice of analgesic agent** depends on the degree of organ dysfunction. **Morphine, hydromorphone, and fentanyl** are all options. Starting doses will need to be determined according to the patient's narcotic requirements. Table 13.3 (in Chapter 13) lists the suggested initial pump settings for IV and subcutaneous PCA in narcotic-naïve patients. However, if the patient has been receiving frequent bolus doses or an infusion of opioids, larger basal and self-administered doses will be necessary. In patients with severe hepatic dysfunction, fentanyl or hydromorphone is recommended as the opioid of choice, using a basal rate that is about half the normal dose, a normal lockout, and a slightly lower than normal self-administered dose. Larger doses may be required if the patient was receiving substantial amounts of opioid prior to initiation of the PCA. **Meperidine is a poor choice** in the ICU setting because of the frequency of renal insufficiency and the potential formation of the neurotoxic metabolite normeperidine. Furthermore, the high incidence of the **development of narcotic tolerance** in the critically ill population resulting from prolonged administration of opioids often leads to the need for rather large doses of drug for adequate analgesia (see Chapter 29), thus increasing the likelihood of toxicity.

   c. If a patient remains alert, but is in pain, it is better to decrease the lockout interval than to increase the bolus dose. Supplemental techniques, such as nerve blocks, transcutaneous electrical nerve stimulation (TENS), or small doses of ketorolac may be considered.

   4. **Transcutaneous electrical nerve stimulation**   TENS may provide useful supplementation therapy in postsurgical pain. It has the important benefits of reducing the total opioid requirement and of offering a very limited side-effects profile (see Chapter 14).

   5. **Self-regulation techniques**   Both pain and anxiety can sometimes be managed in the ICU setting by the use of **self-regulation techniques.** Specific clinical uses include control of anxiety during weaning and analgesia for repeated, painful therapeutic interventions, such as burn debridement or dressing changes. When appropriately applied, these techniques can significantly improve the patient's sense of well-being and decrease the need for supplemental medications. The various techniques are reviewed in Chapter 14.

CASE DISCUSSION

> The patient presented offers a number of therapeutic dilemmas. Her problems include sepsis, respiratory failure, cardiovascular instability, renal failure, and coagulopathy. This clinical scenario poses at least two separate management issues. The first is how to manage her day-to-day (baseline) analgesic and sedative requirements. The other is how to "anesthetize" the patient adequately for daily irrigations and dressing changes at the bedside.

In light of the severity of the patient's ARDS, she requires a high minute ventilation (>25 L/min), an Fio_2 of .60, and a PEEP of 24 with a Vd/Vt of .78. The resulting blood gas is Pao_2 62, $Paco_2$ 52, and pH 7.25. Further increases in ventilation result in auto-PEEP and the significant elevation of mean airway pressure. As such, it was elected to sedate the patient aggressively and paralyze her to decrease airway pressures, as well as her metabolic rate. Sedation included a morphine infusion, which was started at 4 mg/h and titrated to eliminate grimaces associated with suctioning or repositioning during nonparalytic periods. Other options included fentanyl or hydromorphone infusions. Due to limited venous access, intermittent, *scheduled* doses of lorazepam (2 mg IV every 4 h) were administered (rather than a midazolam infusion). Once it was felt that adequate sedation and analgesia were established, the patient was started on an atracurium infusion. This was titrated to maintain a single twitch in the train-of-four (see Chapter 12 for monitoring of neuromuscular blockade). Attempts were made to maintain her core temperature between 36°C and 37.5°C. These maneuvers improved her CO_2 and pH, and also decreased her peak and mean airway pressures.

Peritoneal irrigations were undertaken at the bedside on a daily basis. It was felt that the patient could not be adequately ventilated by the transport or operating room ventilators, so that making daily trips to the operating room was not feasible. The bedside nurse was designated to administer medications and monitor the patient during the procedure, while a second nurse was responsible for assisting the physician. A third nurse was available to act as a "circulating" nurse—to open supplies, procure additional medications, and the like. Approximately 20 min prior to the daily abdominal irrigation, an additional dose of lorazepam (2 mg) was administered. This was repeated as the irrigations commenced. During this 20-min period, fentanyl (200 to 300 µg) was also titrated in. Finally, ketamine, 0.5 to 1.0 mg/kg, was administered just before the onset of the procedure. Repeated, smaller doses were given every 5 to 10 min for the duration of the intervention. Propofol (Diprivan) was not considered because it was felt that the patient would not hemodynamically tolerate any vasodilation the drug might cause. Her baseline blood pressure was 85 to 90/40 to 55 on the dobutamine and norepinephrine.

Although invasive techniques such as an epidural catheter might have been very helpful to the patient, these were felt to be contraindicated by the patient's sepsis and coagulation disorder. This patient also needed profound sedation to facilitate mechanical ventilation, a requirement that would not have been fulfilled by a regional technique. The area of pain generation was too large and the stimulus too profound for TENS application to be practical, and the patient was too obtunded to be able to participate in any form of self-regulation.

In spite of aggressive treatment, the patient died of overwhelming sepsis and MSOF 16 days after admission to the ICU.

SUGGESTED READINGS

American College of Chest Physicians/Society of Critical Care Medicine Consensus Conference: Definitions for sepsis and organ failure and guidelines for the use of innovative therapies in sepsis. *Crit Care Med* 20(6):864–874, 1992.

Barton R, Cerra FB: The hypermetabolism multiple organ failure syndrome. *Chest* 96(5):1153–1160, 1989.

Biebuyck JF: The metabolic response to stress: an overview and update. *Anesthesiology* 73(2):308–327, 1990.

Carrasco G, Molina R, Costa J, et al: Propofol vs. midazolam in short-, medium-, and long-term sedation of critically ill patients: a cost–benefit analysis. *Chest* 103(2):557, 1993.

Lee VC: Non-narcotic modalities for the management of acute pain. *Crit Care Clin* 6(2):451–481, 1990.

Murray MJ: Pain problems in the ICU. *Crit Care Clin* 6(2):235–254, 1990.

Rung GW, Marshall WK: Nerve blocks in the critical care environment. *Crit Care Clin* 6(2):343–368, 1990.

Sinatra RS: Pain management in patients suffering from major organ failure, in Sinatra RS, Hord AH, Ginsberg B, Preble LM (eds): *Acute Pain: Mechanisms and Management.* St. Louis, Mosby, 1992, pp 399–411.

Yeager MP, Glass DD, Neff RK, Brinck-Johnsen T: Epidural anesthesia and analgesia in high-risk surgical patients. *Anesthesiology* 66(6):729–736, 1987.

CHAPTER
23
PAIN MANAGEMENT FOR THE PATIENT WITH BURNS OR INTEGUMENT FAILURE

Sherry Sutton
Harvey N. Himel

Case
   I. Introduction
  II. Neurophysiology of Pain Related to Cutaneous Injury
 III. Factors Influencing the Pain of Acute Cutaneous Injury
     A. Extent of Injury
     B. Mechanism of Injury
     C. Preexisting Illness
     D. Age
     E. Gender
     F. History of Drug Use
     G. Sociocultural Factors
     H. Socioeconomic Background
     I. Educational Level
     J. Psychological Factors
 IV. Phases of Cutaneous Pain
     A. Acute Inflammatory Phase
     B. Healing Phase
     C. Convalescent Phase

406 PART 5 CLINICAL PROBLEMS

    V. Rationale Behind Active Pain Control
        A. Preemptive Pain Control
        B. Metabolic Stress Response
        C. Morbidity and Coping
   VI. Basic Principles of Pain Therapy
        A. Diagnosing the Cause
        B. Nutrition
        C. Covering Exposed Nerve Surfaces
        D. Monitoring Fluctuating Pain Levels
        E. Evaluating Treatment Efficacy
  VII. Selecting an Analgesic Regimen
        A. Pharmacokinetic Alterations in the Burn Patient
        B. Route of Administration
        C. Opioids
        D. Intravenous Sedation
        E. Anesthetic Agents
        F. Nonsteroidal Anti-inflammatory Drugs
        G. Nonpharmacologic modalities
 VIII. Painful Sequelae to Burns
        A. Paresthesias and Dysesthesias
        B. Contractures
        C. Hypertrophic Scars
        D. Keloid Scars
        E. Causalgias
        F. Phantom Limb Pain
   IX. Pressure Sores
    X. Other Chronic Wounds
   XI. Influence of Cutaneous Injury on Pain Management
Case Discussion
Suggested Readings

CASE

A 25-year-old male who had been rescued from a house fire was admitted to the emergency room with second- and third-degree flame burns involving 30 percent of the body surface area, including the face, neck, chest, upper extremities, and back, along with a suspected inhalation injury. His pulmonary injury was evaluated by a radiograph of the chest, serial arterial blood gases with carboxyhemoglobin determinations, and a nasotracheal flexible fiberoptic bronchoscopy. Due to elevated carboxyhemoglobin levels and significant airway edema, the patient was intubated at the time of bronchoscopy. Aggressive fluid resuscitation was initiated upon his arrival in the Burn Unit, and he required in excess of 50 L of crystalloid fluids during the first 24 h after the injury.

I. INTRODUCTION

Cutaneous injuries are often associated with severe pain. Because of the functional and cosmetic implications of cutaneous damage, these injuries carry specific physiologic, pharmacokinetic, and psychological ramifications. Although this chapter addresses multiple types of skin damage, the discussion focuses primarily on burns as an example of severe cutaneous disruption. The issues and principles cited apply to most other integument injuries as well.

II. NEUROPHYSIOLOGY OF PAIN RELATED TO CUTANEOUS INJURY

    A. Most of the **pain of a burn injury** is due to the stimulation of sensory receptors, known as **nociceptors,** that are preferentially sensitive to tissue damage. These nociceptors are prevalent in skin, muscle, and connective tissue, as well as in viscera and other tissues.

        1. There are several types of **cutaneous sensory units** in skin, subcutaneous tissue, and viscera, including:

            a. **myelinated nociceptors,** which respond to noxious mechanical stimuli almost exclusively, and, when stimulated, elicit a sharp, tingling pain; and

            b. **unmyelinated nociceptors,** which are polymodal and respond to mechanical, thermal, and chemical stimuli. The morphology of the unmyelinated nociceptor is not well understood, but it is apparently a "bare" nerve ending. Microneurographic studies have shown that stimulation of a single nociceptor is sufficient to cause pain. The stimulation of unmyelinated nociceptors elicits a dull, burning, or aching pain.

        2. The recent literature confirms that activation of peripheral nociceptors leads to **hyperexcitability in the dorsal horn of the spinal cord,** although nociceptors are not spontaneously active. The sensitization of myelinated nociceptors may occur after thermal injury and it is manifest in:

            a. A decreased threshold of activation after injury.

            b. The increased intensity of a response to a noxious injury.

            c. The emergence of spontaneous activity. It has been speculated that this may be the physiologic correlate of the hyperpathia of persistent pain.

        3. Most burn patients report the onset of their pain as occurring within minutes after the injury, but in cases of alcohol or other drug intoxication, the delay in pain perception has been noted to be as long as 48 h.

    B. The **pain management** for burns bears similarities to that for other traumatic injuries, inasmuch as unrecognized or undertreated pain can patient care and recovery. This issue is faced more directly by burn patients than by other trauma patients, as multiple therapeutic procedures are carried out in the course of treatment. Thus the patient must be provided with adequate pain management to allow him or her to endure **daily wound care.** Inadequate cleansing and debridement allow the accumulation of **surface pseudomembrane** composed of wound exudate, day-old topical wound-care agents, and frankly **necrotic eschar,** all of which increase the risk of life-threatening septic complications. Tolerance to analgesic agents does develop with prolonged exposure. Many clinicians worry about dependence, although this concern is often unwarranted (see Chapter 29).

III. FACTORS INFLUENCING THE PAIN OF ACUTE CUTANEOUS INJURY

A. Extent of Injury

There is an inverse relationship between the **depth of the burn** and the intensity of wound pain at the time of presentation. However, the classic description of **full-thickness (third-degree)** burns as being painless holds true only until the eschar is removed. When the eschar is removed, the nerve fibers in the underlying tissue become exposed and more sensitive to pain. Areas of **partial-thickness (second-degree)** burns, **superficial (first-degree)** burns, and unburned skin bordering the injury may also be painful due to the phenomenon of hyperalgesia. In addition, as peripheral fibers regenerate, the patient once again will experience sensation in very deep full-thickness burns. Regardless of their depth, the open wounds will continue to be painful and hypersensitive, at least until they are completely covered with epithelium. Furthermore, the treatment of deep burns necessitates harvesting of skin for grafting, a procedure that results in an additional unavoidable injury at the donor site that is also painful until it heals. In fact, many patients will complain more of their donor site pain than of their wound pain after skin grafting.

Recent quantitative studies strongly suggest a correlation between the intensity of pain and the extent of the burn injury (i.e., **percent of body surface area burned**), such that patients with larger burns experience greater overall severity of pain.

B. Mechanism of Injury

1. **Chemical burns** and **electrical burns** can be far more penetrating and more painful, although with intact-appearing surface structures, than **scald or flame burns,** most likely because of the nociceptors located in muscle, viscera, and connective tissues.

2. **Low-temperature contact burns** (e.g., from a heating pad) proceed over a longer period and penetrate more deeply, with less pain appreciated, but with a more severe injury resulting.

C. Preexisting Illness

1. **Chronic ischemia** secondary to peripheral vascular disease may render even minimal injuries very painful, will impede healing, and will predispose to secondary infectious complications.
2. **Peripheral neuropathies,** such as that associated with diabetes, can render otherwise painful injuries painless. These relatively insensate tissues, lacking a normal afferent reflex limb, are more prone to burns.

D. Age

Although emotional regression should be anticipated in most severely stressed patients, children will often exhibit obvious age regression following injury. Older adults often display exaggeratedly emotive behaviors, including grief, fear, and a desire for attention. Communication should be modified in such a way that information is presented in a manner appropriate to the current emotional level of function rather than the chronological age. A simple, straightforward, concrete style is much more appropriate than abstract information, even for adults.

E. Gender

Male patients will be less able to verbalize their emotions of fear and grief. They also can display resistance to being in the dependent role of a patient, seeking control through the manipulation of their analgesic regimen.

F. History of Drug Use

A **history of previous drug use** may influence the patient's physiologic and psychological requirements for analgesic and anxiolytic drugs. For example, in the patient with recent significant narcotic exposure, tolerance is likely to predate the injury. Thus the actual dose of narcotic required for adequate analgesia may seem enormous. In these patients, the absolute number of milligrams is unimportant. Rather, the drug should be titrated to the desired effect. Detoxification, if indicated, can be accomplished after the patient has passed the acute phase of injury.

G. Sociocultural Factors

Patients may have learned behavior patterns, based on their cultural background, which influence pain perception. Thus the assessment of pain by observing the verbal and nonverbal behavior of the patient is not a good way to predict pain severity. For example, Asian-Americans often exhibit stoic behavior, rarely complaining of pain, whereas patients with a Southern European heritage tend to be much more emotive and dramatic.

H. Socioeconomic Background

A person's socioeconomic background and level of income have been shown to have an inverse correlation with procedural pain.

I. Educational Level

One's level of education has been inversely correlated with the perception of procedural pain, but directly correlated with one's tolerance of procedural pain.

J. Psychological Factors

    1. Burn victims with extensive injuries are often in a **state of physiologic and emotional disruption,** which may render them less responsive to pain initially.

    2. Stoic and emotive **coping styles,** the two extremes of behavior in pain patients, make pain assessment difficult.

    3. Fear, apprehension, survivor guilt, and the loss of control all serve to intensify the perception of pain as symbolic of the illness.

    4. The **obvious disfigurement** associated with burn trauma as opposed to internal soft tissue injuries or closed fractures serves to magnify the patient's horror of the illness, and can also magnify the perception of pain. Conversely, progress is more readily demonstrated to the patient, which can help to modulate pain treatment needs.

IV. PHASES OF CUTANEOUS PAIN

A. Acute Inflammatory Phase

The inflammatory phase begins with the loss of skin integrity after the application of kinetic energy to the skin, or after the failure of homeostasis of the skin (e.g., burn, abrasion, or ischemic ulcer). The inflammation may be exacerbated by **colonization or infection of retained necrotic tissue** and the release of exotoxin and endotoxin by invading organisms.

B. Healing Phase

The **proliferation of granulation tissue** can further interact with local pain receptors. The mechanical trauma of wound care, as seen with the avulsion of a bandage from a wound, can disrupt adherent eschar and coagulum. Sharp debridement, as well as daily scrubbing of the wound, causes a direct injury to underlying viable (and pain-sensitive) tissue. The successful coverage of the wound, with restoration of the epidermis, leads to the muffling of pain signals.

C. Convalescent Phase

Remodeling of the wound scar is often associated with pruritus and burning pain, followed by a gradual approach to premorbid sensory function. The final level of sensory function obtained is determined by the degree of tissue loss in the wound, the type of tissue chosen to recover the surface, and the degree of success in wound reconstruction.

V. RATIONALE BEHIND ACTIVE PAIN CONTROL

A. Preemptive Pain Control

Because of the profound metabolic, physiologic, and emotional responses to pain, it is easier and more therapeutic to **control pain preemptively** than it is to limit and manage pain and the attendant responses, once they are well established.

B. Metabolic Stress Response

Effective pain management will decrease the profound catabolism and sympathetic overdrive that are seen with significant burns. The metabolic stress response promotes the breakdown of body tissue; increases metabolic rate, blood clotting, and water retention; impairs immune function; and triggers a flight-or-fight alarm reaction. While these reactions may be appropriate in the wild, in the controlled environment of a hospital, they can complicate medical management and increase morbidity and mortality.

C. Morbidity and Coping

Inadequate pain control can lead to anticipatory anxiety, which exacerbates the perception of pain and so creates a need for higher doses for adequate analgesia, decreases the effectiveness of physical and occupational therapy, and prolongs hospitalization. While **reduced morbidity and improved coping** are difficult to document, the humanitarian goal of minimizing a patient's pain remains a valid goal in and of itself.

VI. BASIC PRINCIPLES OF PAIN THERAPY

A. Diagnosing the Cause

1. In addition to the **pain due to the cutaneous injury,** many burn patients have **secondary sources of pain** that contribute to their suffering, including:

    a. **Nonburn injuries,** such as fractures.

    b. **Complications of critical illness,** such as stress ulcerations, or thrombophlebitis.

    c. Pain associated with **management-related devices,** including nasogastric tubes, tight-fitting splints, or improperly secured central venous catheters.

    d. Pain associated with **prolonged bed rest** made manifest as muscle spasm, joint pain and stiffness, and pressure-related ischemic pain.

    e. **Preexisting painful conditions,** such as migraine headaches, osteoarthritis, and degenerative disk disease.

B. Nutrition

For burn patients, nutrition is fundamental to their wound healing, immune competence, and survival.

1. Whenever possible, **enteral feeding** is employed because the use of the gut diminishes the risk of gastrointestinal (GI) bleeding and the septic complications associated with central venous catheters, as well as bacterial overgrowth in the gut, which has been implicated as contributing to nosocomial pneumonias and the sepsis syndrome through the translocation of bacteria and endotoxin across the intestinal wall.

2. **Pain and stress divert blood flow** from the GI tract, decrease peristalsis, and increase interstitial water, all of which impede absorption. Thus good pain management is necessary to maximize gut function and nutrient absorption.

C. Covering Exposed Nerve Surfaces

Covering the exposed bare nerve surfaces greatly diminishes the intensity and frequency of nociceptive input.

1. This can be accomplished with **bandages, cadaver skin allografts, or synthetic skin substitutes.** The latter two coverings are more physiologic,

providing better temperature and insensible fluid retention, and are often used until the wound can be covered by **autologous split-thickness skin grafts.**

2. Nevertheless, bandages do provide sufficient protection so that the most potent analgesia can be reserved for short periods during daily wound care and can be done best with short-acting agents.

D. Monitoring Fluctuating Pain Levels

1. Patients vary significantly in their pain medication requirements over time. This variation is due not only to **interpersonal variation,** but also to the fact that burn pain follows a **nonlinear reduction over time,** unlike the pain seen with most acute injuries. Thus the pain of a full-thickness burn may be much more severe 3 weeks after the injury, as eschar separates to expose the wound and its pain fibers, than it was at the time of the initial injury. Therefore, a pain management plan must be flexible and be constantly reevaluated.

E. Evaluating Treatment Efficacy

1. No caretaker is as effective as the patient is in evaluating pain medication requirements. Pain evaluation can be very challenging, however, particularly when the patient is young, mentally impaired, or otherwise unable to communicate effectively. Numerous studies have shown little correlation between nursing perception of a patient's pain and the patient's self-assessment. Caretakers **tend to undermedicate** more often than they overmedicate, though both misjudgments have been reported. Studies have described undertreatment as related to such factors as fear of respiratory depression, fear of addiction, and underestimation of the severity of pain, as well as absurd misconceptions such as the myth that "burns always hurt."

2. Pain assessment is discussed in detail in Chapter 2.

VII. SELECTING AN ANALGESIC REGIMEN

A. Pharmacokinetic Alterations in the Burn Patient

1. **Plasma protein concentrations** These concentrations are altered in both the resuscitation and recovery phases of burn injury. **Total protein** concentrations are decreased about 30 percent and return to "normal levels" during the convalescent stage, about 1 month after wound reepithelialization. More important, two significant drug-binding proteins have altered concentrations during the resuscitation and recovery phases of burn injury. **Albumin** levels decrease and remain at approximately 50 percent of normal throughout these phases, and **alpha-1 amino acid glycoprotein concentration**

increases two to three times above normal, and remains elevated over these periods. These changes may alter drug binding and the bioavailability of particular medications, such as meperidine and fentanyl.

2. Hepatic function

    a. Although confirmatory studies are lacking, it is believed that **phase I reactions,** including oxidation, reduction, hydroxylation, and demethylation, are impaired.

    b. Phase II reactions (conjugation with acetyl, sulfate, glucuronide, and methyl groups) are believed to be unaltered.

3. Renal function

    a. Renal blood flow in burn patients is **often elevated** to the range of 80 percent higher than normal, and thus a medication with renal clearance will have a decreased half-life in these patients.

    b. It should be noted that **renal insufficiency or failure** can complicate the course of patients with severe burns, whether due to sepsis, inadequate fluid resuscitation, nephrotoxic drugs, or myoglobinuria. In addition, many elderly patients have preexisting renal insufficiency. Hence the dosing interval must be determined according to the existing level of renal function.

B. Route of Administration

The **route of administration** depends on the phase of rehabilitation.

    1. During the **acute inflammatory phase,** the necessary route of administration is intravenous (IV). The **reduced muscle and skin blood flow** render absorption from intramuscular and subcutaneous routes too erratic to be reliable. Similarly, **decreased bowel motility** following trauma makes the oral route ineffective, and also undesirable, during the initial stages following injury, due to the risk of regurgitation. Because the pain is relatively consistent during this phase, a **continuous infusion** can be readily titrated to analgesic need with less hemodynamic alteration than is seen with intermittent boluses.

    2. The **healing phase** spans the period from 2 days after the injury until wound closure is accomplished. Since this phase may last for several days or months, the method used to reduce pain will vary as time passes and both the type and severity of the pain evolve. The goal is to reduce pain as much as possible.

    a. During this phase, the **management of incident pain** (that incurred by dressing changes, physical and occupational therapy sessions, and other prolonged procedures) takes on increasing importance. Many therapists have reported a progressive inability to work with patients who are inadequately medicated, since the patient will come to view the therapist as inflicting pain rather than as assisting in the recovery of function. Minor maneuvers, such as turning, nasogastric tube insertion, endotracheal suctioning, and vascular access procedures, can become intolerably painful to the burn patient during the recovery period. Efforts should be made to involve the patient in his or her own pain control, since staff assessment of the patient's pain is notoriously poor, as noted above.

b. Patient-controlled analgesia (PCA) is usually substituted for the continuous infusion to optimize dosing as recovery occurs. The basal rate should be set higher for the very ill patient who will not be able to activate the control button. As the patient improves, the basal rate of the PCA can be decreased and the patient-activated dose increased to allow the patient to titrate the pain management more effectively. Additional bolus doses of pain medications should be administered for all painful procedures. Since tolerance will develop in these patients, a continuous infusion can be used in addition to the PCA, should the dose required become greater than that which a PCA pump alone can deliver.

c. When a patient is ready to take **oral medications,** 24 h requirements should be calculated (see Chapter 28) and the patient placed on an equianalgesic, around-the-clock, oral maintenance schedule with additional prn doses for episodes of severe pain. Patients should continue to be premedicated prior to planned painful procedures, such as dressing changes.

3. During the **convalescent phase,** patients will continue to require pain medication for therapy sessions, although the potency of the pain medication may decrease (e.g., less potent opioids and nonsteroidal classes of analgesics). The patient should still be allowed to have some choice of analgesic agent whenever possible.

C. Opioids

Medications are used primarily to modulate the perception of pain in the brain. The most commonly used class of drugs for pain relief are the **opioids,** although others may be used.

1. For over 150 years, **morphine** has been advocated in the management of burns. Its analgesic effect can be readily titrated with incremental IV doses. It can also be administered as a continuous infusion and by PCA. Morphine has two pharmacokinetic advantages for use in the burn patient: a low amount of protein binding (about 30 percent) and a major active metabolite that is conjugated in the liver and removed by glomerular filtration. Rapid elimination results so that doses as high as 50 mg/h have been reported in severely burned patients. The only disadvantage of morphine is its long duration, particularly in the presence of renal insufficiency. Any respiratory depression caused by morphine can be rapidly reversed by small amounts (40 to 80 μg IV) of **naloxone.**

2. **Fentanyl** has the advantages of a more rapid onset of action than morphine and less histamine release. It does have an increased incidence of

nausea and vomiting and sedation as compared with morphine, and also is considerably more expensive. Because it is about 85 percent bound to **alpha-acid glycoproteins,** which are commonly increased in burn patients, dose escalation is often necessary to maintain pain control. Doses often associated with general anesthesia are seen in patients on continuous infusions, yet these patients remain easy to arouse. Bolus injections combined with continuous infusions of fentanyl have also been used. Some researchers worry that excessive sedation and/or respiratory depression will occur when fentanyl is used due to its delay in distribution from the peripheral compartment, but this has not been shown to be the case.

3. **Meperidine** usually is not recommended for use in burn patients, because its clearance depends on renal blood flow. As a highly albumin-bound drug, an unwanted increase in free drug is also frequently observed during the resuscitation and recovery phases of patients with severe burns. Finally, the metabolite normeperidine is neurotoxic. If large doses of meperidine are administered and inadequately cleared, seizures can occur.

D. Intravenous Sedation

1. Anxiety alters pain perception dramatically. Conversely, patient anxiety is directly proportional to how well pain control was achieved the first time a procedure was carried out. Therefore, pain *and* anxiety must be well controlled at the onset of burn therapy.

    a. **Lorazepam** is the preferred long-acting benzodiazepine because it is metabolized by conjugation to inactive metabolites. Its half-life is about 10 h in burn patients, and thus it should be administered by intermittent injection, rather than by continuous infusion.

    b. **Midazolam** has rapidly become the benzodiazepine of choice in the Burn Unit. Its short half-life (1.5 to 2 h) allows administration by intermittent bolus, PCA, or continuous infusion. The half-life is lengthened by continuous infusion, increasing to as long as 12 h. It is metabolized to active metabolites that are excreted by the kidney.

E. Anesthetic Agents

The use of **anesthetic agents for sedation** is becoming increasingly popular, particularly for children. These agents have the advantages of rapid onset and, particularly in children, few adverse effects.

1. **Ketamine** (0.25 to 1.0 mg/kg IV every 10 to 20 min) provides rapid sedation and intense analgesia without depression of respiration, and can be useful in patients requiring multiple dressing changes. The adverse effects include tachycardia, hypertension, increased salivation, and hallucinations.

Smaller, more frequent doses will minimize the cardiovascular effects. If clinically significant, salivation can be controlled by pretreatment with a drying agent such as glycopyrrolate. Hallucinations *do* occur in children, as well as in adults, but can be limited or eliminated by the coincident administration of a benzodiazepine. Patients at high risk for untoward hallucinatory experiences include females, the elderly, those with drug abuse histories, and those with psychiatric histories. Though such experiences are reported in only about 5 percent of children under 10 years of age, this figure is probably higher due to underreporting as a result of communication deficits. In this age group, ketamine can be given orally or intranasally, though with less predictability than with IV administration.

2. Case reports of **propofol** for repeated burn dressings of children appear in the literature. Advantages include a short duration of action; little, if any nausea or vomiting after administration; rapid recovery, with no delirium on emergence; and ease of administration as an infusion. Sedation can usually be achieved with 0.5 mg/kg administered over 3 to 5 min followed by bolus doses of 10 to 20 mg as needed, or an infusion of 1.5 to 4.5 mg/kg/h. Propofol does cause **respiratory depression** and should only be administered by individuals trained in airway management, with oxygen and artificial airway equipment immediately available. Other respiratory depressants, such as narcotics or benzodiazepines, will potentiate this effect. **Hypotension** can result, particularly after a bolus dose, and particularly in elderly, debilitated, or hypovolemic patients. Propofol, unlike barbiturates, is **not antianalgesic.**

3. Self-administered nitrous oxide has been reported in a few burn centers, but is not widely accepted due to the complexity of monitoring and scavenging and the risks of staff exposure and abuse potential.

F. Nonsteroidal Anti-inflammatory Drugs

The use of **nonsteroidal anti-inflammatory drugs (NSAIDs)** in the severely burned is controversial due to concerns about the high risk of GI bleeding in this patient population. The NSAIDs do offer some potential benefits that must be considered.

1. Recent studies have shown that NSAIDs **reduce the body temperature and metabolic rate** of burn patients when given IV during the resuscitation phase. The long-term implications of this are unclear.

2. The IV use of NSAIDs after surgery can **reduce opioid requirements** by one-third to two-thirds.

3. Also, NSAIDs are valuable as an adjunct to narcotics during the convalescent phase.

4. The mechanisms of action, dosing, etc., are addressed in detail in Chapter 7.

G. Nonpharmacologic Modalities

1. Transcutaneous electrical nerve stimulation (TENS)

    a. This technique can be used to treat localized pain complaints, whether related to regional burns or to preexisting chronic pain complaints such as low back pain, or to treat secondary sympathetically maintained pain.

    b. It offers the advantages of patient control, ease of administration, and, other than an occasional skin reaction to the electrode patches, virtually no side effects.

    c. The neurophysiologic mechanism of action depends on the intensity and frequency settings, and is discussed in Chapter 14.

2. Self-regulation techniques Such techniques provide a patient-centered coping skill. Some data suggest that systemic endorphin release occurs.

    a. Controlled attention or distraction may use either auditory (music) or visual (movies) foci of attention. Concentration on an external focus promotes muscular relaxation and distraction from painful stimuli as a means of altering the pain threshold. The breathing exercises (e.g., Lamaze) used for the management of labor pain are another example.

    b. Biofeedback uses physiologic measurements such as heart rate, blood pressure, electrographically measured muscle tone, skin temperatures, and galvanic skin resistance to provide objective feedback to the patient regarding the effectiveness of the relaxation exercises. This technique can be very helpful in teaching patients to control muscle tone or regional blood flow, but the equipment can be cumbersome, which limits its application in the critical care setting.

    c. Hypnosis is a technique of inducing a dissociative state through focused concentration, not unlike controlled daydreaming. A trained individual is needed early in the institution of this modality, but patients can be trained in self-hypnosis, or the nursing staff can be trained to facilitate the induction of hypnosis once the patient has learned the technique. (See Chapter 14.)

VIII. PAINFUL SEQUELAE TO BURNS

A. Paresthesias and Dysesthesias

These are generally self-limiting, but their resolution can be accelerated by desensitization therapy, whereby new textures are gradually massaged into the area. If severe, the irritability of injured nerves may be managed with low-dose tricyclic antidepressants (e.g., amitriptyline, 10 to 75 mg qhs) and/or anticonvulsants (carbamazepine, 100 mg tid), titrated to therapeutic levels.

B. Contractures

Contractures are the result of an absolute deficiency of skin and soft tissue or prolonged immobility, and are especially problematic in the face, neck, and extremities. Aggressive management of burn scars includes compression garments, splints, and an exercise program. Refractory contractures can sometimes be softened with corticosteroid injections, but generally require surgical release and reconstruction.

C. Hypertrophic Scars

1. Most wounds heal with a noticeable scar that progresses through an early stage of hyperemia and hypertrophy with thickening and stiffening. These resolve over about 1 year as the scar "matures."

2. Immature wounds can be associated with pruritus, burning pain, sensitivity to cold and/or heat, paresthesia, anesthesia, and dysesthesia. Treatment for all of these is symptomatic, since most of them will resolve in time with scar maturation. The maturation is generally enhanced by compression garment therapy, which decreases the incidence of permanent contractures and improves the final appearance and function of the scar. Pruritus can often be ameliorated by antihistamines. See above for the treatment of paresthesia and dysesthesia.

D. Keloid Scars

Keloid scars are differentiated from hypertrophic scars in that they extend beyond the original borders of the wound. Associated symptoms include itching, burning pain, and stiffness, along with obvious disfigurement. Treatment including various combinations of corticosteroid injection, surgical excision, and low-dose radiation has been described, but all are associated with a high incidence of recurrence.

E. Causalgias

Causalgias are mediated by the sympathetic nervous system, and exhibit nerve damage and sudomotor and vasomotor changes, as well as burning pain. Multiple treatment modalities are available. Early, aggressive treatment of sympathetically maintained pain offers the best chance of resolution. (See Chapter 32.)

F. Phantom Limb Pain

The risk of **phantom limb pain** after amputation is decreased by the use of perioperative epidural local anesthetics (with or without narcotics). If phantom limb pain develops, management includes that described for neuropathic pain. Injection of neuromas into the stump with steroid and local anesthetic can also decrease symptoms. (See Chapter 32.)

IX. PRESSURE SORES

Pressure sores or decubitus ulcers result from anoxic necrosis of cutaneous and possibly subcutaneous tissues. All patients confined to bed for any length of time are at risk.

A. Stage I is characterized by erythema not resolving within 30 min of pressure relief. The epidermis remains intact. Pain is relieved when pressure is removed. This stage is reversible with the immediate and complete removal of pressure until the sore is healed. The site should be washed every 8 h with a mild antibacterial cleanser and left exposed to air. Care should be taken to avoid excessive moisture or dryness of the skin.

B. Stage II is characterized by partial-thickness loss of skin layers involving the epidermis and possibly penetrating into, but not through, the dermis. Clinically, stage II may present with pain, blistering with erythema, and/or induration; the wound base is moist and pink, and free of necrotic tissue. As with stage I, the area should be washed every 8 h with a mild antibacterial cleanser. Subsequently, an adhesive hydrocolloid occlusive dressing should cover the area until it is healed. Care should be taken that the area does not become excessively moist or dry. Once the exposed wound surface is covered with an occlusive dressing, it is less painful, and so most patients do not experience further pain unless they are exposed to further direct pressure on the affected tissues.

C. Stage III is characterized by full-thickness loss extending through the dermis to involve the subcutaneous tissue, and usually presents as a crater, unless this is concealed by overlying eschar. *Stage III wounds must be debrided.* **Mechanical debridement** is performed by applying gauze that is kept moist with normal saline, and changed every 4 h until a clean red tissue base is established. **Enzymes** may be used to supplement this debridement. **Hydrotherapy** is very effective, and should be used daily to facilitate cleaning and debriding. **Surgical debridement** is usually reserved for extensive necrosis. Once debridement is complete, an occlusive moist dressing such as bacitracin ointment should be applied once daily to cover the exposed wound surface and reduce pain. Difficult-to-remove substances such as zinc oxide ointment or paste should be avoided for all pressure sores as the effort needed to remove the paste may extend the sore.

D. Stage IV is characterized by deep tissue destruction extending through the subcutaneous tissue to the fascia, and may involve underlying muscle, joint, and/or bone. This stage often presents as a deep crater. It may include necrotic tissue, undermining, sinus tract formation, exudate, and/

or infection. This stage requires **surgical debridement** of the thick eschar, thoroughly removing all necrotic tissue, followed by reconstruction with either a soft tissue flap or skin graft.

X. OTHER CHRONIC WOUNDS

Other chronic wounds will be painful as a result of several factors, each of which must be addressed separately.

A. Arterial insufficiency will produce ischemic pain in addition to the pain of the ulcer with its exposure of nerve fibers. Coverage of these fibers with a stable epithelium will be facilitated by the correction of the ischemia, if possible, which will often also improve the pain of the ischemia itself. Vasodilators, peridural local anesthetics that provide a chemical sympathectomy, or surgical revascularization may be needed to improve blood flow.

B. Venous insufficiency, while not often surgically correctable, can generally be ameliorated by venous compression garments, which will enhance wound healing and stability.

C. Chronic infection will cause pain in a wound through the release of various endogenous mediators of inflammation (by the host) and toxins (by the infecting organism) into the wound. Eradication of the infection is essential to both wound closure and pain relief.

D. Metabolic abnormalities such as poorly controlled diabetes mellitus generally do not cause wound pain, but may delay wound healing and prolong a patient's pain until healing is complete.

E. A sensory neuropathy may decrease a patient's medication needs, but can itself be a source of pain. Peripheral neuropathies also lead to impaired healing, which has been widely documented, but is poorly understood. (The management of neuropathies is discussed in Chapters 16 and 32.)

XI. INFLUENCE OF CUTANEOUS INJURY ON PAIN MANAGEMENT

A. Skin is a sensory organ that also **regulates temperature,** acts as a **bacterial barrier,** and, to a lesser extent, influences **fluid and electrolyte balance.** A disruption of the integrity of the skin, especially with the more severe examples such as burns or skin disorders such as pemphigus vulgaris, can lead to hypothermia and substantial loss of fluid, electrolytes, and protein, and carries an extremely high risk of secondary infection. The serous drainage from these raw surfaces can also leak medications, accounting in part, perhaps, for the high doses of muscle relaxants, antibiotics, narcotics, and other medications required by these patients.

B. Cutaneous injuries are particularly painful because a complex network of receptors in the deeper skin structures is uncovered by the loss of epidermal integrity. As a result, other injuries or painful conditions may be of secondary importance until the injured integument and exposed nerve endings are covered.

C. The principles of pain management for integument failure and the associated alterations in pharmacokinetics were discussed in earlier sections of this chapter. While managing the pain of coincident noncutaneous injuries, the practitioner needs to keep in mind that unmeasurable insensible losses may lead to the requirement for very large doses of analgesic medications. These drugs should be titrated to effect rather than administered according to the "usual" dosing schedule.

D. Depending on the location, extent, and phase of integument injury, TENS application may not be possible. The use of transcutaneous patches (e.g., fentanyl, clonidine) or subcutaneous infusions of medications (e.g., hydromorphone) may be mechanically impossible or their effects unacceptably unpredictable due to alterations in cutaneous permeability and blood flow.

CASE DISCUSSION

As part of his initial care, the patient's burns were cleansed and evaluated, and bandages impregnated with topical antibiotic ointment were applied. The patient was placed on a continuous-air-flow mattress for comfort and to protect his skin from a pressure injury. The severity of the pulmonary injury necessitated mechanical ventilation, which was not well tolerated by the patient. As a result, pain management and sedation were accomplished with an infusion of morphine and scheduled doses of lorazepam. Dressing changes were managed with fentanyl and propofol boluses. As the patient was hemodynamically hyperdynamic, ketamine was considered undesirable.

On hospital day 3, when the patient's condition was stabilized, his wounds were surgically debrided. By this time, the patient's pulmonary injury was improving and the plan was to wean him from mechanical ventilation after the effects of the general anesthesia had dissipated. It was felt that a PCA would allow the patient better control of his analgesia and level of sedation, so a morphine PCA was started with a basal rate that was approximately half of his previous average hourly requirement. Self-administered doses were available every 6 min. Once extubated, the use of propofol for dressing changes was discontinued.

On hospital day 7, the patient was taken to the operating room where split-thickness skin grafts were applied to the deeply burned areas. It was noted that the patient's pain diminished greatly over the next several days, so the PCA basal rate was weaned accordingly. The patient was ultimately converted to oral oxycodone with acetaminophen (Percocet), with IV opioids only for dressing changes and debridements. Amitriptyline, 50 mg PO, was given at bedtime for sleep and for the burning pain and itching from the second-degree-burn sites. When PO feeding was well established and the patient clinically stable, a scheduled NSAID was added to decrease his narcotic requirements further.

Daily wound care and scar management therapy continued throughout the patient's 35-day hospitalization. On hospital day 30, the patient was fitted with compression garments, and was discharged home 5 days later on an NSAID, acetaminophen with codeine and amitriptyline.

SUGGESTED READINGS

Choinière M, Melzack R, Girard N, et al: Comparisons between patients' and nurses' assessment of pain and medication efficacy in severe burn injuries. *Pain* 40:143–152, 1990.

Kinsella J, Booth MG: Pain relief in burns: James Laing memorial essay 1990. *Burns* 17:391–395, 1991.

Longe RL: Current concepts in clinical therapeutics: pressure sores. *Clin Pharm* 5:669–681, 1986.

Mackersie RC, Karagianes TG: Pain management following trauma and burns. *Crit Care Clin* 6:433–447, 1990.

Marvin J: Pain management in the burn patient: excerpts from a symposium on pain management at Harborview Hospital, Seattle, Washington, July 23, 1986. *J Burn Care Rehab* 8:307–318, 1987.

Marvin J, Heimbach DM: Pain control during the intensive care phase of burn care. *Crit Care Clin* 1:147–156, 1985.

Patterson DR, Questad KA, Boltwood MD: Hypnotherapy as a treatment for pain in patients with burns: research and clinical considerations. *J Burn Care Rehab* 8:263–268, 1987.

Perry S, Heidrich G: Management of pain during debridement: a survey of U.S. burn units. *Pain* 13:267–280, 1982.

Perry SW: Undermedication for pain on a burn unit. *Gen Hosp Psychiatry* 6:308–316, 1984.

CHAPTER 24

PAIN MANAGEMENT AFTER TRAUMA

Roger Cicala
Douglas B. Coursin

Case
   I. Controlling the Pain
      A. Adverse Physiologic Effects of Pain
      B. Rationale Behind Active Pain Control
      C. Basic Principles of Pain Therapy
  II. Parenteral Medications
      A. Narcotic Analgesics
      B. Nonnarcotic Agents
  III. Epidural Analgesia
      A. Catheter Placement
      B. Epidural Narcotic Administration
      C. Epidural Infusion of Local Anesthetics
      D. Combined Narcotic and Local Anesthetic Infusions
      E. Monitoring Practices
  IV. Intrathecal Analgesia
   V. Intrapleural Analgesia
  VI. Peripheral Nerve Blocks
  VII. Other Techniques
      A. Cryoneurolysis
      B. Transcutaneous Electrical Nerve Stimulation
      C. Self-Regulation Techniques
  VIII. Analgesia for Patients with Common Traumatic Injuries
      A. Thoracic and Upper Abdominal Injuries
      B. Orthopedic Injuries
  IX. Summary and Case Discussion
Suggested Readings

CASE

A 53-year-old male with a history of obstructive pulmonary disease was involved in a motor vehicle accident. Injuries included multiple rib fractures on the right with a flail segment, liver lacerations, and fracture of the right femur and tibia. Operative interventions included laparotomy with repair of hepatic fracture, and open reduction and internal fixation of the lower extremity fractures.

I. CONTROLLING THE PAIN

A. Adverse Physiologic Effects of Pain

The **adverse physiologic effects of pain** are numerous (Tables 24-1 and 24-2). Unfortunately, many clinicians fail to recognize the significant detrimental impact that pain has upon the recovery of the trauma patient.

  1. Perhaps the most dramatic consequence of pain is its adverse effect on **respiratory function,** especially in patients who have undergone thoracic or upper abdominal surgical procedures.

   a. Mechanism Painful stimuli from chest wall afferent nerves cause reflex splinting of the intercostal muscles, decreasing ipsilateral lung volumes and promoting atelectasis. Other nociceptive reflex arcs inhibit diaphragm contractility and decrease tidal volume. Because of pain, patients consciously avoid coughing and deep breathing.

Table 24-1 Systemic hormonal changes seen after injury

Increased levels	Decreased levels
Cortisol*	Insulin
Epinephrine*	Testosterone
Glucagon*	Triiodothyronine
Aldosterone*	Progesterone
Renin*	
Prolactin	
ACTH	
Thyroxine	
Growth hormone	
Antidiuretic hormone	

*This increase has been shown to be eliminated or attenuated by some pain control methods.

Data adapted from: Watkins J, Salo M: *Trauma, Stress and Immunity in Anesthesia and Surgery.* London, Butterworth Scientific, 1982.

Table 24-2 Adverse physiologic effects caused or accentuated by pain following injury

Change	Physiologic mediator
Decreased diaphragmatic contractility	Spinal and medullary reflex arcs
Chest wall splinting	Spinal reflex arcs
Tachycardia	Systemic catecholamines, direct sympathetic outflow
Hypertension	Systemic catecholamines, direct sympathetic outflow Renin/Aldosterone
Increased oxygen consumption	Catecholamines, cortisol, glucagon
Hyperglycemia	Catecholamines, glucagon, cortisol
Ileus	Catecholamines, ?others
Splanchnic hypoperfusion	Catecholamines, direct sympathetic outflow
Fluid retention	ADH
Immobility	Spinal reflex arcs, supratentorial motivation

    b. Inspiratory capacity (IC), vital capacity (VC), functional residual capacity (FRC), and arterial oxygen content are all predictably decreased after abdominal surgery or thoracic injury, and remain decreased for at least several days.

  2. Pain stimuli transmitted to the central nervous system (CNS) may initiate brainstem reflexes, including systemic increases in sympathetic nervous system outflow and increased secretion of the catabolic or "stress" hormones (Table 24-1).

    a. Increased sympathetic outflow caused by pain results in an increase in cardiac output, blood pressure, and myocardial oxygen consumption.

    b. Sympathetic outflow and visceral nociception contribute to and prolong postoperative ileus.

    c. Hormone secretion caused by painful stimuli increases blood levels of catecholamines, cortisol, adrenocorticotropic hormone (ACTH), antidiuretic hormone (ADH), glucagon, and aldosterone. In turn, whole body metabolic rate and total body oxygen consumption are increased; sodium and water retention occur; proteolysis, gluconeogenesis, and hyperglycemia develop; bowel function is further depressed; and redistribution of blood flow to muscle tissue results in poor organ perfusion. Splanchnic blood flow is particularly affected, which may further impair hepatic perfusion in patients with liver injury.

  3. Immobility secondary to pain is a predisposing factor for postoperative thrombophlebitis, promotes urinary retention, and further compromises pulmonary function.

B. Rationale Behind Active Pain Control

1. Adequate pain control achieved by any method promotes ambulation and movement, which, in turn, dramatically improves pulmonary function and decreases the incidence of other complications such as venous stasis, thrombosis, and thromboembolism. Although controversial, there is some evidence that adequate pain control may lessen morbidity and mortality.

2. Some methods of pain control can block nociceptive reflex arcs, preventing much of the physiologic derangement normally seen after traumatic injury. Doing so minimizes the adverse effects which pain has on ventilation, attenuates the increase in sympathetic nervous system outflow, and reduces the high circulating levels of stress hormones associated with pain and injury.

C. Basic Principles of Pain Therapy

The basic principles of pain therapy include:

1. Decreasing the production of chemicals which sensitize peripheral nerves to painful stimuli (the mechanism of action of anti-inflammatory agents).

2. Blocking nociceptive neurotransmission at a peripheral nerve or spinal level (usually with regional or spinal local anesthetics), or stimulating descending pain inhibitory pathways from the CNS to attenuate pain transmission at the spinal cord level (one of the mechanisms of action of intrathecally administered narcotic analgesics).

3. Modulating pain perception in the brain (the mechanism of action of systemically administered narcotic analgesics).

4. The factors which should be considered when deciding on an **appropriate pain management plan** include:

a. The type of **environment** in which the patient will be cared for postoperatively and the appropriate treatment options available there.

b. The **anatomic location and severity of the injuries** and any subsequent surgical manipulations or incisions.

c. The presence or **possibility of any serious complications** (especially infectious, pulmonary, or coagulopathic).

d. The patient's **preoperative history,** including the presence of concurrent disease, a history of substance abuse, and the premorbid psychological status and intellectual capabilities of the patient.

e. **Psychosocial implications of the pain;** for example, the pain of traumatic leg amputation versus that of simple leg fracture.

f. Whether regional anesthetic techniques are planned for any **surgical interventions.**

II. PARENTERAL MEDICATIONS

A. Narcotic Analgesics

Narcotics remain the mainstay of acute pain therapy.

   1. Most injectable narcotics can be administered in roughly equipotent doses, and so should be selected on the basis of duration of action and potential side effects (Table 24-3 on page 433).

   2. The most feared side effect of narcotic administration is the occasional occurrence of marked **respiratory depression.**

      a. No substitute for careful patient monitoring exists for preventing this complication.

      b. It is to be noted that hypoxic episodes occur much more frequently in elderly and obese patients and in those with CNS injuries.

      c. Agonist–antagonist medications, such as buprenorphine (Buprenex) or nalbuphine (Nubain), seem to have a ceiling for respiratory depression effects, and for this reason may be somewhat safer than pure narcotic agonists. On the other hand, these medications also have a ceiling effect for analgesic potency, and may not be appropriate for treating severe pain. Dezocine (Dalgan) may be more efficacious than the other agonist–antagonist medications.

   3. **Narcotic analgesics** have other, less commonly recognized **side effects,** which may be particularly pertinent in the trauma patient.

      a. All narcotic agonists may cause nausea and vomiting, although this is most common with meperidine (Demerol). Pure narcotic agonists also depress bowel function and may cause adynamic ileus, which can be a critical problem in catabolic trauma patients who are at increased risk of sepsis. Agonist–antagonist agents such as buprenorphine do not appear to depress bowel function, and, in fact, may reverse the ileus caused by pure narcotic agonists.

      b. Meperidine is excreted primarily by the kidneys, and will have a prolonged half-life in patients with borderline renal function. Normeperidine, a metabolic by-product of meperidine, has a half-life of over 24 h, and may cause symptoms of CNS stimulation, including confusion, sedation, agitation, and seizures. Pentazocine (Talwin) may be associated with psychomimetic effects and dysphoria, and should be avoided for those reasons.

   4. **Routes of narcotic administration**

      a. Because of the variability of muscle perfusion in patients after injury, it is difficult to obtain consistent pain relief using the intramuscular **(IM)** route of administration.

      b. Continuous intravenous (IV) infusions of narcotics maintain predictable steady-state plasma levels of the narcotic agents and thus are more effective than intermittent injections. The major disadvantage of continuous IV infusions of narcotic analgesics is that the rate of infusion must be adjusted by nursing staff until adequate analgesia is obtained.

c. In trauma patients, **patient-controlled analgesia (PCA)** is often not useful, since the patient must be alert and oriented enough to use the device.

d. Alternative methods for the parenteral administration of narcotic agents are being developed, but again, cutaneous blood flow variability may limit their usefulness in trauma patients.

i. The **transdermal** delivery of fentanyl recently was introduced into clinical practice, and appears to yield steady serum levels of narcotic agent without expensive equipment. However, there is an onset delay of up to 24 h after the patch is placed, and a significant serum level remains for some time after the patch has been removed.

ii. A **nasal** spray form of butorphanol is also under development, and should provide rapid onset of analgesia because of the swift uptake of agent from the vascular nasal mucosa. Sublingual forms of other agents are also in clinical trials at this time.

iii. Either form of drug delivery would bypass the need for gastrointestinal absorption, providing alternatives to the injection of narcotic agents in at least some cases.

5. The optimization of narcotic analgesia provides enhanced comfort for the patient postoperatively, but does not in itself correct any of the pulmonary or metabolic sequelae of pain. However, when pain relief is sufficient and the patient is cooperative, secondary improvements in these functions will occur if the patient is able to ambulate and inspire deeply.

B. Nonnarcotic Agents

1. Nonsteroidal anti-inflammatory drugs (NSAIDs) provide good analgesia for musculoskeletal and incisional pain, and are especially effective for the increased pain associated with movement after surgery (see Chapter 7).

a. They are not particularly effective for visceral pain.

b. The majority of NSAIDs are available only in oral dosage form, but several **parenteral alternatives** are available, such as ketorolac tromethamine (Toradol) injectable, and indomethacin (Indocin) as a **suppository.**

c. NSAIDs may be used effectively to relieve postoperative and posttraumatic pain either alone or in conjunction with narcotic analgesics. The combination of narcotics with NSAIDs gives pain control that is superior to that of narcotic analgesics alone, and markedly decreases narcotic requirements.

d. Conversely, NSAIDs have **adverse effects** of their own, including decreased platelet aggregation, sodium retention, gastric irritation, and decreased glomerular filtration rate (GFR), which may limit their usefulness.

Gastric irritation can occur even if injectable or rectal forms of NSAIDs are used. Misoprostol (Cytotec), a synthetic form of prostaglandin E_1, may be administered orally to patients receiving NSAIDs in order to decrease the incidence of gastric side effects. It may cause systemic vasodilation and diarrhea, however. Antacids, H_2-blocking agents, and mucosal coating agents may be administered either IV or via nasogastric tube, and are also effective in preventing gastric irritation.

NSAIDs also interfere with renal prostaglandin synthesis, resulting in **decreased renal blood flow** and GFR. Therefore, they should not be used in patients who may have suffered renal ischemia or injury, or whose renal function is otherwise impaired. NSAID-induced renal dysfunction is especially common in elderly patients.

2. It must also be remembered that trauma patients are under extreme emotional stress and in a frightening environment. Often the request for pain medication is made because the patient is anxious or cannot sleep. The proper use of **anxiolytic, amnestic, and sedative medications** may alleviate these secondary symptoms, and thus decrease the patient's subjective pain complaints.

a. Tricyclic antidepressants have excellent sedative properties, and may also provide some analgesic effect. Amitriptyline (Elavil, 25 to 50 mg orally or 20 mg IM) usually provides excellent sedation lasting 6 to 8 h.

b. Anxiety may be treated with a variety of agents. Most sedative agents (especially benzodiazepines) have respiratory depressant effects, which may be additive with those of narcotic analgesics. Buspirone (Buspar, 10 mg orally) has excellent anxiolytic effects with minimal sedation. Alprazolam (Xanax, 0.5 mg orally) and lorazepam (Ativan, 2 to 4 mg IM) provide more sedation in addition to a potent anxiolytic effect. Midazolam (Versed, 1 to 5 mg IM or IV) has both anxiolytic and sedative properties, and additionally is a more potent amnestic than the other benzodiazepines.

III. EPIDURAL ANALGESIA

A. Catheter Placement

1. Epidural analgesia is most effective if the tip of the catheter is located near the level of the spinal nerve roots innervating the dermatomal area of the most painful stimuli.

a. Analgesia obtained with routine volumes of local anesthetics usually extends four to seven spinal segments both cephalad and caudad to the site of the catheter tip.

b. Analgesia obtained with narcotic agents is effective to some degree over the entire body because of the spread of these agents in the cerebrospinal fluid (CSF), but the most profound analgesic effect is obtained near the site of injection.

2. Epidural catheters may be safely inserted anywhere from the sacral hiatus (caudal insertion) to the C7–T1 interspace.

a. It is useless to attempt to "thread" a catheter from a needle placed in the lumbar region into the thoracic space unless continuous fluoroscopy is used. The vast majority of catheters inserted more than a few centimeters into the epidural space either will curl into a loop or exit the epidural space altogether via an intervertebral foramen.

b. Obviously, only experienced practitioners should attempt cervical or thoracic epidural catheter placements.

3. Whenever feasible, epidural catheters should be placed with the patient awake to allow assessment of possible complications and proper placement of the catheter. Catheters may be placed at the end of surgery while the patient is still undergoing general anesthesia, or in patients who have otherwise altered consciousness, if appropriate informed consent has been obtained beforehand. Fluoroscopic catheter placement should be considered in such cases, to avoid potential neurologic injury.

a. If complications from the patient's injuries or subsequent surgery (especially coagulopathy or sepsis) seem likely, or if injury to the spine or CNS has not been completely ruled out, it is best to delay catheter placement until later in the patient's hospital course.

b. Catheters may be left in place for up to 7 days without unreasonable risk of infection, provided an excellent aseptic technique is used during placement and subsequent dressing changes.

c. If it is necessary that the epidural analgesia be provided for a prolonged period, the catheter should be tunneled subcutaneously for 3 to 5 inches to provide further protection against contamination of the epidural space. This is most simply done by making a small stab incision around the epidural needle insertion site prior to removing the needle. A 14- or 16-gauge, 6-inch-long Angiocath IV needle can then be introduced percutaneously and advanced until the tip enters the incision. The epidural needle is then removed, the epidural catheter passed through the Angiocath, and the Angiocath removed. The stab incision is then closed with a single suture. Obviously, this technique is reserved for cases at low risk of sepsis who require prolonged regional analgesia (e.g., limb reimplantation or myocutaneous free tissue transfer).

B. Epidural Narcotic Administration

1. Epidurally administered narcotics provide pain relief which is superior to that of systemically administered narcotics. Dosage guidelines for epidurally administered narcotic analgesics are shown in Table 24-4 on page 437 and in Chapter 13.

a. Because these agents spread through the CSF prior to becoming absorbed into the spinal cord, effective pain control is provided over a wide area of the body.

b. In addition to spread in the CSF, a significant portion of the agent may be transported via the bloodstream and the CSF to the brain, where it can exert an additional analgesic effect.

   c. Highly lipophilic agents such as fentanyl and sufentanil tend to be rapidly absorbed into the spinal cord. They provide a swift onset of analgesia with a relatively short duration of action. And because they are rapidly absorbed into neural tissue, the lipophilic agents manifest more limited diffusion throughout the CSF and are active in a more limited area of the spinal cord.

   d. Less lipophilic agents, such as morphine, are absorbed into the spinal cord more slowly. They, therefore, have a longer delay in the onset of analgesia, but an extended duration of action. Because of their extensive spread through the CSF, such agents provide more widespread analgesia for patients who have multiple sites of injury.

   2. A number of reports have demonstrated that **depression of respiration** to the point of apnea may occur following the epidural administration of narcotic agents.

   a. Respiratory depression may take place within 1 h after injection, or as long as 24 h after the last epidural dose of narcotics.

   b. This complication is most likely to occur in elderly patients, those with preexisting respiratory disease, and those who also are receiving systemic narcotic or other sedative agents.

   c. Even in patients who do not exhibit clinical signs of respiratory depression, carbon dioxide response curves are depressed to a similar or greater extent after the administration of epidural narcotics than after parenteral narcotics.

   d. Lipid-soluble agents such as fentanyl appear to have a lower incidence of delayed respiratory depression, but the incidence of early respiratory depression is not affected by the choice of agent.

Table 24-3 Equipotent intravenous doses of commonly used narcotic analgesics

Agent	Loading dose (μg/kg)	Duration (hours)	Infusion dose* (μg/kg/h)	Side effects
Meperidine	1.0–1.5	3	250–350	Prolonged in renal failure
Morphine	0.08–0.12	2.5–3	20–30	Histamine release, biliary colic
Pentazocine	0.5–1.0	2–3	NA	Psychological side effects
Butorphanol	0.02–0.04	4	5–7	Narcotic withdrawal, sedation
Nalbuphine	0.08–0.15	5	12–17	Narcotic withdrawal
Methadone	0.08–0.12	12–24	NA	Long half-life
Buprenorphine	0.002–0.004	4–6	0.3	Narcotic withdrawal
Fentanyl	0.5–1.5 μg/kg	<1	0.5–1	Chest wall rigidity?

*Minimum hourly infusion dose may be calculated by the formula (loading dose/2)/half-life of drug.

e. An infusion of naloxone, 1 to 5 µg/kg/h, will reverse and prevent the respiratory depression associated with epidural narcotics without adversely affecting analgesia.

3. The epidural administration of narcotic agents is associated with several **other side effects,** including pruritus, nausea and vomiting, and urinary retention.

   a. The incidence of these side effects is higher when morphine is administered than when lipid-soluble agents, such as fentanyl, are used.

   b. In addition, the use of epidural narcotics depresses bowel function to a degree similar to that seen with systemically administered narcotics. A prolongation of postoperative ileus may be of major importance in trauma patients who are in negative nitrogen balance.

   c. Naloxone infusions are also effective in relieving or preventing narcotic-induced pruritus, and might be effective in reversing the adverse effects of epidural narcotics on bowel function. Naloxone is less effective in treating the nausea or urinary retention associated with epidural narcotics.

4. Patients receiving epidural narcotics tend to have better pain control and to ambulate earlier than those receiving parenteral narcotics, which may decrease the incidence of postoperative complications. However, it has not been clearly demonstrated that epidural narcotic administration is superior to PCA or the continuous infusion of narcotics in this regard. Epidural narcotic agents are *no* more effective than parenteral narcotics in attenuating the endocrinologic and metabolic response to the stress of injury.

C. Epidural Infusion of Local Anesthetics

1. Epidural analgesia using local anesthetic agents provides excellent pain control, and may be effective in patients who have not obtained sufficient relief from epidural narcotics. Bupivacaine, 0.06% to 0.25% (infused at 5 to 14 mL/h), will usually provide effective pain relief in trauma patients, while leaving motor function largely intact.

   a. Additionally, this form of analgesia interrupts the afferent and efferent nociceptive reflex arcs, **attenuating the metabolic and hormonal response** to injury. It must be noted that a maximum reduction in the neuroendocrine changes associated with pain (see Table 24-1) is obtained only if the local anesthetic blockade achieves at least a T6 spinal level, possibly indicating that sympathetic efferent blockade is more important than pain control in attenuating the stress response. **Nitrogen balance** has been shown to improve in patients receiving epidural local anesthetic infusions postoperatively, probably as a result of the decreased release of stress hormones.

   b. Furthermore, epidural local anesthetic agents have been shown to shorten the time until **return of bowel function** after abdominal surgery, presumably because of sympathetic blockade.

   c. In patients with upper abdominal or thoracic incisions, the administration of epidural local anesthetic agents clearly improves **pulmo-**

nary function, and has been shown to be superior to epidural narcotics in this regard.

    d. Epidural analgesia with local anesthetic agents also **decreases the incidence of postoperative thromboembolism** significantly, presumably because of increased peripheral blood flow secondary to sympathectomy, and an apparent attenuation of the hypercoagulable state.

  2. Pruritus, nausea and vomiting, and respiratory depression do not occur with local anesthetic agents. On the other hand, epidural local anesthetics are only effective in those particular regions of the body innervated within four to seven dermatomal levels on either side of the spinal level of the catheter tip, and, therefore, may not be appropriate for patients who have sustained injuries at multiple sites. Additionally, epidural local anesthetics will **interfere with sympathetic outflow,** resulting in vasodilation and possibly hypotension.

D. Combined Narcotic and Local Anesthetic Infusions

  1. In patients whose **site of injury is limited** to the upper abdomen or thorax, local anesthetics seem to provide superior pain relief and improvement of pulmonary function.

  2. Patients with more **generalized injuries** will probably require infusions of narcotic agents to obtain the diffuse analgesia required.

    a. Patients with **multiple extremity injuries** will often require morphine, rather than a lipid-soluble narcotic, because of its more widespread distribution in the CSF.

    b. In patients with **more limited sites of injury,** lipid-soluble narcotics will probably have fewer side effects and a decreased incidence of late respiratory depression.

  3. In most multiple trauma patients, especially those with both trunk and extremity injuries, the epidural administration of a combination of local anesthetic agents and narcotic analgesic agents provides optimal pain control.

    a. The **local anesthetic allows improved ventilation and attenuates the stress response to injury,** while providing excellent analgesia to the most severe sites of pain (usually thoracic and abdominal incisions).

    b. The **narcotic agent provides additional analgesia** with a more widespread area of effectiveness.

    c. Several studies have shown that a **combination** of morphine and bupivacaine, or of fentanyl and bupivacaine, **provides superior relief** as compared with either agent alone.

E. Monitoring Practices

For patients receiving epidural analgesia, the monitoring practices vary from institution to institution.

1. About one-third of hospitals currently allow the use of epidural narcotics on general medical–surgical floors postoperatively. Strict respiratory monitoring protocols must be used in these cases, however.
2. If the patient has limited pulmonary reserve due to obesity or significant lung disease, for example, it is desirable that the patient have either bedside nursing or some form of apnea monitor in place for at least the duration of epidural narcotic administration.
3. Alternatively, some writers advocate the continuous IV infusion of naloxone (1 to 5 µg/kg/h) for patients who are receiving epidural narcotics without bedside nursing.
4. It is probably wise not to allow both epidural and parenteral narcotics to be used concurrently, because of the higher incidence of respiratory depression associated with this practice. Obvious exceptions are the ventilated patient, and possibly the patient receiving close nursing supervision.
5. Low doses of naloxone (40 to 80 µg) should be administered and titrated to effect to reverse the respiratory depression associated with neuraxial narcotics. Excessive doses of naloxone have been associated with severe hypertension, tachycardia, myocardial ischemia, and pulmonary edema.

IV. INTRATHECAL ANALGESIA

A. Very small doses of narcotics administered intrathecally have analgesic effects comparable to those observed when much larger doses of narcotics are administered into the epidural space (see Table 24-4 and Chapter 13).
1. Injection of the narcotic agents directly into the CSF eliminates the need for diffusion of the agent through the dural membranes, resulting in a **rapid onset of action.**
2. Intrathecally administered narcotics undergo very little uptake by the bloodstream, resulting in **lower blood levels** of drug as compared with epidurally administered narcotics.

B. Unfortunately, however, there is some evidence that **delayed respiratory depression** is more common with intrathecally than with epidurally administered narcotics.

C. Catheter systems have been developed for **continuous intrathecal infusions.** Very small (27- to 32-gauge) catheters have been developed, but are currently unavailable due to reports of alleged neuronal injury occurring with the use of such systems.

D. Since equivalent analgesia can be obtained with the epidural administration of narcotic agents, the intrathecal technique offers few advantages for the trauma patient, unless spinal anesthesia is planned for surgery. Inclusion of a small dose (0.25 to 0.5 mg of morphine) in addition

Table 24-4 Analgesic agents and dosages for spinal use*

Narcotics	Epidural bolus	Epidural infusion	Intrathecal bolus
Morphine	3–5 mg	100–400 µg/h	0.1–0.5 mg
Fentanyl	25–100 µg	25–100 µg/h	10 µg
Sufentanil	5–25 µg	5–10 µg/h	
Meperidine	30–100 mg	10–20 µg/h	10–30 mg
Methadone	4–10 mg		
Buprenorphine	0.3–0.5 mg		
Butorphanol	2–6 mg		
Hydromorphone	1–2 mg	3–12 µg/h	

*Volume of injectate can also affect the area of analgesia which is obtained, especially with the more lipid-soluble agents. Routinely, narcotic agents are mixed in concentrations which will yield a delivered volume of 5 to 10 mL per hour for epidural administration.

to the local anesthetic used for spinal anesthesia can provide excellent analgesia for 12 to 24 h postoperatively.

V. INTRAPLEURAL ANALGESIA

A. The intrapleural injection of local anesthetic agents provides excellent **unilateral analgesia** for pain originating from the area innervated by the intercostal nerves, which includes **the thorax and most of the abdominal wall.**

   1. A standard epidural catheter is placed into the pleural space via a percutaneous puncture performed at the midthoracic level, medial to the posterior axillary line.

   a. Catheters are most easily inserted at thoracotomy prior to closing of the incision.

   b. In patients with chest trauma who are not undergoing thoracotomy, intrapleural catheters may also be inserted blindly via a 17- or 18-gauge needle. This technique may result in pneumothorax, however, and in some cases, the catheter has actually been inserted into lung tissue.

   2. Intermittent boluses of 20 to 25 mL of 0.25% or 0.5% bupivacaine with epinephrine every 4 to 6 h provide excellent analgesia. Alternatively, continuous infusions of 0.25% bupivacaine at rates of 10 to 12 mL/h may be utilized.

   a. In patients who are undergoing chest tube drainage of the involved hemithorax, bolus injections should be used and the chest tube clamped for 10 to 15 min after injection. This will allow the local anesthetic sufficient time to diffuse across the pleural membranes before being removed by the pleural suction.

    b. Patients should be in the supine position (with the affected side elevated slightly, if possible) during the administration of intrapleural anesthetic agents to allow for appropriate spread within the pleural cavity.

    c. Intrapleural analgesia may not be effective if blood or fluid is present in the pleural cavity.

  3. Serum bupivacaine concentrations during unilateral intrapleural bupivacaine administration approach levels generally considered to be toxic.

    a. Inclusion of epinephrine 1:100,000 with the local anesthetic solution will dramatically reduce serum bupivacaine levels.

    b. But even with the inclusion of epinephrine, intrapleural infusions should not be used bilaterally because of the risk of bupivacaine toxicity.

VI. PERIPHERAL NERVE BLOCKS

  A. Individual peripheral nerve blocks effectively provide 6 h or more of analgesia to the affected area.

    1. Because repeating blocks several times per day is very labor intensive, single-shot peripheral nerve blocks generally have limited usefulness in posttraumatic pain.

    2. Long-acting local anesthetics infused through a catheter placed near a neural plexus can provide profound analgesia for several days, however.

  B. In patients whose injury is confined to one extremity, plexus analgesia provides superb pain relief with extremely low rates of complications and side effects.

    1. Plexus analgesia may be a useful alternative for patients who have a contraindication to epidural analgesia, such as mild coagulopathy or spinal fracture.

    2. Another advantage of continuous plexus block techniques is that, in addition to analgesia, **sympathetic blockade** to the involved extremity also takes place. This may be particularly beneficial for patients who have undergone peripheral vascular procedures or limb reimplantation.

  C. Plexus analgesia is most appropriate for cases in which interscalene, axillary, or psoas compartment–lumbar plexus blocks will provide complete analgesia to the injured area.

  D. In most cases for which plexus analgesia is appropriate for postoperative pain control, regional blockade is also an appropriate choice for surgical anesthesia.

    1. Cannula over needle catheters for continuous plexus analgesia are marketed by several manufacturers, and provide a simple and effective

tive method of obtaining both operative anesthesia and postoperative analgesia.

  2. Bupivacaine in concentrations of 0.125% to 0.375% is ideally suited for postoperative plexus analgesia, since it affords excellent pain relief while leaving motor function largely intact.

VII. OTHER TECHNIQUES

A. Cryoneurolysis

Cryoneurolysis, the temporary destruction of peripheral nerves by freezing, has been shown to be an effective method for relieving postoperative pain.

  1. Unlike other neurodestructive procedures, cryoneurolysis results in the destruction only of axonal tissue, while the perineurium remains intact. The area innervated by the affected nerve is rendered insensate for a period of 4 to 8 weeks, after which axonal regeneration returns neural function to normal. Complications such as neuritis, which are common with other forms of nerve destruction, are rare following cryoneurolysis.

  2. Most commonly, the technique is performed during surgical exposure.

B. Transcutaneous Electrical Nerve Stimulation

Transcutaneous electrical nerve stimulation (TENS) has been reported to be effective in the relief of postoperative and postinjury pain by some writers, while others have reported results with TENS which were similar to those seen with placebo. Because TENS is entirely noninvasive, and gives a cooperative patient control over its use, it can be a useful adjunctive therapy in some cases (see Chapter 14).

C. Self-Regulation Techniques

Self-regulation techniques (see Chapter 14) can augment the patient's pain management and improve his or her sense of control and well-being. These techniques are particularly useful in patients receiving repeated painful procedures, such as bedside debridements or extensive dressing changes.

VIII. ANALGESIA FOR PATIENTS WITH COMMON TRAUMATIC INJURIES

A. Thoracic and Upper Abdominal Injuries

  1. Patients who have chest wall or abdominal injuries with **moderate to severe pulmonary dysfunction,** and those who are in the process of being

weaned from mechanical ventilation, constitute the group most likely to benefit from invasive pain control techniques.

    a. It has been well documented that patients managed with epidural analgesia have fewer pulmonary complications and require fewer days of mechanical ventilation than do patients managed with parenteral narcotics.

    b. Also, epidural local anesthetic infusions have been shown to provide superior improvement in vital capacity and tidal volume as compared with epidural narcotic infusions.

    c. The intrapleural infusion of local anesthetics provides pain control and improves pulmonary function as effectively as does epidural infusion for those patients who have unilateral injuries or thoracotomy incisions.

  2. In patients who receive thoracotomy or subcostal incisions, **intrapleural catheters** are easily inserted at the time of operation, eliminating the risks of thoracic epidural catheter placement. Since intrapleural infusions may only be used unilaterally, patients who have bilateral thoracic injury or midline upper abdominal incisions should be managed with epidural analgesia.

  3. Epidural catheters should be placed in the midthoracic region to allow the spread of local anesthetic over the spinal nerves to the entire affected area.

    a. Bupivacaine (0.06% or 0.25%, infused at 5 to 14 mL/h) is usually very effective.

    b. Fentanyl (5 to 10 μg/mL) or another lipid-soluble agent may be added to the infusate to provide pain control for other sites of injury or surgical incision. In patients with very widespread causes of pain (such as upper and lower extremity fractures), morphine (30 to 60 μg/mL) may provide superior relief.

B. Orthopedic Injuries

  1. Immobilization, by either external or internal fixation, is the key measure in limiting pain from bony fractures. Early immobilization also minimizes the possibility and severity of fat embolization.

  2. Periosteal and synovial pain respond especially well to **NSAIDs,** and these should be administered either orally or parenterally if the patient has no contraindications to their use.

  3. Epidural or plexus analgesia provides exceptionally good pain relief in patients with isolated upper or lower extremity fractures. Regional analgesia also decreases to some degree the tendency of immobilized extremities to develop deep vein thrombosis.

    a. For example, a block of the femoral nerve at the inguinal ligament is a simple, safe procedure which can provide excellent analgesia for patients with fractures of the femur. Ten milliliters of local anesthetic is deposited just lateral to the pulsation of the femoral artery, 1 cm below the inguinal ligament.

    b. Excellent analgesia is obtained within minutes, allowing for comfortable transportation and movement prior to surgery.

    c. If larger volumes (30 mL) of local anesthetic are injected into the connective tissue sheath surrounding the femoral nerve, sufficient cephalad spread may occur to anesthetize the obturator and lateral femoral cutaneous nerves ("three-in-one" block), providing complete analgesia for the hip and thigh.

    d. A catheter may be left in the femoral nerve sheath to allow the intermittent or continuous infusion of local anesthetics for postoperative pain control. However, psoas compartment blocks of the lumbar plexus are more consistently effective than are three-in-one blocks of the femoral sheath.

IX. SUMMARY AND CASE DISCUSSION

Although traumatic injuries occur more frequently in younger patients, the incidence of trauma in older patients continues to grow. Because older patients often have premorbid disease states such as chronic obstructive pulmonary disease, hypertension, coronary artery disease, or diabetes, they tend to tolerate injury poorly as compared with their younger counterparts. The patient presented in the introductory case example would benefit from an aggressive approach to pain control, especially since this could potentially eliminate the need for postoperative ventilation with its associated risks. Assuming that the patient's spine is intact and coagulation is normal, one approach would be the placement of an epidural catheter and the infusion of a solution of dilute local anesthetic (e.g., bupivacaine, 0.125%) containing a narcotic agent. Other alternatives might be the systemic administration of a narcotic by PCA, continuous plexus block for pain from the lower extremity fracture, or supplementation with ketorolac (Toradol) injections, assuming that renal function and coagulation status are within normal limits.

SUGGESTED READINGS

Craig DB: Postoperative recovery of pulmonary function. *Anesth Analg* 60:46–52, 1981.
Cuschieri RJ, Morran CG, Howie JC, McArdle CS: Postoperative pain and pulmonary complications: comparison of three analgesic regimens. *Br J Surg* 72:495–498, 1985.
Edwards TW: Optimizing opioid treatment of postoperative pain. *J Pain Symptom Mgmt* 5:S24–S36, 1990.
Engquist A, Brandt MR, Fernandes A, Kehlet H: The blocking effect of epidural analgesia on

the adrenocortical and hyperglycemic responses to surgery. *Acta Anaesth Scand* 21:330–335, 1977.

Fincher CW, Peterson RE: Interpleural anesthesia: development and application. *Anesth Rev* 17:11–15, 1990.

Mangano DT, Siliciano D, Hollenberg M, Leung JM, et al: Postoperative myocardial ischemia: therapeutic trials using intensive analgesia following surgery. *Anesthesiology* 76:342–353, 1992.

Naulty JS: The role of intrathecal opiates in the management of acute pain. *Clin J Pain* 5:S16–S27, 1989.

Smyreng T, Gomez MN, Johnson B, et al: Intrapleural bupivacaine—technical considerations and intraoperative use. *J Cardiothoracic Anesth* 3:139–143, 1989.

Woolf CJ, Chong MS: Pre-emptive analgesia—treating postoperative pain by preventing the establishment of central sensitization. *Anesth Analg* 77:362–379, 1993.

CHAPTER 25

ISSUES IN POSTOPERATIVE PAIN CONTROL

John C. Rowlingson
Robin J. Hamill

Case
  I. Introduction
     A. Acute Pain Is Biologically Necessary
     B. Postoperative Pain Is a Form of Acute Pain
     C. Postoperative Pain May Cause Pathophysiologic Consequences
 II. Factors That Influence Postoperative Pain
     A. Pathophysiologic Impact
     B. Site of Surgery
     C. Preoperative Preparation
     D. Patient's Physical and Emotional Status
     E. Intraoperative Management
     F. Effectiveness of the Postoperative Team
III. Evaluation of the Patient
     A. Defining the Diagnosis
     B. History of the Pain
     C. Physical Examination
     D. Laboratory Studies
     E. Standardized Assessment Tests
     F. Behavioral Observation
     G. How the Patient Presents
 IV. Management of Postoperative Pain
     A. Narcotic Analgesics
     B. Regional Analgesic Techniques
     C. Nonnarcotic Analgesics
     D. Sensory Modulation
     E. Psychological/Self-regulation Techniques
  V. Acute Pain Service

VI. Conclusion
Case Discussion
Suggested Readings

CASE

A 36-year-old female is involved in a motor vehicle accident and sustains blunt trauma to her left chest and abdomen. She is taken from the scene by helicopter to the trauma center. In flight, she remains alert and is stable, with a blood pressure of 90/60, a heart rate of 110, and a respiratory rate of 26, while receiving 2 L of intravenous (IV) fluid. A workup in the emergency room reveals a five-segment flail chest (T6–10) and an abdominal tap that is positive for blood. Computed tomography of the abdomen shows a fractured spleen. No evidence of disseminated intravascular coagulation or coagulopathy is evident. She is scheduled for exploratory laparotomy and probable splenectomy in the operating room.

I. INTRODUCTION

A. **Acute pain is a biologically necessary** physiologic response that warns a person that damage to tissue is occurring or is about to occur. Acute pain encourages a person to escape the injurious circumstances.

B. **Postoperative pain** is a form of acute pain, but one that serves a lesser warning function and is less escapable. Its presence *may* **herald the onset of a postsurgical complication.**

C. **Postoperative pain can cause** any or all of **the physiologic consequences listed in Table 3-3.** Because "pain" is a sensory *and* an emotional experience, postoperative pain also **can cause anxiety** (due to its frequency, intensity, severity, possible significance, and the uncertainty about its control) **and suffering** (the *unique* way a given patient interacts physically and emotionally with the pain).

II. FACTORS THAT INFLUENCE POSTOPERATIVE PAIN

A. Pathophysiologic Impact

The pathophysiologic impact of postoperative pain (see Table 3-3 in Chapter 3) involves:

1. **Localized tissue trauma** that results from the incision and the manipulation of tissue.

2. A **local release of chemicals** that augment the sensory input to the central nervous system (CNS) (see Chapter 3).

3. **Segmental reflex responses** occur at the spinal levels of nociceptive input.

4. **Suprasegmental responses** represent the additive effects of multilevel inputs to the CNS.

5. The adverse pathophysiologic consequences of pain influence postoperative morbidity and mortality. **All body systems can be affected,** with the failure of one system often leading to the compromise of another. For instance, if pain causes a paralytic ileus of the bowel and abdominal distension results, it can impair adequate respiratory function and increase the likelihood of atelectasis and pneumonia. Subsequent respiratory failure markedly increases the demand on the cardiovascular system, which could lead to cardiac failure.

6. Because the patient will have an **emotional reaction** to the pain (**the integrative response** involving cognition, affective reaction, and beliefs), one *must* deal with his or her understanding of the pain and the significance it has for him or her. **The patient's attitude** toward the pain will influence the response to all other therapy. For example, the patient's experience with abdominal pain will vary dramatically, depending on whether the etiology is that of an impacted common duct stone or of an ampullary carcinoma.

B. Site of Surgery

The site of the surgery influences the incidence and severity of postoperative pain.

1. The most severe postoperative pain results after procedures on the thorax, upper abdomen, major joints, lower back, and the anorectal area.

2. Of these, the first two are the most likely to compromise pulmonary function.

C. Preoperative Preparation

The **preoperative preparation** by the physicians and nurses can include the provision of crucial information to the patient.

1. The surgeon can explain the reason for the surgery, as well as its risks and benefits.

2. The anesthesiologist will discuss the options for intraoperative and postoperative pain control.

3. Nurses can orient the patient to the hospital ward routine and provide comforting answers to questions on a repeated basis, since they are readily available.

D. Patient's Physical and Emotional Status

The patient's status, both physical and emotional, will have a definite bearing on the response to surgery.

1. Trauma, acute illness, and chronic painful conditions will drain the energy and vigor of the patient, as well as impede the ability to be active and to provide self-care. The patient may be suffering from poor nutrition, diminished physical strength, or emotional fatigue upon admission, which can also influence the capacity for healing and recovery.

2. The patient may have concurrent medical conditions that increase the risks of anesthesia and/or surgery.

3. The perception of the impact of the surgery on the patient's ability to ambulate and function is very important.

4. Trauma and other serious illnesses can provoke nonproductive emotions, such as anxiety, depression, or frustration, that will affect the patient's outlook, participation in rehabilitation, and recovery.

E. Intraoperative Management

The intraoperative management by anesthesia and surgery personnel directly influences the severity of postoperative pain.

1. The use of premedication is part of preemptive analgesia (stopping the pain before it gets started!).

2. Care in placing IVs and securing monitoring lines (e.g., without traction on the skin) will enhance comfort.

3. Performing gentle intubation, taking care when positioning the patient, and managing relaxation to prevent the patient from struggling when lightly anesthetized will minimize musculoskeletal and joint pain.

4. Choosing an anesthetic technique that combines regional with general anesthesia allows the patient to derive benefits from local anesthetics and perispinal or perineural narcotics both intraoperatively and postoperatively.

5. Delicate manipulation of tissue and the judicious placement of drains also can enhance a patient's comfort.

F. Effectiveness of the Postoperative Team

The effectiveness of the postoperative team's approach to pain management will be an accumulation of the pre-, intra-, and postoperative consequences of preparation and treatment.

1. The cause for pain will be much clearer after surgery, and anesthetic or surgical complications will be apparent. This information will have an impact on the patient's overall condition.

2. Poor control of pain will demoralize the patient and put him or her at risk for developing pathophysiologic consequences of acute pain (see Table 3-3, Chapter 3).

3. Inattentive and nonsupportive care by physicians and nurses does not inspire the patient to report his or her pain, symptoms, worries, or attitudes.

III. EVALUATION OF THE PATIENT

A. Defining the Diagnosis

Physicians *must* **evaluate** the patient **to diagnose** the problem. Only after this is done can they hope to prescribe treatment that is based on the mechanism(s) for the pain (see Chapter 2 on the assessment of pain).

B. History of the Pain

The **pain history** is obtained by reviewing the patient's chart and interviewing the patient, when possible. The patient's ability to cooperate with an interviewer can be impaired by the effects of trauma, the medications given to gain control of the patient, the residual effects of general anesthesia, and preexisting physical and mental conditions. The minimal data base should include

1. the description of the pain
2. the location and radiation of the pain
3. the response to treatment thus far.

C. Physical Examination

A physical examination, in which the vital signs are noted, will elicit causes for the pain, which might include

1. ischemia
2. compartment syndrome
3. obstruction of viscera or vessels
4. a cast or other dressing that is too tight
5. pneumothorax, or an
6. infection.

D. Laboratory Studies

Occasionally, **laboratory studies** are helpful. These might include

1. an electrocardiogram for myocardial infarction
2. films of the chest for pneumothorax and pneumonia
3. films for prosthesis dislocation, fractures, bowel obstruction, and the like.

E. Standardized Assessment Tests

Standardized tests, such as the visual analog scale (VAS) or a simple numerical declaration about the pain's intensity, can help to quantitate the pain.

These tests can be repeated to reveal the trend of the pain's response to the therapy provided. (See Chapter 2 for further details.)

F. Behavioral Observation

Observation of behavior is not necessarily reliable, but assessing the patient's level of distress and the nonverbal behaviors will provide insight as to the impression the patient is making on the health care team.

G. How the Patient Presents

The **presentation of the patient** may be influenced by the residual effects of regional or general anesthesia, by analgesic or sedative drugs already given, or by the physiologic effects of the trauma or surgery.

IV. MANAGEMENT OF POSTOPERATIVE PAIN

A. Narcotic Analgesics

Narcotics are the mainstay of treatment.

    1. The dose, drug, and route of administration are chosen according to the severity of the pain, its location, its cause, the risk of potential side effects, and the patient's psychophysiologic condition.

    2. The **advantageous clinical effects** include analgesia, sedation, enhancement of mood, and cough suppression (as in those patients who remain intubated).

    3. Common side effects, no matter by what route the drugs are given, may include itching, nausea, vomiting, dysphoria, sedation, urinary retention, and respiratory depression.

    4. For dosing recommendations, see Chapter 8.

    5. Traditional intramuscular (IM) dosing results in tremendous variations in the blood level of the injected drug achieved *and* clinical effect due to the erratic blood flow to muscles and unreliable uptake of the drug from the IM depot. Muscle blood flow will be influenced by the patient's state of hydration, metabolic status, and cardiac function. Up to 70 percent of patients fail to get adequate relief with strictly scheduled IM dosing, and 80 percent say that the relief does not last long enough.

    6. Patient-controlled analgesia (PCA) provides a method by which the patient can self-administer opioids IV (or epidurally in special situations) to achieve maximal analgesia and minimal side effects.

        a. The patient's pain *must* be under control before the PCA is started. This often requires the careful titration of narcotics intravenously to establish a satisfactory level of analgesia, *after* which PCA is started.

b. The technique helps the patient to maintain his or her minimum effective analgesic concentration (MEAC) of the drug being used, below which level pain is experienced.

c. The result is a marked reduction in the patient's anxiety as to whether he or she will "get enough" medication.

d. The use of PCA reduces the need for negotiation with the nursing staff over medication issues.

e. The patient can treat incidence pain (i.e., pain associated with an activity such as coughing) at the time of its occurrence, and pretreat himself or herself in anticipation of pain related to dressing changes, getting out of bed, and so on.

7. Perispinal narcotic therapy places opioid drugs near the spinal cord site of action (see Chapters 6 and 13).

a. Opioids result in both **pre- and postsynaptic inhibition** of neurons in the dorsal horn, the site of first-level integration of noxious input to the CNS.

b. A small dose of opiate (as compared with systemic dosing), placed in proximity to the site of drug action, results in analgesia that is longer in duration and more intense than with other techniques of administration.

c. The subsequently lower blood level of the opiate should result in a lower incidence of drug-related side effects.

d. The lipid solubility of the opiate drug dramatically influences the onset and duration of action, as well as the incidence of side effects.

e. The **epidural route** of administration has become more prominent than the **subarachnoid route** because catheters are commonly placed for anesthesia, access to all spinal levels is possible, and a lower incidence of side effects has been observed than with subarachnoid techniques.

f. Perispinal narcotics are used **in combination with local anesthetic drugs** so that lower doses or concentrations of each may be used, and to attack the pain based on the different mechanisms of action of the two classes of drug.

g. Table 25-1 lists factors that minimize the risk of life-threatening respiratory depression in patients receiving perispinal narcotics or in combination with local anesthetic drugs.

B. Regional Analgesic Techniques

Regional techniques with local anesthetic drugs can provide effective analgesia temporarily, or more continuously if an infusion is used.

1. The **local anesthetic** drug is chosen based on the site of administration, the duration of effect needed, and the patient's medical history (e.g., the history of an allergic reaction to novocaine).

2. Techniques for regional analgesia are discussed in Chapter 13.

Table 25-1 Factors that decrease the incidence of respiratory depression with perispinal narcotics

- Decreased doses of opioids used in epidural bolus therapy or infusions
- More knowledgeable choices about the particular drug used, based on its lipid solubility and the level of instillation
- The use of low concentrations of local anesthetic drugs with epidural narcotics
- The use of concurrent naloxone infusions in patients who show any narcotic-related side effects
- Awareness of the need to control the administration of other drugs that have sedative side effects
- Application of criteria for choosing the most appropriate patients for these techniques
- Monitoring, especially in the form of increased nursing surveillance
- The use of intensive care units and step-down units for selected patients given the acuity of their condition
- The increase in the number of institutions that have Acute Pain Services to facilitate the provision of the techniques, the personnel to provide the care safely and effectively, and the educational background that is so crucial to everyone involved in the patient's care

3. The **advantages** of regional analgesia include:
   a. A quiet awakening from general anesthesia.
   b. Reduction of the stress response and **"windup"** (the hypersensitization of the CNS response that occurs when intense pain is not treated quickly).
   c. A reduced need for opioids, and thus fewer narcotic-related side effects.
   d. An earlier resumption of normal activity, including ambulation, with the benefits of improved limb blood flow and a reduction in the incidence of deep venous thrombosis (DVT) and embolism.

4. The **disadvantages** of regional analgesia include:
   a. Possible local anesthetic side effects, including sensory or motor block.
   b. The time and personnel necessary to provide repeat blocks and follow-up.
   c. The potential for inadequate training, skill, or enthusiasm among the medical or nursing staff members to apply the techniques and/or manage the patients.
   d. The need for extra equipment, such as epidural catheters, or infusion pumps.

C. Nonnarcotic Analgesics

Nonnarcotic agonist analgesics are another method by which the use of opioid drugs can be minimized (see Chapters 7, 8, 9, and 11 for a more complete discussion).

1. **Narcotic agonist–antagonist** drugs have opioidlike analgesic potential, but have the advantage of limited respiratory depression (ceiling effect). Due to an absence of euphoria and a similar ceiling effect with regard to analgesia, they offer a low risk of abuse. By and large, their analgesic strength is of a moderate degree, and this is of little benefit in the management of pain after major surgery or severe trauma.

Administration of low doses (e.g., nalbuphine [Nubain], 2 to 5 mg IV) in the presence of narcotic agonists will improve some opioid-mediated side effects, such as respiratory depression and sphincter of Oddi spasm, without reversing analgesia.

2. **Nonsteroidal antiinflammatory drugs (NSAIDs)** are indicated for patients in whom inflammation is causative of the pain. The property of these drugs to impair renal and platelet function and to cause gastrointestinal (GI) bleeding is a concern with their use in acutely ill and traumatized patients. Limited dosing schedules (e.g., for the first 48 to 72 h postinjury) decrease the risk of GI side effects.

3. **Adjunctive medications** are used with the goal of decreasing the necessary doses of opiates.

    a. **Antianxiety agents** effectively treat the reactionary agitation and upset that patients suffering from trauma and acute illness may experience as a part of their total "pain" problem. Respect must be shown for the sedative and disorienting side effects of drugs in this class.

    b. **Antihistamines** have sedative effects, and perhaps some nonspecific analgesic effects.

    c. **Phenothiazines** have been used with opioids in the past in the belief that they cause a potentiation of effect. It is likely that they offer little more than sedation.

D. Sensory Modulation

Sensory modulation is based on the concept that hyperstimulation of the nervous system will "drown out" pain messages to the CNS, and thereby prevent the cascade of adverse physiologic consequences mentioned earlier (see Chapter 14 for further discussion). Because the nervous system responds to variations in input, many of these therapies can be of benefit.

1. **Massage** is a simple technique that requires touching the patient. This contact may be very comforting to the patient, as can be the reduction in pain and muscle spasm that results when the skin and muscles are rhythmically kneaded.

2. When transcutaneous electrical nerve stimulation (**TENS**) is used, the literature shows that up to 25 percent of patients need no more than this technique alone, 50 percent will have a decreased need for supplemental narcotics, and 25 percent may not benefit at all. This technique has the dis-

tinct advantages of being noninvasive, of not interfering with other therapies that are being used, and of being patient controlled.

    3. Acupuncture of the classic variety is not used routinely, but is a reputable stimulation therapy.

    4. Alternating hot and cold contrast applications are more commonly used in a formal physical therapy setting than for the treatment of postoperative pain. They do represent another of the noninvasive modalities that require physical contact with the patient, and they can provide analgesia without medication side effects.

E. Psychological/Self-regulation Techniques

These techniques give the patient a sense of control over postoperative and posttrauma pain and its consequences, as well as demonstrate to the patient that his or her opinions and beliefs are worthy and important (see Chapters 5 and 14 for further discussion).

    1. Providing explanations and information to patients and their families is within the therapeutic realm of all health care workers. It is amazing how well people cope with their circumstances when information is shared so that they understand what is possible, happening, or expected.

    2. Hypnosis is a general term for states of focused attention that can be achieved by many individuals under various circumstances. Though it takes training and practice, for patients with longer-term problems, hypnosis can be an effective analgesic and anxiolytic therapy.

    3. Biofeedback and relaxation training are alternative forms of self-regulation that are based on modifying a chosen physiologic parameter, such as heart rate or muscle spasm, with progressive training. This activity, as does hypnosis, takes time and practice, so the patient must be alert, responsive, and interactive.

V. ACUTE PAIN SERVICE

An Acute Pain Service is an alliance of specialists interested in the provision of postoperative pain control that is based on scientific evidence of safety and effectiveness. This coordinated management requires the education of all involved; the creation and application of protocols for patient selection, management, monitoring, and follow-up; and the immediate availability of personnel to deal with changing patient needs or complications of therapy.

VI. CONCLUSION

    A. Not all sensations that are experienced by the patient as "pain" can be treated in the same way.

B. Patients must be systematically evaluated to determine the cause(s) of their pain, and frequently reassessed for their response to therapy. Rigid, inflexible treatment schemes deny the reality of marked individual variations in the need for pain relief.

C. The best treatment for a given patient's pain is that which addresses the etiology for the pain and results in pain relief that is satisfactory to the patient.

D. The overall goals of therapy beyond patient comfort are rapid cooperation with rehabilitative therapy, the restoration of normal activity, a shortening of the hospital stay, and a reduction in costs.

CASE DISCUSSION

The preoperative anesthesia assessment of the patient reveals a past medical history that is negative for significant disease. Her only regular medications include birth control pills, and she had an uneventful appendectomy 15 years earlier under general anesthesia. She weighs 73 kg. To manage the pain related to her flail chest *and* her postoperative pain most effectively, it is explained that a thoracic epidural catheter should be placed before anesthesia is induced. This will provide feedback from her as to the proper and safe location of this important catheter. The placement is done at the T7–8 level, and only a test dose of 4 mL of 1.5% lidocaine with 1:200,000 epinephrine is given through the catheter. This reflects the anesthesiologist's choice *not* to create a marked sympathectomy just prior to an exploratory laparotomy in a patient in whom significant blood loss is a likely event.

The operative procedure is completed, and the patient is stable in the intensive care unit (ICU) after an uneventful splenectomy. She was given 5 mg of preservative-free morphine in the epidural catheter 60 min before the end of the operation. She woke up in the ICU 90 min after her arrival, and was able to indicate that she had "some discomfort" (a level 6 on a 10-point scale). She develops a drop in blood pressure from 115/70 to 85/60 after a test dose of 1.5% lidocaine, but this responds to a 500-mL fluid bolus. She is neurologically intact prior to the initiation of an infusion of 0.125% bupivacaine and hydromorphone (Dilaudid, 6 μg/mL) being started at 8 mL^3/h. Within 30 min, her chest pain is at a 2/10 level, and she is uneventfully extubated 30 min later. Left shoulder pain, felt to be due to pleural irritation by the thoracostomy tube, is managed with supplemental IV doses of ketorolac (Toradol, 15 mg every 6 h, as needed) and dezocine (Dalgan, 2 to 4 mg IV every hour, as needed).

The epidural infusion is continued for the next 3 days, with some variation in the rate of infusion based on her clinical condition and comfort. The catheter is removed on the fifth postoperative day when her chest tube is taken out, and she is taking liquids by mouth on a reliable basis.

SUGGESTED READINGS

Agency for Health Care Policy and Research: Acute pain management: operative or medical procedures and trauma. Public Health Service, Department of Health and Human Services, Rockville, Maryland, 1992.

Austin KL, Stapleton JV, Mather LE: Multiple intramuscular injections: a major source of variability in analgesic response to meperidine. *Pain* 8:47–62, 1980.

Bonica JJ: Postoperative pain, in Bonica JJ (ed): *Management of Pain.* Philadelphia, Lea & Febiger, 1990, pp 461–480.

Cousins MJ, Cherry DA, Gourlay GK: Acute and chronic pain: use of spinal opiates, in Cousins MJ, Bridenbaugh PO (eds): *Neural Blockade in Clinical Anesthesia and Management of Pain.* Philadelphia, Lippincott, 1988, pp 955–1029.

Hord AH, Kohenes C: Postoperative pain: a review of management methods. *Hosp Formul* 24:28–40, 1989.

Merrill DC: Clinical evaluation of FasTENS, an inexpensive, disposable transcutaneous electrical nerve stimulator designed specifically for postoperative electroanalgesia. *Urology* 33:27–30, 1989.

Raj PP, Knarr DC, Vigdorth E, et al: Comparisons of continuous epidural infusion of a local anesthetic and administration of systemic narcotics in the management of pain after total knee replacement surgery. *Anesth Analg* 66:401–406, 1987.

Taenzer P, Melzack R, Jeans ME: Influence of psychological factors in postoperative pain, mood, and analgesic requirements. *Pain* 24:331–342, 1986.

Tyler E, Caldwell C, Ghia JN: Transcutaneous electrical nerve stimulation: an alternative approach to management of postoperative pain. *Anesth Analg* 61:449–456, 1982.

Yeager M, Glass D, Neff R, et al: Epidural anesthesia and analgesia in high risk surgical patients. *Anesthesiology* 66:729–736, 1987.

CHAPTER
26

TRANSPLANTATION

Glenn Murray
Kyle Tipton

Case
  I. General Concerns
     A. Medical History
     B. Physiologic Changes
     C. Immunosuppression
     D. Substance Issues
     E. Cultural and Geographic Factors
 II. Liver Transplantation
     A. Preoperative Status
     B. Intraoperative Management
     C. Immediate Postoperative Course
     D. Longer-Term Course
     E. Posttransplant Pain Syndrome
     F. Specific Modalities
III. Renal Transplantation
     A. Nature of the Pain
     B. Pain Management
 IV. Heart-Lung Transplantation
     A. General Concerns
     B. Treatment Options
  V. Bone Marrow Transplants
Case Discussion
Suggested Readings

CASE

A 47-year-old woman with ethanol-related cirrhosis, currently in rehabilitation and without alcohol intake for 2 years, presents for liver transplantation. The patient also has a 75-pack-a-year history of cigarette smoking, still smokes two packs per day, and has a productive cough. She has required sclerotherapy twice in the past 4 months and now has mild encephalopathy. Her intraoperative course is unremarkable. After induction with thiopental, her anesthetic consists of isoflurane, fentanyl, and small doses of benzodiazepine. Postoperatively, her liver is functioning well and her mental status has cleared enough to warrant weaning from mechanical ventilation. As the ventilatory support is decreased, she becomes increasingly agitated, pointing to her abdominal incision. She has moderate amounts of thick, yellow secretions and requires frequent suctioning.

I. GENERAL CONCERNS

A. Medical History

Some general concerns are widely applicable to transplant patients, regardless of the specific organ involved. These patients have often suffered from a primary disease for a prolonged period prior to the transplant procedure, and this disease course may include multiple hospitalizations and invasive procedures, possibly even prior transplants. For example, the typical preoperative morbidity in a liver transplant "candidate" could include inhospital treatment of ascites, with or without associated spontaneous bacterial peritonitis, hepatic encephalopathy, or gastrointestinal (GI) bleeding. A few patients may have already visited the operating room for procedures such as portosystemic shunts for portal hypertension (despite the increased technical difficulty of subsequent hepatic dissection at the time of transplant) or intestinal operations (primary sclerosing cholangitis associated with inflammatory bowel disease, extensive small bowel resection in patients referred for small bowel transplant). In the renal transplant population, of course, long-term dialysis and accompanying vascular access procedures are common experiences.

Pain management considerations for various transplant patients are given in Table 26-1.

B. Physiologic Changes

Recent studies show long-lasting **physiologic changes** in the neuroaxis following even brief noxious stimuli, causing future stimuli to be perceived as even more intense. This phenomenon, called *windup,* coupled with the anticipatory anxiety regarding even minor invasive procedures that chronically instrumented patients have, makes pain control in this population an even greater challenge.

Table 26-1 Pain management considerations in transplant patients

Liver	Kidney	Heart-lung	Bone marrow
Chronic illness with wide spectrum of severity	Chronic illness	Little specific data—possible epidural	Oral mucositis
Frequent renal dysfunction	Impaired metabolism of meperidine and morphine	Treat as all thoracotomies	Cutaneous rashes with pruritus
Possible encephalopathy	Nephrotoxicity of NSAIDs		
Limitations of regional techniques due to coagulopathy	Coagulopathy (platelet dysfunction)		
Chronic pain (including back pain)			
Minimal narcotic requirements			
Substance use issues			

C. Immunosuppression

Immunosuppression is seen in many of these patients even before their transplants due to long-standing chronic disease and, often, malnutrition. In addition, immunosuppressive therapy after transplantation carries its own threat. The issues which the patient must deal with include:

  1. an increased risk of infection such that even a minor sore throat may have ominous significance;
  2. an alteration of organ function as a result of immunosuppressive therapy, as with the renal insufficiency associated with cyclosporine administration or the osteoporosis of chronic steroid exposure; and
  3. an alteration in self-image as a result of both the presence of a foreign organ and the cushingoid habitus from steroid intake.

D. Substance Issues

Substance issues are not uncommon in this patient population. Some of these patients may have developed narcotic tolerance during the course of their illnesses, or, in isolated cases, have a history of blood-borne hepatitis associated with intravenous (IV) drug use. Ethanol-induced cirrhosis is an accepted indication for liver transplant, as selected patients have been found to have a good recovery without recidivism, provided that adequate time is available for preoperative counseling and abstinence from alcohol. Despite abstinence, patients with a history of substance abuse present unique problems with respect to analgesia.

E. Cultural and Geographic Factors

In addition to the physiologic and psychosocial implications of the disease states described above, **cultural and geographic factors** need to be considered. It should be remembered that many referred patients are treated at transplant centers far from their homes, and face prolonged hospitalizations with only sporadic family support. In the case of international referrals, language and cultural factors may be added to geographic ones.

II. LIVER TRANSPLANTATION

A. Preoperative Status

1. Currently, adult hepatic transplantation encompasses not only a wide range of disorders that lead to end-stage liver disease, but also a broad spectrum of disease severity and functional status, as reflected in the United Network for Organ Sharing Classification. Patients may be relatively stable, living at home on a "waiting list"; may be undergoing inpatient treatment; or may require intensive care for GI bleeding, multiorgan dysfunction, or fulminant hepatic failure. This continuum of illness severity is the basis for prioritizing patients to receive the scarce donor organs, and also has a bearing on the variability of their postoperative recovery.

2. As noted above, some patients may have a history of ethanol or other substance abuse and be undergoing concurrent social and psychiatric, as well as medical, treatment.

B. Intraoperative Management

1. For those patients selected for liver transplantation, a typical anesthetic makes use of a rapidly **titratable inhalational agent** (e.g., isoflurane). Agents given IV are subject to pharmacokinetic variability due to unpredictable rapid blood loss; however, most patients receive substantial doses of **narcotics,** as well as some **barbiturates** and/or **benzodiazepines,** as in other lengthy abdominal procedures.

2. There may be advantages to **early extubation,** but this approach often is not possible in patients with severe encephalopathy or respiratory compromise who may require mechanical ventilation even preoperatively. Typically, patients remain intubated during the first 24 h after their transplant, so that intraoperative narcotics can be given freely and allowed to wear off gradually.

C. Immediate Postoperative Course

The immediate postoperative course is similar to that following other extensive abdominal procedures, although the function of the hepatic graft plays a very significant role.

1. **Nature of the pain**   Despite the extensive and prolonged intraoperative procedure, liver transplant patients seem to experience pain which is not much different from that of patients who have undergone seemingly "minor" upper abdominal operations. In fact, one study compared postoperative pain in liver transplant recipients and in patients recovering from routine cholecystectomy (Eisenach, 1989), and found narcotic requirements and pain intensity to be consistently lower following liver transplant. While the etiology of this finding was not revealed, the difference between these groups appeared to be due to endogenous factors in the transplant group and not to altered morphine pharmacokinetics. The practitioner must keep in mind, however, that pain is a personal experience and that analgesic therapy should be tailored to the patient's needs rather than to a preconceived idea of what the patient "should" need.

2. **Role of graft function**
   a. Recovery from the anesthetic and return to a normal neurologic status have been of particular importance in this patient population in both the assessment of adequate graft function and the timing of extubation. Among the many indicators of a well-functioning graft, recovery of a normal level of consciousness and resolution of hepatic encephalopathy have been among the most basic. In these patients, good graft function and adequate mental status constitute important weaning parameters, which carry as much weight as the more traditional measures of respiratory function alone. The morbidity in patients who are unable to protect their own airways is formidable. Pneumonia or the adult respiratory distress syndrome (ARDS) as a result of aspiration can be a devastating complication in both pretransplant candidates, due to immunologic compromise associated with chronic disease and malnutrition, as well as the inability of the cirrhotic liver to clear mediators of lung injury, and transplant recipients, due to immunosuppressive therapy.

   b. In preoperative patients with significant degrees of encephalopathy, it is prudent to secure control of the airway with endotracheal intubation, and to maintain intubation in postoperative patients until their mental status has cleared. Some practitioners have found it useful to have patients write their names or draw simple figures as part of the weaning process to rule out residual encephalopathy.

   c. Reliance on neurologic status as an indicator of graft function and weaning ability has led to the practice of minimizing narcotic analgesia in the postoperative period. There is also the observation that these patients have relatively less pain than expected, despite the extensive nature of their operation. **Diphenhydramine** (Benadryl) is often used for its antihistaminic and sedative properties, and offers some patients adequate pain control. However, **pain therapy must be individualized,** and the titration of small doses of short-acting, reversible narcotics such as **fentanyl** (Sublimaze) is often of benefit, provided that close attention is paid to the patient's neurologic and airway status.

    d. As in other surgical patients, a fine margin may exist between providing adequate analgesia for incentive spirometry and deep breathing and depressing respiration to unsatisfactory levels. **Vigorous respiratory therapy** and **early mobilization** play an obvious role in minimizing the risk of pulmonary and thromboembolic complications.

    e. Some of the other parameters for early **assessment of graft function** besides recovery of the central nervous system include the appearance of bile in those patients who have external biliary drainage via T-tube, liver chemistries and coagulation studies (prothrombin time, thromboelastogram), serum lactate, and arterial ketone body ratio. Frequent serial assessments are done in the acute postoperative phase.

  3. **Intensive care management**

    a. Although reversal of narcotics or anesthetic drugs is rarely necessary in clinical practice, occasionally the situation arises where an immediate assessment of neurologic status is required (e.g., if there are concerns about intracerebral bleeding or edema). Intensive care physicians should bear in mind the availability of **peripheral nerve stimulators** to assess residual neuromuscular blockade. Use of the nerve stimulator and reversal medications is discussed in Chapter 12. The benzodiazepine/gamma-aminobutyric acid (GABA) antagonist **flumazenil** (Mazicon) has been reported to have a dramatic, although often short-lived, effect in reversal of benzodiazepine sedation or hepatic encephalopathy. **Naloxone** (Narcan), *gently titrated in judicious doses* (40 to 80 μg), can be administered to reverse narcotic sedation and respiratory depression. Large doses, particularly in narcotic-tolerant individuals, can cause severe hypertension and tachycardia.

    b. In addition to the native liver or allograft, altered physiology of other organs is often present in these complex patients. Of these, **renal dysfunction** probably represents the most significant change due to disrupted pharmacokinetics of analgesics and other drugs. Pre- or postoperative kidney dysfunction or failure can have multiple etiologies (e.g., hepatorenal syndrome or acute tubular necrosis). In addition, the use of drugs with nephrotoxicity, including immunosuppressives such as cyclosporine or FK 506 and aminoglycosides, is unavoidable in these patients. Due to reduced muscle mass, serum creatinine level may be an insensitive indicator of renal dysfunction, and a creatinine clearance is preferred. Whenever possible, blood levels of nephrotoxic drugs should be monitored to maximize therapeutic effect while minimizing the risk of toxicity.

D. Longer-Term Course

  1. The longer-term course after liver transplant includes both **medical and psychological considerations.** Good functional recovery with return to

work can be expected after reversal of end-stage liver disease by well-timed transplantation.

2. If the liver shows evidence of good metabolic and synthetic function, then the metabolism of **sedative/analgesic medications** should be normal. Renal clearance may be mildly impaired due to the effect of the immunosuppressive cyclosporine. Hence **patient-controlled analgesia (PCA) or epidural analgesia** is a reasonable alternative for postoperative pain management in stable, well-established transplant recipients who require major surgery, often for problems unrelated to the transplant.

3. If the allograft has evidence of dysfunction, analgesic doses and techniques need to be adjusted to the patient's needs. Although epidural would be contraindicated in the presence of a coagulopathy, PCA might be used with modified doses in the presence of mild to moderate liver dysfunction.

4. When the referral population includes patients with advanced disease and dysfunction of other organs, a finite subset of graft recipients may require prolonged intensive care, with or without mechanical ventilation, as well as return trips to the operating room for laparotomies (abscess drainage, biliary reconstruction) or other procedures (tracheostomy). **Parenteral narcotic analgesic therapy** is more likely to be used for these patients due to the desirability of sedation in the ventilated, critically ill patient and the myriad of painful or noxious triggers these patients are exposed to during their hospitalizations (e.g., tracheal stimulation from artificial airways, nasogastric tubes, repeated vascular access procedures, operative sites, etc.).

E. Posttransplant Pain Syndrome

The posttransplant pain syndrome is a specific subacute or chronic pain entity which has been identified. In nearly 10 percent of liver transplants at our institution, pain is severe enough to warrant a Pain Service consultation. This syndrome of low back or midback pain is without neurologic deficit or radiologic evidence of acute pathology, and does not respond to narcotics, benzodiazepines, or physical therapy. It has been termed posttransplantation pain syndrome by P. Bigeleisen, M.D., who noted its characteristic nature in a series of 34 patients from among 333 transplant recipients in 1988. This syndrome is worth mentioning because a combination of transcutaneous electrical nerve stimulation (TENS) therapy with posterior division nerve block (PDNB, or dorsal ramus block) was effective in treating 79 percent of these patients, despite the failure of conventional treatments.

F. Specific Modalities

Specific modalities utilized for postoperative pain management in liver transplantation are best divided into the acute, subacute, and chronic phases, which correlate with the management course as outlined above.

1. In the **acute postoperative period,** patients generally still have significant residual narcotic from their anesthetic and may continue to be encephalopathic until adequate graft function has been established.

   a. During this period of weaning from the ventilator, small **IV boluses** of narcotic, and occasionally benzodiazepine, are administered as outlined above. Short-acting agents such as fentanyl (25 to 50 μg) and midazolam (0.5 to 1.0 mg) are preferred, and are easily reversed via antagonists if need be. Fentanyl metabolism appears to be minimally altered in this setting. Finally, and perhaps most important, narcotics should not be withheld for fear of deleterious effects on graft function, as there is no evidence that they do harm.

   b. **Regional techniques** are avoided as a rule, secondary to coagulopathy and a generally low narcotic requirement. Concerns regarding immunosuppression are small, but would warrant strict aseptic technique if peridural techniques were indicated.

   c. Additionally, **nonsteroidal anti-inflammatory drugs (NSAIDs)** are avoided secondary to nephrotoxicity, increased coagulopathy, and predilection for GI bleeding. Of note, ketorolac (Toradol), which has become increasingly popular as a "narcotic substitute," should be regarded as simply another NSAID with a benefit/risk ratio identical to all others. The sole characteristic separating this drug from other NSAIDs is its availability for parenteral administration.

2. **Subacute pain management**

   a. Patients with a complicated perioperative course warrant more elaborate treatment regimens. It is not uncommon for the abdomen to be left open at the conclusion of operations for abscess or other infections. These patients can expect multiple procedures over the next days to weeks, ranging from daily (or more frequent) packing changes to repeated journeys to the operating room for sequential wound closure. Both the baseline and the intermittently severe pain associated with procedures must be managed.

   b. For the baseline pain, **IV PCA with hydromorphone** (0.1 mg/mL solution), set at 0.1 to 0.2 mg per dose, a lockout of 6 to 8 min, and a 4-h maximum of 3.0 mg, is a reasonable starting point. Hydromorphone offers a "clean" pharmacokinetic profile (no active metabolites) and a moderate $t_{1/2}$ duration and volume of distribution.

   c. For intercurrent, brief, painful procedures, such as packing changes or minor debridement, **fentanyl** (200 to 300 μg) is chosen because of a similarly clean profile and a rapid redistribution to lipid tissues. This allows a return to preprocedure levels of consciousness and respiration more rapidly than with less lipid soluble agents, while avoiding the chest wall rigidity sometimes seen with rapid fentanyl administration. **Ketamine** (Ketalar, 0.2 to 0.3 mg/kg) would be another choice in this scenario. However, our experience with the drug in this setting is minimal.

3. **Chronic pain management**

   a. For a variety of reasons, many transplant recipients experience pain in the weeks to months following their surgery and after full tissue healing would have been expected. These patients can remain in the hospital, and even in the intensive care unit, for several months as graft or other organ functions stabilize. In this setting, complaints of pain often continue despite the lack of a clear-cut etiology.

      b. It is very important to recognize when the patient has changed from acute pain to a chronic pain model, and to seek the advice of consultants who are well versed in the multidisciplinary approach to chronic pain and before the behavioral component of the pain complaint has become firmly established.

      c. Frequently, these patients exhibit the **classic triad of a chronic pain patient;** that is, increased **anxiety,** a predilection to **depression,** and a **sleep disturbance.** These elements interact in a vicious cycle which is difficult to break. Medications such as narcotics and benzodiazepines are usually not effective in this setting, and may complicate management with issues of drug dependence and tolerance. Regular scheduling of pain medications provides the patient with the assurance that analgesia is available while freeing the patient and caretakers from the disturbing issues of manipulation and control.

      d. Psychological intervention, from simple relaxation and distraction techniques to intensive psychotherapy (see Chapter 14), is paramount for these patients. The simple addition of a radio or television set to the patient's room can provide a great amount of relaxation and distraction. Sleep disturbance can be managed with a small dose of tricyclic (or quadricyclic) antidepressant at bedtime on a regularly scheduled basis (e.g., amitriptyline [Elavil], 10 to 50 mg; doxepin [Adapin], 10 to 20 mg; or trazodone [Desyrel], 50 to 100 mg). These may be titrated upward to effect. If significant psychopathology such as major depression is suspected, formal psychiatric consultation for psychotherapy and/or additional medication management is warranted.

III. RENAL TRANSPLANTATION

As a given, patients undergoing renal transplantation have end-stage renal failure preoperatively and should receive all considerations due such patients, as extensively outlined in Chapter 19. However, a few special considerations shall be outlined, as well as a brief reiteration of general concepts concerning these patients.

A. Nature of the Pain

The nature of the pain involved in renal transplantation is not significantly different from that in other patients undergoing lower abdominal procedures, as the graft is generally heterotopically placed in the pelvis with vascular anastomosis made to the iliac vessels. The ureteral anastomosis may provide an additional component of renal colic-type pain, but this does not seem to pose a clinical problem. The postoperative pain is both visceral and somatic in quality, and is severe enough to warrant intervention with potent opioids.

B. Pain Management

   1. **Hydromorphone** (Dilaudid) **PCA** is an excellent choice for pain management after renal transplantation. **Meperidine** (Demerol) is specifically avoided because normeperidine, a neurotoxic metabolite, is renally excreted and may accumulate if graft function is not optimal. **Morphine** is also avoided secondary to the active metabolite, morphine-6-glucuronide, which is renally eliminated. Also, morphine pharmacokinetics and pharmacodynamics are altered such that overdosage can occur at comparatively minuscule dose. It should again be noted that no narcotic agents have been shown to be clinically deleterious to renal function, allograft or otherwise, although a small decrease in the glomerular filtration rate has been noted with morphine.
   2. The **NSAIDs** can, however, be nephrotoxic and are thus generally avoided.
   3. Many institutions use **epidural narcotic analgesia** for renal transplant recipients with good success. A review of the literature and an unpublished retrospective study of a small sample of these patients at our institution show no clear-cut advantage to epidural analgesia with respect to pain control or the incidence of side effects.

IV. HEART-LUNG TRANSPLANTATION

A. General Concerns

   1. Immunosuppression-related problems in this case are similar to those related to other organ recipients and were discussed above.
   2. The pain after heart or lung transplantation is similar to that experienced by nontransplant patients who have had sternotomies or thoracotomies. Analgesic techniques for these patients are addressed in detail in Chapters 17, 18, and 25.
   3. Little has been written regarding the particular needs of transplant recipients versus other patients who have undergone sternotomy or thoracotomy. The most conclusive statement that can be made is that, particularly in the case of lung transplantation, improved pulmonary mechanics due to effective analgesia are as important in this population as in any group of patients after major thoracic surgery. Given the premorbid status of these patients, adequate analgesia is probably even more important.

B. Treatment Options

1. Unless specifically contraindicated, **thoracic epidural analgesia** with a narcotic and/or low concentrations of local anesthetic provides excellent analgesia. These infusions are usually left in place for 48 to 96 h so that aggressive pulmonary toilet will be tolerated by the patient. This technique is discussed in detail in Chapter 13.

2. Catheter-related infection is a very rare complication. Due to immunosuppressive therapy, however, signs and symptoms of epidural catheter-related infection may be minimal. Localized pain, particularly on injection of medication or saline through the catheter, will be a prominent symptom. Local induration or inflammation may or may not be present. Neurologic deficits related to epidural abscess formation may take several days to occur, and should be considered a late sign, but one that requires immediate neurosurgical consultation. The catheter should be removed if a catheter-related infection is suspected. Aspiration through the catheter for culture prior to removal can offer information that will guide antibiotic therapy. Magnetic resonance imaging is often a more accurate diagnostic test than a computed tomography scan, and should be obtained in any patient in whom epidural abscess is suspected. Successful treatment for epidural abscess depends on surgical drainage and appropriate antimicrobial therapy.

V. BONE MARROW TRANSPLANTS

A. Bone marrow transplant recipients encounter a specific pain problem, **oral mucositis,** which creates a constant, burning pain that can be a management challenge.

1. Initial treatment usually entails a topically applied agent. A "swizzle" of equal parts 2% viscous lidocaine, Maalox, and 1.5 mg/cc benadryl solution are administered frequently in 5 mL aliquots designated for "swish and swallow."

2. More severe irritation often necessitates the use of PCA narcotics. Again, a wise choice is hydromorphone, as outlined above, secondary to the tenuous renal status rendered to these patients by nephrotoxic agents such as aminoglycosides and amphotericin B. A recent study has shown that a modification of the usual PCA regimen which allows patients to titrate their own continuous infusion, as well as a routine PCA bolus dose, may be even more effective than conventional PCA alone.

B. Other troublesome symptoms, such as **cutaneous rashes with pruritus,** can be controlled with a topical lotion of lidocaine 5% and polysporin in equal volumes.

C. **Nausea and vomiting** related to chemotherapy are common in this population. Antiemetic medications such as odansetron (Zofran, 5 to 15 mg) or metaclopromide (Reglan, 1.5 mg/kg) have been used with good response. Lorazepam (Ativan, 1 to 2 mg) and diphenhydramine (Benadryl, 1.5 mg/kg) have also been used to manage persistent nausea. In addition, self-hypnosis and other self-regulation techniques may augment control of nausea.

D. Isolation, anxiety, and prolonged hospitalizations make nonpharmacologic interventions such as supportive counseling, relaxation, and distraction therapy especially important to this population.

CASE DISCUSSION

Adequate postoperative pain management is critical in patients with underlying pulmonary disease so as to facilitate good pulmonary toilet. The patient received diphenhydramine, with inadequate relief. Subsequently, fentanyl (25 to 50 μg) was administered as needed. The patient had some improvement in her symptoms and was readily weaned from the ventilator. The patient was also pretreated with similar doses of narcotic for pulmonary toileting, but secretion retention became clinically significant 3 days after her surgery, requiring increasing concentrations of exogenous oxygen. The patient refused to cough because of pain, but nursing felt that she was receiving more narcotic than she needed, although she was not sedated, and felt that she was demanding medication inappropriately. A pain management consultation was obtained.

The pain management team determined that the patient had been taking oral hydromorphone three to four times per day preoperatively for chronic low back pain. The team recommended providing the patient with a hydromorphone PCA so that she could more readily titrate her analgesic needs in light of her significant tolerance for narcotics. In addition, a TENS unit was applied with some success. The patient was encouraged to pretreat herself before using her incentive spirometer and before beginning her hourly deep breathing and coughing regimen. She used the PCA appropriately, improved her pulmonary function over the next several days to the point of being weaned to room air, and tapered herself to using infrequent doses by 5 days postoperation. At this time, she was converted to oral analgesics. The TENS unit was repositioned over her lower back, as this was now her primary pain complaint, and provided significant relief.

SUGGESTED READINGS

Asonuma K, et al: The clinical significance of the arterial ketone body ratio as an early indicator of graft viability in human liver transplantation. *Transplantation* 51:164, 1991.
Breheny FX: Reversal of midazolam sedation with flumazenil. *Crit Care Med* 20(6):736, 1992.
Eisenach JC, et al: Comparison of analgesic requirements after liver transplantation and cholecystectomy. *Mayo Clin Proc* 64:356, 1989.
Marquez JM, Martin D: Anesthesia for liver transplantation, in Winter PM, Kang YG (eds): *Hepatic Transplantation: Anesthetic and Perioperative Management,* New York, Praeger, 1986, chap 4, p 49.
Matuschak GM, et al: Effect of end-stage liver failure on the incidence and resolution of the adult respiratory distress syndrome. *J Crit Care* 2:162, 1987.
Osborne RJ, Joel SP, Slevin ML: Morphine intoxication in renal failure: the role of morphine-6-glucuronide. *Br Med J* 292:1548, 1986.
Reyes J: Critical complications in liver transplantation, in Carlson RW, Reines HD (eds): *Critical Care State of the Art,* vol 13. Society of Critical Care Medicine, 1992.

Roussaint R, et al: Strategy for prevention of infection after orthotopic liver transplantation. *Transplant Proc* 23(3):1965, 1991.

Starzl TE, et al: Orthotopic liver transplantation for alcoholic cirrhosis. *JAMA* 260:2542, 1988.

Starzl TE, et al: Liver transplantation. *N Engl J Med* 321:1014, 1989.

Tarter RE, et al: The quality of life following liver transplantation: a preliminary report, in Makowka L, Van Thiel DH (eds): *Gastroenterology Clinics of North America,* vol 17. Philadelphia, W. B. Saunders, 1988, pp 207–217.

CHAPTER 27

PAIN MANAGEMENT IN THE PATIENT WITH HIV

Terrance Calder
Michael Frank

Case
 I. Introduction
 II. Organ System Dysfunction in HIV/AIDS
   A. Neurologic Dysfunction
   B. Cardiac Disease
   C. Pulmonary Compromise
   D. Hepatic Disease
   E. Kidney Disease
 III. Specific Pain Syndromes in HIV/AIDS
   A. Causes of Pain Syndromes Related to HIV Infections
   B. Neurologic Manifestations
   C. Rheumatologic Disorders
   D. Oropharyngeal Pain
   E. Chest Pain
   F. Abdominal Pain
   G. Painful Lymphadenopathy
 IV. Special Issues for Pain Management in Patients with HIV
   A. General Pain Management Principles
   B. Medications
   C. Invasive Analgesic Techniques
   D. Transcutaneous Electrical Nerve Stimulation
   E. Psychological Support and Related Therapeutic Options
   F. Physical Therapy
Case Discussion
Suggested Readings

CASE

A 28-year-old female is admitted to the ICU with pancreatitis after taking didanosine for HIV. On admission, she complains of severe abdominal pain, nausea, and vomiting, in addition to burning pain in her legs. Her blood pressure is 105/45, heart rate 124, and respiratory rate 30. Her oxygen saturation on 40% oxygen delivered by face mask is 88%. She is begging for pain relief.

I. INTRODUCTION

The human immunodeficiency virus (HIV) is the cause of the acquired immune deficiency syndrome (AIDS). HIV is spread through exposure to contaminated blood and other body fluids. This most commonly occurs through sexual intercourse, the sharing of intravenous (IV) needles, from mother to baby in utero or at delivery, and during transfusion of blood products. HIV attacks helper T lymphocytes (also known as T_4 or CD_4 cells). The degree of depletion of CD_4 cells provides a rough estimate of the degree of the resulting immunocompromise, with an increase in most opportunistic infections after the CD_4 count drops below 200. In addition to opportunistic infections, patients infected with HIV have an increased risk of certain malignancies, including Kaposi's sarcoma and lymphoma, and also suffer from a variety of rheumatologic/autoimmune disorders. The time course from HIV infection to the development of AIDS is quite variable among patients, and is changing with new therapies. At present, the average time from infection to AIDS-defining illness is about 10 years; once AIDS develops, the median survival is 2 to 3 years. With anti-retroviral therapy and specific therapy for the complications of HIV, many patients are now living longer, but also may be more likely to suffer some of the chronic and disabling effects of the illness including pain.

II. ORGAN SYSTEM DYSFUNCTION IN HIV/AIDS

A. Neurologic involvement is common. Confusion and altered mental status can occur early in the disease process, making both assessment and management of the illness and the associated symptoms more difficult and complicated.

B. Cardiac disease and dysfunction secondary to HIV are rare and usually are not clinically significant problems.

C. Pulmonary compromise is usually acute and temporary, with resolution following treatment of the underlying pneumonia.

D. Hepatic disease is common, but often mild or asymptomatic, even in patients who also have chronic hepatitis B. The dosage of drugs may have to be adjusted if impairment of hepatic metabolism is significantly affected.

E. Kidney disease with acute or chronic insufficiency can occur due to HIV nephropathy or related to medications. Again, dose adjustment may be necessary for those drugs that have primarily renal excretion.

III. SPECIFIC PAIN SYNDROMES IN HIV/AIDS

A. Causes of Pain Syndromes Related to HIV Infections

Little has been written about **pain management in patients with AIDS,** and no controlled studies have been done to assess treatment. In a hospice program in England, it was found that more than half of outpatients with end-stage AIDS have pain. Furthermore, pain has variably been found to be the most common or second most common symptom during admission for an AIDS-related illness, yet management remains unsophisticated, with treatment usually limited to analgesics such as acetaminophen, acetaminophen with oxycodone, ibuprofen, and meperidine. Pain syndromes in HIV are related to the direct invasion of tissues by the virus, side effects of the illness, the complications of therapy, or the subsequent immune incompetence and related infections.

1. HIV itself is thought to contribute directly to the **peripheral neuropathy** and **myositis** seen in AIDS. In addition, it can cause an **aseptic meningitis** with headache and **painful generalized lymphadenopathy.**

2. The complications of HIV are a common cause of pain. These include **acute** (e.g., pneumonia) and **chronic** (e.g., *Mycobacterium avium-intracellulare* hepatitis) **infections, malignancies** with resulting invasion of organs and vascular obstruction, and **autoimmune or poorly understood complications** such as Reiter's syndrome and oral aphthous ulcers.

3. Several of the **drugs** used for HIV or its complications have painful adverse effects. Examples include **ddI** (didanosine, Videx) **and ddC** (zalcitabine, HIVid), commonly used antiretroviral agents, which can cause **pancreatitis** and **peripheral neuropathy.** The most widely used antiretroviral, AZT (azidothymidine, also known as zidovudine, Retrovir), causes a myopathy, which may be painful on presentation.

B. Neurologic Manifestations

1. **Headache** is a common presenting symptom of processes of the central nervous system (CNS), including viral, bacterial, fungal, or mycobacterial meningitis; toxoplasmosis; and primary CNS lymphoma. Headache is also a common adverse effect of AZT. Sinusitis is relatively common in HIV infection, with an increased incidence of *Streptococcus pneumoniae* and *Haemophilus influenzae* infection. In addition, headache can occur for any of the reasons that it does in non–HIV-infected persons, including tension and migraine (see Chapter 16 on headache and Chapter 32 on myofascial

pain). Management includes primary treatment of the underlying cause if possible, (preferably) nonnarcotic analgesics such as acetaminophen or nonsteroidal anti-inflammatory drugs (NSAIDs), short courses of narcotics, and psychological modalities as listed below.

   2. **Peripheral neuropathy** is common and can be due to HIV, secondary to other infections (such as cytomegalovirus or herpes zoster), or an adverse effect of medications, including ddI and ddC, two antiretrovirals. **Treatment,** as always, includes addressing the inciting cause. **Medications** such as NSAIDs, tricyclic antidepressants (TCAs), and membrane-stabilizing drugs can be used in combinations. Some feel that the pathogenesis of neuropathy includes some ischemic injury to the nerves; therefore, treatment that would decrease vasoconstriction might be expected to be useful. This is one rationale for the use of **sympathetic blocks** with local anesthetics (LAs) or systemic medications such as verapamil or phenoxybenzamine. Another reason might be to "reset" the neural pathway responsiveness to the prepain level. Whether or not either theory is accurate, sympathetic blocks have been used successfully to treat neuropathic pain. For upper extremity and facial pain, the stellate ganglion is blocked, and for the lower extremity, a lumbar sympathetic block can be performed. If helpful, these blocks are repeated as long as a staircase improvement in pain is noticed (the interval between blocks increases or the amount of pain that returns lessens). Some immunocompromised patients who developed Guillain-Barré syndrome, a predominantly motor disorder, also had a painful neuropathic component, and were successfully treated with an **epidural infusion** of **LA** (with or without narcotic for additional analgesia). An epidural may also be considered in patients with chronic inflammatory demyelinating polyneuropathy, though serious consideration must be given to the concentration of the LA drug used because patients with demyelinating diseases have exaggerated clinical responsiveness to LAs.

C. Rheumatologic Disorders

   1. **Myositis and myopathy** are seen occasionally, and when due to AZT, discontinuation of the drug is necessary. HIV is also a cause of muscle inflammation, as noted above. Antiretrovirals may help in this situation, but NSAIDs or even steroid therapy may be required. In addition, **arthritis** occurs and is thought to be a reaction to HIV or may be a manifestation of Reiter's syndrome or psoriatic arthritis. The response to NSAIDs is variable and sometimes immunosuppressive therapy must be used. While steroids may be helpful, they have been shown to cause an increase in the incidence of Kaposi's sarcoma and *Pneumocystis carinii* pneumonia.

   2. **Pseudothrombophlebitis** (calf swelling, erythema, cutaneous hyperalgesia, fever) has been reported in AIDS patients. After ruling out other causes, such as deep venous thrombosis, Baker's cyst, and cellulitis, treat-

ment is symptomatic, including NSAIDs and elevation of the legs. The etiology is unclear, but is felt either to be due to a direct viral effect or to be immune mediated.

3. **Low back pain** (see Chapter 32) is a frequent complaint in the general population. When present in the HIV patient, the most common etiologies include disk herniation and postural low back. Other causes include epidural metastasis of lymphoma and, rarely, Kaposi's sarcoma. If the platelet count is extremely low, spontaneous epidural hematoma formation must be considered. Evaluation may include computed tomography or magnetic resonance imaging of the spine. Treatment includes analgesics (NSAIDs and mild narcotics), muscle relaxants, steroids, radiation, and/or surgical decompression, depending on the diagnosis.

D. Oropharyngeal Pain

HIV-infected patients can develop diffuse mucositis as a consequence of infection. Oral ulcers can be secondary to fungal (especially candida) or viral (most commonly, herpes simplex) infection. Viscous lidocaine and saline rinses can provide symptomatic relief. One recipe that has been effective is 2% viscous lidocaine with Maalox and 1.5 mg/mL diphenhydramine, 5 mL administered as a "swish and swallow." Antifungal (topical or systemic) or antiviral therapy should be given, based on culture and biopsy results. **Aphthous ulcers** are common, and often respond to topical steroids (triamcinolone in orobase gel), but when severe, may require short courses of systemic steroids. **Kaposi's sarcoma** frequently involves the oropharynx and can be treated when symptomatic with intralesional chemotherapy or local radiation therapy. Sexually transmitted diseases (e.g., gonorrhea) should also be considered if the patient is still sexually active.

E. Chest Pain

In AIDS, **chest pain** can be secondary to **esophagitis,** generally caused by the same agents mentioned above under oropharyngeal pain. Therapy is the same as for oropharyngeal pain. In addition, it is often a presenting symptom of **pneumonia,** which should be treated with antibiotics, NSAIDs, narcotics if necessary, and possibly transcutaneous electrical nerve stimulation (TENS) placed over the appropriate dermatomes (see Chapter 18). **Herpes zoster** or shingles at this level can present with chest pain and should be treated with acyclovir, since these patients have a higher rate of dissemination and a poorer rate of resolution than do non-HIV patients. Further treatment includes sympathetic and field blocks with local anesthetics to improve blood flow and/or alter neuronal input into the CNS (see Chapter 3). The use of TCAs (e.g., amitriptyline, 25 to 75 mg PO qhs) facilitates sleep while improving the pain threshold, presumably through enhanced CNS serotonin and norepinephrine function. Capsaicin (Zostrix, 0.025% or 0.075%, applied topically four to five times a day) initially causes burning pain through the release of substance P, but ultimately depletes substance P stores and thereby relieves pain. EMLA (eutectic mixture of local anesthetics), an ointment with lidocaine and prilocaine formulated in such a way as to be able to penetrate the epidermis, can be placed on the most painful lesions as another option. The onset of action is approximately 1 h and the duration is at least 1 to 2 h.

F. Abdominal Pain

In AIDS, **abdominal pain** can be secondary to **pancreatitis** caused by drugs or infection, **gastrointestinal (GI) infection** caused by a wide variety of organisms, or **hepatobiliary disease** due to infection, malignancy, or drugs. Specific therapy is directed at the underlying cause. Narcotic analgesics can be used for pain relief, but must be dosed cautiously, since they may have a prolonged half-life in patients with liver disease. **Constipation** may be caused by narcotic use and can result in significant additional discomfort. Patients receiving narcotics regularly should be placed on a bowel regimen if constipation is a problem.

G. Painful Lymphadenopathy

A part of many **systemic mycobacterial and fungal** infections, painful **lymphadenopathy** can also result from **lymphoma** and **Kaposi's sarcoma**. The resulting lymphatic obstruction can cause severe edema and swelling. Treatment is again aimed at the underlying cause. Analgesics and local measures for symptomatic relief, such as elevation and compression with elastic stockings or Ace wraps, are used.

IV. SPECIAL ISSUES FOR PAIN MANAGEMENT IN PATIENTS WITH HIV

A. General Pain Management Principles

The application of **general chronic pain management principles** to patients with AIDS is beneficial given the similarities of complaints to those with other chronic pain conditions (see Chapter 32). The goals here are different than for acute pain management, because the pain is unlikely to be totally relieved. Behavioral changes may become manifest with the pain, and the very diagnosis of HIV may be psychosocially devastating.

B. Medications

1. Aspirin and NSAIDs are useful adjuncts for many pain syndromes, particularly those involving bony or musculoskeletal pain or inflammation. Altered platelet adhesiveness may increase the risk of bleeding in the presence of HIV-induced thrombocytopenia. If the patient has any "raw" surfaces, such as with mucositis, for example, blood loss may be significant. NSAIDs are probably more desirable than aspirin under these circumstances because the antiplatelet effect resolves within 24 h of the last dose, whereas aspirin alters platelet adhesion for 10 days. Gastric irritation is not uncommon with NSAIDs, and tends to be related to the dose and the duration of treatment. Prophylaxis with histamine blocking agents (e.g., cimetidine [Tagamet] or ranitidine [Zantac]) or with topically active agents such as sucralfate (Carafate) or antacids decreases the risk of GI complications. It is also important to consider the patient's renal function. If renal insufficiency is present, the dosing interval should be lengthened to minimize the risk of the toxic accumulation of NSAIDs, as well as the worsening of renal function. Liver dysfunction has little effect on the half-life of NSAIDs. NSAIDs are discussed in detail in Chapter 7.

2. Acetaminophen is an excellent mild analgesic, but lacks peripheral anti-inflammatory effects. Because it can cause direct hepatic injury, it should be used with caution in patients with significant hepatic impairment. Attention must be paid to the total acetaminophen dose when acetaminophen is used in conjunction with acetaminophen-containing opioid preparations (e.g., Percocet). The use of acetaminophen in patients taking AZT initially was felt possibly to interfere with AZT metabolism and to result in neutropenia, but is not currently considered important.

3. Narcotics have been used successfully in the treatment of HIV-related pain syndromes, even in patients with a prior history of drug abuse. The neurologic status of the patient can be affected by opiates, and in a disease with a high incidence of CNS involvement (HIV encephalopathy, infections, tumor), the correct diagnosis may be obscured. More recently, the fentanyl patch has become available and may be a useful adjunct, particularly for patients with severe mucositis or other problems with oral intake. Hydromorphone (Dilaudid) suppositories can also be used. In the final stages of the disease, increased narcotic doses may be required. For a more detailed discussion of the management of terminal disease, see Chapter 28 (terminal care) and Chapter 32 (cancer pain section).

4. For a more complete discussion of **TCAs,** see Chapter 11. By increasing central serotonin, it is felt that pain transmission may be decreased. The sedating side effects of some TCAs may be beneficial in patients whose sleep has been affected. Patients often have a component of depression associated with chronic pain which may be helped by doses of a TCA that are higher than those required for pain control.

5. **Anticonvulsants or membrane-stabilizing drugs** such as phenytoin (Dilantin) and carbamazepine (Tegretol) or the γ-aminobutyric acid **(GABA) agonist** baclofen (Lioresal) have been shown to be effective in patients with neuropathic pain, such as peripheral neuropathy. Each of these medications carries the risk of hepatic and bone-marrow toxicity, so dosing may need to be modified in the face of preexisting liver dysfunction. Serial blood counts, therapeutic drug levels, and liver function tests should be monitored every 2 weeks for the first month of use, and then every 1 to 2 months thereafter.

6. **Steroids** are avoided *when possible,* given that these patients are already immunocompromised. Nevertheless, they *are used* when necessary, and many patients tolerate them quite well. In fact, end-stage patients often benefit from the increased appetite, weight gain, and elevated mood which result.

7. Complicating pain management in AIDS patients is the **polypharmacy** necessary to treat the disease and the symptoms. Drug–drug interaction and the impairment of organ function by underlying disease that affects drug clearance are significant issues. As mentioned above, medications can interfere with disease diagnosis and follow-up monitoring for extended symptoms. Because of underlying disease, patients may be more susceptible to the adverse effects of the medicines.

C. Invasive Analgesic Techniques

1. Thrombocytopenia is not uncommon in HIV, and can be secondary to HIV itself or the involvement of bone marrow by other processes. A low platelet count should be considered a relative contraindication to the use of neuraxial blocks such as **subarachnoid injections.** A bleeding time may be used to guide the decision to proceed, although the best predictor of excessive bleeding is the presence of clinical bleeding at other sites (e.g., urine, nose, IV sites). AZT may increase platelet count, probably by suppressing HIV. Pulse dose steroids may also cause an increase in platelet count, albeit a temporary one. The CNS is involved in the early phase of HIV infection; therefore, the concern that performing a subarachnoid block or an epidural would "seed" the CNS is groundless. Single injections are of limited duration, although intrathecal morphine (0.3 to 0.6 mg) may provide up to 24 h of relief. Subarachnoid catheters are fraught with technical problems at present, as well as a risk of arachnoiditis.

2. An **epidural injection** carries a slightly higher risk of bleeding than does the subarachnoid route because of the larger needle (17 to 19 gauge versus 25 gauge). The placement of a catheter into the epidural space, with its venous complexes, further increases the risk of vascular trauma. Neutropenia also occurs in HIV, often secondary to drugs, and may increase the

concern regarding infection with **indwelling catheters.** Epidural hematomas and abscesses, although rare, can be devastating complications, and usually require surgical decompression. Neuronal recovery may not be complete, even with timely surgical intervention. In appropriate patients with localized pain complaints, epidural catheters and either infusions of low-dose local anesthetic and/or narcotic or intermittent boluses of preservative-free morphine may offer excellent analgesia (see Chapter 13 for dosing). If the patient is at an increased risk of bleeding, the administration of epidural narcotic alone will avoid masking the symptoms of cord compression, as with an epidural hematoma.

3. **Sympathetic blocks** may be indicated for the treatment of some pain complaints, as mentioned above. **Stellate ganglion blocks** are performed with a small-caliber needle, yet carry a risk in the face of a severe coagulopathy. **Lumbar sympathetic blocks** and **celiac plexus blocks** require needle passage through multiple muscle layers, as well as carry the potential for vascular perforation (aorta, vena cava, renal and celiac vessels) and the penetration of viscera, particularly the kidneys. Hematoma formation may cause pain, but is not usually of clinical significance. Retroperitoneal lymphadenopathy may also distort the anatomy, making the latter two injections technically difficult.

4. **Peripheral nerve blocks** and **pleural catheters** have fewer risks associated with them than do neuraxial blocks. These modalities may be options when neuraxial blockade is not appropriate.

D. Transcutaneous Electrical Nerve Stimulation

TENS may be very helpful in the AIDS patient for the treatment of localized pain complaints. It carries minimal risk. Limitations include active skin lesions in the area where electrodes need to be placed and, late in the disease, inadequate cognitive functioning to operate the unit. The application and adjustments of the unit are detailed in Chapter 14.

E. Psychological Support and Related Therapeutic Options

In chronic pain, **psychological support** is frequently essential, not only to help to identify aggravating stressors, facilitate the grieving associated with the diagnosis of a terminal illness, and explore patients' expectations and understanding of their conditions, but also to assist in treatment. Therapy options include **psychotherapy, self-hypnosis, relaxation therapy, and biofeedback.** (See Chapter 14.) The associated alterations in mental status may make self-regulatory techniques impossible.

F. Physical Therapy

Physical therapy and rehabilitation are crucial to help increase the chronic pain patient's activity. Sensory modulation techniques other than TENS, such as massage, can provide both physical relief and emotional comfort.

CASE DISCUSSION

The patient presented has developed pancreatitis, most likely as a reaction to her didanosine (ddI). Clinically, she appears to be hypovolemic and/or septic and suffering from respiratory insufficiency. Volume resuscitation is necessary before significant doses of parenteral analgesics will be tolerated hemodynamically, but small doses of opioid can be titrated intravenously (e.g., 0.5 mg morphine or 25 μg fentanyl every 5 minutes) as fluid is administered. Obviously, stopping the ddI needs to be considered.

Assuming that the patient's respiratory status and hemodynamics improve with fluid replacement, an opioid PCA can be initiated for pain control with little associated risk. If the patient has normal coagulation and is not septic, an epidural infusion of dilute local anesthetic with (or without) opioid might be very helpful, but the patient's immunocompromised state and increased risk of infection need to be considered. Instillation of local anesthetic through a pleural catheter is a safe alternative to epidural analgesia in the coagulopathic or neutropenic patient, and it can offer significant pain relief for upper abdominal pain while diminishing the requirement for narcotic medications. Due to the high blood levels of local anesthetic seen after peripleural administration, dosing should be adjusted if hepatic disease is present. Supplemental analgesic options include TENS applied over the appropriate somatic nerves posteriorly, bedtime sedation with a TCA or benzodiazepine, and anxiolytics as needed. While the epidural may offer temporary relief of the neuropathic leg pain, longer-term therapy will likely include membrane-stabilizing agents such as carbamazepine.

If the patient's pulmonary status deteriorates to the point of requiring intubation, parenteral medications will help to treat the discomfort associated with the endotracheal tube and suctioning, and so on. An opioid infusion and a benzodiazepine, administered either as a scheduled bolus or as an infusion, might be needed if the patient becomes too ill to use the PCA effectively.

SUGGESTED READINGS

Janisse T: *Pain Management of AIDS Patients.* Dordrecht, Klüwer, 1991.
Lebovits AH, et al: The prevalence and management of pain in patients with AIDS: a review of 134 cases. *Clin J Pain* 5(3)245–248, 1989.
Lewis MS, Warfield CA: Management of pain in AIDS. *Hosp Prac* 25(10A):51–54, 1990.

PART SIX

SPECIAL CONCERNS

CHAPTER
28

PAIN MANAGEMENT IN THE TERMINALLY ILL

Sherry T. Sutton
Margot L. White
Richard F. Edlich

Case
I. Components of Care
II. Pathophysiology of Pain in the Terminally Ill
   A. Physiologic Pain
   B. Psychosocial Pain or Grief
III. Factors to Be Considered in Deciding on an Appropriate Pain Management Plan
   A. Legal Concerns
   B. Patient's Wishes
   C. Patient's Environment
   D. Route(s) of Administration of Pain Medication
   E. Adjunctive Therapy
   F. Agents to Be Avoided
   G. Other Concerns
IV. The Family
Suggested Readings

CASE

A 69-year-old female had a 2-year history of multiple myeloma, exhibiting the classic triad of plasmacytosis (greater than 10 percent), lytic bone lesions, and a serum and urine M component. She received the standard treatment of intermittent pulses of an alkylating agent and prednisone administered for 7 days every 6 weeks for 1 year. Cessation of therapy was followed by a relapse that was unresponsive to treatment with VAD therapy (vincristine, doxorubicin, and dexamethasone combination therapy). During chemotherapy, allopurinol was used to prevent urate nephropathy. She complained of constant bony pain, for which she was treated, as an outpatient, with a sustained-action preparation of morphine, 120 mg every 12 h, and oxycodone/aspirin, 5 mg/325 mg, two tablets every 3 h as needed. Doctyl sodium sulfonate, 500 mg per day, was administered as a stool softener. This regimen was successful, until she noticed excruciating pain in her right tibia, the site of a lytic bone lesion. She was admitted to the hospital for localized radiation of her right tibia, complemented by the continued use of the analgesics. During this hospitalization, she developed anorexia, profound fatigue, and lethargy that were associated with pancytopenia. With these additional problems, the patient was told that she was terminally ill and would need continued supportive care.

She and her family requested a consultation with the hospice home health care program. This approach to treatment was coordinated by a multidisciplinary team of health care professionals who were prepared to train family members to be caregivers regarding pain management. Because her pain was refractory to oral opioids, a patient-controlled analgesia (PCA) system was employed, and it successfully relieved her pain. Stool softeners in liquid form were continued.

When she died at home, 18 days later, a member of the health care team provided emotional support and guidance to the bereaved. Follow-up telephone calls to her husband over the next 6 months helped him to adjust to the grieving process.

I. COMPONENTS OF CARE

  A. The care of the terminally ill patient has two main components: psychosocial care and symptom control.
  1. Psychosocial care acknowledges the patient, which includes the family as a unit of care, and sets out to help all whose lives are affected by the patient's illness. Attention is paid to psychological, social, and spiritual needs before and after the patient's death. Recent trends in the care of the dying and the bereaved emphasize the need for improving the quality of life rather than simply prolonging it. By exploring the changes that occur during the dying and bereavement processes and sharing these experiences, personal growth can be enhanced. Kübler-Ross enhanced the general fund of knowledge on grief and illuminated psychosocial thought with a humanistic approach to the experience of dying. She elucidated **five phases of grief** in the dying patient: (1) denial and isolation, (2) anger, (3) bargaining, (4) depression, and (5) acceptance. This concept and the concurrent behaviors in each phase help us to understand and care for those anticipating death.
  2. Symptom control is attained mainly by close attention to drug regimens, particularly those required for the relief of pain. The pain component can be both acute and chronic in nature.
  Acute pain differs from chronic pain in several ways.
    a. Acute pain is most often associated with an event. It has a beginning and an end. Acute pain can serve a biologic function in that, if the cause is removed, the pain will eventually disappear; time is its ally. Acute

pain generally has specific signs and symptoms that may be used to identify it.

      b. Chronic pain can be less clearly associated with a specific event. It continues for such a long period that it is hard to pinpoint exactly when it began and impossible to predict when it will end. Time is not its ally; the pain may worsen over time because psychological, affective, environmental, and circumstantial factors influence the perception of the pain. Chronic pain has less biologic function than does acute pain. There are often few physical findings that can exactly explain chronic pain, although it is almost always related to chronic illness.

  B. The rationale behind active acute and chronic pain control is twofold:

    1. Pain control can allow the dying patient and the bereaved to develop renewed social interests and enthusiasm for life's activities, allowing a sudden or subtle emergence of excitement about the joys of their lives.

    2. Pain management provides the basis for a valid alternative to euthanasia. By providing a level of pain relief that is acceptable to the patient, the agony of terminal illness can be lessened. Aggressive pain management can provide comfort until the end of the patient's life.

II. PATHOPHYSIOLOGY OF PAIN IN THE TERMINALLY ILL

A. Physiologic Pain

Physiologic pain includes the following.

  1. Cancer pain caused by direct infiltration and tissue damage. Mechanisms include:

    a. Necrosis, inflammation, infection, and ulceration.
    b. Invasion of bone and/or periosteum or nerves by tumor.
    c. Obstruction of body organs or ducts.
    d. Occlusion of blood or lymphatic vessels.
    e. Stretching of the peritoneum.

  2. Pain caused by surgery, radiotherapy, and/or chemotherapy.

    a. Postoperative pain.
    b. Neuropathic pain (that due to scarring in the nervous system).
    c. Stump/phantom pain.
    d. Causalgia/reflex sympathetic dystrophy.
    e. Chemotherapy (neuritis, mucositis).
    f. Other conditions that may exacerbate pain: constipation from pain medications, insomnia, and nausea and vomiting.

  3. Arthritic pain from the lower back or degenerative joints.
  4. Somatic pain of the musculoskeletal system.
  5. Visceral pain which emanates from involved organs.

6. Deafferentation pain, such as neuralgias and neuropathies, which usually involve alternate neuronal pathways and usually have a peripheral or central nervous system component.

7. Sympathetically maintained pain which is usually marked by a syndrome of nondermatomal burning and aching, exquisite hypersensitivity to even the slightest cutaneous stimulation, and signs of sympathetic nervous system dysfunction (i.e., temperature change, color change in the distal extremities, swelling).

B. Psychosocial Pain or Grief

Grief represents the intense emotions and physical symptoms of loss. The purposes of grief are to help the dying patient and the bereaved reconcile their loss and to attenuate their attachment to each other. The specific psychological task of this process is to break the emotional tie with the deceased and recreate attachment to living people.

III. FACTORS TO BE CONSIDERED IN DECIDING ON AN APPROPRIATE PAIN MANAGEMENT PLAN

A. Legal Concerns

1. No medical decision can be immune from legal scrutiny; however, physicians should do whatever is necessary to relieve pain and bring comfort to the terminally ill without exaggerated concern for legal consequences. In at least one state, the administration of pain medication in excess of therapeutic dosages is explicitly allowed by law when it is for the relief of intractable pain. To withhold any necessary and desired measures for pain relief in a terminally ill patient out of fear of depressing respiration or of possible legal repercussions is unjustified and unethical. Liability turns on the intent of the physician in administering the medication; administering medication with the intent to kill remains illegal in all states as of this writing.

2. **Principle of double effect**

   a. The ethical and legal implications of administering pain medications may be understood in terms of the principle of double effect, whereby the administration of pain medication for the intended purpose of relieving pain is permissible even though there is a risk of hastening death due to respiratory depression. The bad effect is an unintended result of trying to achieve the good effect, and is, therefore, not culpable. Where the statutory authority has been granted to physicians to administer analgesics in excess of therapeutic doses for the treatment of intractable pain, the prohibition against endangering the patient's health has been eliminated when it is an unavoidable side effect of the medication.

b. A recent court decision in Georgia is significant because the court held that a ventilator-dependent quadriplegic patient who was not terminally ill nonetheless could be allowed to die as he wished by having his ventilator disconnected, and that he had a "right to be free from pain at the time the ventilator is disconnected." This right to be free from pain, the court held, was "inseparable from his right to refuse medical treatment."

B. Patient's Wishes

1. Written advance directive or living will

a. These directives are now accepted in all 50 states and the District of Columbia. The purpose of a living will is to enable a person to provide guidance to both health professionals and family members to cover circumstances of terminal illness and incapacity, when the patient no longer can make decisions or provide instructions. Living wills come in many forms, and may provide instructions directly to the physician or designate someone to make terminal care decisions on behalf of the patient who is terminal and incapacitated. The authority of anyone acting on behalf of the patient extends to decisions about pain medications.

b. Approximately 47 states have provided for living wills under statutes which explicitly grant legal immunity to complying physicians. Where there are no statutes, the courts have accepted living wills as the best evidence of a patient's wishes about treatment. Although they tend to be phrased in generalities and require interpretation, the reliance on advance directives ensures that complex and difficult decisions are more likely to reflect the patient's views. In most states, physicians unwilling to comply with an advance directive for reasons of conscience or personal philosophy must make a reasonable effort to transfer the patient to the care of another physician.

c. Many state statutes governing treatment decisions at the end of life specify that the medications needed for adequate pain management are *not* to be considered life-sustaining treatments which may be withdrawn in the final stages of terminal and irreversible illness. The intent of so-called natural death acts is to encourage the provision of sufficient doses of pain medications to enable dying patients to experience as peaceful and dignified a death as possible. Even where a living will or other patient directive does not specifically request analgesics, it should be presumed to be a fundamental component of palliative care or "comfort" care. Patients who express a preference, directly or through a proxy, for less pain medication in order to experience less cognitive impairment, should have their doses tiltrated accordingly, with frequent review and adjustment as needed.

2. Proxy appointments These are a somewhat newer form of advance directive. Some are provided for directly by statute and others are derived from existing durable-power-of-attorney laws. The authority provided to a health care proxy is not limited to terminal illness or end-of-life decisions. By appointing a proxy or agent (also called a durable power of attorney for health care), a person designates, in writing, another person to make medical decisions whenever the patient is unable to be directly involved because of decisional incapacity, either temporary or permanent. The proxy appointment may include specific written instructions, but even if none exist, the proxy is legally bound to make decisions consistent with the patient's wishes, beliefs, values, and goals.

3. Substituted judgment

a. Ideally, all surrogates are bound by a patient's explicit wishes made known prior to losing capacity. When such wishes are unknown or inadequate, the surrogate (legally appointed proxy or family member) must attempt to make decisions based on what the patient would have decided if competent. It is not a process in which the surrogate or proxy substitutes his or her own judgment for that of the patient, but one of implementing what the patient can be presumed to have wanted under the circumstances, based on the surrogate's evaluation of the patient's beliefs, preferences, and personal values. The decision-making rights remain those of the patient, not the family. Recent case law has stressed that family members, as well as appointed proxies, should be able to make these decisions without recourse to the courts or the appointment of a legal guardian.

b. It is important to elicit the patient's views regarding the relief of pain balanced against any resulting cognitive impairment and other side effects. Patients' surrogates and physicians may place differing values on these questions. Surrogates who are providing consent for pain medication should base their consent as much as possible on how the patient would evaluate his or her quality of life as affected by pain, altered mental functioning, bladder and bowel dysfunction, dependency, and related side effects. Where possible, medications that are severely compromising a patient's mental functioning may be decreased for a brief period in order to enable communication directly with the patient about his or her wishes.

4. Best interest doctrine This is the preferred standard of decision making for an incapacitated patient when the patient's wishes cannot be known because the patient has never had decisional capacity or has never indicated a guiding preference of any kind, or where the patient has no one to speak for him or her and has not indicated any guidelines. The decision is arrived at by weighing the likely benefits and burdens of any proposed treatment or intervention. Pain, for example, would clearly be judged a great burden by most people, particularly if it could be relieved without immediate threat to the patient's life. However, for unconscious patients, the concept of balancing benefits and burdens related to the experience of relief of pain has been viewed by the courts as relatively meaningless. Burdens are more likely to be seen in terms of the loss of dignity of the patient, rather than in terms of pain.

C. Patient's Environment

The type of environment in which the patient will be cared for must be considered.

   1. Hospital   Although life-extending support systems, expert staff, and pain-relieving medications are all available, modern medicine remains unable to cure many illnesses. Many Americans die in hospitals, after prolonged efforts to extend their lives. These efforts, although appropriate for some patients, may be unrealistic, useless, and painful for others. The modern hospice movement was begun, in part, as a reaction to the common overtreatment of dying patients receiving routine hospital care. The aim of the hospice movement has been to allow people who are dying to do so without pain, in peace, and at home, if possible.

   2. Hospice   The hospice is both a philosophy and a system of terminal care. As a philosophy, it reflects late-twentieth-century Western cultural and social values. It confronts the dying process openly and prepares people to experience dying as an inevitable natural phase in the life's cycle. American hospices vary greatly in organizational structure. They can be subdivided into two groups: those with hospital-based beds and those without beds (home care).

   a. Hospital-based hospices can mean alien surroundings that leave the patient with a sense of isolation, depression, and helplessness. For those individuals who do not have the luxury of a home, the hospital-based hospice can be a "lifeboat" of emotional support.

   b. In the **home-based hospices,** patients are often comforted by the familiar surroundings that provide considerable emotional support. This benefit must be weighed against the possibility of inadequate pain relief by family members because they are not trained to administer medications.

   3. Nursing homes   These facilities have the same disadvantages as hospitals, plus the fact that the staff and facilities are not geared to care for the terminally ill patient.

D. Route(s) of Administration of Pain Medication

The choice of a given route should be tailored to the individual.

   1. Transdermal   Only fentanyl is available as a patch, providing doses ranging from 25 to 100 μg/h. The duration of activity of the fentanyl patch is 72 h. The advantages of the transdermal route are that it circumvents potential erratic gastrointestinal absorption and the subsequent first-pass metabolism, is effective when swallowing is difficult, and can be employed in the absence of intravenous (IV) access. It is important to remember that the patient must receive analgesics by another route (usually for at least 12 to 24 h) until sufficient transdermal medication is absorbed to provide adequate pain relief. Additional pain requirements above 100 μg/h can be achieved by additional patches. Whenever the patient's medication requirements are changed, supplemental medications will be needed for 24 h, until the analgesic effects of the additional transdermal medication are achieved.

2. Oral The large doses of narcotics often required by the terminally ill patient can cause severe nausea, which may be uncontrolled by antiemetics. Although the dosage at which the nausea occurs is patient specific, it is often encountered at sustained-release morphine doses of 180 mg/day and at lower dosages with the other narcotics. This route will be of no value in the terminally ill patient who is unable to swallow.

3. Epidural This route does provide an alternative method for the delivery of narcotics, particularly in those patients in whom pain control cannot be achieved by other methods and/or without respiratory depression. However, catheter dislodgment or leaking around and clogging of the catheter can be a challenging problem with this route of administration. In addition, the daily changing of the medication and bag when using a sterile technique requires a skilled caregiver and a compliant and alert patient. While this route of administration causes less sedation than the oral or parenteral route, some patients will prefer these routes over epidural analgesia. Although the epidural route does provide adequate pain control, tolerance to the analgesic still may be encountered and require an increase in the medication dose.

4. Rectal Morphine and hydromorphone are available. Rectal medications are effective in patients unable to take oral medications, but their use is limited by the fact that few dosage strengths are available and that absorption is unreliable.

5. Parenteral

a. Peripheral IV therapy may be employed on a short-term basis, although peripheral access sites may be limited and/or difficult to establish and maintain. Also, sites must be changed every few days and frequent needle sticks may be associated with pain in many patients.

b. A central venous catheter can be inserted for patients in whom long-term therapy is anticipated. The current preferred delivery system is PCA, as it provides the patient with control over the therapy and eliminates the peaks and valleys of intermittent bolus therapy. It is administered as follows:

c. PCA administration

(i.) Calculating the dose
1. Calculate the total daily intake of all pain medications.
2. Convert to morphine equivalent.

3. Convert to parenteral morphine equivalent. (Although historically the ratio of the injectable dose to oral dose for morphine was considered to be 1:6, these data were based on a single dose study. Current practice indicates a ratio of 1:3 to 1:2 to be more accurate for chronic therapy.)
4. Divide by 24 h to calculate the hourly rate in milligrams per hour.

ii. Setting the pump For **ambulatory patients,** the ultimate goal is to achieve pain control with a minimum number of boluses by selecting an appropriate basal rate in order to avoid the pain relief–recurrent pain cycle that results from bolus dosing regimens. When the number of boluses needed increases, the basal rate should be appropriately increased. For **nonambulatory patients,** a high basal rate could cause excess sedation. Thus it is best to leave the basal rate low and allow them greater flexibility in the frequency of boluses.

Example: Patient Jones has been receiving sustained-release morphine (MS Contin), 120 mg every 12 h, and oxycodone, two 5-mg tablets every 3 h, for breakthrough pain:

Oxycodone 5 mg × 2 tablets × 8 doses = 80 mg/24 h

80 mg × conversion factor 0.33 = 26 mg parenteral morphine

240 mg morphine PO ÷ 2 = 120 mg parenteral morphine

146 mg total morphine ÷ 24 = 5.1 mg/h morphine equivalent

While this seems like a large dose, it is important to remember that most terminally ill patients have been on analgesics for months to years. Consequently, most will require large doses to control their pain. For a more conservative approach, the 240 mg of oral morphine may be divided by 3 to yield an 80 mg parenteral equivalent. This method gives a total morphine equivalent of 106 mg ÷ 24 = 4.4 mg/h morphine. The disadvantage of the conservative approach is that the patient may require additional analgesic boluses during the first 24 h.

6. Subcutaneous Morphine at 25 to 60 mg/mL, sufentanil at 50 μg/mL, and hydromorphone at 4 to 10 mg/mL are the only medications whose concentrations are sufficient to provide analgesia by this route. It is important to point out that only the sufentanil, the 25 mg/mL morphine, and the 4 mg/mL hydromorphone are commercially available. More concentrated solutions must be prepared from powder by a pharmacist. Insulin infusion pumps, which can contain a 100-mL reservoir of these analgesic solutions, can be used to provide sufficient analgesia for approximately 6 to 7 days. The volume of medication delivered per hour is the limiting factor; leaking around the subcutaneous sites can begin at 0.7 to 0.8 mL/h, and often 9.0 mL/h is too large a volume to be absorbed.

7. **Intramuscular** Although commonly used, this route has the disadvantages of wide fluctuations in absorption from the depot muscle site, a 30- to 60-min lag to peak effect, and a rapid falloff of action when compared with oral administration. Generally, doses need to be about twice the IV bolus dose amount. Because many patients complain of pain after the injection, this route is not preferred in the terminally ill patient.

E. Adjunctive Therapy

1. **Anticonvulsants** can be useful in neuropathic pain such as that seen with neural plexus invasion or compression.

2. **Anxiolytics** are useful for sleep deprivation, feelings of suffocation (e.g., congestive heart failure, lung cancer), and other physical or emotional conditions that produce anxiety.

3. **Steroids,** as anti-inflammatory medications, are particularly helpful in patients with tumors that cause nerve compression or an increase in intracranial pressure (ICP).

4. **Antidepressants** improve depression, neuropathic pain, and pain-related sleep disturbances, as well as early morning awakening.

5. **Tranquilizing psychotropics** are indicated for agitation, confusion and hallucinations secondary to medications, emotional upheaval, and sedation, and as antiemetics.

6. The **psychostimulants** methylphenidate (Ritalin, 5 to 40 mg/day in divided doses) or dextroamphetamine (Dexedrine, 5 to 30 mg/day in divided doses) occasionally can be administered to increase alertness and create a sense of euphoria in the patient suffering excessive drowsiness from large doses of opioids.

7. **Oxygen** can be used in patients with dyspnea or feelings of suffocation to help manage air hunger.

8. **A bowel regimen** should be provided to all patients on high-dose opioids to prevent constipation. This regimen should be initiated before the constipation becomes clinically significant, and generally starts with a stool softener. While the reported effective dose of docusate sodium (Colace) is closer to 500 mg/day, 100 mg of this drug given orally has traditionally been used.

9. **Nonpharmacologic adjuncts**

   a. **Music,** particularly "easy listening" or the patient's favorite music, has been shown to decrease pain.

   b. **Hypnosis** also has been shown to be effective, even in those patients who are extremely close to death.

F. Agents to Be Avoided

1. Sedative/hypnotic medications (i.e., barbiturates) do not have intrinsic analgesic properties and should be avoided in the management of pain.

2. Narcotic agonist–antagonist medications (e.g., pentazocine [Talwin]) are contraindicated in those patients stabilized on narcotics because they may induce withdrawal symptoms in the terminally ill patient who is likely to be physically dependent on his or her narcotics.

G. Other Concerns

1. In terminal illness, components of both acute **and** chronic pain syndromes may be present.

2. Chronic pain often represents a vicious cycle of physical pain and a resultant emotional response that enhances the perception of the pain. The key to its management is to disrupt and block that cycle.

3. Many terminally ill patients have been receiving pain medications for months to years; therefore, each patient's therapy plan must be individualized and flexible. **There is no need to underutilize analgesics for fear of addiction and dependency in the terminally ill patient.**

4. Analgesic requirements change in terminally ill patients as death approaches. Some require more medication during the last 4 weeks of life; others need only 60 percent of the former daily dose. The focus of care, then, must be the needs of the patient and of those grieving over their impending loss, rather than the disease itself. Pain relief must always be addressed to allow the patient and the bereaved to continue in the grieving process.

5. The patient must be involved in the goals of pain management. The patient and the bereaved are best equipped to describe the effectiveness of pain management, but the caregiver must be aware of the potential for disparate goals and place a priority on the goals of the patient.

6. A multidisciplinary team must work in concert to provide optimum care. This team must include the patient, grieving family members and friends, the physician, counselors, pharmacists, nurses, chaplins, legal counsel, and a funeral director.

IV. THE FAMILY

A. The most distinctive feature of pain management in the home is the role of family caregivers. Family caregivers are critical providers of support for terminally ill patients because they give physical, emotional, social, and economic support and allow terminally ill patients to remain in the comfort of their homes, avoiding institutionalization. Some of the ways in which caregivers are especially involved in pain management include

    1. deciding what medications to give
    2. determining when to administer medications
    3. encouraging patient compliance with the desired treatment
    4. supervising and assisting with patient activities and nonmedication treatments
    5. watching for potentially excessive reliance on medications.

    B. It is important to point out that the family caregiver may experience considerable stress and anxiety regarding pain management and/or home care, particularly when hazardous medications and hi-tech modalities are used. Consequently, caregivers need considerable support to prepare for this new role of helping someone they love die with dignity. An educational program should include an assessment of the caregiver's intellectual and emotional capability to provide appropriate pain management and the cognitive information to facilitate the achievement of adequate pain control. Armed with this information, the trained health professional should then observe the caregiver providing safe pain control. The caregiver should be encouraged to contact the health professional at any time if there are questions about pain management. The caregiver must be alerted to the signs of the impending death of the terminally ill patient. As death approaches, the caregiver should be encouraged to contact family members, as well as a member of the health care team, and ask them to come to the home of the dying patient. When the patient dies, the family members should stay with the deceased as long as they wish. The family members thus can live the first hours after death together, remaining close to the body. Having shared the last hours of life, they do the same for the first few hours after death. These hours are intense and moving, but they appear to afford a beneficial and deeply meaningful experience for the family members, who stay closely united with the deceased. This unity becomes a gesture of the acceptance and demystification of death.

    C. The bereaved should be educated as to the symptoms of the **grief response,** and be assured that these responses are normal. Depressed mood, sleep disturbance, crying, difficulty with concentration, loss of interest, and anorexia and/or weight loss are the most common symptoms. Arrangements also should be made for another family member or a friend to stay with the spouse for the next 24 to 48 h because suicide is a possibility, especially for a spouse who has been married for many years.

    D. Leaving the door open for **future contact** is welcome to the bereaved. There is a need for greater family support at the time of the patient's death. Several studies have reported increased morbidity and mortality among the next-of-kin for a year or longer following a patient's death. Their suffering may become manifest in increased somatic symptoms, drug and alcohol use, hospitalization, and even death. It is to be anticipated that the bereaved family members will continue to reflect on their feelings toward the deceased, to examine their own "wounds," and to attend to the task of continuing life without the deceased. To address the survivor's needs, one hospital began a program in which the family receives a sympathy card from the staff members who had cared for their loved one. Follow-up telephone calls are made to the family throughout the year after the death. A letter is sent from the attending physician explaining the autopsy findings. The response of the families to this follow-up is very positive.

E. Health care professionals who attend to the dying are not immune to discomfort. A dying person poses a threat to the health professional's own human attachments. First, the professional realizes his or her own limitations. Second, the loss of a patient reminds him or her of his or her own past or threatened losses. Because of the repeated stresses presented by these threats, health professionals develop defenses. One approach is to avoid involvement with dying patients in order to minimize personal loss or discomfort.

What can be done to reduce this defensiveness of health professionals? Systematic educational training programs need to be provided to help health professionals deal with their feelings about suffering, disappointment, and death. Ideally, these programs should be instituted early in their formal training, so that repeated exposures to dying experiences can be accompanied by emotional growth. Education about death and dying should be incorporated into the medical school curriculum. Faculty should discuss all aspects of patient death, including anticipation and coping skills, death notification, and guidance of the bereaved. Open discussions of the emotional impact of patient death on health care providers should be an integral part of the education program.

F. When we view the shadow of death, we face our own mortality and appreciate that life is finite. The dying person develops deeper meanings and priorities for his or her life, because he or she no longer can postpone choices. Consequently, the dying patient must have the unrivaled opportunity to examine what makes life meaningful. As we share our insights on dying, we fortuitously discover the joys of unconditional love in a glorious journey through life. For many physicians, problems of living become so complicated and overwhelming that this contemplation of their own deaths may serve as an emotional rebirth, revitalizing their suppressed ambitions and passions, and bringing to their lives new dimensions and meanings.

SUGGESTED READINGS

American Pain Society: Principles of analgesic use in the treatment of acute pain and chronic cancer pain, 2nd edition. *Clin Pharm* 9:601–611, 1990.

Conolly ME: Alternatives to euthanasia. Pain Management. *Issues in Law and Medicine* 4:497–507, 1989.

Cowley LT, Young E, Raffin TA: Care of the dying: an ethical and historical perspective. *Crit Care Med* 20(10):1473–1482, 1992.

Edlich RF, Kübler-Ross E: On death and dying in the emergency department. *J Emerg Med* 10:225–229, 1992.

Meisel A: *The Right to Die.* New York, Wiley, 1989.

Rouse F: Legal and ethical guidelines for physicians in geriatric terminal care. *Geriatrics* 43(8):69–75, 1988.

Wanzer SH, Federman DD, Adelstein SJ, et al: The physician's responsibility toward hopelessly ill patients: A second look. *N Engl J Med* 320:844–849, 1989.

CHAPTER 29

TOLERANCE, DEPENDENCE, AND ADDICTION IN THE ICU PATIENT

Charles G. Durbin, Jr.

I. Demographics and Definitions
II. Alcohol
    A. Acute Intoxication
    B. Chronic Abuse of Alcohol
    C. Prevention and Treatment of Delerium Tremens
    D. Treatment of Alcohol Withdrawal
III. Narcotic Use and Abuse
IV. Stimulant Drug Use
V. Benzodiazepine Use
VI. Marijuana and the Perceptual Distorters
    A. Marijuana
    B. Phencyclidine
VII. Treatment of Chemical Dependence
    A. Patients
    B. Health Care Workers
Suggested Readings

I. DEMOGRAPHICS AND DEFINITIONS

    A. Abuse of alcohol and other drugs is common in modern society. The altered mental states resulting from the recreational and addictive use of legal and illegal mood-altering substances contribute significantly to injuries and deaths in otherwise healthy individuals. At least 50 percent of the fatalities in motor vehicle accidents are the direct result of alcohol or other drug use. As many as 75 percent of patients presenting to a trauma emergency room are under the influence of a mood-altering substance. Mood-altering substances contribute significantly to domestic violence and crime. The incidence of alcoholism, which probably has a genetic basis, in this permissive society, is estimated at 10 to 15 percent of the entire population.

    B. The presence of acute drug intoxication, alcoholism, or drug addiction complicates the management of the injured or critically ill patient. Drug **withdrawal syndromes** must be recognized and appropriately managed during the acute treatment phase. Increased or decreased tolerance may be present and the usual therapeutic drug doses must be adjusted appropriately.

    C. The prolonged therapeutic use of addictive drugs poses significant risks for nonaddicted patients. Narcotic analgesics rapidly induce tolerance, and may result in the development of withdrawal symptoms upon abrupt termination. Benzodiazepine withdrawal also results in a characteristic clinical syndrome, which includes seizures. Caregivers need to recognize these symptoms, and to treat them by gradual withdrawal of the drug to which the person has become tolerant.

    D. An additional concern in critical care units is **drug abuse among the caregivers.** Alcoholism is considered a disease with a heritable, genetic basis. An abnormality in the central nervous system (CNS) dopamine receptor, the d2 allele, has been suggested as the site inducing susceptibility. The incidence of this chronic, progressive, but treatable disease is higher than 10 percent in the general population of the United States. It is not confined to any socioeconomic group, although, as the disease progresses, the social and economic status of the victim is usually reduced. Doctors, nurses, and other caregivers are at the same risk for alcoholism as the general population, and these professional groups may be at a higher risk for prescription drug abuse. The general availability of controlled substances, their daily use in patients who show good clinical results, a feeling of an ability to control the use of drugs, and the knowledge of the alleged dangers even with recreational use allow caregivers to rationalize the occasional self-medication reported or seen in many caregivers. This will progress to abuse and dependence in some individuals. When job performance becomes impaired, this will lead to detection, intervention or arrest, and dismissal, or, in enlightened environments, treatment and rehabilitation of the addicted caregiver. During active addiction, patient care may suffer.

    E. The management of the acutely and chronically intoxicated patient, recognition and prevention of therapeutically induced tolerance, and the risks and treatment of addiction in caregivers are discussed in this chapter. The term *addiction* or *addict* is ambiguous and carries a negative judgmental implication. These words are no longer properly used in medical terminology. The American Psychiatric Society has defined three degrees of impairment induced by mood-altering substances.

1. Intoxication. This refers to the acute impairment induced by an excessive (by societal standards) amount of a mood-altering substance.

2. Abuse. Repeated episodes of intoxication resulting in social, physical, or economic impairment are called abuse.

3. Dependence. When tolerance or physical signs of withdrawal (physical dependence) or significant health problems related to nonmedically prescribed drug use take place over a longer period and persistent use of the drug occurs, this is defined as dependence. A hallmark of dependence is the loss of control of drug use. Tolerence and physical dependence can result when people take medically prescribed narcotics for acute or chronic pain. This can occur over days or weeks. As the acute pain subsides, these patients tend to reduce their use of the medications, and continued use is seldom a problem.

F. The term **addiction** has been used to denote nonmedically induced dependence and has a negative connotation. This term should not be used in a medical context. Substance abuse is a medical disease with a predictable course and outcome. It is treatable, and its sufferers should not be approached judgmentally, as the word **addict** would suggest.

II. ALCOHOL

A. Acute Intoxication

A state of acute intoxication is often the desired effect of social drinking.

1. Alcohol is the most commonly abused drug in American society. This agent affects many areas of the CNS, causing **depression of brain function** similar to the effects of general anesthesia. The presumed mechanism is expansion of cell membranes and interference with membrane protein activities.

2. At **low doses,** higher cortical centers are depressed and the release of inhibitions occurs.

3. At **higher doses,** general CNS depression ensues, and at lethal doses (blood alcohol level [BAL] greater than 0.5 percent), respiratory arrest results. Acutely intoxicated patients often are combative, are uncooperative, have a high pain threshold, and are sensitive to sedative and analgesic drugs. Anesthetic requirements are reduced during acute intoxication.

B. ·Chronic Abuse of Alcohol

The chronic abuse of alcohol results in the **alteration of intercellular electrolytes** (a reduction in potassium and increase in sodium). Brain function may actually be improved in the presence of some alcohol (BAL 0.05 to 0.1 percent).

1. **Withdrawal** of alcohol in the chronic user may result in CNS irritability, autonomic hyperactivity, and seizures. These signs and symptoms are listed in Table 29-1. The rapid metabolism of ethanol results in this syndrome within 24 to 48 h after the induction of abstinence.

2. Classical **delirium tremens (DTs)** usually appears within 72 h after the cessation of chronic drinking, and is heralded by increasing autonomic activity, hallucinations, and seizures. Without treatment, this syndrome carries a 10 to 15 percent mortality rate.

3. The DTs can be **prevented by sedative drugs.** Due to cross-tolerance in this class of drugs, any sedative drug will satisfy the body's need for the drug and prevent withdrawal. Common drugs used to treat alcohol withdrawal are the benzodiazepines, because of their safety (acute lethal overdose is impossible) and lack of acute and chronic organ toxicity. They also raise the seizure threshold and are useful in treating actual seizures. Other sedative drugs have been used to treat or prevent alcohol withdrawal, including the barbiturates and intravenous (IV) ethanol, however, their ease of use and safety have made the benzodiazepines the mainstay of treatment.

4. **Nutritional deficiencies** are common in alcoholics, as much of the daily caloric needs are met by ethanol. Vitamin B_6 and folate deficiencies may produce the degenerative neurologic condition known as Wernicke's encephalopathy. Vitamin and electrolyte replacement, particularly magnesium, may improve this condition, and should be given to any acutely intoxicated patient.

5. The administration of glucose-containing fluids IV may precipitate an acute psychotic condition similar to **Wernicke's encephalopathy;** however, the conditions may not be reversible with vitamin treatment. **Glucose should be avoided** or used cautiously in anyone with a chronic history of alcohol use.

6. A chronic form of alcohol-induced neurologic disease is **Korsakoff's psychosis,** which is associated with a degeneration of specific loci in the brain. This condition is not reversible. Other chronic intellectual abnormalities occur with chronic alcohol use, and these will improve slowly with abstinence.

C. Prevention and Treatment of Delerium Tremens

Controversy exists over whether to give benzodiazepines routinely to all hospitalized patients with a history of chronic alcohol abuse. This is probably unnecessary in that only 1 to 2 percent will develop severe withdrawal. Their hospital stay and complications may be increased with sedative drug administration in patients not needing it. Those who should receive prophylaxis include patients with a history of previous episodes of DTs, patients who cannot be well monitored for the signs of developing DTs, patients with a

Table 29-1   Signs and symptoms of alcohol use and withdrawal

Sign or symptom	Acute intoxication	Early withdrawal, 0–48 h	Impending DTs, 48–96 h
Systolic blood pressure	Decreased	Elevated	Normal or elevated
Diastolic blood pressure	Decreased	Normal	Normal or elevated
Heart rate	Normal or decreased	Elevated	Elevated
Temperature	Normal or decreased	Elevated	Normal
Tremors	Absent	May be present	Marked
Cravings	Absent	Marked	Absent
Paranoia	May be present	Minimal	Marked
Hallucinosis	None	May be present	May be present
Hallucinations	Rare	Rare	Usually present—often auditory or tactile
Disorientation	Marked	Minimal	May be marked
Sleep disorders	Not applicable	Marked	Marked
Seizures	Rare	Occasionally—brief "rum fits"	Characteristic prolonged
Mortality	Occasionally—secondary to overdose	Rare	0.5–15%

very high daily alcohol intake (a fifth of distilled spirits per day or more), and those developing severe tremors several days after abstinence. Sedative drugs should be avoided or used with caution in patients over 60 years of age regardless of their risk factors.

D. Treatment of Alcohol Withdrawal

The treatment of withdrawal should be based on signs and symptoms. These are listed in Table 29-1. Systolic blood pressure elevation is an invariable accompaniment of acute alcohol withdrawal. The degree of elevation in blood pressure and heart rate indicates the severity of the acute withdrawal syndrome. Short-acting benzodiazepines are useful for treating this condition. They should be rapidly tapered over a week to 10 days to avoid oversedation and continued habituation. Longer-acting benzodiazepines can be used to prevent the development of DTs, but are less helpful in full-blown syndromes. Diazepam (Valium) or midazolam (Versed) is useful to treat acute DTs. Concurrent medical problems should be identified and addressed during the treatment of acute and chronic withdrawal.

III. NARCOTIC USE AND ABUSE

A. During the treatment of pain, patients will develop **tolerance** to the effects of narcotics. This may necessitate increasing doses to achieve satisfactory analgesia. Narcotics bind at specific receptors in the spinal cord and brain to exert their effects. Neuronal receptor density rapidly increases when exposed to exogenous narcotics. This occurs rapidly, in several days, and is the explanation for tolerance. Withdrawal of narcotic drugs is associated with a characteristic syndrome, the symptoms of which are listed in Table 29-2. People using narcotics recreationally also experience tolerance and withdrawal. Short-acting narcotics (fentanyl and sufentanil) rapidly induce tolerance, and massive doses may be needed to achieve analgesia after a few days of continuous use. Intermittent dosing and rest periods of several hours may restore sensitivity and retard the development of tolerance.

B. Most patients dislike the sedative and gastrointestinal side effects of the narcotics and will reduce their use spontaneously after the acute pain subsides. Patients accustomed to their use may continue to request narcotics for their mood-altering effects. Gradual withdrawal, over 3 to 5 days, is necessary to prevent an acute, severe abstinence syndrome. Since a principal symptom of narcotic withdrawal is severe pain, the therapeutic use of narcotics often continues despite the resolution of the primary anatomic causes of acute pain. Awareness of this and a plan to taper narcotics will reduce the occurrence of iatrogenic medical addiction. Narcotics are generally felt to be ineffective in treating chronic pain syndromes. Their use for more than several days after the acute injury should alert the caregiver to the potential for withdrawal-induced, continued-use syndromes.

C. Narcotic-addicted persons should not be deprived of needed analgesia—a larger dose than anticipated may be necessary due to tolerance. Withdrawal or maintenance can be considered after the acutely painful period is past.

1. Clonidine (Catapres), a centrally acting, alpha-1 adrenergic blocking drug, has been used to reduce drug cravings and sympathetic overactivity in persons withdrawing from narcotics. It may be helpful in the hospitalized patient habituated to narcotics as well. It has also been effective in preventing relapse in smoking cessation. Clonidine can be applied transdermally with good persistent effects, though oral dosing is more common in drug-withdrawal programs.

Table 29-2 Effects of narcotic use and withdrawal

Sign or symptom	Acute intoxication	Withdrawal
Mental state	Euphoria, sleepiness, lethargy, coma	Anxiety, nervousness, agitation, narcotic cravings
Pain	Absent	Severe diffuse pain in bones and joints, myalgias, "aching all over"
Skin	Cool, dry	Piloerection, profuse sweating
Pupils	Constricted	Dilated
Reflexes	Depressed	Increased
Temperature	Normal	Increased
Gastrointestinal	Nausea and vomiting, constipation	Diarrhea
Blood pressure	Normal	Elevated
Pulse	Low	Elevated
Cardiac	Acute pulmonary edema	Bacterial endocarditis risk
Mortality	From overdose respiratory arrest	None

    2. Beta-blocking drugs can also suppress some of the unpleasant sympathetic manifestations of narcotic withdrawal.

    3. Recognition of the occurrence of tolerance and the need for **gradual detoxification** in most patients will make this problem less of an issue in the patient requiring intensive care.

    4. The **use of regional analgesic techniques and nonnarcotic analgesics** will reduce the incidence of the problem of tolerance and withdrawal.

IV. STIMULANT DRUG USE

    A. Crack cocaine has replaced **amphetamines** as the most frequently abused stimulant drug. Used for the enhancement of mood, this drug has an extreme addiction potential. The user often feels invincible, and because the effect is evanescent and is followed by profound depression, repeated use is needed to maintain the desired state. Other activities of life are abandoned, and drug seeking and use become paramount. The cost rises as use increases.

Stealing and other illegal activities to get more drugs result. Victims stop eating, and this, as well as the hyperactivity, causes profound weight loss. After several days of continued use without sleep, the person collapses (the "crash") for several days. Severe depression with thoughts of suicide follows prolonged use. Crack addicts are often injured in this cycle or suffer medical complications, including cardiac events, and frequently require medical care.

B. The **signs and symptoms of intoxication and withdrawal** are listed in Table 29-3. The diagnosis can be made from the patient's history and/or testing for urinary excretion of cocaine metabolic products.

C. Acute intoxication **treatment** is supportive, and the most significant problem is the profound cravings which accompany the use of this drug. A return to use is the rule, although some treatment programs have been successful in rehabilitating crack addicts. Dopamine-blocking drugs such as bromocriptine seem to reduce the irresistible urge to use this drug.

V. BENZODIAZEPINE USE

A. Believed to have little abuse potential, this class of drugs has been the most commonly prescribed in the past 30 years. Many patients are placed on these **anxiolytic agents,** and maintained on them indefinitely. Rarely do patients spontaneously increase drug dosage.

B. Recently, a characteristic **withdrawal syndrome** has become recognized with this group of drugs. Since they are rather fat soluble, withdrawal is often delayed after stopping the agent. Weeks or months are sometimes necessary to see this syndrome. The primary symptom of withdrawal is

Table 29-3 **Signs and symptoms of cocaine use and withdrawal**

Sign or symptom	Acute intoxication	Withdrawal
Blood pressure	Elevated	Normal
Heart rate	Elevated	Normal
Mood	Feeling of being invincible; chronic use may lead to severe paranoia	Depressed, may be suicidal
CNS	Agitation, may lead to seizures	Slow reaction, sleeps constantly
Gastrointestinal	No appetite	Hungry
Cravings for drug	Continual	Severe, intermittent

extreme anxiety, which may be the reason the drug was prescribed in the first place. The most severe symptom is seizures; these are usually unheralded and may be intractable. Often used as sleep-inducing agents, alteration in sleep during withdrawal is universal. The other symptoms of withdrawal include depression, malaise, tremors, delusions, myalgias, paresthesias, muscle cramps, and severe bandlike, unrelenting headache. Inadvertent withdrawal may occur when patients who are receiving these agents at home therapeutically are hospitalized.

    C. The **abuse** of benzodiazepines is common. Tolerance develops rapidly and enormous doses of drug may be consumed. Toxicity is rare. Death from an overdose is related to the medical complications of coma. Alcoholics often use benzodiazepines instead of alcohol.

    D. The use of benzodiazepines for **sedation in the critically ill** can lead to the same withdrawal syndrome as described above. This is especially true with the short-acting agents such as midazolam. This cause of agitation and delirium in the critically ill must be considered in the differential diagnosis, recognized, and gradual withdrawal of the drug instituted.

VI. MARIJUANA AND THE PERCEPTUAL DISTORTERS

    A. Acute **marijuana** use results in sedation and passivity. Prolonged use results in a lack of interest in any activity, also known as the **amotivational syndrome,** as well as paranoia and depression. Medical concerns with acute use in the injured patient are minimal, and include slightly decreased blood pressure, high pulse rate, and injected conjunctiva. Marijuana smoke has over 200 active ingredients, although **tetrahydrocannabinol** (THC) is found in the greatest quantity and accounts for most of the identified effects. It is an appetite stimulant, and may decrease the nausea and vomiting associated with some forms of chemotherapy. Although THC is a bronchodilator, the smoke from marijuana cigarettes causes bronchoconstriction. Withdrawal from marijuana is uncomplicated, although cravings to get high are common.

    B. **Phencyclidine** (PCP) is related to ketamine and was developed as an animal tranquilizer (hence the street name "tranq" or "animal"). It alters one's perception of the internal and external environment. During use, aggressive behavior, lack of pain response, and hallucinations occur. Recurrent use and cravings for the drug are frequent. Because of the agitated state associated with its use, patients are often injured (or injure others) and present for medical care. Acute intoxication symptoms are listed in Table 29-4. Withdrawal causes depression, anorexia, insomnia, and anergy, but requires no treatment.

Table 29-4 Symptoms of acute phencyclidine intoxication

Mild intoxication	Agitation, analgesia, anxiety, catalepsy, diaphoresis, disorganization, flushing, visual hallucinations, irritability, euphoric mood
Moderate intoxication	Extreme anxiety, excitement, hyperthermia, enhanced reflexes, salivation, mutism, psychosis, rigidity, violence, steriotopy
Severe intoxication	Arrhythmias, catatonia, coma, hallucinations, hypertension, opisthotonus, seizures, death

    C. Other perceptual distorters include cholinergic drugs and plants, hashish, and lysergic acid diethylamide (LSD). These have specific medical implications, and although similar to PCP, are less lethal.

VII. TREATMENT OF CHEMICAL DEPENDENCE

    A. Patients

The most important issue in the treatment of chemical dependence is identification of the problem. Most affected individuals are in a state of denial about the significance and severity of their disease. Caring confrontation, structured treatment, lifelong support programs (Alcoholics Anonymous or Narcotics Anonymous), peer assistance, and a gradual return to society improve the likelihood of the maintenance of abstinence. Referral for treatment after the resolution of the acute illness in patients with chemical dependence should be aggressively pursued.

    B. Health Care Workers

As mentioned previously, **health care providers are subject to chemical dependence** in numbers similar to the population in general. Although alcohol abuse/dependence is the most common problem in health care providers, characteristic patterns of other drug abuse occur in special groups. The IV abuse of narcotics, especially those short-acting agents used for general anesthesia, is the most common addiction problem in anesthesiologists. Nurses who work in intensive care units preferentially abuse narcotics and benzodiazepines. They believe that they can control the use of the drugs owing to their superior knowledge about their clinical use. This falsely justifies the experimentation by medical personnel with legal but regulated drugs. Use rapidly progresses to abuse, and the disease of denial prevents the affected person from seeking help for the addiction. Colleagues cover for poor job performance, and no one is willing or able to address the drug issue. Eventually, the disease evolves to the point that patient care suffers.

        1. The most caring thing one can do is to confront a suffering colleague and succeed in getting him or her to seek treatment for the disease.

Chemical dependence is a treatable disease, and the success rates for health care workers are very high. Often a formal intervention is necessary and very effective in convincing the addicted person to seek help. Involvement of the employer and the presence of a recovering peer in the intervention are important. The signs of chemical dependence in a health care provider (or other person) are listed in Table 29-5.

Table 29-5 Signs of chemical abuse in a colleague

Community life	Withdraws from friends, leisure activities, church and civic organizations
	Inappropriate spending, gambling
	Legal problems, driving under the influence
Family life	Withdrawal
	Domestic arguments
	Illegal behavior in children
	Sexual problems
	Spouse leaves
Physical health	Poor hygiene
	Visits doctors frequently
	Vague complaints
	Medical absence from work, often on Mondays
	Mood swings
Work life	Changes jobs
	Poor job performance
	Poor or compulsive record keeping
	Works overtime voluntarily
	Prescription pattern changes
	Withdraws from colleagues
	Tremulousness
	Drug use at work

2. The details of **addiction treatment** are beyond the scope of this text. Most professional societies have committees or task forces to assist anyone dealing with chemically dependent members, and local help can be obtained from these sources. Treatment rather than punishment is the appropriate approach. The reward of a colleague's life saved is worth the time, money, and effort expended.

3. Drug exposure with abuse potential is considered an **occupational hazard** of some types of medical practice. Education about this problem, the precautions to be taken, and the positive results of treatment are used to reduce the risk of developing chemical dependence. Acceptance by the medical community at large of the disease concept of chemical dependence, rather than its being considered a moral weakness, will go a long way toward reducing the suffering from this disease.

SUGGESTED READINGS

Giannini AJ, Slaby AE: *Drugs of Abuse.* Oradell, New Jersey, Medical Economics, 1989.

Goodwin DW: Genetic influences in alcoholism. *Adv Intern Med* 32:283–298, 1987.

Goodwin DW: Genetic factors in the development of alcoholism. *Psychiatr Clin N Am* 9:427–433, 1986.

Gravenstein JS, Kory WP, Marks RG: Drug abuse by anesthesia personnel. *Anesth Analg* 62:467–472, 1983.

Hallstrom C, Lader M: Benzodiazepine withdrawal phenomena. *Int Pharmacopsychiatry* 16:235, 1981.

Johnson VE: *Intervention: How to Help Someone Who Doesn't Want Help.* Minneapolis, Johnson Institute, 1986.

Morse RM, Martin MA, Swenson WM, Niven RG: Prognosis of physicians treated for alcoholism and drug dependence. *JAMA* 251:743–746, 1984.

Spiegelman WG, Saunders L, Mazze RI: Addiction and anesthesiology. *Anesthesiology* 60:335–341, 1984.

Sullivan E, Bissell L, Williams E: *Chemical Dependency in Nursing.* Menlo Park, California, Addison-Wesley, 1988.

Talbott GD, Gallegos KV, Wilson PO, Porter TL: The Medical Association of Georgia's impaired physician program: review of the first 1000 physicians: analysis of specialty. *JAMA* 257:2927, 1987.

Winokur A, Rickels K, Greenblatt DJ, et al: Withdrawal reaction from long-term, low-dosage administration of diazepam: a double-blind, placebo-controlled case study. *Arch Gen Psychiatry* 37:101, 1980.

CHAPTER
30

PAIN MANAGEMENT IN THE CRITICALLY ILL CHILD

Madelyn Kahana

Cases
 I. Differences Between Children and Adults
 II. Neuroanatomy and Neuropharmacology
     A. Anatomic Framework
     B. Sensory Cortex
     C. Neurohumoral Response
 III. Pain Assessment in Children
     A. Subjective Experience
 IV. Pharmacologic Management of Pain
     A. Nonopioid Analgesics
     B. Opioid Analgesics
     C. Neural Blockade
     D. Peripheral Nerve Blocks
 V. Conclusions
Case Discussions
Final Thoughts
Suggested Readings

CASES

Case 1

A 10-year-old child is involved in a motor vehicle accident as an unrestrained front-seat passenger. Because of hemodynamic instability on presentation to the emergency department, he is taken to the operating room for urgent exploratory laparotomy. His other injuries include second-degree burns of his legs, multiple rib fractures, and a pulmonary contusion. At operation, a splenic laceration is repaired. Postoperative care is continued in the pediatric intensive care unit (ICU). The patient is intubated, but is awake and able to follow simple commands on arrival from the operating room.

Case 2

A 32-week-gestation infant, now several hours old, is brought to the operating room for urgent closure of a ruptured omphalocele. He is intubated because of coexisting hyaline membrane disease and a large ventricular septal defect. The omphalocele repair is accomplished using a silastic silo. Postoperatively, the infant remains intubated, and is returned to the neonatal ICU for staged reduction of the abdominal wall defect.

These two cases illustrate the scope and complexity of the problem of pain management in the critically ill child. Injured and ill children experience pain for a variety of reasons. Pain may be secondary to traumatic injuries, surgical procedures, or underlying disease, or it may accompany invasive procedures performed in the ICU setting. The pathophysiology of pain and the rationale for the ablation of pain are similar in adults and children. This mandates a thorough understanding of the options for pain management and the aggressive use of these options in the pediatric patient population.

I. DIFFERENCES BETWEEN CHILDREN AND ADULTS

The **differences that exist between children and adults** are secondary to the physiologic and behavioral maturation that result from the aging process. Because of these differences, pain historically has been undertreated in neonates and children.

    A. Neonates were once believed to be neurologically incapable of pain perception. **Older children** were undermedicated because of their cognitive and expressive limitations or the fear of opiate addiction. Recent information detailing the neuroanatomy and the physiologic competence of even the smallest child dispels these myths.

    B. Data describing the incidence of in-hospital pediatric opiate addiction are limited. For the adult, physical tolerance to therapeutic opioids is common, while addiction is exceedingly rare. The child should be no different.

II. NEUROANATOMY AND NEUROPHARMACOLOGY

A. Anatomic Framework

Building the anatomic framework for pain transmission begins during the seventh week of gestation and is nearly complete at term. **Nociceptive nerve endings** in the skin of the newborn outnumber those in the adult. Central and peripheral nociceptive pathways are intact though incompletely myelinated at birth, even in the premature infant. Slower conduction velocities in the pathways lacking myelin are compensated by the shorter distances traveled by these nerve impulses. The **laminar arrangement of the dorsal horn** of the spinal cord is present in the fetus by 30 weeks' gestation, as are pain pathways to the thalamus. **Thalamocortical pain fibers** are completely myelinated by 37 weeks.

B. Sensory Cortex

The **sensory cortex** is also structurally well developed in the neonate. In fact, cerebral glucose utilization is higher in the sensory cortex than in any other fetal cortical structure at 28 weeks' gestation.

C. Neurohumoral Response

The **neurohumoral response** to a nociceptive stimulus is well documented in the neonate and child, as is the presence of **neural transmitters** in sufficient concentration to mediate nociceptive neuronal activity. A high density of substance P fibers has been observed in the fetal brainstem, thalamus, and cortex. **Endogenous opioids** are released in the human fetus at birth and in response to fetal distress. In addition, there is now significant evidence that there is an intact humoral stress response to surgical manipulation of the newborn. Elevated levels of catecholamines, growth hormone, glucagon, and cortisone have been noted, as has a prolonged catabolic state. As in the adult, this response is blunted by adequate analgesia and/or anesthesia.

III. PAIN ASSESSMENT IN CHILDREN

A. Subjective Experience

Pain is a **subjective experience** and its assessment depends heavily on patient report.

   1. In the **neonate,** there are only indirect measures of the pain experience. Behavioral and physiologic changes can be measured and pain level inferred. Much of the evidence supporting pain management in the neonate

relies heavily on changes in heart rate, respiratory rate, and blood pressure, and interpretation of the newborn's cry and facial expression.

   2. In the **older child,** direct cognitive measures of pain perception are possible to perform. There are two useful methods of pain assessment for the child capable of communication.

      a. **Self-report methods** of pain evaluation require that the child directly describe his or her attitude toward and perception of pain. Patients must be able to comprehend and communicate verbally to use self-report techniques or questionnaires.

      b. **Projection methods** of pain evaluation use the child's selection of a cartoon face (see Fig. 30-1) or other drawings that best represent his or her feelings. Projection methods require comprehension, but rely on nonverbal communication.

IV. PHARMACOLOGIC MANAGEMENT OF PAIN

A. Nonopioid Analgesics

Mild to moderate pain in the pediatric population can be managed with nonsteroidal antiinflammatory drugs (NSAIDs), acetaminophen, or salicylates. In more severe pain, nonopioids serve as adjuncts to opioid therapy.

   1. There are a number of **NSAIDs** which are safe and effective analgesics in pediatric patients (see Table 30-1). The NSAIDs do not produce respiratory depression and are not associated with physical dependence or addiction. All NSAIDs currently available, except choline magnesium salicylate (Trilisate), reversibly inhibit platelet cyclooxygenase, prolong bleeding time, and occasionally lead to gastritis and ulceration of the small intestine. Except for ketorolac tromethamine (Toradol), NSAIDs are administered enterally. Nephrotoxicity and hepatotoxicity are uncommon with short-term use. There is no information on the use of NSAIDs in the newborn infant, and little on their use in the child younger than 2 years of age. There is no clinical evidence linking NSAIDs other than acetylsalicylate (aspirin) to Reye's syndrome.

   2. As the use of other NSAIDs has increased, the use of **acetylsalicylic acid (aspirin)** has dramatically fallen in pediatric practice. This is due pri-

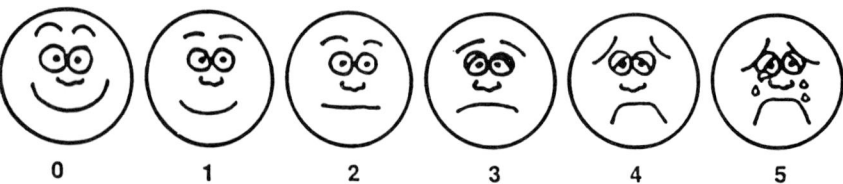

Figure 30-1   Faces pain rating scale

Table 30-1 Nonnarcotic analgesics

Drug	Dose	Interval	Route*
Ibuprofen	4–10 mg/kg	q 6–8 h	PO
Naproxen (Naprosyn, Syntex)	5–7 mg/kg	q 6–8 h	PO
Tolmetin (Tolectin, McNeil)	5–7 mg/kg	q 6–8 h	PO
Choline magnesium salicylate (Trilisate, Purdue Frederick)	10–15 mg/kg	q 8 h	PO
Ketorolac tromethamine (Tordal, Syntex)	First dose: 1 mg/kg Repeat doses: 0.5 mg/kg	q 6 h	IV or IM
Acetaminophen	10–15 mg/kg	q 4 h	PO
	15–20 mg/kg	q 4 h	PR

*PO = by mouth; PR = per rectum; IV = intravenous; IM = intramuscular.

marily to the association between aspirin use and Reye's syndrome. Aspirin administration is now reserved exclusively for specific inflammatory and rheumatic disease processes.

  3. **Acetaminophen** is the most common nonnarcotic analgesic prescribed for children. It is safe and effective for the management of modest pain, even in the newborn. In neonates, acetaminophen is eliminated primarily as the sulfate conjugate instead of as the glucuronide metabolite. Despite this, there are *no* age-related differences in the elimination rate constants for acetaminophen. For all ages, the recommended dose for acetaminophen is 10 to 15 mg/kg every 4 h orally or 15 to 20 mg/kg every 4 h rectally. As with the NSAIDs, there is no respiratory depression, physical tolerance, or addiction associated with acetaminophen use. In addition, coagulation is unaffected by acetaminophen administration. Acetaminophen's weak analgesic properties make it suitable as a sole agent for treating minor pain and discomfort, or as an adjunct to opioid analgesics for patients with more severe distress.

B. Opioid Analgesics

Opioid analgesics continue to be the mainstay of pain management in the critically ill neonate and child. Unlike the NSAIDs and acetaminophen, **physical dependence** on and **tolerance** to opioids occur predictably after 5 to 7 days of regular administration. After such time, effective dose requirements will increase, and narcotic withdrawal symptoms can occur. True addiction in the pediatric population is believed to be rare.

  1. In equipotent doses, all opioids produce **respiratory depression.** The carbon dioxide response curve is both flattened and shifted to the right. In

Table 30-2 Pediatric opiate pharmacokinetics

	Activity*	Fentanyl	Morphine	Meperidine	Methadone
Neonate	Vd, L/kg	5.1 ± 1		5	
	$t_{1/2}$, min	317 ± 70	360 ± 60	140 ± 20	
	CL, mL/kg/min	18 ± 4.4	6.3 ± 1		
Older child	Vd, L/kg	2.1 ± 1		4.17	
	$t_{1/2}$, min	129 ± 20	120 ± 30	180 ± 40	1200 + 60
	CL, mL/kg/min	7.05 ± 1.2	23.8 ± 2		

*Vd = volume of distribution; $t_{1/2}$ = half time; Cl = clearance.

the premature and term newborn infant, respiratory depression may be out of proportion to the dose of opioid administered. Caution, therefore, is recommended in this patient population when adequate spontaneous ventilation is desired. A number of theories have been offered to explain increased respiratory depression in the newborn in response to narcotics. The most plausible thus far is the alteration in the ratio of mu-1 and mu-2 receptors in the newborn. The neonatal predominance of mu-2 receptors would favor significant respiratory depression.

2. The **elimination** half-life of most opioids is prolonged in the newborn, such that the dosing interval is significantly longer than in the older child, and accumulation of narcotics can occur when a continuous infusion is used. At particular risk is the newborn with increased intra-abdominal pressure in whom opioid clearance can approach zero. By the age of 6 months, metabolism and excretion of the opioid analgesics resemble those in the older child and adult (see Table 30-2).

3. The **options for the administration of opiates** to critically ill children parallel those for adults (see Table 30-3). In most circumstances, the **intravenous (IV)** route of administration is preferred. Intermittent dose schedules are effective. However, narcotic infusions are a more effective means to control pain and require a lower total dose of opiate. **Nurse-administered intermittent IV narcotic doses** and **continuous opiate infusions** are effective and useful, even in the nonverbal child. Patient-controlled analgesia **(PCA)** is useful in the older, verbal child.

    a. The **PCA** technique has been successfully used in children as young as 4 years of age, when instructions can be made clear, though school-age children are usually better equipped to handle the self-administration of analgesics.

    b. As in the adult, PCA can be used with or without a background continuous narcotic infusion (see Table 30-4). It offers the child a sense of control and rapid access to IV narcotics. As in the adult, the total dose of

Table 30-3 Opiates in common use in pediatric/neonate ICUs

Drug	Route of administration	Starting dose*†	Duration, h
Morphine	Intermittent IV	0.05–0.1 mg/kg	2–4
	Continuous IV	0.01–0.1 mg/kg/h	N/A
	Intramuscular	0.1–0.15 mg/kg	3–4
	Oral	3 mg/kg	3–4
Meperidine	Intermittent IV	0.8–1.0 mg/kg	2–4
	Continuous IV	0.3–0.6 mg/kg/h	NA
	Intramuscular	1–1.5 mg/kg	3–4
	Oral	1–2 mg/kg	4
Fentanyl	Intermittent IV	1–2 μg/kg	1–2
	Continuous IV	1–2 μg/kg/h	NA
Methadone	Intermittent IV	0.05–0.1 mg/kg	4–12
	Oral	0.1–0.15 mg/kg	4–8
Codeine	Oral	0.5–1.0 mg/kg	4
	Intramuscular	0.5–1.0 mg/kg	4

*Use low-dose recommendations in spontaneously ventilating neonates and be prepared for respiratory depression.
†Before starting an infusion of any narcotic, give a loading IV dose of the same narcotic, sufficient to achieve analgesia.

narcotic is less than that used with standard intermittent nurse-administered IV opiates.

4. A number of opioids are available for use in neonates and children. As stated previously, in equipotent doses, all produce respiratory depression and tolerance. However, certain peculiarities of specific narcotics deserve review when considered for use in small children.

   a. **Morphine,** particularly in large doses, can produce vasodilation and hypotension, and should be used cautiously when the patient's hemodynamic status is questionable.

   b. **Meperidine** has an active metabolite, normeperidine, which is renally cleared. In the infant, decreased clearance leads to the accumulation of normeperidine and can produce respiratory depression and seizures.

Table 30-4 Suggested initial orders for pediatric PCA

Drug: morphine, 1 mg/mL
PCA dose: morphine, 0.01–0.02 mg/kg (10–20 μg/kg)
Lockout: 5–10 min
Infusion: morphine, 0.01 mg/kg/h (10 μg/kg/h)
Maximum dose in 4 h: morphine, 0.25 mg/kg

Therefore, meperidine is not recommended for use in the child younger than 6 months of age.

    c. Fentanyl is commonly used in the critically ill child because of its limited effect on hemodynamics, although bradycardia can occur, particularly when high-dose fentanyl is administered. Chest wall rigidity has been reported in children, even in those receiving low-dose fentanyl. Muscle relaxants may be necessary to facilitate mechanical ventilation should chest wall rigidity occur.

    d. Congeners of fentanyl and **partial opiate agonists** are not commonly used in the ill neonate or child.

    e. Because of its long half-life and oral bioavailability, **methadone** is used primarily to facilitate withdrawal of narcotics in children who have developed physical dependence on opiates.

C. Neural Blockade

    1. Regional anesthetic techniques are not new in the pediatric population. In fact, the first reports of spinal anesthesia in the newborn were found in the *Medical Record* at the turn of the century.

    2. The use of regional analgesia requires a thorough knowledge of both the anatomy and the pharmacology of local anesthetic agents in children. In general, the **volume of distribution** for local anesthetics is larger in the newborn, while the **elimination half-life** is prolonged. This makes a single dose of local anesthetic quite safe, but predisposes the neonate to the accumulation of local anesthetic agents when continuous infusion techniques are employed. In addition, the neonate is challenged by having reduced levels of alpha-1 glycoproteins, which increase the unbound local anesthetic level and contribute to potential toxicity (see Table 30-5).

    3. The **toxicity of local anesthetics** produces central nervous system excitation and hemodynamic instability. Resuscitation equipment should be available when performing any regional technique. With the exception of prilocaine, all currently available local anesthetic agents are safe and effective in even the smallest child. A by-product of prilocaine biotransformation is 6-hydroxytoluidine, which can produce severe methemoglobinemia in the young infant, even when an appropriate dose is used. For that reason, prilocaine is contraindicated in infants younger than 6 months of age.

    4. Central neural blockade with local anesthetic agents is particularly useful when the painful stimulus is below T8. The addition of opiates to central blocks improves the quality of the analgesia, particularly when the origin of the painful process is higher than the midthoracic level.

    a. The most commonly used regional technique for pain management in the child is an **epidural.** This block can be performed safely at any level from the caudal space to the midthoracic level. The level injected is determined in large part by the area of pathology. Recommendations for

Table 30-5 Pharmacokinetic properties of local anesthetics

Drug	VdSS,* L/kg	Plasma protein binding, %	$t_{1/2}$, h	Maximum single dose, mg/kg†	Maximum dose with epinephrine, mg/kg
Lidocaine					
Neonate	1.4–4.9	25	3	7	9–10
Adult	0.2–1.0	55–65	1.6		
Bupivacaine					
Neonate	—	50–70	9	2.0–2.5	2.5–3.0
Adult	0.8–1.6	85–95	2–3		

*VdSS = volume of distribution at steady state.
†This is the *maximum* dose of local anesthetic agent used in neural blockade. It is *not* the maximum IV dose.

drug doses are found in Table 30-6. These refer to children who are older than 6 months.

   b. When using continuous local anesthetic infusion for analgesia in the preterm or term newborn, the accumulation of drug is possible. Single-dose recommendations for **neonates** are the same as those for the older child. Initial infusion rates should be reduced by half and cautiously titrated to effect.

   c. The use of **central neural blockade** frequently eliminates the need for systemic opiates, and produces analgesia without sedation. Ambulation with assistance is possible; bowel function returns rapidly. When using central neural blockade, it is imperative that the bedside nurse assess the level of the block as part of the routine record of vital signs. This will prevent an ascending block from going unnoticed, which could result in unexpected physiologic consequences.

   d. **Warning:** Should narcotics, particularly morphine, be administered in the central neuroaxis, the risk of respiratory depression is real. Remember that this reduction in respiratory drive can occur as late as 16 h after the opioid is given. Appropriate monitoring is imperative throughout the administration period *and* for a drug-specific period after the infusion has been discontinued.

   5. **Lumbar epidural blockade** in infants and children can be accomplished in the same fashion as in the adult. After sterile preparation of the field, an 18- or 20-gauge Touhy needle is introduced into the epidural space by the loss-of-resistance technique. A catheter can then be inserted through the needle for continuous infusion of local anesthetic. It should be noted that the distance from the skin to the epidural space is considerably less in the child than in the adult. In the infant under 1 year of age, the distance is 1 to

Table 30-6 Central neural blockade for acute pain management*

Block	Drug recommended	Dose mg/kg	Duration, h	Notes
Lumbar epidural: single dose	1–1.5% lidocaine	7–9	1–2	Use 1–1.5 mL/segment to be blocked
	0.25% bupivacaine	1.5–2.5	4–8	
	0.125% bupivacaine	1.5–2.5	2–4	
	Preservative-free morphine	0.05–.1 Max:5 mg	8–24	May cause respiratory depression
Lumbar epidural: continuous infusion	0.125% bupivacaine	0.3 mL/kg/h	NA	Fentanyl has much less rostral spread than morphine
	0.1% bupivacaine + fentanyl 2 μg/mL	0.3 mL/kg/h	NA	
Caudal epidural: single dose	1–1.5% lidocaine	7–9	1–2	1 mL/kg of local agent is required for T6–T8 block
	0.25% bupivacaine	1.5–2.5	4–8	
	0.125% bupivacaine	1.5–2.5	2–4	
	Preservative-free morphine	0.05–0.1 Max 5 mg	8–24	
Caudal epidural: continuous infusion	0.25% bupivacaine	0.3 mL/kg/h	NA	Some motor block will occur with 0.25% bupivacaine
	0.1% bupivacaine + fentanyl 2 μg/mL	0.3 mL/kg/h	NA	
Thoracic epidural: single dose	1–1.5% lidocaine	7–9	1–2	0.5–0.7 mL of local anesthetic is needed per segment blocked
	0.25% bupivacaine	1.5–2.5	4–8	
	0.125% bupivacaine	1.5–2.5	2–4	
Thoracic epidural: continuous infusion	0.125% bupivacaine	0.2 mL/kg/h	NA	
	0.1% bupivacaine + fentanyl 2 μg/mL	0.2 mL/kg/h	NA	

*Recommendations for children over 6 months of age.

1.5 cm. In the adult, this distance ranges from 7 to 18 cm. The drug chosen for epidural blockade should be based on the desired effect and duration of action desired (see Table 30-6).

6. In the small child, the **caudal** approach to the epidural space is commonly used. With the patient in the prone or lateral decubitus position, the skin over the sacrum is prepped with antiseptic and a 22-gauge, short-bevel needle is introduced through the sacrococcygeal ligament at the sacral hiatus into the caudal epidural space. The sacral hiatus can be readily identified as the space between the sacral cornua. Entry into the caudal epidural space is marked by a subtle "pop." The needle is then minimally advanced (less than 3 mm), and careful aspiration of the needle performed, to avoid accidental IV or subarachnoid injection. Recall that the dural sac may end as low as the level of S3 in the newborn. The caudal approach can be used as a means for establishing a continuous technique by substituting a Touhy or Crawford needle for the 22-gauge, short-bevel needle. Although there are reports of thoracic-level catheter placement from the caudal approach, the catheter is generally threaded only 2 to 4 cm. The choice of anesthetic solution depends on the desired duration and the level of analgesia required. The addition of narcotics to local anesthetic solutions will enhance the quality of the analgesia and improve the level of analgesia achieved.

7. **Thoracic epidural** anesthesia is achieved in the child as it is in the adult. There are two approaches to the thoracic epidural space: midline and paramedian. Though the catheter can be introduced at virtually any level, the recommended position is T6 or lower. In the paramedian method, the epidural needle is placed 1 cm lateral to midline and advanced cephalad and toward the midline until the lamina is encountered. The needle is then walked off the bony surface into the epidural space, which is recognized by the loss of resistance, as it is at lower spinal levels. The angle of the needle at thoracic levels needs to be significantly more acute than it is in the lumbar area in order to be successful. The choice of local anesthetic or narcotic again depends on the desired effect and duration (see Table 30-6). Because of the propensity of morphine to circulate cephalad in the cerebrospinal fluid and cause delayed respiratory depression, and the decreased distance between the site of injection and the respiratory center in the brainstem, morphine rarely is used in thoracic epidurals.

D. Peripheral Nerve Blocks

A number of **peripheral nerve blocks** are useful in managing pain in the critically injured or ill child. These include intercostal block, intrapleural block, femoral nerve block, and penile nerve block. As with central neural blockade, a thorough knowledge of the pharmacokinetics of local anesthetic agents in the small child is mandatory. (See Table 30-5.)

1. An **intercostal nerve block** is useful in the management of pain that originates in the chest or the upper abdominal wall. The ribs are readily pal-

pated in most children. The intercostal nerve runs in a groove, with the intercostal vessels under each rib. At the midaxillary line, a lateral cutaneous branch of the intercostal nerve innervates the regional skin, and there are anterior cutaneous branches at the sternal termination of each nerve.

    a. Medial to the posterior axillary line, a 23- or 25-gauge needle is inserted at a slightly less than perpendicular angle to the rib. After bony contact with the rib is made, the needle tip is gently "walked" down and then under the rib until bony contact is lost. After aspiration for blood is negative, 1 to 3 mL of local anesthetic is injected. The procedure is repeated until all the necessary intercostal nerves are blocked. (See Table 30-7.)

    b. It must be remembered that the serum levels of local anesthetic for a given dose injected are highest with intercostal nerve blocks. Strict adherence to the maximum dose recommendations for the local anesthetics thus is mandatory. In addition, epinephrine in a concentration of 5 μg/mL (1:200,000) should be added to the anesthetic solution to limit systemic uptake. This technique generally provides excellent analgesia for thoracic pain, and facilitates pulmonary toilet. Its disadvantage is the need for multiple repeated injections, which are distinctly unpopular in the pediatric population.

    2. In 1986, the administration of **intrapleural local anesthesia** was described as an alternative to intercostal blocks. This requires the placement of an epidural catheter into the pleural space, through which local anesthetic can be instilled. This technique obviates the need for repeated needle punc-

Table 30-7 Recommended doses of local anesthetic for peripheral neural blockade

Block	Agent	Dose	Notes
Intercostal	1–1.5% lidocaine with epinephrine 1:200,000	1–3 mL/level	Highest systemic drug levels
	0.25% bupivacaine with epinephrine 1:200,000	1–3 mL/level	
Intrapleural	0.25% bupivacaine with epinephrine 1:200,000	0.4 mL/kg	
	1–1.5% lidocaine with epinephrine 1:200,000	0.4 mL/kg	
Femoral	0.25% bupivacaine with epinephrine 1:200,000	0.4 mL/kg	Max 10 mL
Penile (ring block)	0.25% bupivacaine	1–8 mL	Avoid the use of epinephrine

tures. For best results, the epidural catheter should be placed in the posterior pleural space, under direct vision. Percutaneous catheter placement can be accomplished with the loss-of-resistance technique with the patient in the lateral decubitus position. A 17- or 20-gauge Touhy needle is walked off the superior margin of the sixth or seventh rib along the posterior axillary line and directed toward the vertebral column. A well-lubricated glass syringe filled with 2 mL of air and attached to the Touhy needle is used to signal entry into the pleural space, by emptying during inspiration in the spontaneously ventilating patient. In the mechanically ventilated patient, gentle pressure on the syringe will accomplish the same task. An epidural catheter can then be easily introduced into the intrapleural space. A dose of 0.3 mL/kg of local anesthetic agent is usually sufficient to produce unilateral analgesia for 4 to 8 h. (see Table 30-7.) The quality of the intrapleural block is significantly affected by body position. Standing or sitting can reduce its efficacy substantially. The Trendelenburg position results in Horner's syndrome. The placement of two catheters has been shown to improve the spread of local anesthetic, and hence improve analgesia.

3. Local anesthetic can also be injected directly into an existing **chest tube.** The proposed puncture site of the tube is cleaned with an antiseptic solution, and should be as proximal to the chest wall as possible. Local anesthetic can then be instilled through a 25-gauge needle introduced into the chest tube at an oblique angle. If the chest tube can be clamped distal to the injection site for 10 min, analgesia will be enhanced. Intrapleural administration of local anesthetic solutions is contraindicated when the pleural surfaces are inflamed. Systemic absorption of local anesthetics is enhanced by infection or inflammation, making toxic reactions common. When the pleural space is not infected, the systemic absorption of local agents resembles that of a lumbar epidural block.

4. Blockade of the **femoral nerve** is particularly useful in providing analgesia when there is a midshaft fracture of the femur, or to alleviate phantom limb pain. The femoral nerve is located lateral to the femoral artery at the inguinal ligament and can be easily blocked using the artery as a landmark. Local anesthetic agent is infiltrated lateral to and at the depth of the artery. A volume of 1 to 10 mL is sufficient to establish neural blockade. (See Table 30-7.)

5. In the neonatal nursery, circumcision is a common procedure. A well-performed **penile block** provides excellent local anesthesia and analgesia for even the smallest premature infant. Although dorsal nerve block is easily performed in the older child, there is a safer and equally effective approach for the premature and term newborn. A ring of local anesthetic injected at the base of the penis in the subcutaneous space avoids potential intravascular injection when attempting to locate the dorsal nerves that are superficial to the corpora cavernosa. Alternatively, the surgical site can be wrapped in local-anesthetic–impregnated dressings, taking care to limit the total dose of anesthetic.

CONCLUSIONS

A. Acute pain management in the critically ill or injured child is both a difficult and a pressing health care problem. Caretakers for these especially needy patients must be cognizant of their level of comfort at all stages of therapy.

B. This requires sensitivity and a knowledge base capable of guiding therapy. As stated previously, pain is frequently undertreated in the pediatric patient. With the myriad of choices of available analgesics, there should always be an option that is effective and safe.

CASE DISCUSSIONS

Case 1

In the first case, the patient is a critically injured trauma patient with painful injuries at multiple sites. In addition, he has just undergone an emergency surgical procedure which involved significant blood loss. Before formulating any plan for pain management, it is imperative that the patient's hemodynamic status be assessed and stabilized and a decision be made regarding the continuation of mechanical ventilation. If an invasive procedure is considered (i.e., an epidural), the patient's coagulation status must be examined. For this patient, the need for continued mechanical ventilation is likely because of the presence of a significant pulmonary contusion.

For this discussion, consider the patient's hemodynamic status as stable and his coagulation profile as entirely normal. The options for the management of this child's pain are several. A lumbar or thoracic epidural catheter could be placed, and epidural narcotics could be used. Morphine would be the preferred epidural agent for lumbar administration because of its wide distribution along the neuroaxis. Epidural narcotics would provide excellent analgesia with little sedation. It should be noted at this point that this child did not have a significant head injury. If he had, the placement of an epidural catheter, with its associated risk of dural puncture, could be contraindicated.

The other option for pain management in this patient is the use of parenteral narcotics. For maximum efficacy, using the lowest total dose of opioid, a continuous narcotic infusion with or without PCA as an option could be used. The advantage of this method of pain management is the ease of administration. It also provides analgesia for endotracheal and nasogastric tubes. The disadvantage is the likely occurrence of somnolence, and the potential of delayed return of intestinal motility.

Case 2

The patient in the second case is perhaps somewhat less straightforward. He is a preterm infant with at least two congenital malformations, an omphalocele and a ventricular septal defect. Before defining a plan for the management of this patient, it would be important to identify other congenital malformations that may be present. For this discussion, consider the infant to be normal otherwise. The need for the continuation of mechanical ventilation is clear because of the concomitant hyaline membrane disease, as well as the increased intra-abdominal pressure. If the ventricular septal defect is hemodynamically significant, it too will contribute to the ongoing need for the ventilator.

The best method for managing this patient's pain is with the cautious administration of parenteral opioids. The dosing schedule must take into account the prolonged elimination half-life of opioids in the preterm infant, as well as the further reduction in the clearance of opioids in the infant with increased intra-abdominal pressure. Recall that under these unique circumstances, opioid clearance can fall to zero. If the continuous infusion of narcotics is attempted, the time to recover spontaneous ventilation after discontinuation of the infusion will be prolonged. In anticipation of delayed drug elimination, a narcotic infusion should be stopped well in advance of attempting to wean him from mechanical ventilation. Intermittent narcotic administration may avoid this problem.

FINAL THOUGHTS

Although the problems encountered in the successful management of pain in children are substantial, so are the rewards. Children will be much more cooperative with therapy when they are made comfortable. Children should be allowed to participate in decision making, as their age permits. The child's hospital experience, and that of the family, will be significantly improved when attention to patient comfort measures is not treated in a secondary fashion.

The hesitancy to treat pain, based on either the fear of creating a child drug addict or the notion that treatment is unnecessary in the infant, should be relegated to historical perspective. Neither concern should, in any way, limit the access of the child to appropriate analgesia.

SUGGESTED READINGS

Anand KJS, Hickey PR: Pain and its effect in the human neonate and fetus. *N Engl J Med* 317:1321–1329, 1987.
Lloyd-Thomas AR: Pain management in pediatric patients. *Br J Anesth* 64:85–104, 1990.
McGrath PA: An assessment of children's pain: a review of behavioral, physiological and direct scaling techniques. *Pain* 31:147–176, 1987.
McGrath PJ, Craig KD: Developmental and psychological factors in children's pain. *Pediatr Clin North Am* 36:4, 823–838, 1989.
Yaster M, Maxwell LG: Pediatric regional anesthesia. *Anesthesiology* 70:324–338, 1989.

CHAPTER
31

THE CRITICALLY ILL OBSTETRIC PATIENT

Robert B. Lechner

Case
  I. Normal Pregnant Patient
     A. Physiologic Alterations
     B. Pharmacology
     C. Pain Pathways
 II. Management of Labor Pain
     A. Preoperative Asessment
     B. Treatment Modalities
III. Post–Cesarean Section Pain Management
     A. Subarachnoid technique
     B. Epidural technique
     C. Patient-controlled analgesia
     D. Side effects of neuroaxial opioids
IV. Management of the Critically Ill Pregnant Patient
     A. Pregnancy-Induced Hypertension (Preeclampsia)
     B. Infection
     C. Disseminated Intravascular Coagulation
     D. Cardiac Disease
     E. Neurologic Disease
     F. Blunt Trauma
     G. Surgical Trauma

Case Discussion
Suggested Readings
Appendix

CASE

An 18-year-old G_2P_1 with an intrauterine pregnancy at 28 weeks' gestation is an unrestrained passenger in a motor vehicle accident. She is taken to the operating room for treatment of her subdural hematoma and ruptured spleen, and postoperatively, she is admitted to the intensive care unit (ICU). Her injuries include mild closed-head injury, multiple rib fractures with possible pulmonary contusion, and pelvic and multiple lower extremity fractures. She is ventilated with settings: $FIO_2 = 1.0$, tidal volume = 900, rate = 8, positive end-expiratory pressure = 5 cmH$_2$O (arterial blood gases = pH 7.40, PCO_2 = 30 mmHg, PO_2 = 375 mmHg). Monitors include intracranial pressure (ICP) monitor (ICP = 8 mmHg), A-line (blood pressure = 100/72) mmHg, central venous pressure (CVP) monitor (CVP = 4 mmHg), tokodynamometer (10 contractions/h), and fetal heart rate monitor (fetal heart rate = 120 beats/min). You are consulted by her primary physicians to assist in the management of this patient's pain.

I. NORMAL PREGNANT PATIENT

A. Physiologic Alterations

1. Cardiovascular Cardiovascular consequences of pregnancy appear in the first trimester. Table 31-1 summarizes the changes occurring at term.

   a. During pregnancy, fatigue and systolic flow murmurs become common, but cardiology consultation is usually needed only for patients

Table 31-1 Changes in the cardiovascular system at term

Variable	Change
Blood volume	+35%
Plasma volume	+45%
Red cell volume	+20%
Cardiac output	+40%
Stroke volume	+30%
Heart rate	+15%
Systolic blood pressure	−0–15 mmHg
Diastolic blood pressure	−10–20 mmHg
Mean blood pressure	−15 mmHg
Central venous pressure	No change
Femoral venous pressure	+20 cmH$_2$O

with systolic murmurs greater than grade III, any diastolic murmur, severe arrhythmias, and overt signs of failure.

   b. The gravid uterus can compress the inferior vena cava when the patient assumes the supine position. This results in increased femoral venous pressure and decreased venous return to the heart, and a subsequent decrease in cardiac output. Therefore, **uterine displacement** (usually to the left) or a **semi-Fowler's position** should be maintained whenever possible.

   c. During labor, cardiac output increases 30 to 50 percent, and after delivery, it increases 80 percent over prelabor values.

   2. Pulmonary Respiratory changes also appear in the first trimester; their ultimate levels at term are summarized in Table 31-2.

   a. Elevated levels of progesterone are probably responsible for the **increased ventilatory drive** and result in a compensated respiratory alkalosis. During labor, minute ventilation can increase an additional 300 percent.

   b. Acute hyperventilation resulting in a $P{CO_2}$ of less than 30 torr can result in decreased uterine blood flow and fetal distress.

   c. Hyperbaric oxygen therapy to the pregnant patient can result in congenital abnormalities and retrolental fibroplasia. Administering supplemental oxygen (even 100 percent) for the treatment of maternal hypoxia should not be deleterious to the fetus; however, it is prudent to increase the $FI{O_2}$ only to a level that maintains maternal $P{O_2}$ in the normal range.

   3. Hematologic Changes in hematologic values for the term parturient are listed in Table 31-3. The increased levels of coagulation factors are thought to be responsible for the **hypercoagulable state of pregnancy.** Though prothrombin time (PT) and partial thromboplastin time (PTT) do not change with pregnancy, other assessments of coagulation (e.g., thromboelastography) do.

   4. Gastrointestinal Pregnancy results in increased gastric acid production, delayed gastric emptying, and decreased esophageal sphincter tone. These changes place the parturient at increased risk for reflux and aspiration.

Table 31-2 Changes in the respiratory system at term

Variable	Change
Minute ventilation	+50%
Alveolar ventilation	+70%
Oxygen consumption	+20%
Functional residual capacity	−20%
Arterial $P{O_2}$	+10 torr
Arterial pH	No change
Arterial $P{CO_2}$	−10 torr

Table 31-3 Changes in the hematologic systems at term

Variable	Change
Hemoglobin	−15%
Platelet count	−20%
Leukocyte count	0 to +100%
Factor I (fibrinogen)	+75%
Factor II (prothrombin)	+25%
Factor V	+50%
Factor VII	+100%
Factor VIII	+200%
Von Willebrand's factor	+250%
Factor X	+100%
PT	No change
PTT	No change

5. Hepatic Elevated liver function enzyme levels are often increased in the absence of hepatic insufficiency. At term, cholinesterase, total protein, and albumen-to-globulin ratios are decreased, and may result in a prolonged effect of succinylcholine and increased free drug fractions for drugs usually highly protein bound.

6. Renal By the fourth month of pregnancy, glomerular filtration rate and renal plasma flow increase by 50 to 60 percent with a concomitant decrease in blood urea nitrogen (BUN) and creatinine of 40 percent.

B. Pharmacology

Drugs administered to the pregnant patient will have variable effects on the fetus.

1. The factors mediating these effects include **toxicity of the drug**, its **ability to cross the placenta**, and **fetal metabolism.** Drugs which have low toxicity, are rapidly metabolized (by both parturient and fetus), are highly protein bound, have a high molecular weight, are ionized, and have low lipid solubility will have minimal effects on the fetus.

2. Normal **fetal pH** is lower than maternal, and decreases markedly with fetal stress. Drugs that are weak bases (e.g., local anesthetics) become more ionized at lower pH, and so diffuse across barriers (including the placenta) more slowly. This can result in higher levels of local anesthetics in fetal than in maternal blood **(ion trapping)** as un-ionized drugs cross into the fetal circulation, become ionized, and are unable to diffuse back to the maternal circulation.

3. Local anesthetics, analgesics, sedatives, drugs used to treat pain syndromes, and drugs commonly used in an ICU which affect the fetus are listed in Appendix 31-1.

C. Pain Pathways

1. During the **first stage of labor,** visceral stimuli from uterine contractions are transmitted via Aδ fibers accompanying sympathetic nerves and enter the neuroaxis at levels T10 to L1.
2. During the **second stage of labor,** pain also arises from somatic perineal stimulation, and is transmitted via the pudendal nerve and enters the neuroaxis at levels S2 to S4.

II. MANAGEMENT OF LABOR PAIN

A. Preoperative Assessment

The history and physical examination of the parturient do not significantly differ from those of any patient for whom a regional anesthetic technique is planned. In the parturient, however, fetal status should be assessed and documented prior to any intervention. In the low-risk parturient, the data from continuous electronic fetal monitoring have not been shown to alter fetal outcome; however, the use of such monitoring in the high-risk parturient is strongly recommended.

B. Treatment Modalities

1. **Psychoprophylaxis** Hypnosis, Lamaze techniques, and relaxation techniques can reduce, but not eliminate, the need for intravenous (IV) or regional analgesic techniques. These methods work best in the previously prepared parturient, and have no discernible negative effects on the fetus.
2. **Transcutaneous Electrical Nerve Stimulation (TENS)** units can be useful in the latent stage of labor to provide analgesia with a noninvasive, nonmedication modality, without preventing the onset of the active stage of labor. They can also be useful in providing additional analgesia to "hot spots" (see below). The stimulating electrodes are placed over the regions to which the pain is referred.
3. **Parenteral analgesics** Nonsteroidal antiinflammatory drugs (NSAIDs) should *not* be used during labor, and thus opioids are the most frequently used analgesic drugs. Common regimens include morphine 5 mg IV and 5 mg intramuscularly, fentanyl 25 to 50 μg IV, or butorphanol 2 mg

IV. Butorphanol has the advantage of self-limiting respiratory depression; however, it may produce excessive central nervous system side effects. Meperidine should not be used because prolonged fetal respiratory depression may result due to poor fetal metabolism and excretion of the parent drug and its metabolites.

4. Nitrous oxide is the only currently recommended inhalational analgesic. The Nitronox unit delivers 50 percent nitrous oxide in oxygen via a demand regulator and a tight-fitting face mask that the patient is directed to apply 30 s prior to contractions, and remove as the contraction intensity reduces. Theoretically, this delivery system will discontinue nitrous oxide if the patient loses consciousness, and the patient should awaken as she breathes room air. This treatment modality is most effective in patients who had planned to use psychological methods for childbirth, but request additional analgesia for the transition stage, and in those whose contractions are regular enough to minimize the effects of the 30 s delay between beginning nitrous oxide administration and achieving analgesia.

5. Intrathecal opioids Numerous opioids have been administered into the intrathecal space to provide analgesia. Use of a small needle (27-gauge Quincke, 25-gauge Whitacre, or 24-gauge Sprotte) is associated with an acceptably low post–dural puncture headache rate (0 to 3 percent). Due to their lipid solubility, fentanyl and sufentanil theoretically have the advantage of minimizing cephalad spread, and thus of minimizing respiratory depression. However, it may be preferable to use 0.25 to 0.3 mg of preservative-free morphine, delivered as a single dose, to provide adequate analgesia within 20 min and that lasts 6 to 12 h or until most parturients achieve 8- to 10-cm cervical dilation. At this time, either a pudendal block can be performed or epidural bupivacaine (0.0625% at 8 to 10 mL/h) can be started to provide analgesia for the second stage of labor. In contrast to continuous epidural analgesia with local anesthetics, frequent blood pressure determinations are not necessary until local anesthetic is given.

6. Continuous lumbar epidural analgesia

    a. Prior to placement of the epidural catheter, a 10 to 15 mL/kg bolus of non–dextrose-containing solution should be given, and the maternal blood pressure cuff and continuous electronic fetal monitors placed.

    b. Either the sitting position or lateral decubitus position can be used, since neither has been shown to be superior to the other in improving maternal comfort or fetal status or in reducing the incidence of epidural venous cannulation. Usually, the second or third lumbar interspace is used with the midline or paramedian approach. After the epidural space has been located, the administration of either saline or the test dose of local anesthetic will distend the space and reduce the incidence of venous cannulation when the catheter is inserted. Most commonly, 8 to 10 mL of 0.25% bupivacaine is used to establish a block, though lidocaine can also be used. Using 15 μg of epinephrine to test for intravascular cannulation is controversial, but its specificity and sensitivity are about 90 percent if administered after a contraction.

c. After establishing the block, adequate analgesia can be maintained either by administering intermittent "top up" doses of 8 to 10 mL of 0.25% bupivacaine as a bolus every 60 to 90 min, or by initiating a constant infusion. Commonly used infusion solutions and rates are listed in Table 31-4. Hot spots usually occur in the inguinal region, and may result from direct nerve compression by the descending fetus. Two percent lidocaine with 1:200,000 epinephrine can also be used; however, epinephrine's beta-adrenergic stimulation may result in prolonging labor to a greater degree. As labor enters the expulsive stage, a pudendal block can be performed (usually by the obstetrician) or a "sitting" dose of 1% to 2% plain lidocaine (5 to 10 mL) can be administered via the epidural catheter to provide adequate anesthesia.

d. When establishing a block or administering top-up or sitting doses, maternal and fetal vital signs should be recorded every 3 min seven times, and then twice at 5-min intervals. If a patient receives a constant infusion, then, in addition to the above regimen, vital signs should be determined every 15 to 20 min. The anesthesiologist should evaluate the patient every 60 to 90 min, record vital signs and assess block height, and increase or decrease the infusion as needed.

III. POST–CESAREAN SECTION PAIN MANAGEMENT

Both epidural and subarachnoid anesthetic techniques permit effective postoperative analgesia.

A. Subarachnoid Technique

If the cesarean section is done with a **subarachnoid technique,** 0.25 to 0.3 mg of preservative-free morphine can be mixed with 12.5 to 15 mg of hyperbaric

Table 31-4 Solutions for continuous epidural analgesia

Bupivacaine, %	Fentanyl, μg/mL	Rate, mL/h	Treatment for hot spots
0.0625	2	10–12	5–8 mL of 0.25% bupivacaine
0.125	1	6–8	50 μg of epidural fentanyl
0.125	0	10	50 μg of epidural fentanyl

bupivacaine and administered as a single solution (adding fentanyl to this solution is unnecessary, since the morphine will provide effective analgesia by the time the bupivacaine wears off). This provides excellent operative anesthesia and effective postoperative analgesia for 18 to 24 h.

B. Epidural Technique

If an epidural technique is used, 3.5 to 5 mg of preservative-free morphine can be administered after the fetus is delivered. This provides 18 to 20 h of effective analgesia.

C. Patient-Controlled Analgesia

The subarachnoid and epidural technique both provide pain control superior to that of IV patient-controlled analgesia (PCA), and do so with less narcotic usage (which minimizes the newborn narcotic dose in nursing mothers). Patient satisfaction, however, is equal with all three techniques.

D. Side Effects of Neuroaxial Opioids

Neuroaxial opioids are associated with numerous side effects, such as respiratory depression, urinary retention, pruritus, and the recurrence of herpetic lesions. These can be at least partially prevented by adding 0.8 mg of naloxone (Narcan) to each liter of the patient's maintenance IV fluids. The naloxone may slightly decrease the effectiveness and duration of neuroaxial analgesia, and, therefore, patients may benefit from a second dose of epidural morphine about 12 h after the first dose. At this time, the epidural catheter can be removed, since oral analgesics are usually adequate after the first 24 h postoperatively.

IV. MANAGEMENT OF THE CRITICALLY ILL PREGNANT PATIENT

A. Pregnancy-Induced Hypertension (Preeclampsia)

1. Pathophysiology Despite extensive research, the underlying cause of pregnancy-induced hypertension (PIH), or preeclampsia, remains unknown. The disease is characterized by progressive hypertension, proteinuria, and generalized edema. As the disease progresses, the renal (decreased creatinine clearance), hematologic (decreasing platelet number and function), cardiovascular (intravascular volume depletion, rising hemoglobin, and cardiac failure), hepatic (decreased clotting factors), respiratory (pharyngeal edema), and nervous (headaches, photophobia, visual field changes, intracerebral hemorrhage, and edema) systems can be affected. Variants of preeclampsia include eclampsia (seizures) and the HELLP (Hemolysis of red blood cells, Elevated Liver enzymes and Low Platelets) syndrome. The only "cure" for PIH is delivery of the fetus, after which symptoms usually resolve over the next 24 to 72 h. However, vigilance must be maintained because pulmonary edema and seizures can occur postpartum.

2. **Labor management**

   a. **Coagulopathies** produce the greatest concern when dealing with PIH. Both PT and PTT are usually normal, platelet function can be decreased even if the platelet count is normal, and bleeding time does not correlate well with the ability to maintain hemostasis. Thromboelastography may be the most effective method for determining coagulation status, but it is not always available, and so clinical signs (e.g., spontaneous hemorrhage from IV sites, nasal or oral mucosa) are the best guide for deciding whether to place an epidural catheter.

   b. If other treatment modalities are inadequate, **epidural analgesia** should be considered. If the patient has no clinical signs of coagulopathy, epidural catheters can usually be safely placed. If coagulopathy is present, the decision to place an epidural catheter must be made on an individual basis after the patient has been adequately informed of the possible risks (hematoma formation, with possible permanent paralysis) and benefits (analgesia and improved uterine blood flow).

   c. **Techniques** that decrease the incidence of intravascular cannulation and epidural hematomas should be utilized. These include placing the epidural catheter early before platelet count decreases, using a midline technique, using small needles and catheters, and distending the epidural space with saline prior to placing the catheter. Detection of epidural hematomas can be facilitated by placing the epidural catheter before the patient requires analgesia. This permits a period during which the patient can be observed for signs of hematoma formation (paresthesia and leg weakness). When analgesia is required, local anesthetic requirements (and, therefore, signs mimicking those of epidural hematoma) can be minimized by using epidural opioids.

   d. After placement of the epidural catheter, **epinephrine-containing solutions** should be avoided because of the hypertension that can result if they are administered IV. Fluid administration should be kept to a minimum to limit the risk of pulmonary edema. Epidural blocks should be initiated gradually, because patients with PIH tend to be intravascularly volume depleted and hypotension can be severe if large volumes of local anesthetics are rapidly given.

3. **Post–cesarean section pain management** Subarachnoid anesthesia is contraindicated in PIH because of the risks of hypotension mentioned above. However, epidural analgesia should be initiated slowly, using the above guidelines. Postoperative pain management is the same as for the parturient without PIH.

B. Infection

1. Pathophysiology Chorioamnionitis secondary to prolonged rupture of membranes is the most likely cause of serious infection in the laboring patient.

2. Anesthetic management If the patient has received appropriate antibiotics, and is not in shock, epidural analgesia can be safely initiated. Intrathecal techniques are not recommended because of the theoretical risk of inoculating the subarachnoid space with bacteria. If dural puncture occurs and the patient develops a post–dural puncture headache, placing an epidural blood patch is not recommended because of the risk that the contaminated blood will cause an epidural abscess. Furthermore, possible side effects of epidural blood patch (pain, backache, fever, and neck stiffness) can mask the signs of abscess formation and delay its diagnosis. In these patients, conservative management with analgesics, fluid administration, and caffeine is recommended.

C. Disseminated Intravascular Coagulation

1. Pathophysiology In addition to the causes of disseminated intravascular coagulation (DIC) discussed in Chapter 22, the pregnant patient can develop DIC from placental abruption, intrauterine fetal demise, amniotic fluid embolus, saline abortion, and PIH. As with other cases of DIC, the most important aspect of treatment consists of removing the underlying cause, which, for the pregnant patient, means rapid removal of the uterine contents.

2. Anesthetic management Regional analgesia is not recommended for the patient with DIC. If the patient is stable enough that vaginal delivery is attempted, parenteral narcotics are recommended. When maternal well-being is threatened, operative delivery is usually done with general anesthesia, and postoperative pain is managed with PCA. In the postpartum patient, pain control is less complete with PCA than with neuroaxial opioids; however, the added psychological benefit of controlling one's own medication results in the same degree of patient satisfaction with PCA as with neuroaxial opioids.

D. Cardiac Disease

1. Cardiac failure

a. Pathophysiology Causes of primary heart failure include PIH, viral infections, cardiomyopathy of pregnancy, and preexisting cardiac disease.

b. Anesthetic management Afterload reduction is beneficial, and thus regional techniques for labor are recommended. If a patient is in failure, monitoring with arterial and pulmonary arterial catheters prior to slowly initiating epidural blockade will facilitate fluid management. Tachycardia (resulting from painful stimuli) and Valsalva maneuvers can exacerbate the failure; therefore, epidural analgesia should be initiated as early as possible, and the patient should not push during the second stage of labor. Labor progresses with uterine contractions alone until forceps or vacuum extraction can be accomplished. Anesthesia for the expulsive phase can be accomplished with a saddle block using 25 to 50 mg of hyperbaric lidocaine. The legs should be wrapped to maintain venous return from the lower extremities. Caudal anesthesia with 2% plain lidocaine is an alternative. Caudal anesthesia, however, has a higher failure rate and risks perforation of the sacral plate, which can result in potentially devastating consequences due to intrauterine or direct neonatal administration of local anesthetic.

2. **Aortic stenosis**

   a. Pathophysiology Rheumatic heart disease is the primary etiology. Aortic stenosis results in fixed cardiac output and left ventricular hypertrophy. Tachycardia is poorly tolerated. If afterload is reduced, systemic pressure can fall and result in coronary ischemia and reduced cardiac output, which worsens ischemia and contributes to a catastrophic positive feedback loop.

   b. Anesthetic management Because of the dangers of afterload reduction, regional techniques have not been recommended; however, with careful monitoring (arterial and pulmonary arterial catheters) and slow implementation of blockade, epidural analgesia for labor can be accomplished safely. As with cardiomyopathies, Valsalva maneuvers are poorly tolerated, and anesthetic techniques similar to those listed above for cardiac failure can be used. As oxytocin causes decreased peripheral vascular resistance, if it is administered after delivery, this should be done in small, divided doses.

3. **Mitral stenosis**

   a. Pathophysiology Rheumatic fever is the primary etiology. Mitral stenosis results in underloading of the left ventricle, and eventually can lead to pulmonary hypertension and right ventricular failure. Tachycardia, increased central blood volumes, and reduced afterload are poorly tolerated.

   b. Anesthetic management The principles used in the treatment of aortic stenosis can be applied to the pain management of the patient with mitral stenosis.

4. **Eisenmenger's syndrome**

   a. Pathophysiology Eisenmenger's syndrome consists of pulmonary hypertension and bidirectional or right-to-left shunt with peripheral cyanosis. Decreases in systemic vascular resistance or venous return or increases in pulmonary vascular resistance are poorly tolerated.

b. Anesthetic management Although regional techniques can be used to control labor pain, monitoring with arterial and central venous catheters should be accomplished prior to the slow initiation of epidural analgesia. The application of Ace wraps to the lower extremities as the block is initiated can help preserve venous return. Oxytocin causes decreased peripheral vascular resistance. Therefore, if it is administered after delivery, this should be done in small, divided doses.

E. Neurologic Disease

1. Closed-head injury Pregnant patients who develop closed-head injuries can often maintain their pregnancies and deliver at term. Except for the most profoundly injured patients, analgesia may be required for the pain associated with labor and delivery. If the patient is neurologically stable and has normal ICP, epidural analgesia can be established in the usual manner once the patient begins to respond to contractions. Labor is permitted to continue until the uterus has brought the fetus to a station where forceps or vacuum extraction can be performed, at which time surgical anesthesia with 2% lidocaine is established.

2. Spinal cord lesion Pregnant patients with spinal cord lesions above T8 can develop autonomic hyperreflexia as they enter labor. The hemodynamic fluctuations can be controlled effectively with either epidural or spinal anesthesia. If epidural anesthesia is chosen, a continuous infusion technique with 0.125% bupivacaine is recommended, but if hemodynamic fluctuations continue, higher concentrations can be used. Additional doses for instrumental deliveries are usually not needed.

3. Aneurysm and arteriovenous malformation Pregnant patients with intracerebral vascular lesions are at increased risk for hemorrhage, especially if they perform a Valsalva maneuver during the second stage of labor. To minimize this risk, epidural analgesia is established during the first stage of labor, and surgical anesthesia is established once the patient feels the urge to push. Labor continues, with the uterus providing the force necessary to bring the fetus to a station where instrumental delivery can be accomplished.

F. Blunt Trauma

The pain management of victims of blunt trauma is discussed in detail in Chapter 23. With few exceptions, the principles discussed in that chapter can be applied to the pregnant patient.

1. Since two patients are involved, **monitoring of fetal status** (fetal heart rate and uterine activity) is recommended. As with all obstetric patients, the **supine position should be avoided** whenever possible because the gravid uterus can compress the aorta and vena cava, with resulting decreases in venous return, cardiac output, and uterine perfusion. The deleterious effects of the supine position are more pronounced in the presence of hypovolemia.

2. When administering a field block or other regional technique to a pregnant patient, the monitoring guidelines described for continuous lumbar epidural analgesia in labor pain management should be adhered to. Pain control using field blocks or other regional techniques (provided hypotension is avoided) is preferable to high-dose narcotics, since the former limits fetal exposure to potentially damaging drugs. Appendix 31-1 can be used as a guide when choosing other analgesics, sedatives, and drugs used in the treatment of pain syndromes. Since the fetus does not tolerate hypoxia, **maternal oxygen saturation should be monitored and supplemental oxygen administered as needed.** As discussed above, supplemental oxygen provided to the mother does not place the fetus at increased risk for retrolental fibroplasia.

G. Surgical Trauma

1. After nonobstetric surgical procedures, **monitoring of fetal status** (fetal heart rate and uterine activity) is recommended. This is especially true for lower abdominal procedures, since these are more associated with the onset of **premature labor** than are surgeries in other regions.

2. Since stress may induce premature labor, postoperative stress (including pain) should be minimized. This can be best achieved with **field blocks or other regional techniques.** Infiltration of surgical incisions with .25% bupivacaine (with epinephrine when appropriate) at the conclusion of surgery helps to prevent the development of pain for 6 to 8 h. Continuous epidural (lumbar or thoracic) infusions of dilute bupivacaine solutions can help to maintain the pain-free state for most surgical sites. Though rarely necessary, continuous or intermittent administration of bupivacaine into the axillary sheath can be used to treat severe upper extremity pain.

3. Anesthetic management for these patients is the same as for patients with blunt trauma.

CASE DISCUSSION

The critically ill obstetric patient presents unique problems to the pain management team. These challenges result from two main factors: the physiologic alterations that occur with pregnancy, and the fact that there are two patients (mother and fetus) who can be affected by treatment modalities. When possible, treatments that decrease uterine perfusion or uterine oxygen delivery, or expose the fetus to potentially dangerous drugs, should be avoided.

In the case presented, attention should first be directed to the mother's hemodynamic and pulmonary status, and then to her pain management. To prevent a decrease in uterine blood flow, the supine position should be avoided and systolic arterial pressure should be maintained above 100 mmHg with volume expansion or inotropic agents, and vasoconstrictors should be avoided if at all possible. Oxygen delivery to the uterus can be achieved by keeping the Pao_2 above 100 mmHg. Hyperoxia is neither advantageous nor detrimental. Hemoglobin should be maintained at between 8 and 10 g/dL. Maintaining mixed venous oxygen in the normal range can help ensure adequate oxygen delivery to the fetus.

Adequate hemodynamic function must be given first priority, though pain management cannot be ignored. Pain and stress can be detrimental to uterine blood flow and can provoke premature labor. Adequate analgesia minimizes the risk of either of these problems occurring. Parenteral narcotics can be effective in maintaining adequate pain control. In this patient, however, their use may result in delayed weaning from the ventilator, hypercarbia and hypoxia postextubation from decreased respiratory drive, or withdrawal symptoms in the neonate if labor cannot be prevented.

If no coagulopathy is present, a continuous epidural infusion of bupivacaine with 1 μg/mL of fentanyl would be the preferred method for controlling the pain from her splenectomy and orthopedic injuries. The low concentration of fentanyl is unlikely to have any deleterious effect on the fetus or neonate, and can permit the use of lower concentrations of local anesthetic, and, therefore, minimize deleterious hemodynamic effects. A lumbar epidural catheter has the advantage of being technically easy and safe to place, and would be effective in controlling labor and delivery pain if tocolysis was ineffective. However, a thoracic epidural catheter has the advantage of more effective control of the pain from rib fractures and splenectomy.

SUGGESTED READINGS

Briggs GG, Freeman RK, Yaffe JJ: *Drugs in Pregnancy and Lactation.* Baltimore, Williams & Wilkins, 1990.
Shnider SM, Levinson G: *Anesthesia for Obstetrics.* Baltimore, Williams & Wilkins, 1993.

APPENDIX 31-1 PHARMACOLOGY OF DRUGS IN PREGNANCY

The risk factors (A, B, C, D, and X) are assigned for each drug based on criteria used by the Food and Drug Administration. If the manufacturer has assigned a category, a subscript M appears (e.g., A_M), otherwise the risk factors assigned in *Drugs in Pregnancy and Lactation* are used. The definitions of the risk factors are as follows:
A: Studies in women failed to demonstrate risk to fetus in first trimester, and no evidence for risk in later trimesters exists.
B: Either animal studies failed to show risk to fetus and there are no human studies, or animal studies indicated risk during the first trimester, but this was not confirmed by human studies. No evidence for risk in later trimesters exists.
C: No human studies exist; however, animal studies may have found teratogenic or embryocidal effects. Drugs should only be used if benefits outweigh potential risks.
D: Evidence for human fetal risk exists; drugs should be used only for life-threatening conditions or if safer drugs are ineffective.
X: Drugs cause fetal abnormalities and are contraindicated in pregnant women.

Acetaminophen (Tylenol)   Class: **Analgesic/antipyretic**   Risk factor **B**
At therapeutic doses in first trimester, prior to delivery, or during breastfeeding, there is no apparent risk to fetus.

Alphaprodine   Class: **Narcotic analgesic**   Risk factor C_M
(Risk factor **D** if used in high doses or for prolonged periods.)
Risks include respiratory depression of newborn, and high incidence of sinusoidal fetal heart rate pattern if given during labor.

Amobarbital   Class: **Sedative/hypnotic**   Risk factor **D**
High risk of neurologic, cardiovascular, or skeletal abnormalities.

Aspirin   Class: **Analgesic/antipyretic**   Risk factor **C**
(Risk factor **D** if used in high doses in third trimester.)
Effects include risk of increased postpartum hemorrhage and prolonged or delayed labor due to prostaglandin synthesis inhibition. Chronic usage or high doses are associated with increased risk of stillbirth, intrauterine growth retardation, and teratogenic effects. Low doses (40 to 150 mg/day) are probably safe.

Bupivacaine (Marcaine)   Class: **Local anesthetic**   Risk factor **B**
Several cases of cardiac arrest after use of 0.75% bupivacaine (but not 0.5%) have been reported. Pregnancy increases susceptibility to cardiac toxicity of bupivacaine more than other local anesthetics. Currently most commonly used drug for management of labor pain.

Butorphanol (Stadol)   Class: **Analgesic**   Risk factor **B**
(Risk factor **D** if used in high doses or for prolonged periods.)
Increased risk of sinusoidal fetal heart rate pattern if given during labor.

Carbamazepine (Tegretol)   Class: **Anticonvulsant**   Risk factor C_M
Possible teratogenic effects, but probably fewer than those seen with phenytoin.

Chloral hydrate   Class: **Sedative/hypnotic**   Risk factor C_M
No known teratogenic effects.

Chlordiazepoxide (Librium)   Class: **Sedative**   Risk factor **D**
Use is associated with a fourfold increase in the incidence of severe congenital abnormalities, including neurologic, cardiovascular, and gastrointestinal systems.

Chloroprocaine (Nesacaine)   Class: **Local anesthetic**   Risk factor **A**
Very safe drug due to rapid intravascular metabolism. Chloroprocaine is currently formulated with EDTA, which serves as an antioxidant and may cause severe maternal back spasm.

Chlorpromazine (Thorazine)   Class: **Tranquilizer**   Risk factor **C**
Use is associated with maternal hypotension during labor, and extrapyramidal effects in the newborn.

Clomipramine (Anafranil)   Class: **Antidepressant**   Risk factor **D**
Use is associated with risk of lethargy, hypotonia, cyanosis, hypothermia, respiratory acidosis, and convulsions in newborn.

Codeine   Class: **Narcotic analgesic**   Risk factor **C**
(Risk factor **D** if used in high doses or for prolonged periods.)
Increased risk of cardiovascular, gastrointestinal, or respiratory malformations and respiratory depression at birth.

Desipramine (Norpramin)   Class: **Antidepressant**   Risk factor **C**
Use is associated with neonatal withdrawal manifested as tachycardia, cyanosis, and diaphoresis.

Diazepam (Valium)   Class: **Sedative**   Risk factor **D**
Use of diazepam during the first or second trimester is associated with increased incidence of

cleft lip and/or palate in the fetus. During labor, diazepam can cause hypotonia, lethargy, loss of sucking reflex, and beat-to-beat variability.

Diphenhydramine (Benadryl)   Class: **Antihistamine/antipruritic**   Risk factor **C**
Anecdotal reports have linked diphenhydramine and congenital malformations; however, prospective studies have failed to confirm the association.

Doxepin (Adapin)   Class: **Antidepressant**   Risk factor **C**
Use is associated with neonatal withdrawal symptoms, but not congenital malformations.

Droperidol (Inapsin)   Class: **Tranquilizer/antiemetic**   Risk factor C_M
Prospective studies failed to show an association between droperidol and congenital malformations.

Fenoprofen (Nalfon)   Class: **NSAID**   Risk factor **B**
(Risk factor **D** if used in third trimester or near delivery.)
See ibuprofen.

Fentanyl (Sublimaze)   Class: **Narcotic analgesic**   Risk factor **B**
(Risk factor **D** if used in high doses or for prolonged periods.)
Prospective studies failed to show an association between fentanyl and congenital malformations. Maternal doses of 1 μg/kg have no discernible fetal effects. Higher doses may cause respiratory depression. Prolonged maternal use may result in neonatal withdrawal.

Hydroxyzine (Atarax, Vistaril)   Class: **Tranquilizer**   Risk factor X_M
Prospective studies failed to show an association between hydroxyzine and congenital malformations; however, the manufacturer considers its use contraindicated in the first trimester. Hydroxyzine is probably safe during the last two trimesters.

Ibuprofen   Class: **NSAID**   Risk factor **B**
(Risk factor **D** if used in third trimester or near delivery.)
NSAIDs theoretically may cause closure of the ductus arteriosus *in utero,* and are known to inhibit or prolong labor.

Imipramine (Tofranil)   Class: **Antidepressant**   Risk factor **D**
Anecdotal reports have linked imipramine and congenital malformations; however, prospective studies have failed to confirm the association. Prolonged use can lead to fetal withdrawal *ex utero.*

Indomethacin (Indocin)   Class: **NSAID**   Risk factor **B**
(Risk factor **D** if used after 34 weeks' gestation, for more than 48 h or near delivery.)
Indomethacin may cause closure of the ductus arteriosus *in utero,* with resulting pulmonary hypertension, and is a tocolytic drug.

Ketamine (Ketalar)   Class: **IV analgesic/anesthetic**   Risk factor **B**
Teratogenic in animals. Maternal doses of >2mg/kg during delivery can cause neonatal depression and reduced Apgar scores. Doses of 0.2 to 1.0 mg/kg are considered safe.

Ketorolac (Toradol)   Class: **NSAID**   Risk factor **B**
(Risk factor **D** if used after 34 weeks' gestation, for more than 48 h or near delivery.)
Ketorolac may cause closure of the ductus arteriosus *in utero,* with resulting pulmonary hypertension, and is a tocolytic drug.

Lidocaine (Xylocaine)   Class: **Local anesthetic**   Risk factor **C**
Prospective studies have failed to show an association between lidocaine and congenital malformations. One study linked lidocaine to decreased newborn muscle tone; however, four other studies failed to confirm these findings.

Lorazepam (Ativan)   Class: **Sedative**   Risk factor D_M
No association between lorazepam and cleft lip and/or palate has been reported. Lorazepam may result in the floppy-baby syndrome.

Meclofenamate (Meclomen)   Class: **NSAID**   Risk factor **B**
(Risk factor **D** if used in third trimester or near delivery.)
NSAIDs theoretically may cause closure of the ductus arteriosus *in utero,* and are known to inhibit or prolong labor.

Meperidine (Demerol)   Class: **Narcotic analgesic**   Risk factor **B**
(Risk factor **D** if used in high doses or for prolonged periods.)
Prospective studies failed to show an association between meperidine and congenital malformations. After maternal administration, neonatal respiratory depression is prolonged due to poor neonatal metabolism of meperidine. Prolonged maternal use may result in neonatal withdrawal.

Meprobamate (Miltown, Equanil)   Class: **Sedative**   Risk factor **D**
Numerous reports have linked meprobamate with cardiac, ophthalmologic, and neurologic malformations; however, a large prospective study failed to confirm this association.

Methadone (Dolophine)   Class: **Narcotic Analgesic**   Risk factor **B**
(Risk factor **D** if used in high doses or for prolonged periods.)
Prospective studies failed to show an association between methadone and congenital malformations. Prolonged maternal use results in neonatal withdrawal, increased incidence of sudden infant death syndrome, jaundice, and thrombocytosis.

Metoclopramide (Reglan)   Class: **Antiemetic**   Risk factor B_M
No association between metoclopramide and congenital anomalies has been reported.

Morphine   Class: **Narcotic analgesic**   Risk factor **B**
(Risk factor **D** if used in high doses or for prolonged periods.)
Prospective studies failed to show an association between morphine and congenital malformations. Maternal use results in neonatal respiratory depression (acute usage) or withdrawal (chronic usage).

Nalbuphine   Class: **Narcotic agonist–antagonist**   Risk factor **B**
(Risk factor **D** if used in high doses or for prolonged periods.)
Prospective studies failed to show an association between nalbuphine and congenital malformations. Maternal use can result in neonatal respiratory depression (acute usage) or withdrawal (chronic usage).

Nalorphine   Class: **Narcotic antagonist**   Risk factor **D**
Nalorphine use can cause neonatal respiratory depression. Naloxone is recommended to reverse acute opioid effects.

Naloxone (Narcan)   Class: **Narcotic antagonist**   Risk factor B_M
Naloxone may result in fetal asphyxia if administered maternally in the absence of maternal opioid toxicity immediately prior to delivery.

Naproxen (Naprosyn)   Class: **NSAID**   Risk factor B_M
(Risk factor **D** if used in third trimester or near delivery.)
NSAIDs theoretically may cause closure of the ductus arteriosus *in utero,* and are known to inhibit or prolong labor.

Nortriptyline (Pamelor)   Class: **Antidepressant**   Risk factor **D**
Anecdotal reports have linked nortriptyline and congenital malformations; however, prospective studies have failed to confirm the association.

Oxycodone (Percodan, Percocet)   Class: **Narcotic analgesic**   Risk factor **B**
(Risk factor **D** if used in high doses or for prolonged periods.)
Prospective studies failed to show an association between oxycodone and congenital malformations.

Oxymorphone (Numorphan)   Class: **Narcotic analgesic**   Risk factor **B**
(Risk factor **D** if used in high doses or for prolonged periods.)
Prospective studies failed to show an association between oxymorphone and congenital malformations. Maternal use results in neonatal respiratory depression (acute usage) or withdrawal (chronic usage).

Oxyphenbutazone   Class: **NSAID**   Risk factor **D**
Anecdotal reports have linked oxyphenbutazone and phenylbutazone with congenital malformations, and embryotoxicity has been demonstrated in animals. Its use in pregnancy is not recommended.

Pentazocine (Talwin)   Class: **Analgesic**   Risk factor **B**
(Risk factor **D** if used in high doses or for prolonged periods.)
Prospective studies failed to show an association between pentazocine and congenital malformations. Maternal use results in neonatal respiratory depression (acute usage) or withdrawal (chronic usage).

Pentobarbital (Nembutal)   Class: **Sedative/hypnotic**   Risk factor B_M
Prospective study failed to associate pentobarbital with congenital anomalies. Neonatal withdrawal can occur after chronic use, and pentobarbital may cause hemorrhagic disorders in the neonate.

Phenobarbital   Class: **Sedative/anticonvulsant**   Risk factor **D**
Use of phenobarbital is weakly associated with minor congenital anomalies; however, when combined with other anticonvulsant medicines, a two- to threefold increase in the rate of congenital anomalies is seen. Phenobarbital may cause folate deficiency during pregnancy and hemorrhagic disorders in the neonate. Neonatal withdrawal can occur after chronic use.

Phenylbutazone (Butazolidin)   Class: **NSAID**   Risk factor **D**
Anecdotal reports have linked phenylbutazone and oxyphenbutazone with congenital malformations, and embryotoxicity has been demonstrated in animals. Its use in pregnancy is not recommended.

Phenytoin (Dilantin)   Class: **Anticonvulsant**   Risk factor **D**
Phenytoin usage is associated with multiple skeletal and craniofacial abnormalities, and is also possibly carcinogenic to the fetus. Phenytoin may cause folate deficiency during pregnancy, and hemorrhagic disorders in the neonate.

Ropivacaine   Class: **Local anesthetic**   Risk factor **C**
Ropivacaine is structurally similar to bupivacaine, and preliminary data suggest it has less cardiac toxicity and a favorable potency-to-toxicity ratio. Data concerning risk factors are not currently available; however, they are expected to be the same as for bupivacaine.

Scopolamine   Class: **Antiemetic**   Risk factor **C**
No association between scopolamine and congenital anomalies has been reported.

Secobarbital (Seconal)   Class: **Sedative/hypnotic**   Risk factor D_M
No association between secobarbital and congenital anomalies has been reported. Neonatal withdrawal and hemorrhagic disorders can occur after chronic use.

Sulindac (Clinoril)   Class: **NSAID**   Risk factor B_M
(Risk factor **D** if used in third trimester or near delivery.)

No association between sulindac and congenital anomalies has been reported. NSAIDs theoretically may cause closure of the ductus arteriosus *in utero,* and are known to inhibit or prolong labor.

Tolmetin (Tolectin)   Class: **NSAID**   Risk factor B_M
(Risk factor **D** if used in third trimester or near delivery.)
No association between tolmetin and congenital anomalies has been reported. NSAIDs theoretically may cause closure of the ductus arteriosus *in utero,* and are known to inhibit or prolong labor.

Valproic acid (Depakene)   Class: **Anticonvulsant**   Risk factor **D**
Valproic acid usage is associated with multiple neural tube, cardiac, hepatotoxic, and craniofacial abnormalities. Valproic acid may cause hemorrhagic disorders in the neonate.

CHAPTER
32

CONCOMITANT CHRONIC PAIN SYNDROMES

John C. Rowlingson
Robin J. Hamill

I. Goals of Chronic Pain Management
II. Sympathetic Mediated Pain Syndromes
   A. Syndromes
   B. Etiology
   C. Diagnosis
   D. Treatment
III. Neuralgic Pain
   A. Etiology
   B. Pathophysiology
   C. Diagnosis
   D. Treatment
IV. Phantom Limb and Stump Pain
   A. Phantom Limb Pain
   B. Stump Pain
V. Low Back Pain
   A. Etiology
   B. Diagnosis
   C. Treatment
VI. Arthritis
   A. Prevalent Disease
   B. Manifestations
   C. Osteoarthritis
   D. Rheumatoid Arthritis

    VII. Myofascial pain
        A. Nomenclature
        B. Etiology
        C. Diagnosis
        D. Treatment
    VIII. Cancer Pain
        A. Special Concerns
        B. Acute and Chronic Features
        C. Treatment
Suggested Readings

I. GOALS OF CHRONIC PAIN MANAGEMENT

A. The elimination of pain is usually an achievable goal in the management of acute pain. This same expectation may not be realistic in many chronic pain conditions because of the multiplicity of etiologic factors contributing to the pain. The term chronic implies that some of the discomfort will persist in spite of therapy and the passage of time.

B. The reasonable goals of chronic pain management are:

1. to decrease the chronic pain as much as possible,
2. to help the patient cope with the pain that cannot be taken away so easily,
3. to increase the patient's ability to function, and
4. to encourage the patient to regain as productive a lifestyle as is possible, and yet is realistically compatible with the residual amount of pain.

II. SYMPATHETIC MEDIATED PAIN SYNDROMES

A. Syndromes

There are **multiple names** given to what are now called sympathetic mediated pain (SMP) syndromes. **The two most common are reflex sympathetic dystrophy (RSD) and causalgia.**

1. The former term, RSD, is a "descriptive term referring to a complex group of disorders that may develop as a consequence of trauma affecting limbs, with or without obvious nerve lesion. RSD may also develop after visceral diseases or CNS [central nervous system] lesions or, rarely, without an antecedent event. It consists of pain and related sensory abnormalities, abnormal blood flow and sweating, abnormalities in the motor system, and changes in the structure of both superficial and deep tissues ('trophic changes'). It is not necessary that all components be present" (Consensus Statement on RSD, Sixth World Congress on Pain, 1990).

2. Causalgia is an RSD-like syndrome that is caused by direct injury to major nerves. These patients will have neurologic deficits upon examination, as well as the stigmata of RSD.

3. Shoulder–hand syndrome occurs when RSD pain in the upper extremity causes inhibition of movement such that the patient develops a frozen shoulder. This may occur after myocardial infarction, cerebrovascular accident, cervical radiculopathy, or trauma.

4. Sympathetic motor paresis, or the **movement disorder of RSD,** includes such symptoms as spasms, weakness, tremors, increased tone and reflexes in the involved extremity, focal dystonia, and difficulty in initiating movement. These signs may precede the development of pain and/or the autonomic manifestations of RSD by weeks or months.

5. When associated with CNS damage, RSD is called **mimocausalgia.**

6. Sudeck's atrophy is the subepiphyseal bone atrophy seen with SMP syndromes.

7. Algoneurodystrophy refers to RSD symptoms after minor trauma.

B. Etiology

The **etiology** of SMP syndromes is unclear, but a sensitization of peripheral receptors, and perhaps the nerves to the dorsal horn, appears plausible. See Chapter 3 for a more complete presentation.

C. Diagnosis

The **diagnosis** of SMP is based primarily on clinical findings.

1. Historically, there may be evidence of a traumatic event. This is always true in causalgia, but not so in all cases of RSD.

2. The **physical examination** may be unremarkable (Table 32-1 lists the classic finding)

　　a. The **acute or denervation phase** presents as if the patient has a sympathectomy.

　　b. The **dystrophic or hypersensitivity phase** presents with the classic picture of intense vasoconstriction and reduced blood flow in the affected body region.

　　c. The **atrophic phase** is characterized by detrimental changes that limit the patient's use of the affected body region.

3. Diagnostic tests may contribute to the evaluation once the syndrome is suspected. Radiographs reveal subperiosteal bone resorption. Technetium bone scans reveal increased periarticular uptake in the involved extremity. These findings are nonspecific and reflect only the condition of increased bony turnover.

4. Diagnostic sympathetic blocks with local anesthetics are frequently done to confirm the clinical impression of an SMP syndrome.

Table 32-1 Causalgia and RSD—symptoms and physical findings

Acute phase changes
 Hyperpathia and burning pain, increased blood flow, rubor
 Increased temperature, increased hair/nail growth
 Decreased sweating, soft edema

Dystrophic phase changes
 Hyperpathia and burning pain, decreased blood flow, cyanosis
 Decreased temperature, decreased hair/nail growth
 Increased sweating, brawny edema
 Decreased range of motion of the joints

Atrophic phase changes
 Less hyperpathia and burning pain, more normal blood flow and skin color
 Less temperature change and difference in hair/nail growth, though a difference persists
 Less sweating difference, and some edema remains
 Marked if not irreversible structural changes in the form of tight, thin skin; wasted muscles; osteoporosis; pericapsular fibrosis; and marked limitation of function of the affected extremity

D. Treatment

1. The treatment of the cause of SMP does not constitute its management.

2. One of the primary treatments for SMP is **physical therapy.** There is some suggestion that immobilization after trauma predisposes to the onset of RSD symptoms. **Disuse atrophy** and **pericapsular fibrosis** are also end points for many patients with SMP. Activity is therapeutic and improves blood flow, normalizes the neuronal input into the CNS, and prevents further dysfunction.

3. Injections into the appropriate sympathetic ganglion can be diagnostic, as well as therapeutic. The choice of block is tailored to the patient's physical status, the severity and duration of the syndrome, and the ease of access to medical care. These procedures require an anesthesiologist because of the potential adverse complications (see Chapter 13). The blocks are routinely done with local anesthetic drugs, and selected blocks can be repeated with neurolytic drugs, such as alcohol or phenol, when chemical sympathectomy of long duration is warranted by the patient's clinical response to local anesthetics.

  a. Cervicothoracic block (stellate ganglion) is indicated for SMP symptoms above T8.

  b. Thoracic ganglion block provides sympathectomy of the chest wall and parietal pleura.

  c. Celiac plexus block interrupts afferent input from the abdominal viscera.

  d. Lumbar sympathetic block provides sympathectomy of the ipsilateral lower extremity.

e. **Hypogastric plexus block** denervates the pelvic viscera.

f. **Bier (intravenous regional) block** employs 0.5% lidocaine for sympathectomy and analgesia, heparin to prevent thrombosis, and a sympatholytic drug such as bretylium (1 to 2 mg/kg) or guanethidine (10 to 20 mg) to reduce receptor sensitization. Other agents that have been added include solumedrol 80 mg, ketorolac, and fentanyl.

g. **Peridural blocks** with local anesthetics with or without narcotics can be administered as a single injection or as an infusion. Because of the possible somatic block, epidural or spinal blocks may be of less diagnostic benefit than sympathetic block techniques. Infusion techniques for inpatients can provide continuous sympathectomy, and subsequently allow intensive occupational therapy/physical therapy (OT/PT).

h. **Brachial plexus blocks** can provide sympathectomy to the upper extremity, and can be done via a catheter for continuous effect.

i. **Interpleural local anesthetics** can block sympathetic nerves to the thorax, head, and neck. This technique is a reasonable alternative for patients who are not candidates for other regional sympathetic procedures.

j. **Peripheral nerve blocks** can provide a degree of sympathetic block, as there are sympathetic nerve fibers that travel for variable distances with the somatic nerves. In general, the more distally the block is done, the lower is the likelihood of providing a significant sympathectomy.

4. Many **medications** have been used in the treatment of SMP syndromes. These include low-dose antidepressants (see Chapter 11), nonsteroidal anti-inflammatory drugs (NSAIDs), nifedipine (10 mg tid), clonidine (per os or transdermal patch), calcitonin (per os or intranasal), phenoxybenzamine (up to 40 mg qid), topical nitrates, beta-adrenergic blocking drugs, and pulse steroids (oral).

5. Other modalities include transcutaneous electrical nerve stimulation (**TENS**) over vascular channels to the affected extremity and **alternating hot and cold baths. Self-regulation techniques** such as hypnosis and biofeedback can decrease the stress related to the pain, permit the patient's control of regional blood flow, and facilitate the management of the emotional impact of a traumatic event.

6. **Surgical intervention** is usually reserved for patients who have failed to achieve long-lasting relief from conservative therapy, but who have shown significant short-term relief on multiple occasions. The patient may have an open sympathectomy procedure or, more recently, a fiberoptic scope approach, such as a thoracoscopic ganglionectomy. These procedures offer a substantial advantage over neurolytic injections because they are performed under direct vision and minimize the potential for damage to nontargeted tissue. The short-term results tend to be very good, but, unfortunately, there appears to be a high recidivism rate, with recurrence of some symptoms 3 to 6 months after the procedure.

III. NEURALGIC PAIN

A. Etiology

These pain syndromes are the result of trauma to the nervous system from any of the following:

1. **Mechanical damage,** as by entrapment of a nerve or ischemia.
2. **Toxic damage,** as with lead or arsenic poisoning.
3. **Metabolic disarray,** as with diabetes, alcoholism, or malnutrition.
4. **Inflammatory disease,** as with postherpetic neuralgia.

B. Pathophysiology

Much of the **nervous system function** is inhibitory. This regulation becomes **disrupted** after injury, as does the delicate balance of facilitation and inhibition, because the above-mentioned pathologic processes result in scarring in the nervous system. This scar tissue interferes with the normal transmission of neural input such that neuralgic pain is often described as being spontaneous, paroxysmal, hyperpathic (increased reaction to a stimulus), hyperalgesic (enhanced response to a stimulus which is normally painful), and allodynic (pain from a stimulus that is usually not painful).

C. Diagnosis

1. History taking will often reveal a gradual onset of **pain of two types.** There is commonly a **dull, aching component** that is there all the time and is not influenced by activity. The patient may **also** report **lightning-like episodes of sharp, stabbing pain** that, though transient, are very severe and frightening.
2. **Physical examination** may reveal a sensory or motor deficit or hyper- or hypoesthesia of the skin in the involved area.
3. There are **few laboratory studies** available, though an electromyelogram may document the presence of neuropathic changes in the nervous system.

D. Treatment

1. **Routine analgesics,** such as NSAIDs and even narcotics, may not be highly successful. However, these drugs may offer some diminution of pain and are worth trying if the patient's renal function, hematologic system, and CNS function are intact.
2. Because uninhibited hyperactivity in damaged peripheral nerves contributes to neuralgic pain, **anticonvulsant drugs** have been found to be

highly beneficial. Carbamazepine (Tegretol, 200 to 1000 mg qd), phenytoin (Dilantin, 200 to 600 mg qd), and valproic acid (Depakote, 500 to 1500 mg qd) are used.

   3. **Antidepressant medications** have the physiologic effect of increasing CNS serotonin, an inhibitory neurotransmitter, and this is of benefit alone or in combination with anticonvulsants. Amitriptyline (Elavil, 10 to 100 mg qhs), desipramine (Norpramin, 25 to 75 mg qhs), doxepin (Sinequan, Adapin, 25 to 100 mg qhs), trazodone (Desyrel, 50 to 200 mg qhs), and imipramine (Tofranil, 25 to 75 mg qd) are used.

   4. **Nerve blocks** with local anesthetic drugs may provide temporary relief. If entrapped nerves are causative of the pain, infiltration with steroids may be of benefit. Sympathetic blocks may alter the cutaneous threshold for pain and the sensitivity of peripheral receptors (see Chapter 13).

   5. TENS or other forms of **sensory modulation** may be of benefit, but require the presence of enough normal neural circuitry to allow the stimulation to reach the CNS and exert a physiologic effect.

   6. **Physical and psychological rehabilitation** may enhance a patient's ability to cope with the residual pain.

   7. **Surgical procedures** that relieve nerve entrapment can be highly successful. Procedures that simply cut the nervous system may only translocate the source of pain from a peripheral site to the surgical area.

IV. PHANTOM LIMB AND STUMP PAIN

A. Phantom Limb Pain

Pain that occurs in an absent body part is called **phantom limb pain (PLP)**. A literature review reveals that many therapeutic techniques have been described for this difficult problem. Only a few are effective for more than a year, but nonsurgical approaches are generally better than surgical ones. **Treatment** with antidepressants and anticonvulsants, TENS or other neural stimulation techniques, sympathetic blocks, and psychotherapy can be helpful.

B. Stump Pain

Stump pain is distinct from PLP and is caused by infection, undue pressure on tissues of the stump, or neuromas in the stump. **Focal therapy**—such as surgical incision and drainage of infection, surgical removal or injection of neuromas, TENS, and adjustment of the fit of the prosthesis—may be effective.

V. LOW BACK PAIN

A. Etiology

A minority of patients with chronic low back pain will have **herniated disks, spinal stenosis,** or activity-limiting degenerative **osteoarthritis** as the cause of their complaints. In a majority of the patients (80 to 90 percent), the pain is explained by **postural changes.** Basically, this connotes a shift of the weight-bearing function of the erect spine from the strong column of disks and vertebrae to the more delicate posterior elements (facet joints, the supra- and interspinous ligaments, and the erector spinae muscles). This results in chronic stress and strain on the joints (facet, sacroiliac, hip) and ligaments (interspinous, posterior longitudinal), distortion of the disks, narrowing of the neural foramina, and myofascial pain.

B. Diagnosis

The **diagnosis of chronic low back pain** will follow the distillation of data from an evaluation protocol that encompasses history taking, physical examination, and laboratory study.

    1. The **history** will document the chronic nature of the patient's complaints. It is important to elicit the record of medication use. There is at least a theoretic concern about the effects of chronic NSAID use on coagulation. Long-term use of narcotic analgesics will result in down-regulation of the receptors, and this *must* be taken into account when prescribing opioids for the control of acute pain. Nonspecific cross-tolerance to the sedative effects of medications may become manifest if the patient has taken indirect muscle relaxants, antidepressants, or anticonvulsants regularly.

    2. The findings from the **physical examination** are important to note and compare with past records because these patients may have deficits on neurologic examination that preceded their acute trauma or surgery. For instance, one would be less worried about a potentially epidural injection-related technical mishap based on the complaint of numbness if the sensory deficit was there before the epidural therapy was started.

    3. Laboratory study would not generally be crucial in a patient with chronic low back pain who suffers trauma unless there is the possibility of an acute disk herniation, a fractured vertebrae or spinal fusion, or the like contributing to the patient's current pain problem.

C. Treatment

The mainstay of therapy for chronic low back pain is **conservative therapy,** which generally includes any treatment other than surgery.

    1. Medication management could include NSAIDs, judicious narcotics, antidepressants, baclofen, anticonvulsants, and the nonspecific muscle relaxants.

2. Nerve blocks such as trigger point injections and epidural steroid injections are common in selected patients.

3. Stimulation techniques such as massage, TENS, acupuncture, and passive PT with modalities may diminish pain and reflex muscle spasm.

4. Active PT is crucial to restore range of motion (ROM) and improve overall strength when the patient is capable of cooperating.

5. True to the definition of pain, it must be acknowledged that a patient with chronic pain may have some **emotional overlay** attached to the pain before the acute trauma or surgery that resulted in his or her ICU admission occurred. Eliciting this will help the health care professional to understand the patient more fully and to enhance the care provided. It may be necessary to solicit the services of **psychosocial specialists** in the recovery period for the nonmedication management of depression and untoward anxiety, as well as the traumatic nature of the patient's current situation.

VI. ARTHRITIS

A. Prevalent Disease

Because arthritis is a **prevalent disease,** this is a chronic pain problem that many older patients who present with acute trauma or surgery will have.

B. Manifestations

Given the degenerative changes to joints associated with arthritis, these patients may have very **low activity profiles.** They may then suffer metabolic consequences such as obesity and osteoporosis, neuropathy, and physical deconditioning as a result of prolonged inactivity or bed rest. These factors will influence their ability to cooperate with PT and their being active in the recovery process.

C. Osteoarthritis

Osteoarthritis is noteworthy for the stress put on the articular cartilage.

1. This causes an increase in chondrocytes and the production of synovial fluid, focal erosion, and thickening of the synovium. Eventually, there is a **replacement of cartilage with bone.**

2. The result is **diffuse, aching pain** that is increased with activity and decreased with rest.

3. Treatment that reduces the stress on the joints includes rest, OT/PT, and weight reduction. To control pain, Tylenol or NSAIDs, joint injections, and occasionally surgery are used.

D. Rheumatoid Arthritis

This is an inflammatory synovitis that eventually leads to the destruction of the cartilage and bone of the joints. It is more common in women than in men and in patients between the ages of 35 and 50.

    1. The patients complain of **joint pain, stiffness, fatigue,** generalized weakness, and anorexia. The pain is increased with passive or active motion of the joints.

    2. Treatment may include rest, splinting, exercise, orthotics, and surgery (if intolerable pain is present or function is markedly impaired). The pain is managed with NSAIDs, antidepressants, steroids, immunosuppressive drugs, and agents that influence the progression of the disease, such as gold.

VII. MYOFASCIAL PAIN

A. Nomenclature

Many names have been used to refer to the syndrome of pain complaints that derive from the muscles and their supporting tissues. They include fibromyositis, muscular rheumatism, fibromyalgia, and the myofascial pain syndrome (MPS).

B. Etiology

Myofascial pain may be the primary cause of pain after injury to muscles, soft tissue, bones, or joints, **or** may be a **secondary** consequence of pain from a distant site that causes postural alteration and/or chronic stress/strain on musculoskeletal structures.

C. Diagnosis

The **diagnosis** is made when the following history and physical changes are revealed.

    1. Characteristic symptoms include complaints of widespread musculoskeletal pain that is steady, deep, and aching in nature, and is associated with reflex muscle spasm that contributes to morning stiffness and decreased ROM. The patient may also complain of sleep disturbance due to pain and moderate to marked activity disruption.

    2. The patient is likely to have **trigger points** on physical examination.

    3. There are no confirmatory **diagnostic tests.**

D. Treatment

The **treatment** may include any of the following.

1. NSAIDs, muscle relaxants, baclofen, and antidepressants (particularly amitriptyline to increase the amount of non–rapid-eye-movement [REM] stage 4 sleep during which even the muscles rest at night).
2. Trigger point injections with saline or local anesthetic drugs, with or without corticosteroids.
3. Physical therapy, massage, heat and/or ice, and TENS used in a sequential program to stretch muscles, decrease muscle spasm, increase ROM, improve strength, and restore normal posture.
4. Psychological techniques to minimize stress and tension, identify circumstances that aggravate the pain, and utilize self-regulation strategies.

VIII. CANCER PAIN

A. Special Concerns

Though a thorough discussion of cancer pain is beyond the scope of this section, it is important to recognize the **special concerns** and issues patients with cancer-related pain have when they present for surgery or after trauma.

B. Acute and Chronic Features

Cancer pain represents **a combination of acute and chronic pain features.** Pain directly due to the cancer process (e.g., metastases to bone, nerve compression or infiltration, bowel obstruction) usually presents as an acute problem. Pain due to cancer therapy (e.g., neuritis after radiation, neuralgic pain after surgery) often presents as chronic pain. The diagnosis of cancer intensifies the **emotional impact** of pain, so attention must be given to the psychosocial aspects of the disease.

C. Treatment

Treatment considerations *must* take into account the patient's quality of life, his or her physical and emotional condition, the probable life expectancy, the source(s) and severity of the pain, and the risk/benefit ratio. **Special features** of the patient's treatment include the following:

 1. The **chronic use of opioids** will result in down-regulation of opioid receptors, such that enormous doses of narcotics may be needed to gain control of acute traumatic or postoperative pain.

2. **Agonist-antagonist drugs and pure antagonist drugs** to treat excessive opiate side effects **should be used with great caution** in these patients because precipitating withdrawal is a very real and potentially life-threatening possibility. **Amphetamines** and an effective **bowel regimen** to counteract, respectively, the sedation and constipation seen with high doses of narcotics can significantly improve patient comfort.

3. The patient's **coagulation status** may be influenced by NSAIDs, malnutrition, chemotherapy, or radiation.

4. **Nerve blocks** with local anesthetic drugs and, occasionally, neurolytic agents (alcohol, phenol) are very beneficial in reducing some of the pain so that the total dose of narcotics and adjunctive medications can be decreased and the undesired side effects, such as sedation, attenuated.

5. These patients may have **implanted infusion devices** that will require attention during their postoperative or posttrauma care.

SUGGESTED READINGS

Bickerstaff DR, Kanis AJ: The use of nasal calcitonin in the treatment of post-traumatic algodystrophy. *Br J Rheum* 30:291-294, 1991.

Boissevain MD, McCain GA: Toward an integrated understanding of fibromyalgia syndrome. I. Medical and pathophysiological aspects. *Pain* 45:227-238, 1991.

Boissevain MD, McCain GA: Toward an integrated understanding of fibromyalgia syndrome. II. Psychological and phenomenological aspects. *Pain* 45:239-248, 1991.

Bonica JJ: Cancer pain, in Bonica JJ (ed): *The Management of Pain.* Philadelphia, Lea & Febiger, 1990, pp 400-460.

Bonica JJ: Causalgia and other reflex sympathetic dystrophies, in Bonica JJ (ed): *The Management of Pain.* Philadelphia, Lea & Febiger, 1990, pp 220-243.

Chabal C, Jacobson L, Mariano A, et al: The use of oral mexiletine for the treatment of pain after peripheral nerve injury. *Anesthesiology* 76:513-517, 1992.

Eisenach JC, Rauck RL, Buzzanelli C, et al: Epidural clonidine analgesia for intractable cancer pain: phase I. *Anesthesiology* 71:647-652, 1989.

Foley KM: Pain syndromes in patients with cancer. *Med Clin North Am* 71:169-184, 1987.

Hord AH, Rooks MD, Stephens BO, et al: Intravenous regional bretylium and lidocaine for treatment of reflex sympathetic dystrophy: a randomized, double-blind study. *Anesth Analg* 74:818-821, 1992.

Kesler RW, Saulsbury FT, Miller LT, et al: Reflex sympathetic dystrophy in children: treatment with transcutaneous electrical nerve stimulation. *Pediatrics* 82:728-732, 1988.

Portenoy RK, Foley KM, Inturrisi CE: The nature of opioid responsiveness and its implications for neuropathic pain: new hypotheses derived from studies of opioid infusions. *Pain* 43:273-286, 1990.

Robertson DR, George CF: Treatment of post herpetic neuralgia in the elderly. *Br Med Bull* 46:113-123, 1990.

Rowlingson JC, Hamill RJ: Treatment of low back pain. *Int Anesth Clin* 29:57-68, 1991.

Schwartzman RJ, Kerrigan J: The movement disorder of reflex sympathetic dystrophy. *Neurology* 40:57-61, 1990.

Sola AE, Bonica JJ: Myofascial syndromes, in Bonica JJ (ed): *The Management of Pain.* Philadelphia, Lea & Febiger, 1990, pp 352-367.

CHAPTER 33
NURSING ISSUES

Ann Gill Taylor

I. Nurses' Role in Pain Treatment in Critical Care Environments
   A. Pain Control as a Multidisciplinary Process
   B. Specific Nursing Considerations
II. Options to Prevent and Control Pain
   A. Pain Control Options
   B. Pharmacologic Options—The Mainstay of Pain Control
III. Common Clinical Dilemmas in Critical Care
   A. The Hemodynamically Unstable Patient
   B. The Chemically Dependent Substance Abuser
   C. The Withholding of Analgesics and Sedatives as a Part of Plans for Special Procedures
   D. Patients Who Are Unable to Communicate
IV. Summary
Suggested Readings

Pain is ever-present in critical care environments. Some pain is associated directly with injury or disease, such as that of acute myocardial infarction, a distended abdomen, or metastatic cancer. Other pain is often the result of procedures and tasks carried out by nurses and physicians that involve debridement, suctioning, physiotherapy, or dressing and position changes. The growing awareness that pain has negative consequences with regard to a patient's stay in an intensive care unit (ICU) has prompted attention to how health care professionals might lessen the pain and suffering indigenous to these environments.

I. NURSES' ROLE IN PAIN TREATMENT IN CRITICAL CARE ENVIRONMENTS

A. Pain Control as a Multidisciplinary Process

1. The **key players** involved in controlling pain include physicians, nurses, the patient, and the patient's family members, with each having a unique contribution to make.

2. **Other players** include the clinical pharmacist, pain psychologist, social workers, and respiratory, occupational, and physical therapists.

B. Specific Nursing Considerations

1. The **focus of nursing care** is on the restoration of the functional abilities of the patient, as well as on treating the underlying pathologic processes and sustaining life.

2. **Nursing interventions** generally compensate for the patient's inability to
   a. self-regulate fluid and food intake, hygiene, elimination, rest, and activity;
   b. communicate; and
   c. control events within the critical care environment.

3. Implementation of the teacher-role component of nursing practice through **patient and/or family member instruction** about pain treatment alternatives, potential risks, dosage adjustments, and adjunctive therapies is basic to all other pain-related interventions. Teaching emphasizes what the patient is likely to experience when undergoing procedures and care-related tasks. It includes specific methods of pain assessment nurses will use, the level of patient participation required, the importance of preventing pain versus treating established pain (Chapter 32), and the concept that unrelieved pain must be communicated to health professionals if relief is to be achieved.

4. **Nursing goals** in treating pain include:
   a. Effectively and accurately assessing pain for severity and meaning.
   b. Preventing pain whenever possible.
   c. Relieving pain to the patient's satisfaction.
   d. Modulating pain.
   e. Enhancing the patient's tolerance of pain.
   f. Sustaining patients emotionally.

These nursing goals can be consistently achieved only through a well-formulated team plan, as outlined in Fig. 33-1. Pain assessment is detailed in Chapter 2.

II. OPTIONS TO PREVENT AND CONTROL PAIN

A. Pain Control Options

1. **Continuous intravenous** (IV) administration of opioids and/or nonsteroidal anti-inflammatory drugs (NSAIDs) or **nurse-controlled analgesia** can be used when the patient is unstable and/or unable to use **patient-controlled analgesia** (PCA) (Chapter 13). Occasionally, PCA can be used after initial loading dosages are given by a nurse or physician.

2. Augment analgesia with appropriate **anxiolysis, or sedation.**

3. **Perispinal analgesia** in the form of epidural/spinal opioids and/or local anesthetics can be injected intermittently or infused continuously (Chapter 13).

4. **Intermittent or continuous neural blockade** (Chapter 13).

5. **Physical agents** such as massage and the application of heat or cold (Chapter 15).

6. **Transcutaneous electrical stimulation (TENS)** (Chapter 14).

7. **Cognitive-behavioral interventions** such as relaxation, distraction, and guided imagery, can be taught as soon after admission as is practical. These interventions tend to improve mood and reduce pain intensity, anxiety, and the amount of medication required for pain control (Chapter 14).

B. Pharmacologic Options—The Mainstay of Pain Control

1. The most widely accepted approach to pain control is the administration of **narcotic and nonnarcotic analgesics,** preferably in a continuous IV drip or on a regular, around-the-clock basis, titrating the dosage to achieve the desired level of pain control, while evaluating safety and effectiveness. A flow sheet such as shown in Fig. 33-2, can be used to document this.

2. A nurse's responsibility in **assessing patient response** to prescribed analgesics necessitates

    a. a knowledge of the pharmacology and pharmacokinetics of analgesics (Chapter 6),

    b. a knowledge of reversal agents and their application in the event of rapid changes in a patient's condition that warrant reversal of narcotics and/or sedative agents.

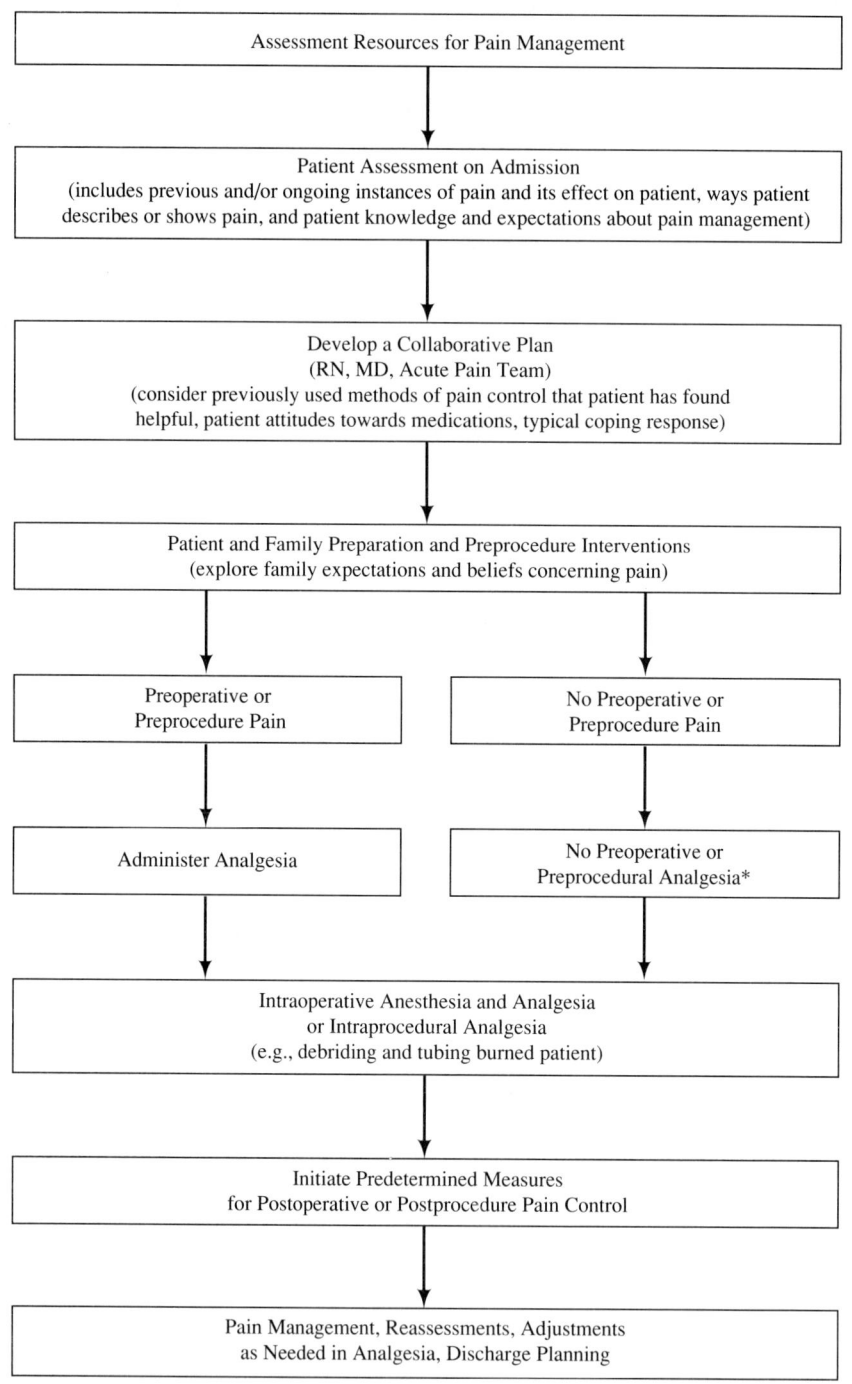

Figure 33-1. Flow chart depicting development of plan for systematic pain treatment from admission through all phases of hospitalization. (Adapted from AHCPR Pain Guideline, 1992.)

*Current research on use of preoperative epidural opioid analgesia in reducing postoperative pain provides some evidence that opioids given preoperatively reduce the hyperexcitability of the CNS that is caused by the intraoperative stimuli such as the incision, thus reducing the amount of postoperative pain.

Patient _____ Date _____

Pain rating scale used to evaluate effectiveness and safety of analgesics _____
Analgesic(s) prescribed _____

Time	Pain	Analgesic/s ordered	R	P	BP	Level of arousal	Other (side effects and other pain relief measures)	Plan and comments

Figure 33-2. Pain flow sheet.

of rapid changes in a patient's condition that warrant reversal of narcotics and/or sedative agents.

    c. familiarity with the literature about the pharmacologic control of pain in order to support recommendations for any changes, and

    d. skill in communicating, both orally and in writing, with other health professionals the observations and conclusions drawn from serial pain assessments. Nurses commonly have data to support suggestions for specific changes in drugs, the route of administration, dosage, and the time interval based on their systematic pain assessments.

  3. Nurses' concerns about maximum narcotic dose

    a. There is no specific answer as to a maximal or optimal dose in terms of milligrams of an opioid analgesic. The dosage to be used is the one that controls the pain *to the patient's satisfaction* with minimal side effects.

    b. Undertreatment with opioid analgesics occurs because nurses, physicians, patients, and families have firm, but unwarranted, fears about the risk of addiction, which lead to the administration of insufficient pain medication.

    c. Many factors go into a health care professional's interpretation of a patient's pain, including the professional's own pain experience, assumptions about how much pain *should* result from a procedure or injury, and his or her perception of the patient's personality style (e.g., the straight-shooter versus the complainer or the manipulator), as well as, perhaps, a desire to deny the severity of pain associated with a particular procedure, such as wound debridement.

III. COMMON CLINICAL DILEMMAS IN CRITICAL CARE

A. The Hemodynamically Unstable Patient

Clinical scenario: A 50-year-old male, 12 h after the resection of a large, abdominal, malignant tumor, was admitted to the ICU secondary to a large intraoperative blood loss and hypotension. The patient had been maintained comfortably on IV morphine sulfate, 1 mg to 2 mg/h, since his return from the operating room, but during the night, he became febrile and hypotensive. The nurse, noting the drop in his blood pressure in conjunction with mild tachycardia, decreased urinary output, and fall in the central venous pressure (CVP), stopped the morphine sulfate infusion. The patient remained alert and oriented, with complaints of pain. His body language revealed bracing, splinting of the abdomen and chest with shallow respiration, and facial grimacing. His response to the question about his pain was tantamount to a report of 8 on a 10-point scale on which 0 is no pain and 10 is the worse possible pain. Once the nurse had increased the IV fluid rate to raise the patient's blood pressure, the physician was notified and orders for a stat complete blood count and blood cultures were obtained. The nurse then reassessed the pain relief options.

1. **Nursing diagnoses** For this patient, nursing diagnoses were:
   a. Fluid volume deficit related to blood and fluid loss.
   b. Alteration in cardiac output related to sepsis.
   c. Altered comfort/pain.
2. **Nursing actions**
   a. **Diagnosis of fluid volume deficit** This diagnosis requires, first, an assessment for fluid losses evident from postoperative nursing documentation, the hematocrit, and fluid intake/output. Vital signs are then reviewed to detect a downward trend in blood pressure and evidence of mild tachycardia; from physical examination, any evidence of dryness of the patient's mouth and decreased skin turgor should be noted.

   The patient's fluid status is monitored via urinary (Foley) catheter to reveal hourly urine output, and the CVP is determined by measurements from the CVP line. The fluid volume and titrating are then increased to maintain normotension. Monitoring is also conducted for complications of uncorrected fluid volume deficit, which may include hypotension due to decreased vascular volume; poor tissue and organ perfusion due to compensatory vasoconstriction and shunting, that is, increased risk of renal failure if hypovolemia is untreated; and the likelihood that pain may be used as the vasopressor to keep the blood pressure up.

   b. **Diagnosis of alteration in cardiac output** This diagnosis **requires** an investigation into the etiology of decreased cardiac output, such as blood cultures or evaluation of hematocrit; the readiness to initiate and titrate vasopressors in conjunction with the administration of fluids and/or blood; and an alertness to the effect of pain on the blood pressure. The fact that there may be a need to return the patient to surgery to correct the source of bleeding should be anticipated.

c. Diagnosis of altered comfort/pain This diagnosis necessitates, first, a pain assessment using the agreed-upon tool and documentation of the pain on a flow sheet (Fig. 33-2), and which is based on the awareness that the analgesic options available to the hypovolemic patient are limited. Pain treatment must coincide with fluid resuscitation. *Note:* **The sympathetic stimulation caused by pain should *not* be used as a vasopressor in a hemodynamically unstable patient.**

The narcotic infusion is reinitiated once the fluid intake has been increased. While narcotics administered by IV infusion have a negligible effect on patients as compared with the use of intermittent boluses of the drug, narcotics in any form will affect the blood pressure. Attention must be paid to adequate loading of the narcotic at the beginning of the infusion and to the maintenance of analgesic blood levels. Orders for vasopressors to maintain the blood pressure and to permit adequate analgesia administration, if necessary, should be requested.

Although epidural analgesia can be very effective, the epidural route may not be immediately accessible in many critical care situations because of the need for anesthesiologists to insert epidural catheters. Epidurally administered narcotics have virtually no hemodynamic effect. However, local anesthetics, which need to be used at the time of catheter insertion to test and confirm the catheter position, can cause vasodilation and a decrease in blood pressure through blockade of sympathetic outflow from the spinal cord. In a hemodynamically marginal patient, the physician may choose to deliver continuous epidural narcotics without local anesthetic. More stable patients frequently receive a combination of the two drugs.

Analgesia can be augmented using nonnarcotic medications, such as the injectable NSAID ketorolac tromethamine (Toradol), which has limited adverse hemodynamic effects in critically ill patients.

One must be alert to the consequences of not identifying and treating pain, including an impaired level of breathing, decreased ventilation, decreased depth of cough, the failure to use the incentive spirometer effectively, pneumonia (a potential result of the foregoing factors), decreased gastrointestinal motility, decreased mobility, and heightened emotional distress due to a stress response to major surgery and potential complications (Chapter 4). However, in hemodynamically unstable patients, attention must first be given to the hypotension, using volume and vasopressors, if necessary, to help maintain the blood pressure, and then to the resumption of pain and sedative medications.

3. Other considerations

a. Although less likely to have an impact on acute pain in hemodynamically unstable patients, nonpharmacologic modalities may be used as adjuncts to the opioid analgesics, for example, selecting a cognitive-behavioral intervention (relaxation, distraction, or imagery) that has been taught preoperatively.

b. A physical comfort agent such as TENS or a massage can help the patient to relax. Both are noninvasive, nonmedication techniques with few or no hemodynamic consequences.

B. The Chemically Dependent Substance Abuser

Clinical scenario: A 25-year-old male with a history of sickle cell disease was admitted to the ICU following a motorcycle accident that left him a paraplegic and in need of extensive surgery to repair his injuries. The patient had a history of substance abuse (cocaine, heroin, and meperidine), and of involvement with the police regarding drug-related charges. After 3 weeks in the ICU, his lacerations and skin grafts began to heal, and he began to comprehend the reality of his spinal cord injury. His pain medications were reduced, yet some nurses believed that the dosage and frequency should be decreased even further. These nurses contended that because of his paraplegia, there should be decreased input of some noxious stimuli, and that because his wounds were healing, he should have been experiencing less pain than earlier in his hospitalization. The patient, on the other hand, continued to use abusive language; to demand specific foods, cigarettes, Cokes, and narcotics; and to threaten to get drugs from external sources, if not from the nurses. The nurses began to feel manipulated and bullied by a drug-seeking individual, while the patient contended that he was being tortured by a group of uncaring health professionals.

1. Nursing diagnoses   For this patient, nursing diagnoses were:
   a. Altered comfort/pain.
   b. Chemical dependence.
   c. Acute grief related to trauma and the resulting paraplegia.
   d. Personality disorder with an associated inadequate or dysfunctional coping style.

(Only the diagnosis of altered comfort/pain is addressed here. Diagnoses pertaining to the spinal cord injury are not the focus of this discussion.)

2. Nursing actions
   a. Diagnosis of altered comfort/pain
      i. this diagnosis requires the nurse to, first, obtain a **pain history and assessment.** A history of substance abuse may confer a certain degree of opioid tolerance (Chapter 29) and the likelihood that the patient with such a history will require substantially higher dosages of pain medications than the usual trauma patient (Chapter 24). In some cases, as in this scenario, patients may also suffer from physical dependence and/or addiction. The patient's history and a review of previous medical records should help to define the extent of dependence.

      ii. The nurse must set aside the patient's antisocial history, which was well established before his injury, and give validity to his current pain complaints. Every effort should be made to define the mechanism of the pain, and to treat it. **Drug dependency should not be "treated" (i.e., detoxification of drugs should not be attempted) in the acute setting.** Rather, the patient should be dosed adequately to achieve analgesia, regardless of the number of milligrams required.

iii. Trends in pain medication utilization and the impact on the pain intensity level must be assessed and documented. Withdrawal signs and symptoms may begin within 8 to 12 h after the last opioid dose, and become most intense in 36 to 48 h. One must observe for lacrimation, piloerection (goose bumps), diaphoresis, irritability, restlessness, tachycardia, diarrhea, and other symptoms that reflect a sympathetic response and possible withdrawal in patients with suggestive histories or behaviors or high dosage requirements (Chapter 29).

iv. Time-contingent administration of long-acting opioids should be utilized to keep blood serum levels of opioid consistent. Administration using PCA infusion, although controversial for substance-abuse patients, can help to give the patient some control, remove the potential for conflict over the patient's demand for drugs, and reduce the nurses' reinforcement of the patient's pain behaviors. Regular scheduling of pain medications, rather than an as-needed (prn) scheduling, also helps to limit conflict. The patient knows when the drug is to be given, and the nurse is less likely to feel manipulated and hence to act out his or her anger by punitively withholding or delaying the medication. All staff members working with the patient need to be consistent and punctual with the dosing if this approach is to be effective. Adjunct medications to the PCA opioid administration may include the infusion of a peridural local anesthetic and the use of NSAIDs.

v. Breakthrough pain should be treated at the time of wound examination with a larger dose of opioid than is provided via the PCA, or with a bolus through the PCA. It must be recognized that the choice of opioid drug used to treat the pain will influence the pain level, but will have little influence on the addiction problem.

vi. Remember that **paralysis** due to spinal cord injury or to the use of paralytic agents does not always have an analgesic effect. Central pain and muscle spasms are likely to be responsive to nonnarcotic medications, such as muscle relaxants, tricyclic antidepressants, and anticonvulsants (Chapter 11). The neural injury pain reported by the spinal-cord-injured patient described in the scenario may be relieved by barbiturate-like drugs, and not by opioids. The pathophysiology of central pain caused by a cord lesion is unknown.

b. Other pain treatment options Psychological intervention can be very helpful in defining the patient's agenda; in dealing with issues related to the spinal cord injury, the attendant losses, and lifestyle changes; and in allowing the patient to feel "heard." Pain tolerance will be lowered by fear, anxiety, anger, and unresolved grieving related to the nature of the injury. The use of self-selected relaxation techniques should be encouraged, especially for procedures or control of muscle spasms. TENS may also help the patient by increasing the sense of control over who is "calling the shots" in the pain treatment.

3. Other considerations

a. Communication should be established and maintained using the framework of a **contract** developed with the patient by a staff member who has some authority over the way that events will transpire.

b. The contract empowers the patient and ensures that a sufficient level of opioid analgesia will be provided, that a preset schedule will be maintained, and that timing and dose changes can be negotiated only with a designated staff member.

c. The consequences of any suspicion that the patient is obtaining drugs from any other source should be included in the contract.

d. The **responsibility of health care professionals** in the critical care environment is to treat the patient's traumatic injuries and acute pain, not the addiction problem, which remains an unresolved diagnosis in the ICU. Referral can be made for treatment after the acute crisis has been resolved.

C. The Withholding of Analgesics and Sedatives as a Part of Plans for Special Procedures

> Clincal scenario: A 69-year-old male with a history of malignant pleural effusion resulting from disseminated oat-cell lung cancer was admitted to the ICU because of respiratory failure requiring intubation and mechanical ventilation. The patient's prognosis was poor, and the family concurred with the health care team's goal of palliative therapy and comfort measures. Morphine sulfate, 2 mg/h, and midazolam, 1 mg/h, by continuous IV infusion, were started after appropriate loading doses and prior to the insertion of a chest tube for drainage of the pleural effusion. Two days later, a therapeutic pleurodesis with tetracycline and lidocaine was done to prevent fluid reaccumulation. Increases in analgesia (morphine sulfate, 10 mg/h) and an anxiolytic agent (midazolam, 4 mg/h) were ultimately required to control his pain and anxiety and to permit sleep and rest.
>
> Once the respiratory failure was resolved, the team addressed weaning from mechanical ventilation and adjustment of the pain medication for discharge. Both the analgesic and anxiolytic drugs were titrated downward, concurrent with the initiation of oral forms of these drugs. Though the patient was still sedated, his pain was controlled and extubation was successful, thus making discharge to home possible.

1. Nursing diagnoses
For this patient, nursing diagnoses were:

  a. Altered comfort/pain.

  b. Ineffective gas exchange related to altered pulmonary volumes and function; pain and distress.

  c. Sleep deprivation related to pain.

(Only the diagnosis of altered comfort/pain is addressed here.)

2. Nursing actions

  a. Diagnosis of altered comfort/pain

  i. This diagnosis requires the nurse to titrate the prescribed analgesic to achieve the desired pain relief, considering that **short-acting opioids** such as morphine sulfate, fentanyl (Sublimaze), sufentanil (Sufenta), and alfentanil (Alfenta) may be used for painful procedures. The opioid is administered using PCA or continuous infusion to maintain an analgesic blood serum level, and the patient is observed for the effects of accumulation, such as increasing sedation.

    ii. An **opioid antagonist** such as naloxone (Narcan) should be available at bedside to be used judiciously. Doses of 0.04 to 0.08 mg IV can increase the respiratory rate adequately without causing reversal of the analgesia. These doses may be repeated every 20 min, or can be supplemented with a dose of naloxone 0.4 mg intramuscularly for a more sustained effect.

    iii. Remember that the physician may consider a scheduled **NSAID,** such as ketorolac tromethamine (Toradol) IV or ibuprofen (Motrin) PO, that will act at the site of the incision to block prostaglandin synthesis (Chapter 7). This will have a significant analgesic effect without respiratory depression, and will minimize narcotic requirements.

    iv. Low-dose narcotics provide excellent analgesia with little risk of significant sedation or respiratory depression. Epinephrine-contained **local anesthesics** intrapleurally may be administered prior to the removal of the chest tube in order to reduce pain. Also, local anesthetic intercostal nerve blocks may be done by an anesthesiologist to control pain in a patient with a flail chest, thus eliminating splinting and enhancing weaning from mechanical ventilation.

  b. Other pain treatment options Cognitive-behavioral interventions such as relaxation, distraction, and imagery can be used to reduce anxiety. Physical comfort agents, such as massage, a heating pad, or an ice pack, may be perceived as effective by the patient.

3. Other considerations

  a. Improved pulmonary toilet and adequate sleep are contingent upon sufficient pain relief to ensure that the patient begins to move, cough, and use the incentive spirometer after intubation.

  b. Patients can benefit from sedatives such as midazolam (Versed), lorazepam (Ativan), or low-dose tricyclic antidepressants at bedtime to facilitate restful sleep. Dose and interval requirements vary, based on the patient's age, weight, history of alcohol use, and severity of agitation. Efforts should be made to minimize sleep disruptions during the night, with a goal of maintaining as normal a wake–sleep cycle as is possible.

  c. Combination therapy using a benzodiazepine such as midazolam and an opioid may result in additive central nervous system (CNS) or respiratory depressant effects.

D. Patients Who Are Unable to Communicate

> Clinical scenario: A 55-year-old, non–English-speaking man found beaten and unconscious on the street was admitted to the ICU. He had been seen previously in the outpatient clinic, and was known to have end-stage renal disease and chronic obstructive pulmonary

disease (COPD). Intubation was avoided for several days following admission, but eventually had to be performed. The observation and assessment of functional patterns and human response patterns revealed characteristics that ranged from distress and increased tension, fearfulness, restlessness, irritability, and facial tension to a decreased level of consciousness from time to time. Orders included haloperidol (Haldol) according to the level of agitation, the benzodiazepine lorazepam to treat anxiety, and morphine sulfate infusion to control the pain.

1. Nursing diagnoses For this patient, nursing diagnoses were:

    a. Impaired verbal communication related to cultural differences (non–English speaking).

    b. Altered comfort/pain.

    c. Anxiety related to situational crises and change in environment.

(Other diagnoses pertaining to end-stage renal disease and COPD are not considered here, except as these relate to the management of pain, restlessness, and irritability.)

2. Nursing actions

    a. Diagnoses of impaired verbal communication and altered comfort/pain require the nurse to, first, obtain a **pain history and assessment.** However, the non–English-speaking status of this patient is a major factor impeding the likelihood of getting an accurate verbal report of pain level. Thus **the patient's nonverbal behavior** must be **observed,** especially during procedures and other times of stimulation, because this is probably the best way to assess pain in patients unable to communicate verbally. Careful attention is required to differentiate among anxiety, agitation, and restlessness without pain; delirium; and pain in response to noxious stimuli. For those unable to communicate verbally (Chapter 2), a simple, modified measurement scale and approach to assessing pain can be used. The patient's response to the opioid, anxiolytic, and neuroleptic drugs ordered can be assessed to aid in defining the extent and type of distress the patient is experiencing. A **translator** may be required to establish a mechanism of communication for any non–English-speaking patient. Such an action acknowledges that attention to the preferences and needs of patients whose education or cultural traditions impede effective communication is important.

    b. Diagnosis of altered comfort/pain This diagnosis additionally requires the nurse to consider the patient's decreased renal clearance when administering opioids, particularly morphine and meperidine, due to the production of active metabolites. It must be kept in mind that while the initial loading dose may need to be large, subsequent doses may need to be smaller or given less frequently than for a patient with normal renal function. Monitoring should be conducted to note any increased sensitivity to the respiratory depressant effect of the opioid morphine sulfate, because long-standing respiratory problems lead to increased sensitivity to the respiratory depressant effect of opioids. The continuous infusion of morphine sulfate will decrease variations in blood levels and permit more aggressive pain management once the patient is intubated. Intubation lessens concerns about the respiratory depressive effect of the opioid. The nurse might suggest to the physician the continuous infusion of a shorter-acting, more potent, easy-to-reverse opioid such as fentanyl or alfentanil if morphine sulfate is assessed as causing too many side effects or judged to be ineffective in pain management.

c. Diagnosis of anxiety related to situational crises and change in the environment This diagnosis requires the nurse to administer the prescribed benzodiazepine lorazepam (0.5 mg to 1.0 mg) at regular intervals to control anxiety (peak effect is in 2 to 4 h). The patient is monitored for the sedative effect of lorazepam, and, if necessary, a shorter-acting benzodiazepine, such as midazolam, which has a peak effect in 0.5 to 1 h, is recommended. The patient is then monitored for the combined therapy effect of the opioid and the benzodiazepine, acknowledging that these may result in additive CNS or respiratory depressant effects, particularly in any patient with long-standing respiratory problems. Agitation in this patient can be controlled with the neuroleptic haloperidol as ordered. This drug causes minimal sedation or respiratory depression. Guidelines for IV use are given in Chapter 11.

3. Other considerations Other patient populations with no verbal skills or poor communication skills that affect health care professionals' assessment of pain include:

    a. Neonates and children without adequate verbal skills.
    b. Individuals who are developmentally delayed.
    c. Psychotic patients.
    d. Patients with Alzheimer's disease or dementia.
    e. Patients with a decreased level of consciousness.
    f. Intubated patients on mechanical ventilation.
    g. Patients receiving paralytic agents or with neuromuscular disorders, such as cervical cord injuries, Guillain-Barré syndrome, or closed-head injuries.

IV. SUMMARY

    A. Key factors to be considered by nurses in monitoring the effectiveness of pain control include
        1. patient comfort and satisfaction with pain management;
        2. range and appropriateness of pain control options available, and who will coordinate their implementation;
        3. how to apply the available options; and
        4. how to minimize side effects and complications related to pain

control, along with contingency plans to avert or treat such side effects as nausea, vomiting, urinary retention, and respiratory depression, as well as a range of analgesic doses to combat varying pain intensities.

B. The optimal application of pain control in acutely and critically ill patients depends on communication and information sharing among all health team members.

C. The quality of pain control is influenced by the training, expertise, and experience of nurses and other health team members. Clarity about each member's contribution to pain control ensures successful team collaboration.

D. A periodic review of pain management procedures will likely reveal evidence of ways to enhance the efficacy of pain treatment in nursing units.

SUGGESTED READINGS

Acute Pain Management Guideline Panel: *Acute Pain Management: Operative or Medical Procedures and Trauma. Clinical Practice Guideline.* AHCPR Pub. no. 92-0032. Rockville, Maryland, Agency for Health Care Policy and Research, Public Health Service, U.S. Department of Health and Human Services, February 1992.

Bellinger K, Romelfanger M, Algren CL, Hogan PC: Nursing and pain management, in Weiner S (ed): *Innovations in Pain Management,* vol 1. Orlando, Florida, Deutsch Press, 1990.

Donovan MI: Acute pain relief. *Nurs Clin North Am* 25:851-861, 1990.

Eland JM: Pain in children. *Nurs Clin North Am* 25:871-884, 1990.

Litwack K (ed): Pain and post anesthesia management. *Crit Care Nurs Clin* 3:1-158, 1991.

McCaffery M, Beebe A: *Pain: Clinical Manual for Nursing Practice.* St. Louis, Mosby, 1989.

Puntillo KA (ed): *Pain in the Critically Ill: Assessment and Management.* Gaithersburg, Maryland, Aspen, 1991.

Wild L, Coyne C: The basics and beyond: epidural analgesia. *Am J Nurs* 92:27-34, 1992.

PART SEVEN

APPENDIXES

APPENDIX
A
PAIN TERMINOLOGY

Acute pain pain that follows a bodily injury and disappears with the healing of that injury. Acute pain is self-limited, and is associated with tissue damage and the attendant autonomic changes, such as hypertension, tachycardia, and diaphoresis.

Allodynia pain due to a stimulus which does not normally provoke pain.

Analgesia alteration in the **perception** of nociceptive stimuli such that the sensation no longer is painful.

Antalgesia alteration of the **production** of a nociceptive stimulus.

Cancer pain can be acute, chronic, or intermittent in nature and is related to the presence of active malignant disease or the antineoplastic treatment. Also has a component that is not directly related to tissue changes or treatment, but is expressed by the patients as "pain," e.g., fear, constipation, worry about financial ruin.

Causalgia a syndrome of burning pain, allodynia, hyperpathia, and autonomic dysfunction, including pseudomotor and vasomotor abnormalities, and, ultimately, dystrophic changes **following major nerve trauma.**

Chronic pain includes three different kinds of pain: (1) pain of a nonmalignant etiology that persists beyond the expected healing time, usually lasts longer than several months, and generally is not associated with increased autonomic activity (see acute pain); (2) pain that is related to chronic degenerative disease; and (3) recurrent or persistent pain that has no identifiable organic basis.

Deafferentation pain associated with damage to the peripheral nerves or spinal pathways and can be of traumatic (phantom limb pain after amputation, causalgia, spinal cord injuries), infectious (postherpetic neuralgia, AIDS, tabes dorsalis), or metabolic or inflammatory (diabetic peripheral neuropathy, Guillain-Barré syndrome) etiology.

Dysesthesia   an unpleasant abnormal sensation, whether spontaneous or evoked, resulting from normal stimuli.

Hyperesthesia   abnormally increased sensitivity to touch, pain, or other sensory stimuli. For example, a light touch in sympathetically maintained pain can cause severe pain.

Hyperpathia   excessive response to a stimulus; e.g., pain that persists after the stimulus has stopped.

Myofascial pain   a syndrome of focal pain in a muscle or the related tissues, stiffness, muscle spasm and decreased range of motion, and decreased exercise tolerance. Often, trigger points, hyperirritable foci in the muscle body that produce a nonneurologic, deep, aching or burning pain upon palpation, are present.

Neuropathic pain (neuralgia)   pain resulting from direct injury to or dysfunction within neural elements; e.g., diabetic peripheral neuropathy, postcerebrovascular accident (CVA) syndrome.

Nociception   the perception of pain, signaling real or impending damage to the tissue.

Nociceptors   peripheral sensory receptors that preferentially detect noxious physical or chemical stimulations that give rise to transmissions that are interpreted as pain.

Pain   an unpleasant sensory and emotional experience associated with actual or potential tissue damage, or described in terms of such damage.

Paresthesia   abnormal sensation, whether spontaneous or evoked, such as tingling, burning, or itching.

Phantom limb pain   pain felt in an absent part of the body.

Reflex sympathetic dystrophy (RSD)   a syndrome of burning pain, allodynia, hyperpathia, and autonomic dysfunction, including pseudomotor and vasomotor abnormalities after what may be a very minor injury and **without major nerve injury.**

Stump pain   pain at the site of amputation of a body part.

Sympathetically maintained pain (SMP)   refers to syndromes in which abnormal activity of the sympathetic nervous system causes a severe, debilitating pain that is classically burning in nature and is associated with an exquisite tenderness to light touch (hyperpathia).

APPENDIX B

COMMON DRUGS, DOSES, AND METABOLISM

	Class*	Dose	Route	Metabolism/excretion**	Comments
Acetaminophen (Tylenol)	Analgesic	10–15 mg/kg q4h	PO, PR	H	Hepatic toxicity
Alfentanil (Alfenta)	Narc ag	8–50 µg/kg q30–60min **Infusion:** 0.5–3.0 µg/kg/min	IV	H	Rapid onset, short $t_{1/2}$; excellent for infusions, 90% protein bound
Amitriptyline (Elavil)	TCA	10–75 mg qhs	PO (IM)	Hm/renal 18%	Caution in seizures, glaucoma MAO inhibitors
Aspirin	NSAID	**Antiplatelet:** 325 mg/d **Anti-inflammatory:** max 4000 mg/d	PO, PR	H/R 30% as salicylic acid	Hepatic toxicity, renal insufficiency, platelet dysfunction, hypersensitivity, Reye's syndrome, >80% protein bound
Atracurium (Tracrium)	NM blocker	**Intubation:** 0.4–0.5 mg/kg **Infusion:** 5–10 µg/kg/min	IV	Hoffman elimination	Histamine release. Laudanosine accum. with large doses or infusions
Baclofen (Liorisol)	Musc relax	20–80 mg/d (dd—tid)	PO	R	Abrupt withdrawal can cause seizures. Decrease dose in renal failure
Benztropine (Cogentin)	Antichol Antihist	1–2 mg/d	PO, IV, IM		Hyperthermia, tachycardia, urinary retention
Bretylium (Bretylol)	Sympatholytic	**Bier block:** 1–2 mg/kg	IV	R (100%)	Hypotension, enhance digoxin-induced dysrhythmias
Buprenorphine (Buprenex)	Narc ag-antag Partial ag	0.05–0.3 mg	IV (dd) IM	H/feces	Ceiling effect—resp. depression; can induce withdrawal in narcotic-dependent patients. 96% protein bound

Drug	Class	Dose	Route	Metabolism	Comments
Butorphanol (Stadol)	Narc ag–antag	0.5–2.0 mg 1.0–4.0 mg	IV IM	H	See **buprenorphine** 80% protein bound
Carbamazepine (Tegretol)	Anticonvulsant	100 mg q8h (max 1200 mg/d)	PO	H (98%)/bile	Enzyme induction, blood dyscrasias, increased LFTs 60–85% protein bound
Chloral hydrate (Notec)	Sedative	250–1000 mg q6–8h	PO, PR	Hm	Can accumulate in renal failure and hepatic insufficiency. High levels can cause cardiac dysrhythmias
Chlorpromazine (Thorazine)	Maj tranq Sedative	25–50 mg q1h 2 mg q2min (max 25 mg)	IM IV	Hm	Active metabolites, hypotension, lower seizure threshold, rarely used 90% protein bound
Choline Mg trisalicylate (Trilisate)	NSAID	50 mg/kg/d dd q8–24h	PO	H	see **aspirin** Reversible platelet dysfunction Doesn't cause bronchospasm
Cimetidine (Tagamet)	H₂ blocker	37.5–50 mg/h 300 mg q6–8h	IV infusion PO, IM, IV	R (100%)	Use half dose in renal insufficiency; can decrease WBC, platelets 20% protein bound
Codeine	Narc ag	0.5 mg/kg q4–6h	PO, SQ, IM, IV	Hm	Constipation common, decrease dose in elderly and patients with hepatic dysfunction. No first-pass effect
Cyclobenzaprine (Flexoril)	Musc relax	10–20 mg tid	PO, IM	H	Extensive first-pass metabolism, structurally similar to TCA 95% protein bound

*Narc ag = narcotic agonist, TCA = tricyclic antidepressant, NSAID = nonsteroidal anti-inflammatory drug, NM blocker = neuromuscular blocker, antag = antagonist, Maj tranq = major tranquilizer, Musc relax = muscle relaxant, Antihist = antihistamine, Antichol = anticholinergic.
**H = hepatic metabolism, Hm = hepatic with active metabolites, R = renal excretion, dd = divided doses.

	Class*	Dose	Route	Metabolism/ excretion**	Comments
Dantrolene (Dantrium)	Musc relax	**Spasm:** 100–150 mg q2h **Malignant hyperthermia, NMS:** 1–2 mg/kg q5–10 min to max 10 mg/kg then 4–8 mg/kg/d × 3 d	PO IV	Hm	Muscle weakness
Dextroamphetamine (Dexadrine)	CNS stimulant	5–10 mg qAM†	PO	H/45% urine	Used for opioid potentiation, treatment of opioid-induced sedation, especially in cancer patients taking large doses of opioids. Reverses antihypertensive effect of adrenergic blockers. †May repeat dose midday if needed
Dezocine (Dalgan)	Narc ag–antag	5–20 mg q3–6 h 2.5–10 mg q2–4h	IM IV	H/67% urine	See **buprenorphine**
Diazepam (Valium)	GABA ag Sedative Anxiolytic	2–10 mg q3–4h	IV, PO	Hm	Active metabolites (30% oxazepam) confusion, paradoxical excitation Propylene glycol base → hypotension
Diclofenac (Voltaren)	NSAID	75–150mg q8–12h	PO	H	Reversible platelet dysfunction See **aspirin**, 99% protein bound
Diflunisal (Dolobid)	NSAID	500 mg q8–12h	PO	H	See **aspirin**, reversible platelet dysfunction 98% protein bound
Diphenhydramine (Benadryl)	Antihist	10–50 mg (max/d = 400 mg)	IM, IV, PO	H	85% protein bound

Drug	Class	Dose	Route	Metab	Comments
Doxacurium (Nuromax)	NM blocker	Intubation: 0.05–0.08 mg/kg	IV	R	Hypotension, dysrhythmias
Doxepin (Adapin)	TCA	30–50 mg qhs (titrate up to 150 mg bid if needed)	PO	H	Active metabolites 85% protein bound
Droperidol (Inapsine)	Maj tranq	Sedation: 2.5–5.0 mg Opioid adjunct: 0.2–0.3 mg/kg q4h Antiemetic: 0.625–1.25 mg	IV IV IV	H	Drowsiness, extrapyramidal effects, hypotension, possible neuroleptic malignant syndrome Lowers seizure threshold
Etodolac (Lodine)	NSAID	200–400 mg q6–12h	PO	H	See **aspirin**, reversible platelet dysfunction 99% protein bound
Etomidate (Amidate)	IV anesthetic Sedative	0.3–0.4 mg/kg	IV	H	Not analgesic, causes adrenal suppression
Famotidine (Pepsid)	H₂ blocker	20–40 mg q24h 20 mg q12h	PO IV	R	See **cimetidine**
Fentanyl (Sublimaze)	Narc ag	10–100 µg prn 50–100 µg prn 25–100 µg/h q24h	IV IM Transdermal	H	80% protein bound High lipid solubility Slower clearance in elderly
Flumazenil (Mazicon)	GABA antag	0.2 mg q1min (max 1 mg)	IV		Can precipitate benzo withdrawal, seizures

*Narc ag = narcotic agonist, TCA = tricyclic antidepressant, NSAID = nonsteroidal anti-inflammatory drug, NM blocker = neuromuscular blocker, antag = antagonist, Maj tranq = major tranquilizer, Musc relax = muscle relaxant, Antihist = antihistamine, Antichol = anticholinergic.
**H = hepatic metabolism, Hm = hepatic with active metabolites, R = renal excretion, dd = divided doses.

	Class*	Dose	Route	Metabolism/excretion**	Comments
Haloperidol (Haldol)	Maj tranq	**Mild agitation:** 0.5–2 mg q20min **Moderate agitation:** 2–5 mg q20min prn **Severe agitation:** 10–20 mg q20min prn **Maintenance once calm:** 0.5–3 mg q6–24h	IM	H	See **droperidol**
Hydromorphone (Dilaudid)	Narc ag	2–4 mg q4–6h 3 mg q6–8h 200–300 µg q6–10h	PO, SQ, IM PR Epidural	H (87%), R (13%)	Lipid solubility >MS, <fentanyl
Hydroxyzine (Atarex, Visteril)	Antichol/antihist	50–100 mg	PO, IV	H	If given too rapidly IV, can cause hypotension, tachycardia, hemolysis
Ibuprofen (Motrin)	NSAID	400–800 mg q6h	PO	H (99%)	See **aspirin**, reversible platelet dysfunction, 99% protein bound
Indomethacin (Indocin)	NSAID	75–150 mg/d dd q6–8h	PO, PR (IV neonates)	H (90%), R (10%)	See **aspirin**, reversible platelet dysfunction, 90% protein bound
Ketamine (Ketalar)	Hypnotic Analgesic	**Induction GA:** 1–3 mg/kg 4 mg/kg **Sedation, maint of GA:** 0.25–1 mg/kg q5–30min	IV IM IV	H (96%)	Sympathomimetic—causes HTN, tachycardia. Can increase ICP. Increased salivation. Hallucinations can be minimized with use of benzodiazepine

Drug	Class	Dose	Route	Metabolism**	Comments
Ketorolac (Toradol)	NSAID	10–30 mg q6–18h 30 mg load then 10–15 mg IV q6–18h	PO IV,‡ IM	H (40%), R (60%)	See **aspirin**. Use longer dosing interval in elderly, renal insufficiency. 99% protein bound ‡IV not FDA approved, but causes no hemodynamic changes.
Levorphanol (Levo-Dromoran)	Narc ag	2–3 mg q6–8h	PO, IV, SQ	H	Potency = morphine, > meperidine. Less nausea, constipation than either 40–50% protein bound
Lorazepam (Ativan)	GABA ag	0.05 mg/kg q4–6h	IV, IM, PO SL	H	Propylene glycol vehicle, 85% protein bound, sedation, resp depression
Mefenamic acid (Ponstel)	NSAID	250 mg q6h	PO	H/R	Parent drug and metabolites excreted in urine. See **aspirin**. Reversible platelet dysfunction
Meperidine (Demerol)	Narc ag	0.5–1.0 mg/kg	IV (dd), IM	HM (90%), R (10%)	Active metabolite accumulates in renal failure, causes CNS excitement (seizures). First-pass effect 50%, protein binding 40–80%
Metaclopromide (Reglan)	GI stimulant Antiemetic	10–15 mg q6h 10 mg q6h	PO IV	H (80%), R (20%)	>50% first-pass metabolism, can cause extrapyramidal symptoms. <20% protein bound
Methadone (Dolophine)	Narc ag	2.5–10 mg	IV, IM, PO	H	$t_{1/2}$ about 24h, accumulates, 75% protein bound. No first-pass effect
Methohexital (Brevital)	Barbiturate	Sedation: 5–10 mg/kg 20–35 mg/kg	IV PR	H (99%)	Rectal bioavailability 17%
Methylphenidate (Ritalin)	CNS stimulant	5–10 mg qAM§	PO	H (99%)	See **dextroamphetamine**. §May repeat (Ritalin) dose midday if needed. 15% protein binding

*Narc ag = narcotic agonist, TCA = tricyclic antidepressant, NSAID = nonsteroidal anti-inflammatory drug, NM blocker = neuromuscular blocker, antag = antagonist, Maj tranq = major tranquilizer, Musc relax = muscle relaxant, Antihist = antihistamine, Antichol = anticholinergic.
**H = hepatic metabolism, Hm = hepatic with active metabolites, R = renal excretion, dd = divided doses.

	Class*	Dose	Route	Metabolism/ excretion**	Comments
Metocurine (Metubine)	NM blocker	**Intubation:** 0.2–0.4 mg/kg	IV	R (30–40%)	Mild histamine release, hypotension, protein binding
Midazolam (Versed)	GABA ag	0.07–0.08 mg/kg 0.2 mg/kg 0.2–0.6 mg/kg	IV IM Intranasal PO	H (99%)	Water soluble, otherwise see **lorazepam**. Signif first-pass effect. Uremia increases free fraction. Protein binding 95%
Misoprostol (Cytotec)	GI mucosal protectant	200 µg q6h	PO	Various active metabolites	Use 100 µg dose if 200 µg not tolerated. Dose-related diarrhea. Parent compound inactive. Protein binding of active metabolite 90%. Potential abortifacient
Mivacurium (Mivacron)	NM blocker	**Intubation:** 0.07–0.2 mg/kg	IV	Plasma cholinesterase	Hypotension, vasodilation, tachy- or bradycardia
Morphine	Narc ag	**Sedation/pain:** 0.1–0.2 mg/kg prn **Infusion:** 0.01–0.06 mg/kg/h **Epidurally:** 0.03–0.05 mg/kg q12–24h	IV (dd), IM	H (90%)	Active metabolite Resp depression, esp. in renal failure. 35% protein bound
Nabumetone (Relafen)	NSAID	1000 mg q12–24h	PO	H	Activated in liver. See **aspirin**. Reversible platelet dysfunction
Nalbuphine (Nubain)	Narc ag-antag	0.1–0.2 mg/kg	IV (dd), IM	H (>90%)	See **buprenorphine**. 2–5 mg IV can reverse narc-induced resp depression, biliary spasm

Drug	Class	Dose	Route	Metabolism**	Comments
Naloxone (Narcan)	Narc antag	1–10 μg/kg q2min 0.01 mg/kg 1–10 μg/kg/h	IV, IM IM (neonate) Infusion	H (95%)	Reverse opioid-induced resp depression, sedation Lower doses treat itching, nausea, urinary retention from epidural narcotics; higher range for resp depression. Aggressive use may cause HTN, tachycardia, myocardial infarction. First-pass effect
Naltrexone (Trexan)	Narc antag	50 mg q24h	PO	Hm (95%)	Due to longer half-life, used to Rx side effects of epi morphine. Do not use until after naloxone challenge has been done (0.2 mg then 0.6 mg IV) due to risk of withdrawal. Significant first-pass metabolism. 20% protein bound
Odansetron (Zofran)	Antiemetic	**Cisplatin use:** 0.15–0.18 mg/kg q2h × 3 doses **Noncisplatin use:** 4 mg q6h or 8 mg q8h	PO, IV, IM	H (90%)	Most often used in conjunction with chemotherapy. Very expensive. 70% protein bound
Oxycodone (Percocet, Tylox)	Narc ag	5 mg q6h	PO	H	Avail with ASA or acetaminophen. No first-pass effect
Pancuronium (Pavulon)	NM blocker	Intubation: 0.1 mg/kg	IV	Hm (35%), R (65%)	Tachycardia. Protein binding <10%. Avoid in patients with creatinine clearance < 10 mL/min

*Narc ag = narcotic agonist, TCA = tricyclic antidepressant, NSAID = nonsteroidal anti-inflammatory drug, NM blocker = neuromuscular blocker, antag = antagonist, Maj tranq = major tranquilizer, Musc relax = muscle relaxant, Antihist = antihistamine, Antichol = anticholinergic.
**H = hepatic metabolism, Hm = hepatic with active metabolites, R = renal excretion, dd = divided doses.

	Class*	Dose	Route	Metabolism/excretion**	Comments
Pentazocine (Talwin)	Narc ag–antag	50–100 mg q3–4h 30 mg q3–4h	PO IV, IM, SQ	H (95%)	Can induce withdrawal in narcotic-dependent patients; high lipid solubility
Pentobarbital (Nembutal)	Barbiturate	**Sedation:** 100 mg q2min (max 500 mg) **Barb. coma:** Load 5–35mg/kg **Infusion:** 1–4mg/kg/h	IV, PO	H/R	Resp depression, myocardial depression, increased venous compliance, hypotension. Propylene glycol vehicle induced hypotension, anaphylaxis. Enzyme induction. 5% protein bound
Phenobarbital (Luminal)	Barbiturate	**Sedation:** 30–120 mg qd (dd) **Infusion:** <2 mg/kg/h	PO, IM, IV	H (80%), R (20%)	See pentobarbital Propylene glycol based → hypotension
Phenylbutazone (Butazolidin)	NSAID	100 mg q6–8h	PO	Hm (95%)	High toxicity profile (can cause bone marrow suppression). Tends to accumulate. See **aspirin**. 95% protein bound
Phenytoin (Dilantin)	Anticonvulsant	100 mg q8–12h Titrate dose to: 15–20 μg/mL (blood)	PO, IV	H	Blood dyscrasias, liver and renal dysfunction. Contains propylene glycol → hypotension
Pipecuronium (Mivacur)	NM blocker	**Intubation:** 0.07–0.085 mg/kg	IV	H (60%), R (40%)	Bradycardia, hypotension, hypertension. Adjust dose if creatinine clearance is decreased. Protein binding 32%

Drug	Class	Dose	Route	Metabolism**	Comments
Piroxicam (Feldene)	NSAID	20 mg q24h	PO	H (95%)	See aspirin. Reversible platelet dysfunction. 99% protein bound
Prochlorperazine (Compazine)	Maj tranq Sedative	Acute agitation: 10–20 mg q1–4h prn Prolonged Rx: 10–20 mg q4–6h	IM, PR PO	H	High incidence of extrapyramidal effects, antiemetic
Promethazine (Phenergan)	Antihist Sedative	25–50 mg	PO, PR IV, IM	H	See prochlorperazine. Significant first-pass effect. 93% protein bound
Propofol (Diprivan)	Gen anesthetic	Induction GA: 1.5–2.5 mg/kg Infusion: 25–100 μg/kg/min	IV	H (99%)	Bolus can cause hypotension. Intralipid vehicle can add significant calories if used as an infusion. 97% protein bound
Propoxyphene (Darvon)	Narc ag	32–65 mg q4h	PO	Hm (99%)	Weak agonist, active metabolite, higher risk of toxicity in renal or hepatic disease. 10% protein bound.
Ranitidine (Zantac)	H₂ blocker	150 mg q12h or 50 mg q6–8h Continuous infusion: 300 mg q24h	PO IV, IM	H (30%), R (70%)	See cimetidine. High doses can cause abnormal liver function tests. 15% protein bound. No supplementation necessary with dialysis
Salsalate (Disalcid)	NSAID	500 mg q4h (max 3000 mg/d)	PO	Hm, sm intestine	See aspirin. Hydrolyzed to salicylic acid. 80% protein bound. Reversible platelet dysfunction
Scopolomine (Transderm-Scop)	Antichol Antiemetic	Amnesia: 0.3–0.6 mg q6–8h Antiemesis: 1.5 mg patch q3d	IV Transdermal	H (99%)	Some patients may need higher doses. Good for amnesia in unstable patients. May be used in ophthalmologic preparation

*Narc ag = narcotic agonist, TCA = tricyclic antidepressant, NSAID = nonsteroidal anti-inflammatory drug, NM blocker = neuromuscular blocker, antag = antagonist, Maj tranq = major tranquilizer, Musc relax = muscle relaxant, Antihist = antihistamine, Antichol = anticholinergic.
**H = hepatic metabolism, Hm = hepatic with active metabolites, R = renal excretion, dd = divided doses.

	Class*	Dose	Route	Metabolism/excretion**	Comments
Secobarbital (Seconal)	Barbiturate	**Sedation:** 100–300 mg (1–2 h before procedure) Peds: 2–6 mg/kg **Agitation:** 30–50 mg q5min (max 500 mg)	PO IV	Hm (99%)	See **pentobarbital**. 50–60% protein bound
Sodium salicylate	NSAID	325–650 mg q4–6h	PO	H (90%)	See **aspirin**. Reversible platelet dysfunction. Doesn't cause bronchospasm. 80–90% protein bound
Succinylcholine	NM blocker	**Adults:** 1–1.5 mg/kg **Neonates, infants:** 2 mg/kg **Children:** 2.5–4 mg/kg	IV IV IM	Pseudocholinesterase	Hypo- or hypertension, brady- or tachycardia, trigger malignant hyperthermia, increase intraocular pressure, hyperkalemia, myoglobinuria
Sucralfate (Carafate)	GI mucosal protectant	1 g q6h	PO	Not absorbed	Binds to ulcer crater. Requires acid for activation. Minimal bioavailability (< 5%)
Sufentanil (Sufenta)	Narc ag	0.2–0.8 µg/kg qh	IV	H, sm intestine	Signif hepatic extraction. 93% protein bound
Sulindac (Clinoril)	NSAID	150–200 mg q12h	PO	Hm	See **aspirin**. Inactive parent compound. Reversible platelet dysfunction. 93% protein bound

Drug	Class	Dose	Route	Metabolism**	Comments
Thiopental (Pentothal)	Barbiturate	**Agitation:** Load 2–5 mg/kg Infuse 1–5 mg/kg/h **Sedation:** 25 mg/kg **ICP control:** 100–500 mg bolus **Barb coma:** Load 20 mg/Kg (×1h) Infuse 3–10 mg/kg/h	IV PR IV IV	H (primary) R (secondary)	See **pentobarbital**. 60–95% protein bound.
Trazadone (Desyrel)	TCA	50–600 mg qd (dd higher doses)	PO	H	Fewer anticholinergic effects than amitriptyline, doxepin. 90% protein bound
d-Tubocurarine (Curare)	NM blocker	**Intubation:** 0.6 mg/kg	IV	40% bile/45% R	Histamine release, hypotension. 50% protein bound
Valproic acid (Depakote)	Anticonvulsant	15 mg/kg/d [serum] = 50–150 μg/mL	PO	H (98%)	Can cause bone marrow suppression and altered platelet function. 91% protein bound
Vecuronium (Norcuron)	NM blocker	**Intubation:** 0.1 mg/kg	IV	Hm§, spontaneous deacetylation	Bradycardia when admin. with fentanyl. §Long-acting metabolite. 30% protein bound.

*Narc ag = narcotic agonist, TCA = tricyclic antidepressant, NSAID = nonsteroidal anti-inflammatory drug, NM blocker = neuromuscular blocker, antag = antagonist, Maj tranq = major tranquilizer, Musc relax = muscle relaxant, Antihist = antihistamine, Antichol = anticholinergic.
**H = hepatic metabolism, Hm = hepatic with active metabolites, R = renal excretion, dd = divided doses.

INDEX

Page numbers followed by *f* denote figures; page numbers followed by *t* denote tables.

A-*alpha* nerve fibers, 31*f*, 32
Abdominal pain, 439–441, 474
A-*beta* nerve fibers, 31*f*, 32
Absorption of drugs, 87–88
Accessory muscles of inspiration, 323
Acetaminophen, 104, 105*t*, 106, 113
   dosage, 107*t*, 574*t*
   hepatic metabolism, 362, 363*t*
   HIV/AIDS medication, 475
   metabolism, 574*t*
   pain management in children, 510, 511*t*
   for posttraumatic headaches, 275
   risk of use during pregnancy, 537
Acetic acids, dosage and dosage forms, 107*t*
Acetylcholine, physiology, 194–195
Acetylsalicylic acid, 104, 105*t*
   antiplatelet effect, 112
   dosage, 106*t*, 574*t*
   forms to reduce gastric irritation, 110
   for HIV/AIDS-related pain, 475
   impact of coagulopathy on, 385–386
   induced hepatitis, 113
   metabolism, 574*t*
   for pericarditis, 310
   platelet abnormalities caused by, 377*t*, 378
   for posttraumatic headaches, 275
   risk of use during pregnancy, 537
   for tension headaches, 274
Acid-base imbalance, 202
Acidic nonsteroidal anti-inflammatory
     agents, by classes, 104, 105*t*, 106
Acidosis, 41*t*
Acquired cardiac dysfunction, 391
Acquired immunodeficiency syndrome
     (AIDS) (*see* HIV/AIDS)
Active metabolites, 89–90
Acupuncture, 236, 237*f*, 240, 248, 452
Acute anterior poliomyelitis, 291
Acute blunt trauma, 311
Acute epidural hematoma headaches, 277–278
Acute hypokalemia, 202
Acute inflammatory
     polyradiculoneuropathy, 288–289
Acute intoxication, 497, 499*t*, 501*t*–502*t*
Acute pain, 28–29, 30*t*, 444
   adverse effects, 34, 35*t*
   characteristics, 56*t*
   chronic and, compared, 29, 30*t*, 56*t*
   defined, 571
   in terminally ill patients, 482–483
Acute pain control
   acute pain service, 452
   corticosteroids for, 108
   nonsteroidal anti-inflammatory drugs for,
     104, 109–110, 114
   in terminally ill patients, 483

Acute pain syndromes, 491
Acute pancreatitis, 366–367
Acute pulmonary hypertension pain, 328
Acute renal failure (ARF), 340–341
Acute splenic enlargement, 383
Acute subdural hematoma headaches, 278
Acute tubular necrosis (ATN), 340
Acute vascular occlusion, 311–312
Acyclovir, 90*t*, 473–474
Adapin (*see* Doxepin)
Adaptive devices, 263
Addiction, 496–497, 506
Additive interactions, 99
A-*delta* nerve fibers, 31*f*, 32
Adenosine triphosphate (ATP), 158
Adjunctive medications, 104–106, 451
Adjunctive therapy, 490
Administration routes, 414–415
Administration techniques
   epidural analgesia, 214–216, 217*t*–218*t*
   general issues, 208–209
   parenteral techniques, 211–212, 212*t*–213*t*, 214
   peripheral nerve blocks, 225–227
   plexus blocks, 225
   regional analgesia, 209–211
   subarachnoid (spinal) analgesia, 219–221
   sympathetic nerve blocks, 221–224
   trigger point injections, 227
Adolescents, attitudes of, 61*t*, 62–63
Adrenal medulla, stimulation, 43
alpha-Adrenergic blocking agents, 285
beta-Adrenergic blocking drugs, 547
Adrenocortical hormones, 256*t*
Adrenocorticotropic hormone (ACTH), 42, 45, 426*t*, 427
Adult respiratory distress syndrome (ARDS), 42–43
   in multiple system organ failure, 391, 394
   pathophysiology, 324–325, 325*t*, 326
   in pretransplant patients, 459
   respiratory failure caused by, 320*t*
   uncomplicated, pain, 328
Advil (*see* Ibuprofen)
A-esters (local anesthetic), structure of, 160*f*
Affective principles, 57
Afrin nasal spray, 274–275
Afterload failure, 302
Agitation, 48–49
Agonist-antagonists (*see also* Agonists;
     Antagonists)
   analgesic effects, 131
   for cancer pain, 554
   narcotic
     contraindicated in terminally ill
       patients, 491
     dosage, 575*t*–576*t*, 580*t*–581*t*

587

Agonist-antagonists *(continued)*
  metabolism, 575t–576t, 580t–581t
  for pancreatitis pain, 367
  for postoperative pain management, 451
  risk of use during pregnancy, 537–541
  for neurologic disease pain, 296–297
  opioid, 131f, 132–135
    classification, 122, 123t
    for renal disease, 352–353
    for renal insufficiency, 350t–351t, 352–353
    for respiratory failure, 332
Agonists *(see also* Agonist–antagonists)
  dosage and metabolism, 574t, 576t–577t, 579t–581t, 583t–584t
  gamma-aminobutyric acid (GABA), 576t, 579t–580t
  narcotic, 574t, 577t, 579t–581t, 583t–584t
  opioid
    classification, 122, 123t
    gastrointestinal effects, 140–141
    for neurologic disease pain, 296–297
    for renal disease, 349, 350t–351t, 352
    for renal insufficiency, 349, 350t–351t, 352
    respiratory effects, 139
Airway management, 192–194, 281, 295
Airway obstruction, upper, 320t
Airway resistance, 323
Albumin, 87t, 162
Alclofenac, 104, 105t, 106
Alcohol, for sympathetic nerve blocks, 222–223
Alcohol abuse, 495–498, 499t
Alcoholics, 496, 503
Alcohol withdrawal, 282–283, 498–499, 499t, 500
Aldosterone, 44, 426t–427t
Alfenta *(see* Alfentanil)
Alfentanil, 119f, 120
  cardiovascular disease effects, 313
  cardiovascular effects, 137
  classification, 122, 123t
  distribution, 128t
  dosage, 436, 437t, 574t
  elimination, 128
  intracranial pressure effects, 280
  metabolism, 362, 363t, 574t
  for multiple system organ failure, 396
  protein binding, 128, 128t
  receptor subtype, 121, 122t
  for respiratory failure, 332t
  structure, 119f
Algesic mediators, 34
Algoneurodystrophy, 545
Alkaline phosphatase, 362t
Alkanoic acids, by classes, 104, 105t, 106

Allergic purpura, 376
Allergic reactions, succinylcholine, 198
Allodynia, defined, 571
Alpha$_1$-acid glycoprotein, 87t, 162
Alpha-adrenergic blocking agents, 285
Alphaprodine, 537
Alprazolam, 431
Altered drug clearance, 99
Altered receptor binding, 88, 97–98
Altered responsiveness, 98
Alveolar dead space, 321
Alveolar gas equation, 322
Amantadine, 287, 292
Ambulation, of critically ill patient, 263–264
Amidate *(see* Etomidate)
Amide local anesthetics, 362, 363t
B-Amides, structure of, 160f
Amikacin, 93f, 94
Aminoglycoside antibiotics, 202
p-Aminophenols, 104, 105t, 106
Amitriptyline
  administration, 185
  for amyotrophic lateral sclerosis, 287
  for chronic pain in transplant patients, 463
  for diabetic neuropathy, 289
  dosage, 574t
  for herpes zoster, 473–474
  metabolism, 574t
  for multiple sclerosis, 287
  for neuralgic pain, 549
  for pancreatitis pain, 367
  pharmacokinetic characteristics, 185t
  for postherpetic neuralgia, 292
  for posttraumatic headaches, 275
  for reflex sympathetic dystrophy, 293
  for spinal cord compression, 285
  for tension headaches, 274
  for vasculitic neuropathy, 291
Amnesia, general anesthesia induced, 144
Amobarbital, risk of use during pregnancy, 537
Amphetamines, 501, 502t, 554
Ampicillin, 377t
Amrinone, 308
Amyloidosis, 375
Amyotrophic lateral sclerosis (ALS), 287
Anafranil (clomipramine), 538
Analgesics/analgesia *(see also* Nonnarcotic analgesics), 510, 511t
  administration routes *(see also* Administration techniques), 297–298, 315–317
  agents, 107–109
  antipyretic, 537
  cardiovascular effects, 50
  defined, 571
  dosage, 574t

INDEX **589**

epidural (see Epidural analgesia)
general anesthesia induced (see also Inhalation anesthesia/analgesia), 144, 154–155
inhalation (see Inhalation anesthesia/analgesia)
intracranial pressure effects, 280–281
intrapleural analgesia, 437–438
intrathecal, 436, 437t
metabolism, 574t
for myocardial infarction, 308
narcotic
   for pancreatitis pain, 366
   for postoperative pain control, 448–449, 450t
   for postoperative pain management, 448–449
   for trauma pain, side effects, 429–430
narcotic-addicted person's needs, 500–501
for neurologic disease pain, 296–298
nonnarcotic (see Nonnarcotic analgesics)
patient-controlled (see Patient-controlled analgesia)
peridural (see Peridural analgesia)
regional (see Regional analgesia)
for respiratory failure, 331, 332t–333t
risk of use during pregnancy, 537–541
routes in respiratory failure, 334–335, 336t
spinal (see Spinal analgesia)
techniques, 385–386, 476–477
for tetanus, 295
thoracic epidural, 465
for traumatic injuries, 439–441
withholding of, 564–565
Anaprox (naproxen sodium), 106t
Anasarca, 259
Anatomic dead space, 321t
Anatomic framework in children, 509
Anectine (see Succinylcholine)
Anesthetics/anesthesia
   administration (see also Administration techniques), 316–317
   for cutaneous injury pain, 416–417
   general, 144, 145t, 154–155, 315, 583t
   local
      amide, 362, 363t
      carbonated solutions, 167
      cardiovascular disease effects, 315
      dosage, 165, 166t, 217, 218t
      epidural (see Epidural local anesthetics)
      ester, 357
      eutectic mixture, (EMLA), 473–474
      for herpes zoster, 473–474
      interpleural, 547
      isomers, duration and toxicity, 162t, 163
      for multiple system organ failure, 396–397
      narcotic combined, 217, 218t, 435, 449, 450t
      for neurologic disease pain, 297
      neuromuscular blockade potentiation with, 202
      peridural (see Peridural local anesthetics)
      perispinal, 216, 217t, 449, 450t
      pharmacology
         action, 158, 159f, 166, 167t, 168
         chemical properties, 159, 160f, 160t, 161f, 162t, 163
         chiral forms, 160f, 162t, 163
         equipotent concentrations, 159, 160t
         ionization, 160, 161f
         lipid solubility, 159, 160f, 160t
         modification of onset of action, 166–167, 167t, 168
         opiate, combinations, 168
         peak blood levels, 163, 164f, 165
         physical properties, 159, 160f, 160t, 161f, 162t, 163
         protein binding, 160t, 162
         safety, applications to improve, 165, 166t
         stereoisomers, 160f, 162t, 163
         structure, 159, 160f–161f
         toxicity, 162t, 163–165
      for respiratory failure, 332, 333t
      in pregnancy, risk of, 537–541
      in respiratory failure, routes, 334–335, 336t
      trace exposure, 151–152
   volatile, 202
Aneurysm malformation in pregnant patients, 534
Anger, pain threshold influenced by, 28, 29t
Angina, persistent, 305
Angina decubitus, 303–304
Angina pectoris, 303–304
Angiotensin converting enzyme (ACE) inhibitor therapy, 111, 112t
Angiotensin II, 44
Ankles, positioning of, for contractures, 260t
Anorexia, immobility negative effect, 256t
Ansaid (flurbiprofen), 104, 105t–106t
Antacid/aspirin compounds, 110
Antagonism, pharmacodynamics and, 99
Antagonists (see also Agonist–antagonists)
   for cancer pain, 554
   dosage, 577t, 581t
   gamma-aminobutyric acid (GABA), 577t
   metabolism, 577t, 581t
   narcotic, 313–314, 537–541, 581t
   opioid, 122, 123t, 135–136
   risk of use during pregnancy, 537–541

Antalgesia, defined, 571
Antianxiety agents, 451
Antibiotics, 93f, 94, 274–275
Antibodies to receptor sites, 98
Anticholinergics
  adverse effects, 178, 184
  common medications, 178–179
  contraindications, 178
  dosage, 574t, 578t, 583t
  excessive activity, 184
  indications, 178
  metabolism, 574t, 578t, 583t
Anticholinesterase, 203, 294
Anticoagulant-induced bleeding, 379–380
Anticoagulation, 209–210
Anticonvulsants (*see also specific drugs*), 185
  adverse effects, 186
  common medications, 186–187
  dosage, 575t, 582t, 585t
  for HIV/AIDS-related pain, 476
  indications, 186
  metabolism, 575t, 582t, 585t
  for neuralgic pain, 548–549
  for postherpetic neuralgia, 292
  for reflex sympathetic dystrophy, 293
  risk of use during pregnancy, 537–541
  for terminally ill patients, 490
Antidepressants (*see also specific drugs*)
  for neuralgic pain, 549
  pain threshold influenced by, 28, 29t
  for pancreatitis pain, 367
  risk of use during pregnancy, 537–541
  for sympathetically mediated pain, 547
  for terminally ill patients, 490
  tricyclic, 183–184, 185t
Antidiuretic hormone (ADH), 44, 426t–427t
Antiemetics, 537–541, 579t, 581t, 583t
Antihemophiliac factor, 382
Antihistamines
  adverse effects, 178
  common medications, 178–179
  contraindications, 178
  dosage, 574t, 577t–578t, 583t
  indications, 178
  metabolism, 574t, 577t–578t, 583t
  for postoperative pain management, 451
  risk of use during pregnancy, 537–541
Anti-inflammatories (*see* Corticosteroids; Nonsteroidal anti–inflammatory drugs)
Antipruritics, 537–541
Antipsychotic drugs, 333–334
Antipyretics, 537–541
Antispasticity agents, 284–285
Anuric acute renal failure, 340–341
Anxiety, 28, 29t, 41t, 48, 49f, 50–51
Anxiolytics, 28, 29t, 490, 576t
Aortic insufficiency, 312–313

Aortic stenosis, 312–313, 533
Apnea, prolonged, 198
Arachidonic acid derivatives, 31
Arduan (*see* Pipecuronium)
Areflexia, general anesthesia induced, 144
Arrested grief response, 58, 59t
Arsenic poisoning, 290
Arterial insufficiency, wound pain from, 421
Arteriolar constriction, 45–46
Arteriovenous malformation, 534
Arthritic pain, physiologic, 483
Arthritis, 551–552
Arthropan (choline salicylate), 106t
Aryl acetic acids, 104, 105t, 106
Ascending pain pathways, 32, 33f, 34
Aspirin (*see* Acetylsalicylic acid)
Asthma, 113, 154–155
Asthma/bronchospasm, 320t
Atarax (*see* Hydroxyzine)
Atelectasis/secretions, 320t
Atenolol, 90t, 273
Ativan (*see* Lorazepam)
Atracurium
  cardiovascular side effects, 201t
  clearance, 200t, 201
  dosage, 199t, 574t
  histamine release, 201t
  for intubation, 281
  metabolism, 574t
  for renal disease, 350t–351t, 354
Atrophy, respiratory failure caused by, 320t
Autogenics training, 242
Autonomic hyperreflexia, 285
Axilla, positioning for contractures, 260t
Azapropazone, 104, 105t, 106, 113
Azidothymidine (AZT), 471, 475
Azotemia, renal failure associated, 341

Back pain, low, HIV/AIDS related, 473
Baclofen, 188
  administration, 189
  for amyotrophic lateral sclerosis, 287
  dosage, 574t
  metabolism, 574t
  for multiple sclerosis, 287
  pharmacokinetic parameters, 189
  for spinal cord compression, 284–285
  for thalamic pain syndrome, 286
Bacterial overgrowth, 48
BAL (British antilewisite), 289–290
B-amides (local anesthetics), structure of, 160f
Barbiturates, 173
  administration, 175
  adverse effects, 174
  common medications, 175t, 176
  contraindications, 174–175, 491
  dosage, 579t, 582t, 584t–585t

hemodynamic function effects, 145t
hepatic metabolism, 362, 363t
indications, 174
intracranial pressure effects, 280
for intravenous anesthesia, 152–153
for liver transplant patients, 458
for multiple system organ failure, 398–399
pharmacokinetic parameters, 174, 175t
Barrier integrity, drug distribution and, 89
Bed rest, problems with prolonged, 393
Behavior, patient, pain assessment and, 16–17
Behavioral accommodation, 55, 56t
Behavioral assessment, patient, 18
Behavioral observation, 448
Benadryl (*see* Diphenhydramine)
Benoxaprofen, 104, 105t, 106
Benzodiazepines, 170
　abuse, 502–503
　adverse effects, 171
　for alcohol withdrawal, 282–283, 498–500
　for anesthetic-induced seizures, 165
　for anxiety following injury, 431
　common medications, 172–173
　contraindications, 171–172
　hepatic metabolism, 362, 363t
　indications, 171
　intracranial pressure effects, 280–281
　for intubation, 281
　for liver transplant patients, 458, 462
　for multiple system organ failure, 397–398
　for neurologic disease pain, 297
　pharmacokinetic parameters, 172t
　for renal disease, 353
　for respiratory failure, 333, 334t
　for spinal cord compression, 284–285
　tolerance, 503
　withdrawal symptoms, 502–503
Benzomorphan derivatives, 120
Benztropine, 334, 574t
Benzylisoquinoline alkaloids, 118
Best interest doctrine, 486–487
Beta-adrenergic blocking drugs, 547
Beta-blocking drugs, 308, 501
Beta-endorphins, 42–43, 121, 122t
Bicarbonate, 167t
Bier (IV regional) blocks, 223–224, 547
Bile stasis, 392
Biliary colic, 365
Biliary dilatation, 392
Biliary pain, 363
Biliary spasms, 140–141
Bioavailability, 94
Biofeedback, 242, 418, 452, 477, 547
Biopharmaceutics, 88, 89t–90t
Bleeding, from spinal analgesia, 219
Bleeding diatheses, 383
Bleeding disorders, 381t, 383–384

Bleeding time, hemostasis screening test, 376t
Blocadren (nadolol), 273, 276t
Blockades, 6–7, 202, 514, 515t–516t, 517
H_2-Blockers, 377
beta-Blocking drugs, 308, 501
Blocks
　administration (*see* Administration techniques)
　Bier (intravenous regional), 223–224
　brachial plexus, 224–225, 547
　celiac plexus (CPB), 222–223
　cervical plexus, 225
　cervicothoracic, 221–222, 546
　dorsal ramus, 461
　hypogastric plexus, 547
　lumbar plexus, 225
　lumbar sympathetic (LSB), 222, 477, 546
　peridural, 547
　plexus (*see* Plexus blocks)
　stellate, 221–222, 546
　sympathetic, 316, 477
　thoracic ganglion, 546
Blood alcohol level (BAL), 497–498
Blood flow, 88, 99–100
Blood levels, peak, of anesthetics, 163, 164f
Blood pressure (BP), 145t, 282, 501t–502t, 524t
Blood volume, increased in pregnancy, 524t
Blunt trauma, in pregnant patients, 534–535
Bolus administrations, 316
Bone marrow infiltration, 383
Bone marrow transplants (*see also* Transplantation), 457t, 465
Bone pain, 342–343
Botulism, 294
Bowel edema, 48
Bowel ischemia, 48
Bowel motility, decreased, 48
Bowel regimens, 490, 554
Brachial plexus blocks (*see also* Plexus blocks), 224–225, 547
Bradycardia, opioid, 137
Bradykinin, 31, 45
Brain abscess, headache from, 276–277
Breathing, factors controlling, 324
Bretylium, 574t
Bretylol (bretylium), 574t
Brevital (*see* Methohexital)
Brief psychotherapy, 243
British antilewisite (BAL), 290
Bronchiectasis pain, 327
Bronchoconstriction, 503
Buffered aspirin (*see also* Acetylsalicylic acid), 110
Bufferin (buffered aspirin), 110
Bupivacaine
　anesthetic duration, 162t, 163

Bupivacaine *(continued)*
  bicarbonate to adjust pH of, 167*t*
  cardiac toxicity, 164–165
  for chest pain, 311
  distribution, 87*t*
  dosage, 166*t*, 217, 218*t*, 516*t*, 518*t*
  for epidural analgesia, 217, 218*t*, 529*t*
  equipotent concentration, 160*t*
  intrapleural injection of, 437–438
  lipid solubility, 159, 160*f*, 160*t*
  for multiple system organ failure, 396
  for patient-controlled analgesia, 217, 218*t*
  for peripheral nerve blocks, 226–227
  pharmacokinetic properties, 515
  for plexus blocks, 224–225
  protein binding, 87*t*, 160*t*, 162
  for respiratory failure, 333*t*
  risk of use during pregnancy, 537
  for spinal analgesia, 217*t*–218*t*, 220–221
  structure of, 160*f*
  for sympathetic nerve blocks, 222–223
  toxicity, 162*t*, 164–165
  for traumatic injuries, 440
  use in children and neonates, 515
Buprenex *(see* Buprenorphine)
Buprenorphine
  agonist-antagonist properties, 133
  analgesic effects, 133
  classification, 122, 123*t*
  distribution, 133
  dosage, 211, 212*t*, 433*t*, 436, 437*t*, 575*t*
  equipotent IV dosage and side effects, 433*t*
  metabolism, 133, 575*t*
  for parenteral administration, 211, 212*t*
  for renal disease, 350*t*–351*t*, 352–353
  respiratory depression from, 133
  for respiratory failure, 332
  side effects, 133–134, 429
  for spinal use, 436, 437*t*
  structure, 131*f*
  for trauma pain, 429
  withdrawal, 133–134
Burns *(see also* Cutaneous injuries), 202
BuSpar (buspirone), 431
Buspirone, 431
Butazolidin *(see* Phenylbutazone)
Butorphanol
  abuse potential, 133
  agonist-antagonist properties, 132–133
  analgesic effects, 132
  classification, 122, 123*t*
  dosage, 211, 212*t*, 433*t*, 436, 437*t*, 575*t*
  equipotent IV dosage and side effects, 433*t*
  gastrointestinal effects, 140–141
  hepatic metabolism, 362, 363*t*
  intramuscular injection, 132
  metabolism, 575*t*
  parenteral administration, 211, 212*t*
  for the pregnant patient, 527–528
  receptor subtype, 121, 122*t*
  for renal disease, 350*t*–351*t*, 352–353
  respiratory depression from, 132
  for respiratory failure, 332
  risk of use during pregnancy, 537
  side effects, 133
  for spinal use, 436, 437*t*
  structure, 131*f*
  withdrawal, 133
Butorphanol nasal spray, 430
Butyrophenones
  adverse effects, 180, 184
  cardiovascular disease effects, 314
  common medications, 181*t*, 182
  contraindications, 181
  indications, 180
  pharmacokinetic parameters, 181*t*
  for renal disease, 353
  for respiratory failure, 334

Cachectin, 45
Cafergot (ergotamine), 273
Caffeine, 275
Calcitonin, 547
Calcium channel blockers, 202
Cancer pain, 36, 483, 553–554, 571
Cannulation pain, dialysis associated, 346
Capsaicin, 292, 474
Carafate *(see* Sucralfate)
Carbamazepine
  administration, 187
  for diabetic neuropathy, 289
  distribution, 87*t*
  dosage, 575*t*
  for HIV/AIDS-related pain, 476
  inducer of drug metabolism, 100*t*
  metabolism, 575*t*
  for neuralgic pain, 548–549
  pharmacokinetic parameters, 187
  protein binding, 87*t*
  for reflex sympathetic dystrophy, 293
  risk of use during pregnancy, 537
  for vasculitic neuropathy, 291
Carbenicillin, 377*t*
Carbocaine *(see* Mepivacaine)
Carbohydrate metabolism, 48
Carbonated local anesthetic solutions, 167
Carbon dioxide production (V_{CO_2}), 46, 47*f*, 50
Carboxylic acids, 104, 105*t*, 106
Cardiac disease *(see* Cardiovascular disease and pain)
Cardiac ischemia pain *(see also* Cardiovascular disease and pain), 303–304
Cardiac-muscle oxygen transport, 303–304
Cardiac output, 145*t*, 524*t*

INDEX   **593**

Cardiac pain (*see* Cardiovascular disease and pain)
Cardiovascular disease and pain
 case study, 302, 317
 clinical manifestation of pain, 302–305
 dysfunction in HIV/AIDS, 470
 painful syndromes, 305–312
 pain management with preexisting disease, 312–317
 in pregnant patients, 532–534
Cardiovascular system
 adverse effects of
  acute pain, 34, 35*t*
  anticholinergics, 178
  antihistamines, 178
  barbiturates, 174
  benzodiazepines, 171
  chloral hydrate, 177
  immobility, 256*t*
  local anesthetics, 164–165
  tricyclic antidepressants, 184
 effects of
  metabolic stress response (MSR), 45–46
  narcotic use and withdrawal, 501*t*
  opioid use, 136–137, 138*f*, 138*t*
  pain and anxiety management, 50
  pregnancy, 524*t*, 525
Caregivers (*see also* Nursing issues)
 attitudes, 4–5, 46, 54
 chemical dependence in, 504, 505*t*, 506
 family, 491–493
 professional, 493
 for terminally ill patients, 491–493
Carpal tunnel syndrome, 345–346
Carprofen, 104, 105*t*, 106
Catabolic activity, accelerated, 256*t*
Catecholamines, 43, 306, 427*t*
Catheters
 placement techniques
  for epidural analgesia, 215–216, 430–431
  for traumatic injuries, 440–441
 pleural
  for administration of analgesic and sedative agents in ICU, 316
  impact of coagulopathy on, 386
  for neurologic disease pain, 298
  related infection in heart-lung transplant patients, 465
Cauda equina syndrome, 215
Caudal epidural blockade, 515, 516*t*, 517
Causalgia, 292–293, 544–545, 571
 sequelae to burns, 419
 symptoms and physical findings, 546*t*
Ceftazidime, 90*t*
Celiac plexus block (CPB), 222–223
Central compartment, 90, 91*f*, 92

Central nervous system (CNS)
 adverse effects of
  acute pain, 34, 35*t*
  anticholinergics, 178
  anticonvulsants, 186
  antihistamines, 178
  barbiturates, 174
  benzodiazepines, 171
  chloral hydrate, 177
  cocaine use and withdrawal, 502*t*
  tricyclic antidepressants, 184
 infections of, headaches from, 276–277
 physiologic effect of pain, 426*t*–427*t*
 spontaneous bleeding, 384
 stimulants, 576*t*, 579*t*
Central neural blockades, 6–7, 514, 515*t*–516*t*
Cerebral blood flow (CBF), 147, 148*f*–149*f*, 279
Cerebral metabolic rate (CMR), 139–140, 148*f*–149*f*
Cerebral metabolic rate of oxygen ($CMRO_2$), 155
Cerebral perfusion pressure (CPP), 279
Cerebral-spinal-fluid (CSF), 275–277
Cervical plexus blocks (*see also* Plexus blocks), 225
Cervicothoracic (stellate) blocks, 221–222, 546
Character disorders, 61*t*, 62–63
Chemical abuse (*see also* Drug abuse), 504, 505*t*, 506, 562–564
Chemicals, affect on pain receptors, 31
Chemotherapy, physiologic pain of, 483
Chest, positioning for contractures, 260*t*
Chest pain (*see also* Cardiovascular disease and pain), 311, 473–474
Chest wall compliance, 322–323
Chest wall restriction, 320*t*
Chest wall splinting, 427*t*
Children (*see also* Neonates; Pediatric patients)
 attitudes of, 61*t*, 62–63
 differences between, and adults, 508–509
 narcotic effects in, 126
 pain assessment in, 509, 510*f*
 pain management in critically ill, 507–521
  case studies, 508, 520–521
 pharmacologic management of pain
  neural blockade, 514, 515*t*–516*t*, 517
  nonopioid analgesics, 510, 511*t*
  opioid analgesics, 510, 511*t*–513*t*, 514
  peripheral nerve blocks, 517, 518*t*, 519
 risk of opiate addiction in, 508
Chiral forms of local anesthetics, 160*f*, 162*t*, 163
Chloral hydrate
 dosage, 575*t*

Chloral hydrate *(continued)*
  inducer of drug metabolism, 100*t*
  metabolism, 575*t*
  for renal disease, 350*t*–351*t*
  risk of use during pregnancy, 537
Chloral hydrate (NOCTEC), 176–177
Chloramphenicol for tetanus, 295
Chlordiazepoxide
  for alcohol withdrawal, 283
  for renal disease, 350*t*–351*t*, 353
  risk of use during pregnancy, 537
Chloroprocaine
  bicarbonate to adjust pH of, 167*t*
  dose, maximum, 166*t*
  protein binding, 162
  for respiratory failure, 333*t*
  risk of use during pregnancy, 537
  structure of, 160*f*
Chlorpromazine
  administration, 183
  for alcohol withdrawal, 283
  dosage, 575*t*
  metabolism, 575*t*
  for renal disease, 350*t*–351*t*, 353
  for respiratory failure, 333
  risk of use during pregnancy, 537
  for tetanus, 295
Cholecystectomy for biliary colic, 365
Choline magnesium salicylate, 510, 511*t*
Choline magnesium trisalicylate, 104, 105*t*–106*t*, 113, 575*t*
Cholinergic crisis, 294
Choline salicylate, 106*t*
Chronic extremity hypoperfusion, 312
Chronic infection, wound pain from, 421
Chronic pain, 28–29, 30*t*
  versus acute pain, 56*t*
  characteristics, 56*t*
  defined, 571
  nonsteroidal anti-inflammatory drugs for, 103
  in terminally ill patients, 483
Chronic pain syndromes
  arthritis, 550–551
  cancer pain, 553–554
  goals of management, 544
  low back pain, 550–551
  myofascial pain, 552–553
  neuralgic pain, 548–549
  phantom limb pain, 549
  stump pain, 549
  sympathetic mediated pain, 544–546, 546*t*, 547
  in terminally ill patients, 491
Chronic pancreatitis, 367–368
Chronic pulmonary hypertension, 328
Chronic renal failure (CRF) (*see also* Renal failure), 341

Chronic subdural hematoma headaches, 278
Chronotropy, 45–46
Cimetidine
  dosage, 575*t*
  gastric irritation reduced with, 111
  for HIV/AIDS-related pain, 475
  inhibitor of drug metabolism, 100*t*
  metabolism, 575*t*
Ciprofloxacin, 100*t*
Circuitry of pain, 30–31, 31*f*, 32, 33*f*, 34
Citanest (*see* Prilocaine)
Clearance (Cl), 94–96
Clinoril (*see* Sulindac)
Clomipramine, 538
Clonidine, 500, 547
Closed-head injuries, 534
Closing capacity (CC), 329–330
Clostridium botulinum, 294
Clostridium tetani, 294
C nerve fibers, 31*f*, 32
Coagulation cascade, 375, 376*f*
Coagulation factors
  acquired disorders, 379–380, 381*t*
  congenital disorders, 378–379
  Factor VIII-related von Willebrand's factor (VIII:vWF), 374
  normal, 375, 376*f*
  screening tests for, 376*t*
Coagulopathies
  impact on pain management, 384–386
  in multiple system organ failure, 392, 394
  in pregnancy-induced hypertension (PIH), 531–532
Cocaine use and withdrawal, 501, 502*t*
Codeine, 118
  classification, 122, 123*t*
  dosage, 211, 212*t*, 575*t*
  metabolism, 575*t*
  parenteral administration, 211, 212*t*
  risk of use during pregnancy, 538
  structure, 119*f*
  use in pediatric/neonate ICU, 512, 513*t*
Cogentin (benztropine), 334, 574*t*
Cognitive assessment, 258
Cognitive modulation of cardiac pain, 305
Cognitive principles, 57
Collagen vascular diseases, 202
Compartments, pharmacokinetic model, 90, 91*f*, 92
Compazine (*see* Prochlorperazine)
Compliance curve of the lung, 322
Compromised absorption, 48
Computed tomography (CT), 276–277, 283–284
Concomitant chronic pain syndromes (*see* Chronic pain syndromes)
Connective tissue, 375
Constipation, 256*t*, 501*t*

Continuous arteriovenous hemofiltration (CAVH), 345
Continuous drug infusion, 93f, 94–96
Continuous IV administration, 316
Continuous venovenous hemofiltration (CVVH), 345
Contractions, sustained, 198
Contractures
 immobility negative effect, 256t
 positioning to prevent, 258–259, 260t
 sequelae to burns, 419
Controlled attention or distraction, 418
Coping with pain
 background factors, 55
 energy for, 58
 individual difference factors, 60–61
 morbidity and, 411–412
 motivation for, 58
 psychology of pain factor, 60–61
 sensitizers, 60–61
 skills training, 71–72
 strategies, 55
 styles, 60–61
Corgard (timolol), 273
Corrective information, 55, 56t
Cortical reaction, 34, 35t
Corticosteroids
 as analgesic agent, 108
 anti-inflammatory effects, 108
 excessive, 375
 nonsteroidal anti-inflammatory drugs (NSAIDs) versus, 108
 for reflex sympathetic dystrophy, 293
 therapy, 108
Corticotropin releasing factor (CRF), 42, 45
Cortisol, 42–43, 426t–427t
Costochondritis, chest pain, 310
Coughing, 147, 193
Coumadin (see also Warfarin), 379–380, 381t
Crack cocaine use, 501, 502t
Cravings, 499t, 502t
Critical patients (see Intensive care unit: patients)
Crushing pain of pericarditis, 309–310
Cryoneurolysis, 439
Cryoprecipitate, 379, 381–382
Cryotherapy, 266, 267t
Curare (see Tubocurarine)
Cushing's syndrome, excessive, 375
Cutaneous injuries
 analgesic regimens for, 413–418
 arterial insufficiency induced pain, 421
 basic principles of pain therapy, 412–413
 case study, 406, 422–423
 chronic infection induced pain, 421
 factors influencing the pain of, 408–410
 influence on pain management, 421–422

 metabolic abnormalities, healing delayed by, 421
 neuropathies induced pain, 421
 neurophysiology of pain related to, 407–408
 phases of pain, 410–411
 pressure sores, 420–421
 rationale behind pain control, 411–412
 sequelae to, 418–420
 suggested readings, 423
 venous insufficiency induced pain, 421
Cutaneous rashes, with pruritus, 465
Cyclobenzaprine, 189, 575t
Cyclosporine, metabolism, 89t
Cytotec (see Misoprostol)

Dalgan (see Dezocine)
Dantrium (see Dantrolene)
Dantrolene
 administration, 189–190
 for amyotrophic lateral sclerosis, 287
 dosage, 576t
 metabolism, 576t
 for multiple sclerosis, 287
 neuromuscular blockade potentiation with, 202
 pharmacokinetic parameters, 189
 for spinal cord compression, 284–285
 for thalamic pain syndrome, 286
Darvon (see Propoxyphene)
Dead space, 321
Dead space to tidal volume (V_D/V_T) ratio, 321–322
Deafferentation pain, 484, 571–572
Debridement, 408, 411, 420–421
Decongestants, for sinus headaches, 274–275
Decubitus ulcers, 256t, 258–259
Deep heat, 264–266
Deep massage, 262, 451
Dehydration, MSR activator, 41t
Delirium tremens (DTs), 282, 498–499, 499t
Delta receptors, 32, 121, 122t
Demerol (see Meperidine)
Depakene (see Valproic acid)
Depakote (see Valproic acid)
Dependence, 497, 510–511
Depolarization, 158
Depolarizing agents, 195–198
Depression, 18, 28, 29t, 252–253
Deprol (meprobamate), 295, 539
Descending circuits of pain, 34
Desipramine, 538, 549
Desyrel (trazodone), 463, 549, 585t
Devices, adaptive, 263
Dexamethasone, 283
Dexedrine (dextroamphetamine), 490, 576t
Dextroamphetamine, 490, 576t
Dextromethorphan, 122, 123t

Dezocine
  agonist-antagonist properties, 134–135
  analgesic effects, 134–135
  classification, 122, 123t
  dosage, 576t
  hepatic metabolism, 362, 363t
  metabolism, 135, 576t
  for multiple system organ failure, 396
  physical dependence, 134–135
  for renal disease, 350t–351t, 352–353
  respiratory depression from, 134–135
  for respiratory failure, 332
  side effects, 135, 429
  for trauma pain, 429
Diabetes, 305
Diabetic neuropathy symptoms, 289
Dialysis, 90t, 344–346
Dialysis dementia, 346
Diaphragm, 323
Diaphragmatic breathing, 258
Diaphragmatic contractility, 427t
Diarrhea, 501t
Diastolic blood pressure (DBP), 499t
Diathermy, 265–266
Diatheses, bleeding, 383
Diazepam
  for alcohol withdrawal, 283, 500
  for anesthetic-induced seizures, 165
  cardiovascular disease effects, 314
  distribution, 87t
  dosage, 576t
  intracranial pressure effects, 280–281
  metabolism, 89t, 576t
  for multiple system organ failure, 398
  pharmacokinetic characteristics, 172t, 173
  for posttraumatic headaches, 275
  protein binding, 87t
  for renal disease, 350t–351t, 353
  for respiratory failure, 334t
  risk of use during pregnancy, 538
  for spinal cord compression, 284–285
  for tension headaches, 274
  for tetanus, 295
  for thalamic pain syndrome, 286
Diclofenac, 104, 105t, 106
  dosage, 107t, 576t
  gastric irritation reduced with, 110
  injectable dosage guidelines, 107t
  metabolism, 576t
Didanosine (ddI), HIV/AIDS medication, 471
Diethyl ether, 146
Diflunisal, 104, 105t, 106, 113
  dosage, 576t
  gastric irritation reduced with, 110
  metabolism, 576t
Difluorophenyl derivatives, 104, 105t, 106
Digitoxin, 90t, 377

Dilantin (see Phenytoin)
Dilaudid (see Hydromorphone)
Diltiazem, 87t
Diphenhydramine
  administration, 179
  for bone marrow transplant patients, 466
  dosage, 577t
  for haloperidol extrapyramidal reactions, 334
  hepatic metabolism, 362, 363t
  for liver transplantation pain, 459
  metabolism, 577t
  pharmacokinetic parameters, 179
  for renal disease, 350t–351t, 353
  risk of use during pregnancy, 538
Diphenyl derivatives, 119f
Diprivan (see Propofol)
Dipyridamole, 87t
Dipyrone, 104, 105t, 106, 107t
Disalcid (see Salsalate)
Discomfort, pain threshold and, 28, 29t
Discrepant enantiomeric processing, 98–99
Disopyramide, 87t
Disordered perception, 282
Disorientation, 499t
Disseminated intravascular coagulation (DIC), 377, 392, 532
Distraction techniques, 241, 463
Distribution, drug (see also specific drugs), 87t, 88–89, 94
Diversion, pain threshold and, 28, 29t
Divided dosing, 211
Dobutamine, 93f, 308
Dobutrex (dobutamine), 93f, 308
Dolobid (see Diflunisal)
Dolophine (see Methadone)
Dopamine, 43, 93f
Dorsal horn, 31f, 32, 509
Dorsal ramus blocks, 461
Dorsolateral funiculus, 32, 33f, 34
Double effect, principle of, 484–485
Down-regulation of receptors, 98
Doxacurium
  cardiovascular side effects, 201t
  clearance, 200t
  dosage, 199t, 577t
  histamine release, 201t
  metabolism, 577t
Doxepin
  administration, 185
  dosage, 577t
  metabolism, 577t
  for neuralgic pain, 549
  for pain in transplant patients, 463
  pharmacokinetic characteristics, 185t
  risk of use during pregnancy, 538
d-propoxyphene (see Propoxyphene)

Draw-your-pain tests for pain assessment, 22f, 24
Dressler's syndrome, 311
Droperidol
  administration, 182
  cardiovascular disease effects, 314
  dosage, 577t
  hepatic metabolism, 362, 363t
  metabolism, 577t
  pharmacokinetic characteristics, 181t
  for renal disease, 350t–351t, 353
  risk of use during pregnancy, 538
Drug abuse (see also Chemical abuse)
  among intensive care unit caregivers, 496
  amphetamines, 501, 502t
  butorphanol, potential, 133
  degree of impairment induced by, 497
  in intensive care unit patients, 500, 501t
  intravenous, 325t
  nalbuphine, potential, 134
  signs of, 500, 501t, 504, 505t, 506
  in transplant patients, 457
Drugs (see also specific drugs)
  absorption, 87–88
  addictive, in intensive care unit patients, 496
  administration, pharmacokinetic models, 92, 93f, 94
  associated pain, 344
  clearance, altered, 99
  distribution, 88–89
  dosages of common, 574t–585t
  effects, with hepatic failure, 369–370
  elimination, 88, 90t, 100t
  hepatic metabolism, 362, 363t
  interactions, 88, 99
  intoxication, 496
  metabolism, 87–88, 89t, 90, 100t, 574t–585t
  monitoring, 150–151
  protein binding, 87t
  risk factors of, used during pregnancy, 536–541
d-tubocurarine (see Tubocurarine)
Duchenne type muscular dystrophies, 295–296
Duodenal ulcers, 110–111
Dural puncture (see also Postdural puncture headache), 214–215
Duranest (see Etidocaine)
Dynorphin, 43, 120–121, 122t
Dysequilibrium syndrome, 346
Dysesthesia, 572
Dysrhythmias, 137

Economic implications of pain management, 6–7
Edema, 258–259, 341

Edematous bowel wall, 88
Edrophonium, 203
EDTA (ethylenediaminetetraacetate), 290
Ehlers-Danlos syndrome, 375
Eisenmenger's syndrome, 533–534
Elavil (see Amitriptyline)
Elbow, positioning for contractures, 260t
Elderly, 126–127, 139
Electrolyte balance, 51
Electrolyte homeostasis, 46, 48
Electrolytes, wasting, 46
Electrotherapy, 266–267, 267t, 268
Elimination linearity, 92
Elimination of drugs (see also specific drugs), 88, 90t, 92, 94
Elimination organ, damage to, 100
Elimination rate constant (Ke), 94–96
Emergent/triage phase, 65
Emotional age, 61t, 62–63
  case examples, 75–81
Emotional arousal, 57
Emotional effects
  of metabolic stress response (MSR), 48–49
  of pain and anxiety management, 51–52
  of post operative pain management, 445–446
Emotional status, 445–446
Emotional trauma, 247–248
Enalapril, 89–90
Enalaprilat, 89–90
Enantiomeric processing, discrepant, 98–99
Encephalitis, 276–277
Encephalopathy, 346
Endocarditis, 310
Endocrine system, 34, 35t, 42–45
Endogenous opioids, effects, 43
Endorphins, 45, 120
beta-Endorphins, 42–43, 121, 122t
Endotracheal tube suctioning, 330
End-stage renal disease (ESRD), 341
Energy for coping, psychology of pain factor, 58
Energy metabolism, 48
Enflurane, 145t, 148f–149f, 197
Enkephalins, 43, 120–121, 122t
Enolic acids, by classes, 104, 105t, 106
Enteral administration, 315–316
Environment, for terminally ill patients, 487
Environmental support, 65–66
Enzyme induction, 100t
Enzyme inhibition, 100t
Epidural abscess, 215
Epidural analgesia (see also Spinal analgesia)
  anatomy, 214
  catheter placement, 215–216, 430–431
  for coagulopathies, 531
  complications, 215
  continuous lumbar, 528–529

Epidural analgesia *(continued)*
  contraindications, 215
  description, 214
  dosage, 216, 217t–218t
  drugs, 216, 217t–218t
  indications, 214
  intrathecal, 335–336, 336t
  monitoring practices, 435–436
  narcotic, 335–336, 336t, 432, 433t, 434–435
  for neurologic disease pain, 297
  for posttrauma pain, 431–432, 433t, 434–436
  for the pregnant patient, 528–531
  for renal dysfunction, 356
  in respiratory failure, 335, 336t
  spinal analgesia versus, 214, 218–219
  for terminally ill patients, 488
Epidural hematoma, 215
Epidural injection for HIV/AIDS-related pain, 476–477
Epidural local anesthetics
  dosage, 217, 218t
  metabolic effects, 50–51
  narcotic combined, 217, 218t, 435
  respiratory effects, 50
  routes in respiratory failure, 335, 336t
  for trauma pain, 434–435
Epidural narcotics
  for chest pain, 311
  for hepatic disease pain management, 369–370
  metabolic effects, 51
  for renal transplantation patients, 464
  respiratory effects, 50
  for trauma pain, 432, 433t, 434
Epiglottitis, 320t
Epinephrine
  dosage, 518t
  increased levels after injury, 426t, 427
  in local anesthetic solutions, 166t, 167
  for peripheral nerve blocks, 226–227, 518t
  for the pregnant patient, 528, 529t
  release, 43
  for spinal analgesia, 217t–218t, 220–221
Epsilon-aminocaproic acid (EACA), 379–380
Equanil (meprobamate), 538, 549
Ergotamine, 273
Erythromycin, 89t, 100t, 295
Esimil (guanethidine), 293
Ester local anesthetics, 357, 160f
Ethanol, inducer of drug metabolism, 100t
Ethylenediaminetetraacetate (EDTA), 290
Etidocaine
  anesthetic duration, 162t, 163
  equipotent concentration, 160t
  lipid solubility, 159, 160f, 160t
  protein binding, 160t, 162
  for respiratory failure, 333t
  stereoisomers, 162t, 163
  structure of, 160f
  toxicity, 162t
Etodolac, 104, 105t, 106, 107t, 109, 577t
Etomidate
  dosage, 577t
  hemodynamic function effects, 145t
  intracranial pressure effects, 280
  for intravenous anesthesia, 153
  for intubation, 281
  metabolism, 577t
  for multiple system organ failure, 398–399
  for renal disease, 350t–351t, 353
Etoposide, 87t
Eutectic mixture of local anesthetics (EMLA), for herpes zoster, 473–474
Exertional angina, 305
Experiences, past, 28, 29t
Expiration, 323–324
Expiratory reserve volume (ERV), 47f
External locus of control (LOC), 60
Extreme temperatures, 41t
Extremities, acute pain and, 34, 35t
Extrinsic pathway, 375
Extubation, for liver transplant patients, 458

Factors, coagulation *(see* Coagulation factors; Hemostatic function)
Family caregivers *(see* Caregivers)
Famotidine, 111, 577t
Fatigue, pain threshold influenced by, 28, 29t
Fear, 28, 29t, 41t, 48–49
Feldene *(see* Piroxicam)
Femoral nerve blocks, 517, 518t, 519
  peripheral, 227
Fenamate, 104, 105t–106t
Fenclofenac, 104, 105t, 106
Fenoprofen, 104, 105t–106t, 538
Fentanyl, 119f, 120
  bioavailability, 127
  cardiovascular effects, 137, 138f, 313
  for children and neonates, 512, 512t–513t, 514
  classification, 122, 123t
  clearance, 127, 512t
  for cutaneous injury pain, 415–416
  distribution, 126, 128t
  dosage, 577t
    for central neural blockades, 516t
    for epidural analgesia, 217, 218t
    equipotent IV, 433t
    for parenteral administration, 211, 212t
    for patient-controlled analgesia, 213t, 217, 218t
    for spinal use, 436, 437t

epidural administration, 335, 336t, 432, 433t, 434
  bolus injection of analgesia, 217t
  for patient-controlled analgesia, 218t
  solutions for continuous analgesia, 529t
gastrointestinal effects, 140–141
hepatic metabolism, 362, 363t
for hepatic tumor pain management, 364
for HIV/AIDS-related pain, 475
intracranial pressure effects, 280
for liver transplant patients, 459–460, 462
metabolism, 126, 577t
for multiple system organ failure, 395–396
neurophysiologic effect, 140
parenteral administration, 211, 213t
  for patient-controlled analgesia, 213t, 217–218, 401
peridural administration, 316
potency, 126
for preexisting cardiac disease, 316
for the pregnant patient, 527–528, 529t
protein binding, 127, 128t
receptor subtype, 121, 122t
for renal disease, 350t–351t, 352
respiratory effects, 139
for respiratory failure, 331, 332t
risk of use during pregnancy, 538
for spinal analgesia, 217t–218t, 220–221
structure, 119f
tolerance to, 500
transdermal administration, 127, 370, 430, 487–488
for traumatic injuries, 440
Fetal pH, 526–527
Fibrin degradation product (FDP), 374, 376t, 378
Fibrinogen, 376t
Fibrinolysis, 375
Fibrinolytic system, 381
Fibrinous pericarditis, 311
Fibromyalgia, 552–553
Fibromyositis, 552–553
First-order kinetics, 92
First-pass effect, 89, 94
Flexeril (see Cyclobenzaprine)
Flow-dependent metabolism, 89t
Flow-independent metabolism, 89t
Flufenamic acid, 104, 105t, 106
Fluid balance, 51
Fluid retention, 46, 48, 427t
Flumazenil, 173, 460, 577t
Fluphenazine, 289, 291–292
Flurazepam, 353
Flurbiprofen, 104, 105t–106t
Focus of attention, 241
Forced expiratory volume (FEV$_1$), 50
Fresh frozen plasma (FFP), 379–382
Fresh whole blood, 382

Function, decreased, consequence of pain, 252–253
Functional abilities, 18
Functional mobility, 263–264
Functional residual capacity (FRC), 47f, 329–330, 426, 427t
Furosemide, for myocardial ischemia, 307

Gallamine, 90t, 355
Gamma-aminobutyric acid (GABA)
  dosage, 576t–577t, 579t–580t
  for HIV/AIDS-related pain, 476
  for liver transplantation patients, 460
  metabolism, 576t–577t, 579t–580t
Gastric ulcers, 110–111
Gastrointestinal (GI)
  acute pain effects, 34, 35t
  anticonvulsants adverse effects, 186
  chloral hydrate adverse effects, 177
  immobility, negative effects on function, 256t
  metabolic stress response (MSR) caused alterations, 48
  morbidity, 111
  mucosal protectants, 580t, 584t
  muscle relaxants adverse effects, 188
  narcotic use and withdrawal effects, 501t–502t
  opioids effects, 140–141
  pain and anxiety management effects, 51
  physiologic alterations in pregnant patients, 525–526
  prostaglandin-inhibiting agents complications, 110–111
  stimulants, 579t
  tract in multiple system organ failure, 391
General anesthetics (see Anesthetics/anesthesia: general)
Gentamycin, 90t, 93–94
Glasgow coma scale, 18
Glucagon, 43–44, 426t, 427, 427t
Glucose, contraindicated in alcoholics, 498
Glycoprotein, alpha$_1$-acid, 87t, 162
Graft function, 459–460
Granulation tissue, 411
Grief, psychosocial, 484
Grief response, 58, 59t, 492
Grief work, 70–71
Grieving process, 58
Growth hormone (GH), 42, 44, 426t, 427
Guanethidine, 297
Guillain-Barré syndrome, 288–289, 320t

Haldol (see Haloperidol)
Half-life ($t_{1/2}$), 94–96
Hallucinosis, 282, 499t
Haloperidol
  administration, 181–182

cardiovascular disease effects, 314
dosage, 578t
extrapyramidal reactions, 334
metabolism, 578t
pharmacokinetic characteristics, 181t
for renal disease, 350t–351t, 353
for respiratory failure, 334
Halothane, 145t, 147, 148f–149f, 197
Halothane hepatitis, 147
Hand, positioning for contractures, 260t
Hand pain, dialysis associated, 345
Hanging drop technique, 216
H_2-blockers, 377, 575t, 577t, 583t
Headaches, 273–278, 471–472
Head injuries, 139–140, 278–282
Healing, delayed, 252–253
Heart-lung transplantation (see also Transplantation), 457t, 464–465
Heart rate, 145t, 499t, 502t
Heat, as a modality, 264–266, 267t
Hemarthroses, 383–384
Hematologic systems in pregnant patients, 525, 526t
Hemodialysis (HD), 344–346, 349
Hemodynamically unstable patient, 560–562
Hemodynamic function, 144, 145t
Hemophilia A, 378–379
Hemophilia B, 379
Hemostasis screening tests, 375, 376t
Hemostatic failure, 374, 386–387
Hemostatic function (see also Coagulation factors)
  abnormal, 375–377, 377t, 378–381, 381t, 382–383
  normal, 374–375, 376f
Henderson-Hasselbalch equation, 161
Heparin
  anticoagulant-induced bleeding, 380
  disseminated intravascular coagulation therapy, 381
  induced thrombocytopenia, 380
  low-dose subcutaneous, 380
  for myocardial infarction, 308
  platelet abnormalities caused by, 377
  subcutaneous, 385–386
  test in acquired bleeding disorder, 381t
Hepatic blood flow, 369
Hepatic clearance, 369
Hepatic disease, 381
Hepatic dysfunction, 369, 394, 470
Hepatic enlargement, 383
Hepatic failure, 362, 362t–363t, 369–370
Hepatic function in burn patients, 414
Hepatic metabolism, 362, 363t
Hepatic pain, 363
Hepatic physiologic alterations, 526

Hepatic tumors, 364
Hepatitis, 113, 364–365
Hepatobiliary disease, 361, 370–371
Hepatobiliary pain, 363
Hepatobiliary system
  anatomy of hepatobiliary pain, 363
  anatomy of pancreatic pain, 366
  pain syndromes related to, 363–369
Heroin, 118, 122, 123t
Herpes zoster, 291–292, 473–474
Heteroaryl acetic acids, 104, 105t, 106
Hips, positioning for contractures, 260t
Histamine release, 137, 138f, 145t, 201t
Histamines, 31, 45
HIV/AIDS (human immunodeficiency virus/acquired immunodeficiency syndrome)
  introduction, 470
  invasive analgesic techniques for, 476–477
  medications, 475–476
  organ system dysfunction in, 470
  pain management principles, 474
  pain syndromes in, 471–474
  physical therapy, 478
  psychological support, 477–478
  psychotherapy for, patients, 477
  transcutaneous electrical nerve stimulations for, 477
Hoffman elimination, 201–202, 354–355
Hormonal changes, systemic, 426t
Hospice environment, 487
Hospital environment, 487
Hot and cold baths, 547
Hot and cold contrast applications, 452
Human immunodeficiency virus (HIV) (see HIV/AIDS)
Human tetanus immunoglobulin, 295
Hydralazine, 282
Hydrocortisone, 89t
Hydromorphone, 118, 131
  classification, 122, 123t
  dosage, 211, 212t–213t, 436, 437t, 578t
  epidural administration, 217t, 335, 336t
  for hepatic disease pain management, 370
  hepatic metabolism, 362, 363t
  for HIV/AIDS-related pain, 475
  for liver transplant patients, 462
  metabolism, 578t
  for multiple system organ failure, 395, 399, 401
  parenteral administration, 211, 212t–213t
  for patient-controlled analgesia, 213t, 401
  for renal disease, 350t–351t, 352
  for renal transplantation patients, 464
  in respiratory failure, 332t, 335, 336t
  for spinal use, 436, 437t
  suppositories, 370
  for terminally ill patients, 487–489

INDEX   601

Hydroxyzine, 178
  administration, 179
  for alcohol withdrawal, 283
  dosage, 578*t*
  metabolism, 578*t*
  pharmacokinetic parameters, 179
  risk of use during pregnancy, 538
Hyperbilirubinemia, 369
Hypercoagulable state of pregnancy, 525, 526*t*
Hyperesthesia, 572
Hyperglycemia, 427*t*
Hyperkalemia, 197, 340–341
Hypermagnesemia, 202, 341
Hyperpathia, defined, 572
Hyperphosphatemia, 341
Hypersensitivity, 97
Hypersplenism, 377
Hypersulfatemia, 341
Hypertension, 137–138, 341, 427*t*, 530–532
Hyperthermia, MSR activator, 41*t*
Hypertrophic scars, 419
Hyperuricemia, 341
Hypervolemia, 340–341
Hypnosis
  characteristics of, 243–245
  for cutaneous injury pain, 418
  for HIV/AIDS patients, 477
  for postoperative pain management, 452
  for pain management in patients with renal dysfunction, 357
  for sympathetically mediated pain, 547
  for terminally ill patients, 490
Hypnotic capacity, 63–64, 75–81
Hypnotic medications, 353, 491, 537–541, 578*t*
Hypocalcemia, 341–342
Hypocalcemic tetany, 295
Hypogastric plexus blocks, 547
Hypoperfusion, 111, 112*t*, 312, 427*t*
Hypoproteinemia, 341
Hyposensitivity, 97
Hypotension, 137
Hypothermia, 41*t*, 202
Hypovolemia, 41*t*, 256*t*
Hypovolemic shock, 136
Hypoxemia, 325
Hypoxia, MSR activator, 41*t*

Ibuprofen, 104, 105*t*, 106, 113
  distribution, 87*t*
  dosage, 106*t*, 578*t*
  gastric irritation reduced with, 110
  metabolism, 578*t*
  pain management in children and neonates, 510, 511*t*
  platelet abnormalities caused by, 377*t*
  protein binding, 87*t*
  risk of use during pregnancy, 538

Idiopathic thrombocytopenia purpura (ITP), 377
Ileus, after injury, 427*t*
Imagery, characteristics of, 241–242
Imidazole antifungal agents, 377*t*
Imidazole salicylate, 104, 105*t*, 106
Imipramine, 538, 549
Immobility, 252–255, 256*t*, 427, 427*t*, 428
Immunologic system, 34, 35*t*, 45
Immunosuppression, 457
Inapsine (*see* Droperidol)
Incisional pain, 320*t*
Incision irrigation, 225
Increased intracranial pressure (ICP)
  headaches, 277–278
  head injury induced, 278–282
Inderal (*see* Propranolol)
Index of pain, 55
Individual difference factors, 58–59
Individualized parameters, 91*f*, 94–96
Indocin (*see* Indomethacin)
Indoleacetic acids, 104, 105*t*, 106
Indomethacin, 104, 105*t*, 106, 113
  distribution, 87*t*
  dosage, 107*t*, 578*t*
  metabolism, 578*t*
  for pericarditis, 310
  platelet abnormalities caused by, 377*t*
  protein binding, 87*t*
  for renal colic, 347
  risk of use during pregnancy, 538
Indoprofen, 104, 105*t*, 106
Indwelling endotracheal tube, 330
Infantile paralysis, 291
Infection, 209–210, 325*t*, 532
Infectious pericarditis, 309
Inflammation, corticosteroids for, 108
Inflammatory myopathies, 295–296
Inguinal peripheral nerve blocks, 227
Inhalation anesthesia/analgesia, 145–148, 148*f*, 149, 149*f*, 150–152
Inhalation injury, 325*t*
Injury (*see* Trauma)
Inocor (amrinone), 308
Inotropic agents, 308
Inotropy, increased, 45–46
Insomnia, 28, 29*t*
Inspiratory capacity (IC), 426, 427*t*
Inspiratory reserve volume (IRV), 47*f*
Insulin, 43–44, 426*t*, 427
Insulin-like growth factor (IGF), 44
Integrative response, 41*f*, 42
Integument failure (*see* Cutaneous injuries)
Intensity theory of cardiac muscle pain, 304
Intensive care unit (ICU)
  pain management in, 4–6
  patients
    implications of pain in the, 4–5

pharmacodynamics for, 97–99, 100t
pharmacokinetic concerns, 87t, 88, 89t–90t
pharmacokinetic models for, 90, 91f, 92, 93f, 94–96
Intercostal muscles, 323
Intercostal nerve blocks, 226, 517, 518t, 519
Intercostal nerves, 309
Interleukin (IL), 45
Interleukin-1 (IL-1), 42, 45
Intermittent drug infusion, 93f, 94–96
Internal locus of control (LOC), 60
Interpersonal influence model, 65–66
Interpleural local anesthetics, 547
Interstitial fluid, increased, 48
Interventions
  iatrogenic, 99, 100t
  psychological, 65–67, 68t
Intervention strategies, 75–81
Intoxication, 497
  phencyclidine (PCP), 503, 504t
Intra-aortic counterpulsation balloon (IACB), 308
Intrabursal peripheral nerve blocks, 227
Intracranial blood flow, 147
Intracranial pressure (ICP) increased (see also Head injuries), 278–282
  opioid associated effects, 139–140
Intrahepatic dysfunction, 362t
Intramuscular (IM) administration of analgesic and sedative agents in ICU, 316
  difficulty of, after injury, 429
  disease-related alterations in absorption, 88
  of drugs, 88, 429
  of pain medication for terminally ill patients, 490
  parenteral administration techniques, 211, 212t
  for postoperative pain management, 448
  for trauma pain, 429
Intraocular pressures, increased, 198
Intraoperative management, 446, 458
Intrapleural analgesia (see also Analgesics/analgesia), 437–438
Intrapleural nerve blocks, 517, 518t, 519
  peripheral, 226
Intrapsychic factors, case examples, 75–81
Intrarenal, 340
Intrathecal analgesia (see also Analgesics/analgesia)
  for posttrauma pain, 436, 437t
  in respiratory failure, 335, 336t
Intrathecal opioids, 528
Intravenous (IV) anesthesia/analgesia (see also Analgesics/analgesia;

Anesthetics/anesthesia)
  barbiturates, 152–153
  dosage, 577t
  etomidate, 153
  ketamine, 153–154
  metabolism, 577t
  for multiple system organ failure, 398–399
  propofol, 154
  in respiratory failure, 334–335
Intravenous (IV) bolus, 355
Intravenous (IV) drug abuse (see also Drug abuse), 325t
Intravenous (IV) injections and infusions, 88, 211, 212t–213t, 416, 429
Intravenous (IV) regional (Bier) blocks, 223–224
Intrinsic pathway, 375
Introversion, pain threshold and, 28, 29t
Intubation, 193, 281
Ionic currents, 158
Ionic gradients, 158
Ionization of local anesthetics, 160, 161f
Ion trapping, 526–527
Ischemia, 41t, 305, 312
Ischemic heart disease, 312
Isoflurane, 145t, 147, 148f–149f, 197, 458
Isoproterenol, 89t

Joint mobilization, 262
Joint pain, 342–343, 345

Kaposi's hemorrhagic sarcoma, 376
Kappa receptors, 32, 121, 122t
Keloid scars, sequelae to burns, 419
Ketalar (see Ketamine)
Ketamine
  cardiovascular disease effects, 315
  for cutaneous injury pain, 416–417
  dosage, 578t
  hemodynamic function effects, 145t
  intracranial pressure effects, 281
  for intravenous anesthesia, 153–154
  for liver transplant patients, 462
  metabolism, 578t
  for multiple system organ failure, 398–399
  for neurologic disease pain, 297
  for renal disease, 350t–351t, 353
Ketoconazole, 100t
Ketoprofen, 104, 105t–106t
Ketorolac tromethamine, 104, 105t, 106, 109, 354, 370, 510, 511t
  for chest pain, 310–311
  dosage, 107t, 579t
  injectable dosage guidelines, 107t
  for liver transplant patients, 462
  metabolism, 579t
  for multiple system organ failure, 397
  for pericarditis, 310

platelet function and, 113
risk of use during pregnancy, 539
for spinal cord compression, 283
for subarachnoid hemorrhage headaches, 277
Kidney dysfunction, in HIV/AIDS, 470
Kidney transplantation (*see also* Transplantation), 457*t*, 463–464
Knees, positioning for contractures, 260*t*
Korsakoff's psychosis, 498
Kyphoscoliosis, 320*t*

Labetalol, for blood pressure control, 282
Laboratory studies, 18–19, 447
Labor pain (*see* Pregnancy)
Laryngoscopy, 281
Laryngospasm, 147, 193
Lasix (furosemide), 307
Late dialysis periarticular syndrome, 345
Lateral spinothalamic tract, 32, 33*f*, 34
Laudanosine, 202, 354–355
Lead poisoning, 290
Leukopenia, 145–146
Leukotrienes, 31
Levo-Dromoran (levorphanol), 119, 579*t*
Levorphanol, 119, 579*t*
Librium (*see* Chlordiazepoxide)
Lidocaine
 bicarbonate to adjust pH of, 167*t*
 for blood pressure control, 282
 for bone marrow transplant patients, 465
 cardiac toxicity, 164–165
 for central neural blockades, 516*t*
 for children and neonates, 515
 distribution, 87*t*
 dosage, 166*t*, 516*t*, 518*t*
 equipotent concentration, 160*t*
 intracranial pressure effects, 281
 for intubation, 281
 lipid solubility, 159, 160*f*, 160*t*
 metabolism, 89*t*
 for multiple system organ failure, 396
 for oropharyngeal pain, 473
 peak blood levels, 163, 164*f*
 for peripheral nerve blocks, 226–227, 518*t*
 pharmacokinetic properties, 515
 for plexus blocks, 224–225
 protein binding, 87*t*, 160*t*, 162
 for respiratory failure, 333*t*
 risk of use during pregnancy, 539
 for spinal analgesia, 217*t*–218*t*, 220–221
 structure of, 160*f*
 for sympathetic nerve blocks, 222–223
 systemic toxicity, 163–164
Linear elimination, 92
Linear kinetics, 94
Lioresal (*see* Baclofen)

Lipid solubility, of local anesthetics, 159, 160*f*, 160*t*
Lipolysis, 48
Lithium salicylate, 104, 105*t*, 106
Liver disease test, 381*t*
Liver P450 function, 100*t*
Liver transplantation (*see under* Transplantation)
Living will for terminally ill patients, 485
Loading dose, 93
Local anesthetics (LA) (*see* Anesthetics/anesthesia: local)
Lockout period (LOP) (*see also* Patient-controlled analgesia), 213*t*, 214, 218*t*
Locus of control (LOC), 60, 247
Lodine (*see* Etodolac)
Loin pain hematuria syndrome, 347
Lopressor (*see* Metoprolol)
Lorazepam
 administration, 172–173
 for alcohol withdrawal, 283
 for anxiety following injury, 431
 for bone marrow transplant patients, 466
 cardiovascular disease effects, 314
 for cutaneous injury pain, 416
 dosage, 579*t*
 metabolism, 579*t*
 for multiple system organ failure, 398
 pharmacokinetic characteristics, 172*t*, 173
 for renal disease, 350*t*–351*t*, 353
 for respiratory failure, 334*t*
 risk of use during pregnancy, 539
Loss of control, 18
Loss of resistance technique, 216
Low back pain, 550–551
L-thyroxine, elimination, 90*t*
Lumbar epidural analgesia, continuous, 528, 529*t*
Lumbar epidural blockade, 515, 516*t*, 517
Lumbar plexus blocks (*see also* Plexus blocks), 225
Lumbar puncture (LP), 275–277
Lumbar sympathetic block (LSB), 222, 477, 546
Luminal (*see* Phenobarbital)
Lung abscess pain, 328
Lung surface tension, 323
Lymphadenopathy, 474
Lysergic acid diethylamide (LSD), 503–504
Lysine acetyl salicylate, 104, 105*t*, 106

Magnesium salicylate, 104, 105*t*, 106
Magnesium wasting, 46
Magnetic resonance imaging (MRI), 283–284
Maintenance dose, 93
Malabsorption, 48

Malignant hyperthermia (MH), 145t, 151, 197–198
Manager-of-recovery, 58, 71, 75–81
Mannitol for spinal cord compression, 283
Manual therapies, 262
Marcaine (*see* Bupivacaine)
Marfan's syndrome, 375
Marijuana, 503
Massage, 262, 451
Masseter spasm, 198
Massive transfusion test, 380, 381t
Matrix assessment, 72–73, 73t–74t, 75–81
Mazicon (*see* Flumazenil)
McGill Pain Questionnaire, 23
Mean arterial pressure (MAP), 148f, 279
Meaning of pain, 59, 75–81
Meclofenamate, 104, 105t–106t, 539
Meclomen (*see* Meclofenamate)
Meditation, 241
Medullary reflex arcs, 426, 427t
Mefenamic acid, 104, 105t–106t, 109, 113, 579t
Membrane stabilization, 158
Membrane-stabilizing drugs for HIV/AIDS, 476
Meningitis, headaches secondary to, 276–277
Mental isolation, 28, 29t
Mental state, narcotic use and, 501t
Meperidine, 119f, 120, 433t
   bioavailability, 125
   cardiovascular effects, 137–138, 313
   classification, 122, 123t
   contraindicants, 464, 527–528
   for cutaneous injury pain, 416
   distribution, 87t, 128t
   dosage, 211, 212t–213t, 217, 218t, 433t, 436, 437t, 579t
   elimination half-life of, in children, 512t
   for epidural analgesia, 217, 217t–218t, 335, 336t
   gastrointestinal effects, 140–141
   hepatic metabolism, 362, 363t
   metabolism, 89t, 125–126, 579t
   for multiple system organ failure, 396
   for pancreatitis pain, 366
   parenteral administration, 211, 212t–213t
   plasma levels, 125
   protein binding, 87t, 126, 128t
   receptor subtype, 121, 122t
   for renal disease, 349, 350t–351t, 352
   respiratory effects, 139
   for respiratory failure, 332t, 335, 336t
   risk of use during pregnancy, 539
   structure, 119f
   for trauma pain, side effects, 429
   use in pediatric/neonate ICU, 512, 513t
Mepivacaine
   anesthetic duration, 162t, 163
   bicarbonate to adjust pH of, 167t
   dosage, maximum, 166t
   equipotent concentration, 160t
   lipid solubility, 159, 160f, 160t
   for multiple system organ failure, 396–397
   for peripheral nerve blocks, 226–227
   for plexus blocks, 224–225
   protein binding, 160t, 162
   stereoisomers, 162t, 163
   structure of, 160f
   toxicity, 162t
Meprobamate, 295, 539
Meptazinol, receptor subtype, 121, 122t
Mercury poisoning, 289–290
Metabolic abnormalities, 421
Metabolic acidosis, 340–341
Metabolic function, immobility and, 256t
Metabolic stress response (MSR)
   cardiovascular effects, 45–46
   definition, 41f, 40
   electrolyte homeostasis caused by, 46, 48
   emotional effects, 48–49
   fluid retention caused by, 46, 48
   gastrointestinal alterations, 48
   metabolic manifestations, 48
   pain as an initiator, 41–42
   pain treatment sites, 49f
   precipitating factors, 41t
   respiratory effects, 46, 47f
Metabolism of drugs (*see also specific drugs*), 87–88, 89t, 90, 100t
Metabolites, 89–90, 124–126, 129
Methadone, 119
   bioavailability, 129
   classification, 122, 123t
   distribution, 87t
   dosage, 211, 212t, 433t, 436, 437t, 579t
   elimination half-life of, in children, 512t
   epidural administration of, 332t, 335, 336t
   equipotent IV dosage and side effects, 433t
   hepatic metabolism, 362, 363t
   metabolism, 579t
   for parenteral administration, 211, 212t
   protein binding, 87t
   for renal disease, 350t–351t
   in respiratory failure, 332t, 335, 336t
   risk of use during pregnancy, 539
   side effects, 129
   for spinal use, 436, 437t
   structure, 131f
   use in pediatric/neonate ICU, 512, 513t, 514
Methohexital, 175t, 176, 579t
Methoxyflurane, 148f–149f, 150
Methyldopa, 377
Methylphenidate, 490, 579t
Metoclopramide, 465–466, 539, 579t
Metocurine
   cardiovascular side effects, 201t

clearance, 199, 200t
dosage, 199t, 580t
histamine release, 201t
metabolism, 580t
for renal disease, 350t–351t, 355
for tetanus, 295
Metoprolol, 89t, 100t, 308
Metubine (see Metocurine)
Midazolam
  administration, 173
  for alcohol withdrawal, 500
  for anesthetic-induced seizures, 165
  for anxiety following injury, 431
  cardiovascular disease effects, 314
  for cutaneous injury pain, 416
  dosage, 580t
  intracranial pressure effects, 280–281
  metabolism, 580t
  for multiple system organ failure, 397
  pharmacokinetic characteristics, 172t, 173
  for renal disease, 350t–351t, 353
  for respiratory failure, 334t
Migraine, 273
Migraine headaches, 273
Miltown (meprobamate), 295, 539
Minimal alveolar concentration (MAC), 146–147, 148f–149f
Minipress (prazosin), 293
Minnesota Multiphasic Personality Inventory (MMPI), 23
Minute ventilation of the lung, 322
Miosis, opioid associated effect, 140
Misoprostol, 111, 430–431, 580t
Mitral regurgitation, 312–313
Mitral stenosis, 312–313, 533
Mivacron (see Mivacurium)
Mivacur (see Pipecuronium)
Mivacurium, 199t–200t, 201, 201t, 580t
Mobility, 258–259, 260t, 263–264
Modalities, 264–266, 267t, 268
Model-dependent parameters, 95
Model-independent parameters, 95
Mood, 28, 29t, 502t
Mood-altering substances, 496–497
Morphinan derivatives, 119
Morphine, 118, 119f, 433t
  bioavailability, 124
  cardiovascular effects, 137, 138f, 313
  for central neural blockades, 516t
  classification, 122, 123t
  contraindicants, 464
  for cutaneous injury pain, 415
  distribution, 128t
  dosage, 211, 212t–213t, 217, 218t, 433t, 436, 437t, 516t, 580t
  elimination half-life of, in children, 512t
  epidural administration of, 217, 217t–218t, 335, 336t
  gastrointestinal effects, 140–141

hepatic metabolism, 362, 363t
intramuscular injection, 124
intravenous injection, 123–124
metabolism, 89t, 124–125, 580t
for multiple system organ failure, 395, 399
for myocardial infarction, 308
for myocardial ischemia, 306–307
oral, 124
for patient-controlled analgesia, 213t, 401
peridural administration of, 316
protein binding, 128t
receptor subtype, 121, 122t
for renal disease, 350t–351t
respiratory effects, 139
in respiratory failure therapy, 331, 332t, 335, 336t
risk of use during pregnancy, 539
for spinal analgesia, 217t–218t, 220–221
structure, 119f
for terminally ill patients, 487–490
use in pediatric/neonate ICU, 512, 513t
Morphine metabolites, 124–125
Morphine-6-glucuronide, 124–125
Morphine sulfate, 280, 349, 352
Morphine-3-glucuronide, 124
Mortality, 499t, 501t
Motivation, 58, 252–253
Motor function, 256t
Motor neuron lesions, 286–293
Motrin (see Ibuprofen)
Multiple-compartment pharmacokinetic model, 90, 91f, 92
Multiple sclerosis (MS), 286–287
Multiple system organ failure (MSOF), 42–43, 50
  adult respiratory distress syndrome effect, 325
  case discussion, 401–402
  introduction, 390
  pain management, 394–401
  pain syndromes associated with, 392–393
  pathophysiology, 390–392
Mu receptors, 32, 121, 122t
Muscle atrophy, 256t
Muscle-contraction headaches, 273–274
Muscle function, normal, 254
Muscle relaxants, 188–190, 354, 574t–576t
Muscle relaxation, progressive, 242
Muscles of respiration, 323
Muscle spasms, 41f, 40, 46
Muscle-strength grading system, 262t
Muscular dystrophies, 295–296
Muscular rheumatism, 552–553
Musculoskeletal function, 254
Musculoskeletal system, 252–253
Music for terminally ill patients, 490
Myalgias, 198
Myasthenia gravis, 202, 293–294, 320t
Myasthenic crisis, 293–294

Myasthenic syndrome, 202
Myelinated nociceptors, 407
Myelography, 283–284
Myocardial depressant factors (MDFs), 391
Myocardial depression, 394
Myocardial infarction, 305, 307–308
Myocardial ischemia, 305–307
Myocardial-muscle oxygen transport, 303–304
Myocardial oxygen consumption (MVo_2), increased, 45–46
Myocardial oxygen supply, 303–304
Myocardial pain, 305
Myofascial pain (MFP), 35–36, 572
Myofascial release, 262
Myoglobinuria, 198
Myopathy, HIV/AIDS related, 472
Myositis, HIV/AIDS related, 472

Nabumetone, 104, 105t, 106, 107t, 109, 580t
Nadolol, 90t, 273
Nalbuphine
  abuse potential, 134
  agonist-antagonist properties, 134
  analgesic effects, 134
  classification, 122, 123t
  dosage, 211, 212t, 433t, 580t
  equipotent IV dosage and side effects, 433t
  hepatic metabolism, 362, 363t
  metabolism, 134, 580t
  parenteral administration, 211, 212t
  for renal disease, 350t–351t, 352–353
  respiratory depression from, 134
  for respiratory failure, 332
  risk of use during pregnancy, 539
  side effects, 134
  structure, 131f
  for trauma pain, side effects, 429
Nalfon (fenoprofen), 104, 105t–106t, 538
Nalline (see Nalorphine)
Nalorphine, 121–122, 122t–123t, 131f, 539
Naloxone
  antagonist properties, 135
  cardiovascular disease effects, 313–314
  classification, 122, 123t
  for cutaneous injury pain, 415
  dosage, 581t
  intracranial pressure effects, 280
  for liver transplantation patients, 460
  metabolism, 135–136, 581t
  risk of use during pregnancy, 539
  side effects, 135–136
Naltrexone, 122, 123t, 136, 581t
Naphthylalkanone, 104, 105t, 106
Naprosyn (see Naproxen)
Naproxen, 104, 105t, 106
  distribution, 87t
  dosage, 106t, 510, 511t
  pain management in children, 510, 511t
  protein binding, 87t
  risk of use during pregnancy, 540
Naproxen sodium, 106t
Narcan (see Naloxone)
Narcotic abuse (see Drug abuse)
Narcotic agonist (see Agonists: narcotic)
Narcotic agonist-antagonists (see Agonist-antagonists: narcotic)
Narcotic analgesics (see Analgesics/analgesia: narcotic)
Narcotic antagonists (see Antagonists: narcotic)
Narcotics (see also Anesthetics/anesthesia; Opiates; Opioids)
  administration techniques (see Administration techniques)
  for biliary colic, 365
  cardiovascular disease effects, 313–314
  for chest pain, 310
  dosage, 575t, 578t–579t
  gastrointestinal effects, 51
  hemodynamic function effects, 145t
  for hepatic tumor pain management, 364
  for HIV/AIDS-related pain, 475
  impact of coagulopathy on, 384–385
  intracranial pressure effects, 280
  for intubation, 281
  for liver transplant patients, 458, 462
  and local anesthetics combined, 435
  metabolism, 575t, 578t–579t
  nonsteroidal anti-inflammatory drugs versus, 104, 108–109
  peridural, 121–122
  perispinal drug effects, 216, 217t
  for respiratory failure, 331, 332t
  risk of use during pregnancy, 537–541
  for spinal cord compression, 283
  for tetanus, 295
  use and withdrawal (see also Drug abuse), 500, 501t
Nasogastric suctioning, 88
Nausea, 48, 140–141, 501t
Neck, positioning for contractures, 260t
Necrosis, 483
Necrotizing fasciitis, 113
Negative emotional arousal, 57
Negative nitrogen balance, 42, 48
Nembutal (see Pentobarbital)
Neonates (see also Children; Pediatric patients), 136, 139, 507–521
Neoplastic spinal cord compression, 283
Neospinothalamic system, 32, 33f, 34
Neostigmine, 203
Nerve blocks (see also specific blocks)
  administration (see Administration techniques)
  Bier (intravenous regional), 223–224, 547

for cancer pain, 554
in children and neonates, 514, 515t–516t, 517
femoral, 227, 517, 518t, 519
inguinal peripheral, 227
intercostal, 226, 517, 518t, 519
intrapleural, 226, 517, 518t, 519
for low back pain, 550–551
for multiple system organ failure, 400
for neuralgic pain, 549
penile, 517, 518t, 519
peripheral (*see* Peripheral nerve blocks)
posterior division (PDNB), 461
ring, 517, 518t, 519
sympathetic, 221–224
Nerve fibers, 31f, 32
Nesacaine (*see* Chloroprocaine)
Neural blockade (*see* Nerve blocks)
Neuralgic pain, 36, 548–549, 572
Neural impulses, afferent, 42
Neural injury, 219–220
Neural transmitters, 509
Neuraxial opioids, 530
Neuroanatomy, 509
Neuroendocrine axis, 42–45
Neurohumoral response, 509
Neuroleptic drugs, 333–334
Neurologic disease (*see* Neurologic injury and disease)
Neurologic dysfunction, 392, 470
Neurologic injury and disease
  alcohol withdrawal syndrome, 282–283
  case study, 272
  headaches, 273–278
  head injury and increased intracranial pressure, 278–282
  motor neuron lesions, 286–293
  neuromuscular junction disorders, 293–296
  pain management in the presence of, 296–298
  in the pregnant patient, 532–534
  spinal cord compression, 283–286
Neurolytic drugs, 222–223
Neurolytic procedures for pancreatitis pain, 367–368
Neuromax (*see* Doxacurium)
Neuromuscular blocking agents
  cardiovascular disease effects, 315
  dose and metabolism, 574t, 577t, 580t–582t, 584t–585t
  for multiple system organ failure, 399
Neuromuscular blocking agents (NBM) classes
  depolarizing, succinylcholine, 195–198
  nondepolarizing, 195, 198–200, 200t–201t, 202
  monitoring, 202

need for other agents with, 192
physiology, 194–195
reversal, 203
uses, 192–194
Neuromuscular electrical stimulation, 267
Neuromuscular junction disorders, 293–296
Neuropathies
  acute inflammatory polyradiculoneuropathy, 288–289
  diabetic, 289
  pathogenesis of generalized, 288
  peripheral (PNS), 288, 472
  physiologic pain, 483
  renal failure associated, 343
  toxic, 289–290
  vasculitic, 290–291
  wound pain from, 421
Neuropharmacology in children, 509
Neurophysiologic effects of opioids, 139–140
Newborns (*see* Neonates)
Nifedipine, 293, 347, 547
Nitrates for myocardial infarction, 308
Nitroglycerin, metabolism, 89t
Nitroglycerin IV for myocardial ischemia, 307
Nitrous oxide (*see also* Anesthetics/anesthesia), 145, 145t, 146, 528
Nociceptive function, 327
Nociceptive nerve endings, 509
Nociceptive reflex arcs, 426, 427t
Nociceptors, 30, 31f, 407, 572
Noctec (*see* Chloral hydrate)
Nonacidic nonsteroidal anti-inflammatory agents, 104, 105t, 106, 107t
Nonanalgesic respiratory failure therapy, 333, 334t
Noncompetitive blockers, 195–198
Nondepolarizing agents, 195, 198–200, 200t–201t, 202, 295
Noninfectious pericarditis, 309
Nonlinear elimination, 92
Nonlinear kinetics, 94
Nonnarcotic analgesics (*see also* Analgesics/analgesia), 430–431, 450–451, 510, 511t
Nonoliguric acute renal failure, 340–341
Nonopioid analgesics (*see also* Analgesics/analgesia; Nonnarcotic analgesics), 510, 511t
Nonpharmacologic adjuncts, 357, 490
Nonpharmacologic modalities, 418
Non-Q-wave myocardial infarction, 307–308
Nonsteroidal anti-inflammatory drugs (NSAIDs) (*see also specific agents*)
  in acute pain situations, 104, 109–110, 114
  as adjunctive medication, 104–106

Nonsteroidal anti-inflammatory drugs *(continued)*
  adverse reactions, 110–112, 112*t*, 113–114
  as analgesic agent, 107–109, 114
  analgesic effects, central and peripheral, 109, 114
  anti-inflammatory effects, 108
  available in the United States, 106*t*–107*t*
  for biliary colic, 365
  for cancer pain, 554
  for chest pain, 311
  in children and neonates, 510, 511*t*
  classes, 104, 105*t*, 106
  contraindications, 464, 527–528
  corticosteroids versus, 108
  for cutaneous injury pain, 417
  dosage, 106*t*–107*t*, 217, 218*t*, 574*t*–580*t*, 582*t*–584*t*
  for epidural analgesia, 217, 218*t*
  general considerations, 103–104
  for hepatic tumor pain management, 364
  for HIV/AIDS-related pain, 475
  impact of coagulopathy on, 386
  injectable, 107, 109
  for liver transplant patients, 462
  for low back pain, 550–551
  metabolism, 574*t*–580*t*, 582*t*–584*t*
  for multiple system organ failure, 397
  for myofascial pain syndrome, 552–553
  narcotics versus, 104, 108–109
  nephrotoxicity, 111, 112*t*
  for neuralgic pain, 548
  platelet abnormalities caused by, 377*t*, 378
  for postoperative pain management, 451
  for posttrauma pain, 430–431, 439–440
  for posttraumatic headaches, 275
  prostaglandin production effects, 107–109
  for pulmonary disorders, 327–329
  for reflex sympathetic dystrophy, 293
  for renal disease, 353–354
  risk of use during pregnancy, 537–541
  for spinal cord compression, 283
  for sympathetically mediated pain, 547
  for tension headaches, 274
  therapeutic use, 109–110
Nonsurgical procedures, associated with multiple system organ failure, 393
Norcuron (*see* Vecuronium)
Norepinephrine (NE), release, 43
Normeperidine, 126, 396, 429, 464
Normocytic, normochromic anemia, 341
Norpramin (desipramine), 538, 549
Norpropoxyphene, 129
Nortriptyline, 540
Noscapine, 118
Nosocomial pneumonia, 48
Novocaine (*see* Procaine)
Nubain (*see* Nalbuphine)

Numbness, 283–284
Numeric pain intensity scale, 20*f*, 21–22
Numorphan (*see* Oxymorphone)
Nuromax (*see* Doxacurium)
Nursing home environments, 487
Nursing issues
  common clinical dilemmas, 560–567
  pain control as a multidisciplinary process, 556
  pain control options, 557
  pain flow sheet, 559*f*
  pharmacologic options, 557, 559*f*
  role in pain treatment, 556–557, 558*f*
  specific nursing considerations, 556–557, 558*f*
  systematic pain treatment flow chart, 558*f*
Nutritional deficiencies in alcoholics, 498

Obesity, respiratory failure caused by, 320*t*
Obstetric complications, ARDS risk factor, 325*t*
Occipital peripheral nerve blocks, 227
Occupational therapist, 254
Occupational therapy, 254–255, 256*t*
Oddi's sphincter spasms, 140–141
Oliguric acute renal failure, 340–341
Omeprazole, 100*t*
Ondansetron, 465, 581*t*
One-compartment pharmacokinetic model, 90, 91*f*
Opiates (*see also* Analgesics/analgesia; Anesthetics/anesthesia; Narcotics; Opioids; *specific drugs*)
  local anesthetic combinations, 168
  pharmacokinetics in children, 512*t*
  pharmacology
    agonist-antagonist, 131*f*, 132–135
    cardiovascular effects, 137, 138*t*
    clinically useful, 122, 123*t*, 124–127, 128*t*, 129, 131*f*, 130
    dynorphines, 120
    enkephalins, 120
    gastrointestinal effects, 140–141
    mechanism of action, 120–121, 122*t*
    neurophysiologic effects, 139–140
    peridural, 121–122
    prohormones, 120
    receptors, 120–121
    relative potency, 120–121
    respiratory effects, 139
    structure, 118, 119*f*, 120
Opioids (*see also* Opiates)
  agonist-antagonists, 131*f*, 132–135
    classification, 122, 123*t*
    for renal disorders, 350*t*–351*t*, 352–353
  agonists
    classification, 122, 123*t*
    gastrointestinal effects, 140–141

for neurologic disease pain, 296–297
pure, for renal disease, 349, 350t–351t, 352
respiratory effects, 139
antagonists, 122, 123t, 135–136
for cancer pain, 553–554
for children, 511, 512t–513t, 514
for cutaneous injury pain, 415–416
elimination half-life of, 512t
endogenous in neonates, 509
for multiple system organ failure, 394–396
parenteral administration, 211, 212t
for the pregnant patient, 527–528
receptor subtypes, 121, 122t
Oral
absorption of drugs, 88, 94
administration of drugs, 88, 93f, 94, 96, 488
Oral mucositis, 465
Organ system dysfunction, 393
Oropharyngeal pain, HIV/AIDS related, 473
Orthopedic injuries, 440–441
Orthostatic hypotension, 137, 256t
Orudis (ketoprofen), 104, 105t–106t
Osteitis fibrosa, 342
Osteoarthritis, 551–552
Osteomalacia, 342
Osteoporosis, 256t, 342
Oxazepam, 353
Oxicams, 104, 105t, 106, 107t
Oxycodone, 131, 489, 540, 581t
Oxygen, 164–165, 306–307, 490
Oxygen consumption (Voo$_2$), 46, 47f, 50, 427t
Oxymetazoline, 274–275
Oxymorphone, 122, 123t, 395, 540
Oxyphenbutazone, 104, 105t, 106, 540

Pabalate (*see* Sodium salicylate)
Packed red blood cells (PRBCs), 382
Pain
acute (*see* Acute pain)
chronic (*see* Chronic pain)
circuitry (*see* Circuitry of pain)
consequences of, 252–253, 253f, 254
in critically ill patients, 4–5
defined, 14, 28, 55, 572
drug-associated, 344
gastrointestinal effects, 51
immobilization as a cause, 253–254
labor (*see* Pregnancy)
meaning of, 59
metabolic stress response (MSR) activator, 41t
narcotic use and withdrawal effects on, 501t
physiologic effects, 426t–427t, 428
psychological assessment, (*see* Psychology of pain)
types (*see also specific types*), 28–29, 30t, 34–36
understanding, 28
Pain and immobilization cycle, 252, 253f
Pain assessment
barriers to, 15
components of the pain experience, 16
defined, 14
goals, 14–15
matrix model for (*see* Matrix assessment)
patient assessment (*see* Patient assessment)
pediatric patients (*see* Pediatric patients)
physiologic data, 16
psychological data, 16–17
requirements of tools for, 15–16
suggested readings, 25
techniques
affective measures, 23
desirable characteristics, 19
drawings, 22f, 24
faces, for children, 510f
McGill Pain Questionnaire, 23
Minnesota Multiphasic Personality Inventory (MMPI), 23
numerical scales, 20f, 21–22
pain flow sheet, 559f
verbal scales, 20f–21f
visual analog scale (VAS), 19, 20f, 21
Pain behavior, 55, 56t
Pain consultants, 67
Pain control (*see also* Pain management), 428
Pain evaluation (*see* Pain assessment)
Painful lymphadenopathy, HIV/AIDS related, 474
Pain history, 23, 447
Pain intensity scales (*see* Pain assessment: techniques)
Pain management
benefits of, 5–6
economic implications of, 6–7
education, 69, 70t, 71–72
impact, 49f, 50–52
of preexisting cardiac disease on, 312–317
with occupational therapy, 254–255, 256t
with physical therapy, 254–255, 256t
technology evaluation, 7
Pain mechanisms, 27–28, 29t–30t, 31f, 32, 33f, 34, 35t, 36–37
Pain pathways, 27–28, 29t–30t, 31f, 32, 33f, 34, 35t, 36–37
Pain rating scales (*see* Pain assessment: techniques)
Pain receptors, circuitry, 30, 31f, 32, 33f, 34
Pain syndromes (*see also specific syndromes*)
acute, 491

chronic, (see Chronic pain syndromes)
HIV/AIDS related, 471–474
multiple system organ failure related, 392–393
Pain terminology appendix, 571–572
Pain therapy
  basic principles, 428
    for cutaneous injuries, 412–413
  epidural analgesia, 431–432, 433t, 434–436
  intrapleural analgesia, 437–438
  intrathecal analgesia, 436, 437t
  parenteral medication, 429–431
  peripheral nerve blocks, 438
Pain threshold, 28, 29t
Pain treatment, psychology of pain factor, 55–56
Pain treatment sites, 49f
Paleospinothalamic system, 32, 33f, 34
Pamelor (nortriptyline), 540
Pancreatic carcinoma, 368–369
Pancreatic pain, 366
Pancreatitis, 325t, 366–368
Pancuronium
  cardiovascular effects, 201t, 315
  clearance, 199, 200t
  dosage, 199t, 581t
  histamine release, 201t
  metabolism, 581t
  for renal disease, 350t–351t, 355
Papaverine, 118
Para-aminosalicylic acid (PAS), 377
Paradoxical excitation, 171
Paraldehyde, 283
Paranoia, 499t
Paravertebral peripheral nerve blocks, 226
Parenteral administration techniques, 211–212, 212t–213t, 214, 316, 488
Parenteral medications (see also specific medications)
  analgesics for the pregnant patient, 527–528
  dosing and intervals, 211, 212t
  narcotic analgesics, 429–430, 461
  nonnarcotic agents, side effects, 430–431
  opioids, 50, 211, 212t
  for terminally ill patients, 488
Paresthesias, 283–284, 418, 572
Parietal pleura, 327
Partial thromboplastin time (PTT), 113, 376t
Passive range of motion (ROM), 261t
Pathophysiologic impact of postoperative pain, 444–445
Patient assessment, 17–19, 69, 73, 74t
  analgesic technique decisions and, 208–209
Patient attitudes, 46, 54, 58, 59t, 60–61, 61t, 62–64

Patient behavior, pain assessment and, 16–17
Patient/caretaker relationship, 64–66, 69
Patient characteristics, 72, 73t, 75–81
Patient-controlled analgesia (PCA)
  for bone marrow transplants, 465
  for chest pain, 311
  for cutaneous injuries, 415–416
  dosage, 488–489
  economic implications, 6
  epidural analgesia dosage, 217, 218t
  for hepatic disease pain, 370
  impact of coagulopathy on, 384–385
  for liver transplantation, 461–462
  for multiple system organ failure, 400–401
  parenteral administration techniques, 212, 213t, 214
  pediatric, 512, 513t
  for postoperative pain, 448–449
  for pregnant patients, 530
  for pulmonary disorders, 328
  pump for analgesic and sedative agents in ICU, 316
  for renal dysfunction, 356
  for renal transplantation, 464
  setting the pump, 213t, 214, 316, 488–490
  for terminally ill patients, 488–490
  for trauma pain, 430
Patient presentation, post operative pain management and, 448
Patients who are unable to communicate, 16, 566–567
Pavulon (see Pancuronium)
Peak blood levels of local anesthetics, 163, 164f
Peak drug concentration, 93f, 94–96
Pediatric patients (see also Children; Neonates)
  introductory comments, 23
  pain assessment, 23–24, 509–510, 510f
  pain in, 30
Penicillamine, 289–290
Penicillin G, 274–275, 295, 377t
Penicillins, 90t, 377
Penile nerve blocks, 517, 518t, 519
Pentapeptide enkephalins, 120
Pentazocine, 120
  agonist-antagonist properties, 132
  analgesic effects, 132
  classification, 122, 123t
  dosage, 433t, 581t
  elimination, 90t
  equipotent IV dosage and side effects, 433t
  metabolism, 132, 581t
  receptor subtype, 121, 122t
  for renal disease, 350t–351t, 352–353
  respiratory depression from, 132
  for respiratory failure, 332
  risk of use during pregnancy, 540

structure, 131f
for trauma pain, 429
withdrawal, 132
Pentobarbital
administration, 176
dosage, 582t
intracranial pressure effects, 280
metabolism, 582t
for multiple system organ failure, 398–399
pharmacokinetic characteristics, 175t
risk of use during pregnancy, 540
Pentothal (see Thiopental)
Pepcid (famotidine), 111, 577t
Peptides, endogenous, 120
Perceived control, 57–58
Perceived suffering, degree of, 57
Perception, disordered, 282
Percocet (see Oxycodone)
Percodan (see Oxycodone)
Perfusion, 88, 321
Pericarditis, 308–310
Pericardium, anatomy, 308–309
Peridural analgesia (see also Analgesics/analgesia)
administration in ICU, 316–317
in multiple system organ failure, 399–400
respiratory effects, 50–51
side effects and complications, 399–400
Peridural blocks, 547
Peridural local anesthetics (see also Anesthetics/anesthesia)
cardiovascular effects, 50
gastrointestinal effects, 51
hormone levels effected by, 51
for neurologic disease pain, 297
for preexisting cardiac disease, 316–317
Peridural narcotics, 121–122
Peridural techniques, impact of coagulopathy on, 385
Peripheral compartment, 90, 91f, 92
Peripheral nerve blocks
administration techniques, 225–227
in children, 517, 518t, 519
drugs and dosage for acute pain, 518t
for hepatic disease pain, 370
for HIV/AIDS-related pain, 477
impact of coagulopathy on, 386
for pain of neurologic diseases, 298
for posttrauma pain, 438
for sympathetically mediated pain, 547
Peripheral nerve stimulation, 203, 460
Peripheral neuropathies (PNS), 288, 472
Peripheral pain receptors, 30, 31f
Perispinal drug effects, 216, 217t
Perispinal narcotic therapy, 449, 450t
Peristalsis, altered, drug absorption and, 88
Peritoneal dialysis (PD), 344–345

Phantom limb pain (PLP), 549
defined, 572
sequelae to burns, 419–420
Phantom pain, 483
Pharmacodynamics, 97–99, 100t
Pharmacokinetics
alterations in burn patients, 413–414
disease-related alterations, 88, 89t–90t
influences on serum drug concentrations, 87t, 88
models, 90, 91f, 92, 93f, 94–96
Pharmacologic management of pain, in children and neonates
neural blockade, 514, 515t–516t, 517
nonopioid analgesics, 510, 511t
opioid analgesics, 511, 512t–513t, 514
peripheral nerve blocks, 517, 518t, 519
Pharmacology
drugs used during pregnancy, 536–541
of local anesthetics (see under Anesthetics/anesthesia: local)
Phases of recovery, case examples, 75–81
Phenacetin, 104, 105t, 106
Phenanthrenes, 118
Phencyclidine (PCP), 503, 504t
Phenergan (see Promethazine)
Phenobarbital
administration, 175
dosage, 582t
inducer of drug metabolism, 100t
metabolism, 582t
pharmacokinetic characteristics, 175t
risk of use during pregnancy, 540
Phenol for sympathetic nerve blocks, 222–223
Phenothiazines (see also Tranquilizers)
adverse effects, 182
cardiovascular disease effects, 314
common medications, 183
contraindications, 182
indications, 182
pharmacokinetic parameters, 182–183
for postoperative pain management, 451
for renal disease, 353
for respiratory failure, 333
Phenoxybenzamine, 293, 547
Phenylbutazone, 104, 105t, 106, 113
dosage, 582t
inducer of drug metabolism, 100t
metabolism, 582t
platelet abnormalities caused by, 377t
risk of use during pregnancy, 540
Phenylpiperidine derivatives, 119f, 120
Phenytoin
administration, 186–187
for diabetic neuropathy, 289
distribution, 87t
dosage, 582t
elimination, 90t

inducer of drug metabolism, 100*t*
metabolism, 89*t*, 582*t*
for neuralgic pain, 548–549
neuromuscular blockade resistance with, 202
pharmacokinetic parameters, 186
protein binding, 87*t*
for reflex sympathetic dystrophy, 293
risk of use during pregnancy, 540
for thalamic pain syndrome, 286
for vasculitic neuropathy, 291
Phonophoresis, ultrasound for, 266
Phrenic nerves, 309
Physical examination, 17–18
pediatric patients, 23
post operative pain management and, 447
Physical therapist, 254
Physical therapy modalities, 267*t*
Physical therapy (PT)
consultation and referrals, 255, 256*t*
evaluation and treatment, 255
for HIV/AIDS patients, 477
for low back pain, 550–551
for neuralgic pain, 549
pain management with, 254–255, 256*t*
for reflex sympathetic dystrophy, 293
for sympathetically mediated pain, 546
Physiologic accommodation, 55
Physiologic changes
in pregnant patients, 523–526
in transplant patients, 456
Physiologic dead space, 321
Physiologic pain in terminally ill patients, 483
Physiologic reflexes, failing, 98
Physiologic responses, 55
Pipecuronium
cardiovascular side effects, 201*t*
clearance, 199, 200*t*
dosage, 199*t*, 582*t*
histamine release, 201*t*
metabolism, 582*t*
for renal disease, 350*t*–351*t*, 355
Piroxicam, 104, 105*t*, 106
dosage, 107*t*, 582*t*
metabolism, 582*t*
renal toxicity reduced with, 111
Pirprofen, 104, 105*t*, 106
pK$_a$, 160*t*, 161
Plasmapheresis, 90*t*
Plasma protein concentrations in burn patients, 413–414
Plasma volume, increased in pregnancy, 524*t*
Plateau waves, 279
Platelets
abnormalities, 377*t*, 378

coagulopathy therapy, 382
function
impaired in multiple system organ failure, 392
nonsteroidal anti-inflammatory drugs and, 112–113
normal hemostatic, 374
Pleuritic disease, 320*t*
Pleuritic pain, 309, 329
Plexus blocks
administration techniques, 222–225
brachial, 224–225
celiac, 222–223, 546
cervical, 225
for HIV/AIDS-related-pain, 477
lumbar, 225
for neurologic disease pain, 298
for sympathetically mediated pain, 546–547
Pneumonia
pain, 327–328
in pretransplant patients, 459
respiratory failure caused by, 320*t*
Pneumothorax pain, 329
Polypeptides, 45
Polysporin, 465
Ponstel (*see* Mefenamic acid)
Poppy plant, 118
Positioning and splinting, 46, 258–259, 260*t*, 329
Positive emotional arousal, 57
Positive end expiratory pressure (PEEP), 394
Postcardiac-injury syndrome, 311
Post-cesarean section pain management (*see also* Pregnancy), 529–530
Postcommissurotomy syndrome, 311
Postdural puncture headache (PDPH)
differential diagnosis, 275
epidural analgesia complication, 215
spinal analgesia complication, 220
symptoms, 275
treatment, 220, 275
Posterior division nerve block (PDNB), 461
Posthepatic dysfunction, 362*t*
Postherpetic neuralgia (PHN), 291–292
Postoperative pain, physiologic, 483
Postoperative pain management, 34, 35*t*
acute pain service for, 452
case study, 444, 453
factors that influence, 445–446
for liver transplant patients, 458–459
narcotic analgesics for, 448–449, 450*t*
nonnarcotic analgesics for, 450–451
nonsteroidal anti-inflammatory drugs for, 109
patient evaluation, 447–448
physical status and, 445–446
psychological techniques for, 452

regional analgesic techniques for, 449–450
self-regulation techniques for, 452
sensory modulation for, 451–452
suggested readings, 453
team effectiveness, 446
Postpericardiotomy syndrome, 311
Postpolio syndrome, 291
Postrenal renal failure, 340
Poststroke central pain, 286
Posttransplant pain syndrome, 461
Posttraumatic headaches, 275
Posttriage/stabilization phase, 65
Potassium wasting, 46
Potent vapors, 146
p-aminophenols, 104, 105t, 106
Prazosin, 293
Prednisone
 elimination, 90t
 for inflammatory myopathies, 296
 for pericarditis, 310
 for postherpetic neuralgia, 292
 for temporal arteritis headaches, 276
Preeclampsia, 530–532
Prefunctional activities, 263
Pregnancy
 case study, 524, 535–536
 critically ill patient management, 530–535
 labor pain management, 527–529
 normal patient, 523–527
 pharmacology of drugs in, 536–541
 post-cesarean section pain management, 529–532
 suggested readings, 536
Pregnancy-induced hypertension (PIH), 530–532
Prehepatic dysfunction, 362t
Preload failure, 302
Premorbid emotional status, 18
Preoperative pain, 109
Preoperative preparations, 445
Prerenal renal failure, 340
Pressure sores, 420–421
Prilocaine
 contraindicated in infants, 514
 for multiple system organ failure, 396–397
 stereoisomers, 162t, 163
 structure of, 160f
Problem-solving skills, 60
Procainamide, 90t, 93f
Procaine
 dosage, maximum, 166t
 equipotent concentration, 160t
 lipid solubility, 159, 160f, 160t
 protein binding, 160t, 162
 for respiratory failure, 333t
 structure of, 160f
Procardia (*see* Nifedipine)

Prochlorperazine
 administration, 183
 for alcohol withdrawal, 283
 dosage, 583t
 metabolism, 583t
Progesterone, decreased levels after injury, 426t, 427
Prognostic indicators
 case examples, 75–81
 for matrix assessment, 73, 74t
Progressive muscle relaxation, 242
Prohormones, 120
Prolactin, 42, 426t, 427
Prolixin (fluphenazine), 289, 291–292
Promethazine
 administration, 183
 for alcohol withdrawal, 283
 dosage, 583t
 metabolism, 583t
Proopiocortin, 120
Proopiomelanocortin, 42
Propagated impulse, 158
Propanolol, 293
Propionic acids, 104, 105t, 106, 106t
Propofol
 cardiovascular disease effects, 315
 for cutaneous injury pain, 417
 dosage, 583t
 hemodynamic function effects, 145t
 intracranial pressure effects, 281
 for intravenous anesthesia, 154
 for intubation, 281
 metabolism, 583t
 for multiple system organ failure, 398–399
 for renal disease, 350t–351t, 353
 respiratory depression from, 417
Propoxyphene, 119
 distribution, 129
 dosage, 583t
 intravenous administration, 129
 metabolism, 89t, 129, 583t
 for respiratory failure, 332
 side effects, 129
 structure, 129, 131f–130
Propoxyphene enantiomer, 99
Propranolol
 distribution, 87t
 elimination, 90t
 inhibitor of drug metabolism, 100t
 metabolism, 89t
 for migraine, 273
 for posttraumatic headaches, 275
 protein binding, 87t
Prostacyclin, 44
Prostaglandin inhibitors, 110–111, 112t
Prostaglandins, 31, 107–109
Prostaglandin synthesis, 44
Prostigmin (neostigmine), 203

Protamine, anticoagulant-induced bleeding, 380
Protein binding
　of drugs, 87t, 126–127, 128t
　of local anesthetics, 160t, 162
Protein deficiency, immobility effect, 256t
Proteinuria, renal failure associated, 341
Proteolysis, 48
Prothrombin time (PT), 113
　hemostasis screening test, 376t
Protizinic acid, 104, 105t, 106
Proxy appointments, in terminally ill patients, 485–486
Pruritus, 343–344, 465
Pryazoles, 104, 105t, 106
Pseudocholinesterase, 196
Pseudomembrane, surface, 408
Pseudothrombophelebitis, HIV/AIDS related, 472–473
Psychological assessment of pain (*see* Psychology of pain)
Psychological intervention, 65–67, 68t, 241, 463
Psychological rehabilitation, 549
Psychological support, 477
Psychological techniques, 452
Psychology of pain
　background factors, 46, 54–56, 56t
　case examples, 75–81
　individual difference factors, 58–61, 61t, 62–64
　process factors, 56–58, 59t
　treatment factors, 64–70, 70t, 71–72, 73t–74t, 75
Psychoprophylaxis for pregnant patients, 527
Psychosocial issues, 24, 482, 484
Psychotherapy, 243, 477
Psychotropics, tranquilizing, 490
Pulmonary dysfunction, in HIV/AIDS, 470
Pulmonary edema, 306–307, 320t, 325
Pulmonary embolism
　pain, 310, 328–329
　respiratory failure caused by, 320t
Pulmonary function, deterioration of, 394
Pulmonary hygiene, 255, 257
Pulmonary hypertension, 328
Pulmonary mechanics, 322–324
Pulmonary nerves, 326
Pulmonary system
　adverse effects of acute pain on, 34, 35t
　innervation of the, 326t
　physiologic changes during pregnancy, 525t
Pulmonary volume, 46, 47f
Pulse, narcotic use and withdrawal effects, 501t
Pulse steroids, 547

Pump failure, 302
Pupils, narcotic use and withdrawal effects, 501t
Purpura, 375–376, 383
Pychostimulants for terminally ill patients, 490
Pyranocarboxylic acid, 104, 105t, 106

Quadriplegia, 320t
Quinidine, 87t, 377
Quinine, 377

Radiation therapy, 283
Radiotherapy, physiologic pain of, 483
Range of motion (ROM), 254, 259, 261, 261t, 262, 262t
Ranitidine
　dosage, 583t
　gastric irritation reduced with, 111
　for HIV/AIDS-related pain, 475
　metabolism, 583t
Receptor binding, altered, 88
delta Receptors, 32, 121, 122t
Recombinant tissue plasminogen activator (rTPA), 380
Recovery continuum status, 58
Rectal administration of pain medication, 488
Red cell volume, increased, 524t
Reduced sympathetic tone, morphine-induced, 137
Reflexes, effects of narcotic use and withdrawal on, 501t
Reflex sympathetic dystrophy (RSD), 544–545, 546t
　defined, 572
　diagnosis, 545, 546t
　movement disorder of, 545
　stages, 292–293, 545, 546t
　symptoms, 292–293, 546t
　syndromes, 544–545
　treatment, 293, 546–547
Refractory angina, 306–307
Regional analgesia (*see also* Analgesics/analgesia)
　advantages, 209
　complication sources, 210–211
　contraindications, 209–210
　disadvantages, 209
　for liver transplant patients, 462
　for postoperative pain, 449–450
　toxicity in children and neonates, 514
　volume of distribution in children, 514, 515t
Reglan (*see* Metoclopramide)
Regression, 61t, 62–63, 65–66
Reimplantation vascular pain, 312
Relafen (*see* Nabumetone)

INDEX 615

Relaxants, skeletal muscle, 188–190
Relaxation-induced reactions, 247
Relaxation techniques, 357, 463
Relaxation therapy for HIV/AIDS patients, 477
Relaxation training, 242, 452
Renal blood flow in MSOF, 391–392
Renal colic, 347
Renal disease
 case study, 340, 358–359
 drug elimination and, 90, 126
 loin pain hematuria syndrome, 347
 renal colic, 346
 suggested reading, 359
Renal dysfunction, 394
Renal failure, 340–346
Renal function in burn patients, 414
Renal hypoperfusion, 111, 112t
Renal insufficiency, 111, 112t
 determination of extent, 347–348
 drug choices, 349, 350t–351t, 352–355
 effect of, on drug choices for pain, 348–349
 hemodialysis, impact of, 349
 technique choices, 355–358
Renal osteodystrophy (ROD), 342–343
Renal system, acute pain and the, 34, 35t
Renal transplantation (see also Transplantation), 457t, 463–464
Renin, 44, 426t–427t
Repressing avoiders, 60–61
Residual volume (RV), 47f
Resisted range of motion (ROM), 261t
Respiratory depression
 barbiturates adverse effects, 174
 benzodiazepines adverse effects, 171
 in children and neonates, 510–511
 factors that decrease the risk of, with perispinal narcotics, 450t
 narcotic analgesic side effect, 429
 opioid-agonist-antagonist induced, 131–136, 139
 propofol induced, 417
 respiratory failure caused by, 320t
 tricyclic antidepressants, adverse effect of, 184
Respiratory drive control, 324
Respiratory failure (see also specific disorders)
 adult respiratory distress syndrome (ARDS), pathophysiology, 324–325, 325t, 326
 analgesia/anesthesia routes, 334–335, 336t
 case study, 319–320
 management, 331, 332t, 333, 333t–334t
 pain, 326t, 327–330
 pathophysiology, 320t–321t, 322–324
 suggested readings, 336–337
 therapy, 330–331, 332t, 333, 333t–334t
Respiratory function
 factors effecting
  immobility, 256t
  metabolic stress response (MSR), 46, 47f
  pain, 426t–427t
  pain and anxiety management, 50–51
  pregnancy, physiologic alterations, 525t
  positioning to enhance, 259
  therapeutic intervention, 255, 257–258
Respiratory muscle weakness, respiratory failure caused by, 320t
Respiratory pattern, factors controlling, 324
Respiratory therapy, for liver transplantation patients, 460
Responsiveness, altered, 98
Rest, 28, 29t, 305–306
Retrovir (azidothymidine (AZT)), 471, 475
Reye's syndrome, aspirin use and, 510–511
Rheumatoid arthritis, 551–552
Rheumatologic disorders, HIV/AIDS related, 472–473
Rifampin, inducer of drug metabolism, 100t
Ring blocks, 517, 518t, 519
Ritalin (see Methylphenidate)
Ropivacaine, 159, 160f, 160t, 162, 162t, 163, 540

Sadness, pain threshold influenced by, 28, 29t
Salicylates, 104, 105t
 dosage, 106t
 elimination, 90t
 pain management in children, 510, 511t
Salsalate, 104, 105t, 106, 113
 dosage, 106t, 583t
 metabolism, 583t
 renal toxicity reduced with, 111
Schönlein-Henoch purpura, 376, 383
Scopolamine
 administration, 179
 dosage, 583t
 metabolism, 583t
 pharmacokinetic parameters, 179
 risk of use during pregnancy, 541
Screening tests, hemostatic, 375, 376t
Secobarbital
 administration, 175
 dosage, 584t
 metabolism, 584t
 pharmacokinetic characteristics, 175t
 risk of use during pregnancy, 541
Seconal (see Secobarbital)
Secretions of body fluids, drug elimination through, 90

Sedatives (*see also specific drugs*)
  administration routes, 315–317
  for alcohol withdrawal, 282–283
  analgesic, 461
  anticholinergics, 178–179
  anticonvulsants, 185–187
  antihistamines, 178–179
  barbiturates, 173–174, 175*t*, 176
  benzodiazepines, 170–171, 172*t*, 173
  butyrophenone tranquilizers, 180, 181*t*, 182
  cardiovascular disease effects, 314
  chloral hydrate (NOCTEC), 176–177
  contraindicated in terminally ill patients, 491
  dosage, 575*t*–577*t*, 583*t*
  intracranial pressure effects, 280–281
  metabolism, 575*t*–577*t*, 583*t*
  phenothiazine tranquilizers, 182–183
  for renal disease, 353
  for renal insufficiency, 350*t*–351*t*, 353
  risk of use during pregnancy, 537–541
  skeletal muscle relaxants, 188–190
  tricyclic antidepressants, 183–184, 185*t*
  withholding of, for special procedures, 564–565
Segmental responses, 41*f*, 40
  reflex, 444
  spinal reflex, 34
Seizures
  alcohol use and withdrawal, 282, 499*t*
  local anesthetic induced, 163–165
  neuromuscular blocking agents for, 194
Self-administered doses (SADs) (*see also* Patient–controlled analgesia), 213*t*, 214, 218*t*
Self-regulation skills training, 71–72
Self-regulation techniques (*see also specific techniques*)
  characteristics of, 240–245
  for cutaneous injury pain, 418
  impact of coagulopathy on, 386
  limitations and caveats, 245–248
  for neurologic disease pain, 298
  for postoperative pain control, 452
  for postoperative pain management, 452
  for posttrauma pain, 439
  for sympathetically mediated pain, 547
  types, 240–245
Sensory modulation, 451–452
Sepsis, in multiple system organ failure, 393–394
Sepsis syndrome, 48, 390
Septic shock, naloxone for, 136
Serax (oxazepam), 353
Serotonin, 31, 45
Serum bilirubin, in hepatic dysfunction, 362*t*

Serum creatinine levels, 111, 112*t*
Serum drug concentrations, 86, 87*t*, 88, 89*t*–90*t*
Serum inorganic F⁻ levels, 148*f*–149*f*
Shivering, 194
Shock, ARDS factor, 325*t*
Shoulder-hand syndrome, 544–545
Shunt, respiratory failure factor, 321
Sick euthyroid syndrome, 44–45
Sigma receptors, 32, 121, 122*t*
Silent ischemia, 305
Sinequan (*see* Doxepin)
Sinus headaches, 274–275
Skeletal muscle relaxants, 188–190
Skeletal muscle rigidity, 140
Skin, narcotic use effects on, 501*t*
Sleep, effect on pain threshold, 28, 29*t*
Sleep disorders, alcohol abuse sign, 499*t*
Sodium channel, 158, 159*f*
Sodium nitroprusside, 282, 285
Sodium retention, 46
Sodium salicylate, 113
  dosage, 106*t*–107*t*, 584*t*
  metabolism, 584*t*
Somatic pain, physiologic, 483
Somatomedins, 44
Somatosensory evoked potential (SSEP), 19
Somatostatin, 43–44
Specificity theory, of cardiac muscle pain, 304
Sphincter of Oddi spasms, 366–367
Spinal analgesia (*see also* Analgesics/analgesia; Epidural analgesia), 214, 218–221
Spinal cord, cardiac pain modulation in, 305
Spinal cord compression, 283–286
Spinal cord injury (SCI), 284–285
Spinal cord lesions, 534
Spinal dorsal horn, 31*f*, 32, 407
Spinal epidural abscess, 284
Spinal epidural hematoma, 284
Spinal headaches (*see* Postdural puncture headache)
Spinal opiate receptors, 121–122
Spinal opiates, 369–370
Spinal reflex arcs, 427*t*
Splanchnic hypoperfusion, 427*t*
Splenic enlargement, acute, 383
Splinting and positioning, 46, 258–259, 260*t*, 329
Splints, specialized, 263
Spontaneous abreaction, 247–248
Spontaneous CNS bleeding, 384
Stadol (*see* Butorphanol)
Staff (*see also* Caregivers), 66, 72–73, 73*t*–74*t*
Standardized assessment tests, 447–448
Starvation, 41*t*

Steady state, 92–93, 95
Stellate blocks, 221–222, 546
Stereoisomers, 160f, 162t, 163
Sternotomy, 311
Steroids
  for multiple sclerosis, 287
  pulse, 547
  for spinal cord compression, 283
  for terminally ill patients, 490
Stimulant drug use, 501, 502t
Stimulation-induced analgesia (see also specific analgesia)
  acupuncture, 236, 237f, 240
  transcutaneous electrical nerve stimulations, 230–234, 235t, 236
Streptokinase, 380
Stress inoculation training, 242–243
Stress management, 262
  relaxation in, 263
Stroke volume, increased in pregnancy, 524t
Stump pain, 483, 549, 572
Stunned myocardium, 306–307
Subarachnoid analgesia (see Spinal analgesia)
Subarachnoid hemorrhage headaches, 277
Subarachnoid injections, 476, 529–530
Subcutaneous injections, 88, 211, 212t–213t
Sublimaze (see Fentanyl)
Substance abuse (see Chemical abuse; Drug abuse)
Substance P, secretion, 45
Substantia gelatinosa, 32
Substituted judgment, 486
Succinylcholine
  actions, 196
  advantages, 196
  cardiovascular side effects, 201t
  clearance, 196, 200t
  complications, 196–198
  dosage, 199t, 584t
  histamine release, 197, 201t
  intracranial pressure effects, 281
  metabolism, 584t
  for renal disease, 350t–351t, 354
  uses, 196
Sucralfate
  dosage, 584t
  for HIV/AIDS-related pain, 475
  metabolism, 584t
  use in ulcer healing, 110–111
Suctioning, endotracheal tube, 330
Sudeck's atrophy, 544–545
Sufenta (see Sufentanil)
Sufentanil, 120
  bolus injection, 217t
  cardiovascular effects, 137–138, 313
  classification, 122, 123t
  distribution, 127, 128t

  dosage, 584t
    for parenteral administration, 211, 212t–213t
    for patient-controlled analgesia, 217, 218t, 223
    for spinal use, 217, 218t, 436, 437t
  hepatic metabolism, 362, 363t
  intracranial pressure effects, 280
  metabolism, 127–128, 584t
    for parenteral administration, 211, 212t–213t
    for patient-controlled analgesia, 213t, 217, 218t
  potency, 127
  protein binding, 127–128, 128t
  receptor subtype, 121, 122t
  for renal disease, 350t–351t, 352
  for respiratory failure, 332t, 335, 336t
  structure, 119f
  tolerance to, 500
Sulfonamides, 377
Sulindac, 104, 105t, 106
  dosage, 107t, 584t
  metabolism, 584t
  renal toxicity reduced with, 111
  risk of use during pregnancy, 541
Superficial heat, 265
Suprascapular peripheral nerve blocks, 227
Suprasegmental responses, 41f, 40–42
  post operative pain management and, 445
  reflex, 34, 35t
Suprofen, 104, 105t, 106
Surgery, physiologic pain of, 483
Surgery site, post operative pain and, 445
Surgical access, 194
Surgical decompression, 283
Surgical intervention, 547
Surgical procedures, 393, 549
Surgical therapy, for pancreatitis pain, 368
Surgical trauma, in pregnant patients, 535
Sustained-release dosage forms, 94
Symmetrel (amantadine), 287, 292
Sympathetically maintained pain (SMP), 34–35, 484, 572, 544–546, 546t, 547
Sympathetic blockade, 50
Sympathetic blocks, 316, 477
Sympathetic nerve blocks, 221–224
Sympathetic nervous system, 32, 33f, 34
Sympatholytic drugs, 293, 574t
Sympathy, pain threshold and, 28, 29t
Symptom control, 482–483
Symptom relief, pain threshold and, 28, 29t
Synergism, 99
Systemic inflammatory response syndrome (SIRS), 390
Systemic lupus erythematosus, 377
Systemic narcotics, 50, 384–385
Systemic toxicity, 163–164, 215

Systemic vascular resistance (SVR), 145*t*, 147
Systolic blood pressure, 499*t*

Tachycardia, 138, 427*t*
Tachyphylaxis, 97
Tagamet (*see* Cimetidine)
Talwin (*see* Pentazocine)
Technology evaluation, 7
Tegretol (*see* Carbamazepine)
Temperature, 499*t*, 501*t*
Temporal arteritis headaches, 276
Tenormin (atenolol), 258*t*, 273
Tenoxicam, 104, 105*t*, 106, 107*t*
Tensilon (edrophonium), 203
Tension headaches, 273–274
Terminally ill patients, pain management for
   adjunctive therapy, 490
   administration of medication, 487–490
   agents to avoid, 491
   components of care, 482–483
   the family and, 491–493
   legal concerns, 484–485
   pathophysiology of pain, 483–484
   patient's environment, 487
   patient's wishes, 485–487
   psychosocial care, 482
   psychosocial pain or grief, 484
Testosterone, decreased levels, 426*t*, 427
Tetanus, 154–155, 294–295
Tetracaine, structure of, 160*f*
Tetracycline, for tetanus, 295
Tetrahydrocannabinol (THC), 503
Thalamic pain syndrome, 286
Thalamocortical pain fibers, 509
Thallium poisoning, 290
Thebaine, 118
Theophylline, 89*t*, 93*f*, 202
Therapeutic drug monitoring, 86
Therapeutic intervention
   cognitive assessment, 258
   daily living activities, 263
   functional mobility, 263–264
   modalities, 264–266, 267*t*, 268
   pain and pain perception decreasing strategies, 262–263
   positioning and splinting, 46, 258–259, 260*t*, 329
   prefunctional activities, 263
   range of motion activities, 259, 261, 261*t*–262*t*
   relaxation, 262
   respiratory function, t, 257–258
Thiazides, 377
Thiopental
   administration, 176
   for anesthetic-induced seizure, 165
   for blood pressure control, 282
   dosage, 585*t*
   intracranial pressure effects, 280
   for intubation, 281
   metabolism, 585*t*
   for multiple system organ failure, 398–399
   pharmacokinetic characteristics, 175*t*
   for renal disease, 350*t*–351*t*, 353
Third spacing of fluid, 88
Thoracic epidural analgesia, 465
Thoracic epidural blockade, 515, 516*t*, 517
Thoracic ganglion blocks, 546
Thoracic injuries, 439–441
Thoracotomy, 311
Thorazine (*see* Chlorpromazine)
Threshold for pain, 28, 29*t*
Thrombin time (TT), 376*t*
Thrombocytopenia, 377, 380
Thrombotic disorders (*see also* Hemostatic failure; Hemostatic function), 382–384
Thrombotic thrombocytopenia purpura (TTP), 378
Thromboxanes, 31, 44
Thrombus formation, 256*t*
Thyroid hormone metabolism, 44–45
Thyroid stimulating hormone (TSH), 44–45
Thyrotropin-releasing-hormone (TRH), 44–45
Thyroxine levels, 426*t*, 427
Tiaprofenic acid, 104, 105*t*, 106
Ticarcillin, 377*t*
Tidal breathing, 46, 47*f*
Tidal volume (TV), 47*f*
Tietze's syndrome, 310
Tilt table, 264
Timolol, for migraine, 273
Tissue, normal hemostatic function, 374
Tissue plasminogen activator recombinant (rTPA), 380
Tissue plasminogen activator (TPA), 307–308
Titratable inhalational agents, 458
Tobramycin, 90*t*, 93*f*, 94
Tofranil (imipramine), 538, 549
Tolectin (*see* Tolmetin)
Tolerance
   benzodiazepine, 503
   in children and neonates, 510–511
   in intensive care unit patients, 496, 500
   pharmacodynamics and, 97
Tolfenamic acid, 104, 105*t*, 106
Tolmetin, 104, 105*t*, 106
   dosage, 107*t*
   pain management in children, 510, 511*t*
   risk of use during pregnancy, 541
Topical nitrates, 547
Toradol (*see* Ketorolac)
Toxic neuropathies, 290

Tracheal obstruction, 320t
Tracheobronchial tree, innervation of, 326t
Tracheobronchitis pain, 327
Tracrium (see Atracurium)
Trandate (labetalol), 282
Tranquilizers
  adverse effects, 180, 182, 184
  butyrophenone (see Butyrophenones)
  common medications, 181t, 182–183
  contraindications, 181–182
  dosage, 575t, 577t–578t, 583t
  indications, 180, 182
  metabolism, 575t, 577t–578t, 583t
  pharmacokinetic parameters, 181t, 182–183
  phenothiazine (see Phenothiazines)
  psychotropics, 490
  risk of use during pregnancy, 537–541
Transaminases, in hepatic dysfunction, 362t
Transcutaneous electrical nerve stimulations (TENS), 267–268
  application of, 233–234, 235t, 236
  cardiac pain modulation, 305
  for chest pain, 311
  complications, 232–233
  contraindications, 232
  for cutaneous injury pain, 418
  for HIV/AIDS-related pain, 477
  impact of coagulopathy on, 386
  indications, 231–232
  introduction, 230–231
  for low back pain, 550–551
  modes of stimulation, 234, 235t, 236
  for multiple system organ failure, 401
  for myofascial pain syndrome, 552–553
  for neuralgic pain, 549
  for neurologic disease pain, 298
  for pancreatitis pain, 367
  for postoperative pain management, 451–452
  for posttransplant pain syndrome, 461
  for posttrauma pain, 439
  for the pregnant patient, 527
  for reflex sympathetic dystrophy, 293
  for renal dysfunction, 357–358
  for sympathetically mediated pain, 547
  understanding the unit, 233, 235t
Transdermal administration of medications, 487–488
Transderm-Scop, (see Scopolamine)
Transfusions, 377, 380, 381t
Transmural infarction, 307–308
Transplantation
  bone marrow transplants, 457t, 465–466
  case study, 456, 466
  general concerns, 456–457, 457t, 458
  heart-lung transplantation, 457t, 464–465
  liver transplantation, 457t, 458–462
  psychological intervention for chronic pain, 463
  renal transplantation, 457t, 463–464
Trauma, 34, 35t
  adult respiratory distress syndrome (ARDS) factor, 325t
  adverse physiologic effects, 426, 426t, 427, 427t, 428
  analgesia for common injuries, 439–441
  case study, 426
  controlling the pain, 426t–427t, 428
  cryoneurolysis, 439
  epidural analgesia, 430–432, 433t, 434–436
  intrapleural analgesia, 437–438
  intrathecal analgesia, 436, 437t
  pain therapy principles, 428
  parenteral medications, 429–431
  peripheral nerve blocks, 438
  rationale behind active pain control, 428
  self-regulation techniques, 439
  transcutaneous electrical nerve stimulations, 439
Traumatic spinal cord compression, 284–285
Trazodone, 463, 549, 585t
Treatment factors
  goals and objectives, 64–65
  interpersonal influence model, 65–66
  psychological intervention, levels, 67, 68t
  psychological intervention models, 65–67
  self-regulation training model, 66–67
Tremors, 282, 498, 499t
Tremulousness, 282, 498, 499t
Trexan (see Naltrexone)
Tricyclic antidepressants (TCA)
  adverse effects, 184
  common medications, 185t
  contraindications, 184
  dosage, 574t, 577t, 585t
  for hepatic tumor pain management, 364
  for herpes zoster, 473–474
  for HIV/AIDS-related pain, 475
  indications, 183–184
  metabolism, 574t, 577t, 585t
  pharmacokinetic parameters, 185t
  for reflex sympathetic dystrophy, 293
  for thalamic pain syndrome, 286
Trigger point injections, 227
Triiodothyronine, 426t, 427
Trilisate (see Choline magnesium trisalicylate)
Trough drug concentration, 93f, 94–96
Tubocurarine
  cardiovascular effects, 201t, 315
  clearance, 199, 200t
  dosage, 199t, 585t
  histamine release, 201t

Tubocurarine *(continued)*
  metabolism, 585*t*
  for renal disease, 350*t*–351*t*, 355
  for tetanus, 295
Tumor necrosis factor (TNF), 42, 45
Tylenol *(see* Acetaminophen)
Tylox *(see* Oxycodone)

Ultrasound, as a heat modality, 265–266
Understanding, pain threshold and, 28, 29*t*
Unmyelinated nociceptors, 407
Urokinase, anticoagulant-induced bleeding, 380

Vagal afferents, cardiac pain modulation, 305
Valium *(see* Diazepam)
Valproic acid
  administration, 187
  for diabetic neuropathy, 289
  distribution, 87*t*
  dosage, 585*t*
  metabolism, 585*t*
  for neuralgic pain, 548–549
  pharmacokinetic parameters, 187
  protein binding, 87*t*
  risk of use during pregnancy, 541
  for vasculitic neuropathy, 291
Valvular heart disease, 312–313
Vascular pain, 311–312
Vasculitic neuropathy, 290–291
Vasculitis, 384
Vasoactive intestinal peptide (VIP), 42
Vasoconstriction, 266
Vasodilation, 266
Vasopressin release, 42
Vasospasms, 41*f*, 40
Vecuronium
  cardiovascular effects, 201*t*, 315
  clearance, 200*t*
  dosage, 199*t*, 585*t*
  histamine release, 201*t*
  intracranial pressure effects, 281
  metabolism, 585*t*
  for renal disease, 350*t*–351*t*, 355
Venoconstriction, 45–46
Venous capacitance, decreased, 45–46
Venous insufficiency, wound pain from, 421
Venous pressure in pregnancy, 524*t*
Ventilation, 192–194, 394

Ventilation and perfusion (V/Q) mismatch, 321
Ventilatory drive, increased, 525*t*
Ventricular ectopy, 306
Verapamil, 87*t*, 89*t*
Verbal scales for pain assessment, 20*f*–21*f*
Versed *(see* Midazolam)
Vessels, normal hemostatic function, 374
Victim of injury, 58, 71, 75–81
Visceral function, inhibited, 41*f*, 40
Visceral pain, physiologic, 483
Vistaril *(see* Hydroxyzine)
Visual analog scale (VAS), 19, 20*f*, 21
Vital capacity (VC), 47*f*, 329–330
  decreased after injury, 426, 427*t*
Vitamin K, 379, 381*t*
Voltaren *(see* Diclofenac)
Volume of distribution (Vd), 94–96
Vomiting, 48, 140–141, 501*t*
Von Willebrand's disease, 374, 376*t*, 379

Warfarin *(see also* Coumadin), 87*t*, 89*t*
Weakness, spinal cord compression symptom, 283–284
Wide dynamic range (WDR) neurons, 34–35
Wigraine (ergotamine), 273
Windup, 456
Withdrawal seizures, 282
Withdrawal signs and symptoms
  for alcohol, 282, 498, 499*t*
  for cocaine, 502*t*
  for narcotics, 500, 501*t*
Wound care, 408, 411
Wound margins infiltration, 225
Wrist, positioning for contractures, 260*t*
Written advance directive, 485
Wygesic *(see* Propoxyphene)

Xanax (alprazolam), 431
Xylocaine *(see* Lidocaine)

Zalcitabine (ddC), 471
Zantac *(see* Ranitidine)
Zero-order kinetics, 92
Zidovudine, 471
Zofran (ondansetron), 465, 581*t*
Zomepirac, 104, 105*t*, 106
Zostrix (capsaicin), 292, 474

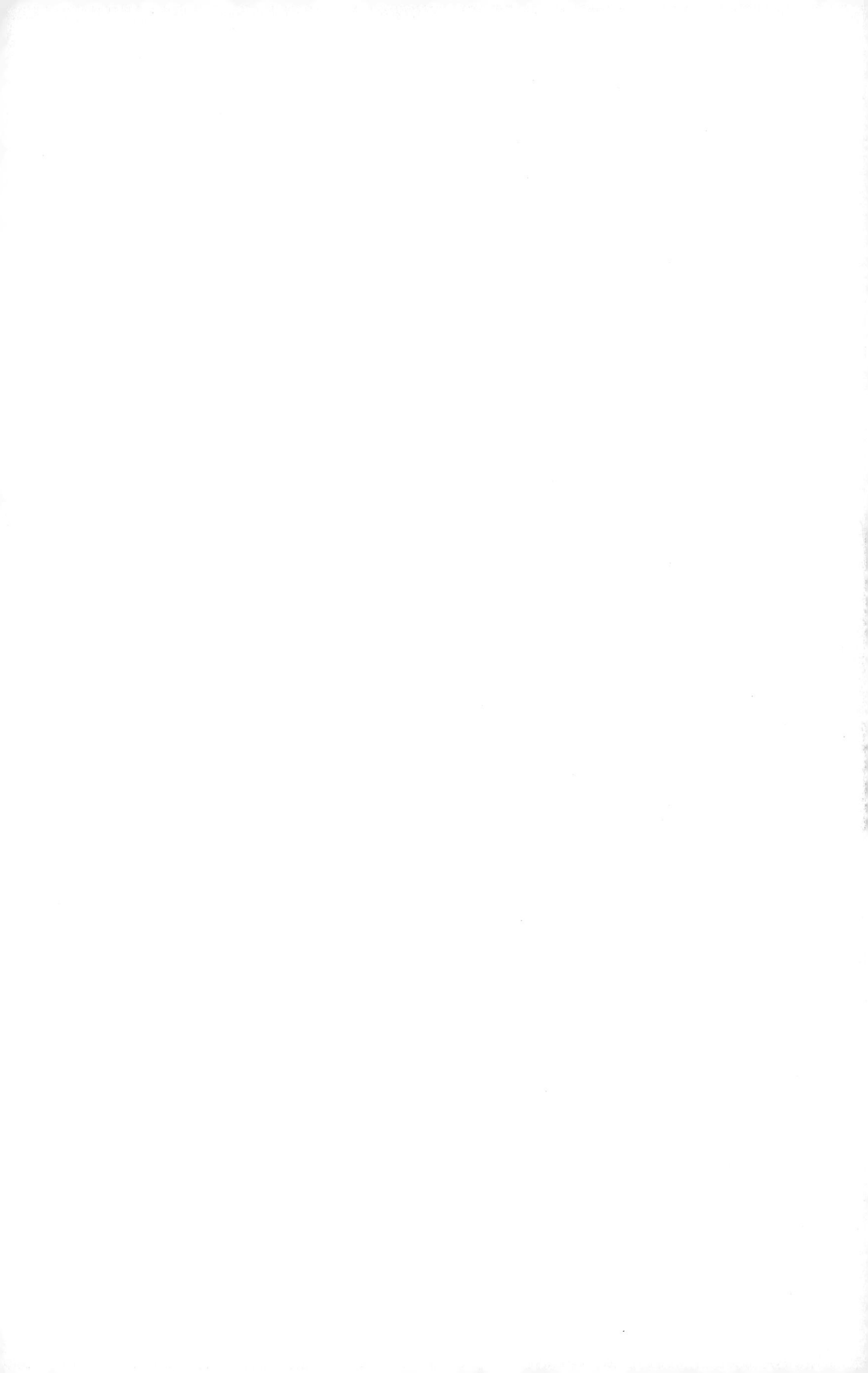